D1616710

Methods in Cell Biology

VOLUME 48

Caenorhabditis elegans: Modern Biological Analysis
of an Organism

Series Editors

Leslie Wilson
Department of Biological Sciences
University of California, Santa Barbara
Santa Barbara, California

Paul Matsudaira
Whitehead Institute for Biomedical Research and
Department of Biology
Massachusetts Institute of Technology
Cambridge, Massachusetts

Methods in Cell Biology

Prepared under the Auspices of the American Society for Cell Biology

VOLUME 48

Caenorhabditis elegans: Modern Biological Analysis
of an Organism

Edited by

Henry F. Epstein

Department of Neurology
Baylor College of Medicine
Houston, Texas

and

Diane C. Shakes

Department of Biology
University of Houston
Houston, Texas

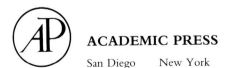

ACADEMIC PRESS

San Diego   New York   Boston   London   Sydney   Tokyo   Toronto

Cover photograph (paperback edition only): Immunofluorescence image of 28-cell stage *Caenorhabditis elegans* embryo stained for actin, DNA, and P granules using rhodamine-coupled secondary antibody. See Chapter 16, Figure 1 for further details. Photograph from Evans *et al,* 1994; reprinted with permission of Cell Press.

This book is printed on acid-free paper. ∞

Academic Press, Inc.
A Division of Harcourt Brace & Company
525 B Street, Suite 1900, San Diego, California 92101-4495

United Kingdom Edition published by
Academic Press Limited
24-28 Oval Road, London NW1 7DX

International Standard Serial Number: 0091-679X

International Standard Book Number: 0-12-564149-4 (Hardcover)

International Standard Book Number: 0-12-240545-5 (Paperback)

PRINTED IN THE UNITED STATES OF AMERICA
95 96 97 98 99 00 EB 9 8 7 6 5 4 3 2 1

CONTENTS

PART II   Neurobiology

PART III   Cell Biology and Molecular Biology

PART IV   Genomics and Informatics

CONTRIBUTORS

Numbers in parentheses indicate the pages on which the authors' contributions begin.

Donna G. Albertson (339), MRC Laboratory of Molecular Biology, Cambridge CB2 2QH, England

Philip Anderson (31), Department of Genetics, University of Wisconsin, Madison, Wisconsin 53706

Leon Avery (225, 251), Department of Biochemistry, University of Texas Southwestern Medical Center, Dallas, Texas 75235

David L. Baillie (147), Institute of Molecular Biology and Biochemistry, Simon Fraser University, Burnaby, Canada V5A 1S6, British Columbia

Cornelia I. Bargmann (225), Programs in Developmental Biology, Neuroscience, and Genetics, Department of Anatomy, The University of California, San Francisco, California 94143

Philip S. Birchall (339), MRC Laboratory of Molecular Biology, Cambridge CB2 2QH, England

Alan Coulson (533), The Sanger Centre, Hinxton, Cambridge CB10 1RQ, United Kingdom

Richard Durbin (583), The Sanger Centre, Hinxton, Cambridge CB10 1RQ, United Kingdom

Lois G. Edgar (303), Department of Molecular, Cellular, and Developmental Biology, University of Colorado, Boulder, Colorado 80309

Mark Edgley (147), Department of Medical Genetics, University of British Columbia, Vancouver, British Columbia, Canada V6T 1Z3

Frank H. Eeckman (583), LBL Human Genome Center, Berkeley, California 94611

Henry F. Epstein (437), Departments of Neurology, Biochemistry, and Cell Biology, Baylor College of Medicine, Houston, Texas 77030

Anthony Favello (551), Genome Sequencing Center, Washington University School of Medicine, St. Louis, Missouri 63108

Andrew Fire (323, 451), Department of Embryology, Carnegie Institution of Washington, Baltimore, Maryland 21210

Rita M. Fishpool (339), MRC Laboratory of Molecular Biology, Cambridge CB2 2QH, England

John T. Fleming (3), Department of Pediatrics/Hematology Oncology, Massachusetts General Hospital, Boston, Massachusetts 02114

Lucinda L. Fulton (571), Genome Sequencing Center, Washington University School of Medicine, St. Louis, Missouri 63108

Timothy N. Gannon (205), Department of Psychology, University of British Columbia, Vancouver, British Columbia, Canada V6T 1Z4

Ed Grossman (607), Beckman Institute for Advanced Science and Technology, Urbana, Illinois 61801

David H. Hall (395), Department of Neuroscience, Albert Einstein College of Medicine, Bronx, New York 10461

Robert K. Herman (123), Department of Genetics and Cell Biology, University of Minnesota, St. Paul, Minnesota 55108

LaDeana Hillier (551, 571), Genome Sequencing Center, Washington University School of Medicine, St. Louis, Missouri 63108

Linda S. Huang (97), California Institute of Technology, Pasadena, California 91125

Chau Huynh (533), Department of Molecular and Cell Biology, University of California at Berkeley, Berkeley, California 94720

Curt Jamison (607), Community Systems Laboratory, National Center for Supercomputing Applications, University of Illinois, Urbana-Campaign, Urbana, Illinois 61801

Carl D. Johnson (187), NemaPharm, Inc., Cambridge, Massachusetts 02139

Yuko Kozono (533), Division of Rheumatology, University of Colorado, Denver, Colorado 80262

Michael Krause (483, 513), Laboratory of Molecular Biology, National Institute of Diabetes, Digestive, and Kidney Diseases, National Institutes of Health, Bethesda, Maryland 20892

Steven W. L'Hernault (273), Department of Biology, Emory University, Atlanta, Georgia 30322

James A. Lewis (3), Division of Life Sciences, University of Texas at San Antonio, San Antonio, Texas 78249

Feizhou Liu (437), Department of Biochemistry, Baylor College of Medicine, Houston, Texas 77030

Shawn Lockery (251), Institute of Neuroscience, University of Oregon, Eugene, Oregon 97403

Craig Mello (451), University of Massachusetts Cancer Center, Biotech II, Worcester, Massachusetts 01605

David M. Miller (365), Department of Cell Biology, Vanderbilt University Medical Center, Nashville, Tennessee 37232

Ronald H. A. Plasterk (59), Netherlands Cancer Institute, Division of Molecular Biology, 1066 CX Amsterdam, The Netherlands

Kevin Powell (607), Digital Library Initiative, Grainger Engineering Library, Urbana, Illinois 61801

David Raizen (251), Department of Biochemistry, University of Texas Southwestern Medical Center, Dallas, Texas 75235

James B. Rand (187), Program in Molecular and Cell Biology, Oklahoma Medical Research Foundation, Oklahoma City, Oklahoma 73104

Catharine H. Rankin (205), Department of Psychology, University of British Columbia, Vancouver, British Columbia, Canada V6T 1Z4

Donald L. Riddle (147), Division of Biological Sciences, University of Missouri, Columbia, Missouri 65211

Thomas M. Roberts (273), Department of Biological Sciences, Florida State University, Tallahassee, Florida 32306

Ann M. Rose (147), Department of Medical Genetics, University of British Columbia, Vancouver, British Columbia, Canada V6T 1Z3

Bruce R. Schatz (607), National Center for Supercomputing Applications, Beckman Institute, University of Illinois, Urbana-Campaign, Urbana, Illinois 61801

Geraldine Seydoux (323), Department of Embryology, Carnegie Institution of Washington, Baltimore, Maryland 21210

Diane C. Shakes (365), Department of Biology, University of Houston, Houston, Texas 77204

Laura M. Shoman (607), Graduate School of Library and Information Systems, University of Illinois at Urbana-Champaign, Champaign, Illinois 61820

Ratna Shownkeen (533), The Sanger Centre, Hinxton, Cambridge CB10 1RQ, United Kingdom

Paul W. Sternberg (97), Howard Hughes Medical Institute, Research Laboratories, California Institute of Technology, Pasadena, California 91125

Benjamin D. Williams (81), Department of Genetics, Washington University School of Medicine, St. Louis, Missouri 63110

Richard K. Wilson (551, 571), Genome Sequencing Center and Department of Genetics, Washington University School of Medicine, St. Louis, Missouri 63108

PREFACE

The choice of the title "Modern Biological Analysis of an Organism" is intended to emphasize the diverse and continuously evolving methodology and scope of *Caenorhabditis elegans* research. The volume is designed to serve the rapidly expanding community of *C. elegans* researchers, both those dedicated to understanding the biology and genetics of the worm and the growing number of people who would like to use *C. elegans* for particular experiments relevant to their favorite biological question. In addition, this volume is intended to serve readers of the *C. elegans* literature who are looking for a single source book that provides detailed explanations of current *C. elegans* methods.

For an introduction to the field, we recommend the 1988 work "The Nematode *Caenorhabditis elegans*," edited by William B. Wood, which reviews the accomplishments and results generated in the first 25 years of concentrated research efforts on *C. elegans*. This first book provides reviews of major areas of *C. elegans* research and sources of frequently used *C. elegans* information, such as the neuronal "wiring diagram," the cell lineage, and mutant strain lists. As a methods volume, our *C. elegans* book is designed to complement rather than supersede the earlier volume. Our emphasis is on methods rather than on areas of biological investigation, and data lists from the previous volume have been supplanted by directions for obtaining the latest updates over the Internet.

The research approaches of both our book and the 1988 volume originated with Sydney Brenner, then at the Medical Research Council of Molecular Biology in Cambridge, England. Brenner had the foresight to recognize the tremendous potential of *C. elegans* as an experimental organism and pioneered research on its genetics and neurobiology. Brenner and his fellow *C. elegans* researchers at the MRC provided a training environment for many of the principal investigators in the field, and Brenner himself is largely responsible for promoting the multidisciplinary and integrative character of *C. elegans* research.

Newcomers to the *C. elegans* field frequently remark upon the frequent use of the word "community" by *C. elegans* researchers. There is a great deal of communication among laboratories, and a tradition of sharing dominates the field. These exchanges include mutants and DNA clones, databases and DNA sequences, physical DNA and genetic linkage maps, and prepublication data publicized in the "Worm Breeder's Gazette" (although one of us has reservations about nonrefereed communications). This philosophy of sharing is tied to the dominant theme of considering the integrated organism and its life cycle in analyzing specific pathways, stages, structures, and cell types. Because *C. elegans* is a multicellular organism with characteristic nervous, muscle, digestive, and reproductive systems, research in the field involves a wide range of biological disciplines including informatics, neurobiology, pharmacology, psychology, and the triad molecular, cell, and developmental biology.

This volume is divided into four sections that evolved as the book was assembled. The diversity of the chapters and sections serves to emphasize the multitude of biological approaches currently employed in *C. elegans* as well as the evolution of the field from one centered almost exclusively around genetics and neurobiology to one that also sits at the forefront of genomics research.

In the first section, the chapters deal with basic culture methods and the classical strength of the *C. elegans* system, namely its use as a genetic organism. The chapter by Lewis and Fleming on basic culture methods will be useful to new investigators as well as to those who want to employ large-scale culturing methods. The chapter by Huang and Sternberg manages to put much of *C. elegans* research in perspective as the authors explain the methods by which genetics can be used to dissect regulatory pathways. For those interested in classical genetic methods, three chapters (mutagenesis techniques, mosaic analysis, and genetic balancers) uniquely integrate a vast amount of useful information that had not until now been pulled together into single articles. Finally, chapters by Williams and Plasterk describe new approaches of combining molecular and classical genetic techniques that greatly expand the power of *C. elegans* genetic analysis.

In the second section, the breadth of the current research in *C. elegans* neurobiology is revealed. The earlier triumphs of the field, the elucidation of the complete *C. elegans* "wiring diagram" based on the reconstruction of transmission EM serial section and the collection of a vast number of neurological mutants, provide the groundwork for many of these new approaches. Chapters on laser ablation and electrophysiology show how the function of single neurons can be analyzed in the context of the entire worm. The other chapters describe methods by which *C. elegans* is being employed in neuropharmacological studies as well as those of learning and memory.

The third section provides a compilation of a wide variety of techniques that are useful for analyzing cell biological problems in *C. elegans*. Chapters on sperm and blastomere culture describe the method for handling two general cell types that are particularly amenable to cell biological analysis. Other chapters deal with general microscopy techniques and the localization and analysis of both mRNA and protein in *C. elegans* embryos and worms. Also included are chapters on transformation techniques and methods for analyzing transcription and translation, two areas that were still in development when the 1988 volume was written but which have now become standard techniques in the field.

The final section is devoted to the ever-growing importance of genomics and the use of computer databases in *C. elegans* research. For those interested in *C. elegans* as a model organism in genomics research, the methodology underlying the large-scale genomics research is described. For the growing number of people who need access to this genomic information and other *C. elegans* information, two chapters describe the most widely used *C. elegans* databases. The tremendous success of ACeDB, originally developed for *C. elegans,* has led to its adoption by genomic researchers in other systems. WCS is a broader database that contains not only the information in ACeDB but also additional information and added mechanisms of information exchange.

At some level a scientific methods volume is always a "snap-shot" in time, but we hope that the nature of most of the chapters is such that the volume will continue to be a useful reference source for years to come. Nevertheless, we have also listed *C. elegans* information sources in the appendixes, which readers can consult for up-to-the-minute information.

In closing, we sincerely thank the various chapter authors who agreed to contribute to this important community resource as well as the many reviewers whose valuable comments helped ensure that this book would serve as a useful resource for *C. elegans* aficionados as well as newcomers to the field. As editors, we strived to have each chapter reviewed by both *C. elegans* and non *C. elegans* researchers to ensure that the chapters would be accessible and useful to a wide audience.

Henry F. Epstein
Diane C. Shakes

ACKNOWLEDGMENTS

We acknowledge the following persons who critically reviewed the various chapters: Chris Bauer, Kate Beckingham, Hugo Bellen, Alan Coulson, Anne Delcour, Monica Driscoll, Bonnie Dunbar, Patrick Dunne, Gregor Eichele, Arnold Eskin, George Fox, Richard Gibbs, Andy Golden, Richard Gomer, Iva Greenwald, Wade Harper, Ralph Hecht, David Hirsh, Sandra Honda, Kenneth Kemphues, Deborah Kimbrell, James Kramer, Michael Krause, Steve L'Hernault, Don Moerman, James Priess, Mary Rayborn, Gary Ruvkun, Amy Sater, Tim Schedl, Heinke Schnabel, Robert Schwartz, Michael Siciliano, Michael Stern, Susan Strome, Kevin van Doren, Michael Wagner, Samuel Ward, and Richard Wilson.

PART I

Genetic and Culture Methods

CHAPTER 1

Basic Culture Methods

James A. Lewis* and John T. Fleming[†]

* Division of Life Sciences
University of Texas at San Antonio
San Antonio, Texas 78249
† Department of Pediatric Hematology/Oncology
Massachusetts General Hospital
Boston, Massachusetts 02114

METHODS IN CELL BIOLOGY, VOL. 48

I. Life Cycle of *Caenorhabditis elegans*

The nematode *Caenorhabditis elegans* is a small, rapidly growing organism that can easily be raised in the laboratory on the bacterium *Escherichia coli.* Because *C. elegans* is a self-fertilizing hermaphrodite, it is possible to readily grow large quantities of the organism in swirling liquid cultures and also possible to propagate severely incapacitated mutants. The rapidity of growth and the ability to self-fertilize necessitate special measures to establish a synchronous culture.

A. Nematode Stages as Seen under the Dissecting Microscope

A single adult hermaphrodite produces both sperm and oocytes. The number of offspring is limited by the number of sperm and can be increased by mating with a male, whose sperm preferentially fertilize the oocytes. A single hermaphrodite produces about 280 hermaphrodite progeny by self-fertilization and more than 1000 male and hermaphrodite progeny when mated with males. Fertilized eggs are carried and develop internally for several hours. The exact period increases with the age of the hermaphrodite. Eggs are continuously fertilized and laid over a several-day period by the adult hermaphrodite. Each egg develops into an L1 larvae over a span of 14 hours at 25°C from the point of fertilization until hatching (Fig. 1). Eggs grossly appear as 30×50-μm oblate ellipsoid bubbles resting on the agar surface of a petri plate (Fig. 2). Self-fertilized XX hermaphrodites produce exclusively hermaphrodite progeny except for rare XO males ($<1/500$) produced by meiotic nondisjunction (Hodgkin *et al.,* 1979). Males and hermaphrodites occur in equal numbers among outcross progeny of a hermaphrodite. The best way to ensure continuous production of males of defined genotype is to propagate a homozygous strain bearing a *him* (*h*igh *i*ncidence of *m*ales) mutation. Up to 37% of the progeny from a strain carrying *him-8* will be males.

Newly hatched larvae grow quickly through a series of four molts to become adult animals (Fig. 1). On the agar surface of a petri plate, a nematode is constrained by its movement to lie on its side so the "sides" apparent to the observer are actually the dorsal and ventral surfaces of the organism. Worms of all stages, except those undergoing molting, move through waves of alternate dorsal and ventral muscle contraction propagating either forward or backward along the length of the body in a sinusoidal wave. Although the size and shape of the animal do not change markedly until the L4 stage, numerous postembryonic cell divisions and cell deaths are taking place internally (Sulston and Horvitz, 1977). Overt distinguishable differences between male and hermaphrodite larvae first appear during the L3 stage. L3 males have a slightly more swollen tail region. By the L4 stage, nascent formation of the hermaphrodite vulva in the midventral region and the bulbous swelling of the male tail preceding the formation of copulatory rays are much more apparent. By the L4 stage, the hermaphrodite also begins to be distinguished by its larger size and by retention of a whiplike

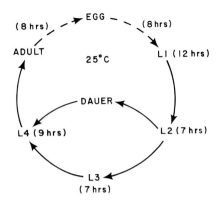

Fig. 1 Life cycle of *Caenorhabditis elegans*. The duration of each developmental state during growth at 25°C on petri plates seeded with *Escherichia coli* strain OP50 is given in parentheses. The solid arrows represent molts. Molting times were determined by monitoring pharyngeal pumping in synchronized populations. Wild-type dauer larvae obtained from starved populations initiate pharyngeal pumping 3–4 hours after being placed in food and reach the L4 stage after an additional 8 hours. The 8 hours from egg to L1 is the interval between egg laying and hatching (the time from fertilization is 14 hours; Wood *et al.*, 1980). The entire life cycle requires 3 days at 25°C. Reprinted with permission from Riddle (1988).

tail. By the adult stage, the larger hermaphrodite has a distinct vulva and eggs begin to accumulate in the anterior and posterior uteri flanking the vulva. The hermaphrodite gut has an enlarged and darkened appearance as it has become a factory for producing stores of material such as vitellogenin for developing oocytes. In the adult stage, the male has a smaller, sleeker appearance. In addition to the fully formed copulatory rays that appear as a fan-shaped flap or triangular spade on the tail (Fig. 2), the male is also readily distinguishable by its behavior. Adult hermaphrodites graze on a lawn of bacteria with relatively little movement. Males are much more active and back up and change direction frequently. A male explores any object that it encounters with its tail and will even chase its own head backward in circles! Although egg laying ceases around day 5, both males and hermaphrodites live mean life span's of 17.7 and 19.9 days at 20°C, respectively (Johnson and Wood, 1982).

Under conditions of starvation and overcrowding, adult hermaphrodites die off and a special third-stage juvenile, the dauer larva, accumulates in cultures (Riddle, 1988). The dauer larva with its sealed mouth and tough cuticle (Fig. 3) can survive several months as an arrested, quiescent developmental stage, particularly if stock plates are stored at 16°C. On reintroduction to food, dauers resume development in a synchronous manner (Fig. 1).

For some purposes, it may be desirable to sex larvae before any overt secondary sexual characteristics are distinguishable under the dissecting microscope. Newly hatched males and hermaphrodites can be distinguished by differential interference contrast optics as described in Fig. 4.

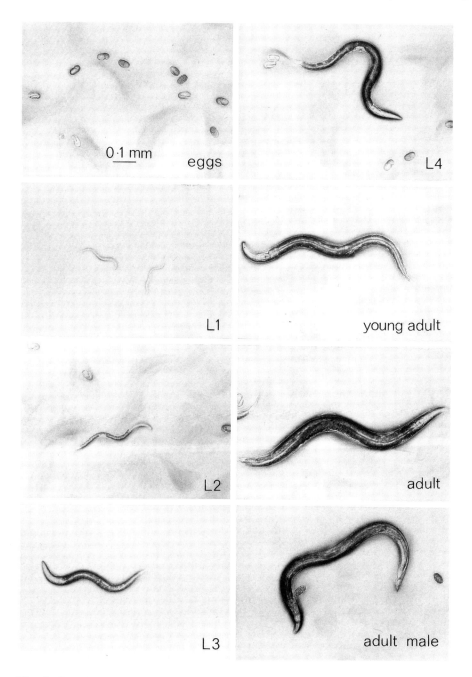

Fig. 2 Eggs, larvae, and adults of *Caenorhabditis elegans*. All panels except bottom right show hermaphrodites. Bright-field photomicrographs taken as described by Sulston and Hodgkin (1988). Reprinted with permission from Wood (1988). Photographs by J. Sulston.

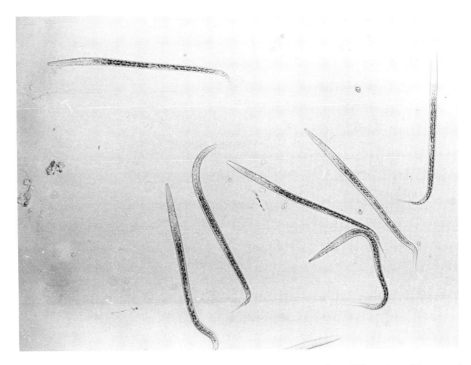

Fig. 3 Bright-field photomicrograph of dauer larvae. Worms are about 400 μm long. Photograph by K. Helmer.

B. Growth Parameters at 16, 20, and 25°C

The growth parameters of the *C. elegans* life cycle at 16, 20, and 25°C are given in Table I. *C. elegans* grows rapidly and is most fecund at 20°C. Growth at 16 and 25°C provides some control over the rate of growth and the facility to work with temperature-sensitive mutants. Hirsh *et al.* (1976) found growth at 25°C to be 2.1 times faster than at 16°C and about 1.3 times faster than at 20°C at all stages of the life cycle. To arrest development temporarily, nematodes may be refrigerated at 6 to 8°C for up to 15 hours (Sulston and Horvitz, 1977).

II. Preparation of Petri Plates for Culturing Nematodes

The observation and genetic manipulation of nematodes are easiest if worms are grown on the hardened agar surface of a petri plate with a limited supply of *E. coli* as food. As too luxuriant a growth of bacteria can inhibit the observation, mating, and growth of nematodes, Brenner (1974) devised the method of seeding NGM plates with the *E. coli* strain OP50 whose growth is limited on NGM

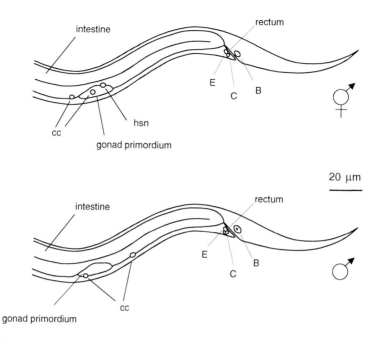

Fig. 4 Anatomical differences between the young hermaphrodite and the young male that can be most readily distinguised by differential interference contrast microscopy. The distinguishing characteristics are position of a left coelomocyte (cc), occurrence of hermaphrodite-specific neurons (hsn), and large size of the B and C cell nuclei in males. Males also differ at hatching in having cephalic companion neurons in the head but these are only readily apparent in older males (Sulston and Horvitz, 1977).

medium by its auxotrophy for uracil. *C. elegans* can be grown on defined synthetic medium in the absence of bacteria but it grows much more poorly and is more expensive to maintain.

A. Pouring Petri Plates

To prepare NGM medium, 3 g of NaCl, 2.5 g of Bacto-peptone, and 17 g of agar are autoclaved in 1 liter of water. After the medium is cooled to 55°C, the following are added in order with swirling, using sterile technique: 1 ml of cholesterol (5 mg/ml in EtOH, flammable!), 1 ml 1 M CaCl$_2$, 1 ml 1 M MgSO$_4$, and 25 ml of 1 M KH$_2$PO$_4$, pH 6.0 (see Section VIII). Plates are usually poured about half-full to facilitate long-term storage of nematodes and the agar surface is flamed to remove air bubbles that allow worms to burrow in the agar. Plates poured by machine, for example, a Brewer Automatic Pipetter (Sepco), will be free of air bubbles and have a uniform height, minimizing the refocusing required in switching between plates under a dissecting microscope. Further additions to

Table I
Growth Parameters of the *Caenorhabditis elegans* Life Cycle[a]

Temperature (°C)	Embryogenesis (h)	Molts (h posthatch)				First eggs laid (h posthatch)
		L1–L2	L2–L3	L3–L4	L4–adult	
16	29[b]	24	39	54.5	74.5	94–97
20	18[b]	15	24	34	46	59–60
25	14	11.5	18.5	26	35.5	45–46

[a] Based on Hirsh *et al.* (1976, Fig. 2).
[b] Calculated by multiplying 25°C embryongenesis time by 20 and 16°C growth rate factors of 1.3 and 2.1, respectively.

the cooled medium can be made immediately before pouring plates, such as the addition of concentrated levamisole hydrochloride to select for drug-resistant mutants. The fungal inhibitor nystatin can also be added to facilitate the long-term storage of stock plates but should not be used in stock plates made for routine growth and observation of worms, as the growth and behavioral characteristics of worms maintained in the presence of this inhibitor are not completely normal. Nystatin can be conveniently and inexpensively prepared by grinding a Mycostatin oral tablet (500,000 units, nystatin U.S.P.; No. 58053, obtainable directly from Bristol Myers–Squibb Pharmaceutical or a local distributor) with 1 ml of H_2O in a mortar and pestle. The slurry is then mixed with 7 ml of EtOH, further ground, and transferred to a capped glass test tube for storage at $-20°C$ in the dark. One milliliter of slurry is added to each liter of medium just before pouring stock plates.

Plates can be stored for months at 4°C either before or after seeding with OP50. Many investigators store plates sealed upright in the plastic bags that the plates originally came packaged in. Temperature fluctuation can cause problems with condensation. We find it convenient to store plates upright in a medium-sized cardboard box lined inside with aluminum foil and covered by a well-fitting foil flap for a top. Disposing of any fungally contaminated plates is best done by sealing them with a thin strip of Parafilm to prevent the scattering of spores around the laboratory.

B. Sterile Precautions

Most medium preparation and growth of worms on plates and in liquid can be done using standard microbiological sterile techniques. If available, a laminar-flow hood would aid preparation of starter cultures for large-scale cultivation of worms and makes it easier to avoid mold when humidity is high; however, a hood is not absolutely necessary. The spread of contamination is facilitated by the forced air systems in constant-temperature incubators. Wrapping critical plates, such as stock plates or starter plates for liquid culture, with a single strip of stretched Parafilm helps preserve sterility and retards desiccation. Worms can crawl from plate to plate under conditions of high humidity, for example, inside a covered box. Otherwise, cross-contamination should not be a problem.

C. Seeding Plates with Bacteria

Plates are seeded with bacteria according to their intended use. Large 9-cm plates can be spread with 3 drops each of an overnight OP50 culture (see Section VIII for minimal medium recipe; OP50 is available from the *Caenorhabditis* Genetics Center, University of Minnesota—St. Paul). Smaller 3.5- or 5-cm plates commonly used for genetics may be spotted with drops of bacteria or painted with a tic-tac-toe grid by using a 1-ml serological pipet and allowing surface tension to draw only a thin layer of OP50 culture out of the pipet tip, lifting the pipet at the end of each stroke. A grid is especially useful for scoring the progeny of a mating on a 5-cm plate as worms prefer the edges of a bacterial lawn and are maximally dispersed along the inside and outside edges of a grid. For a similar reason, large or small plates for mating nematodes are prepared by painting a small Z-shaped mark in the center of each plate. Nematodes mating in a small spot of bacteria tend to burrow. Plates should be incubated overnight at room temperature or about 8 hours at 37°C before adding any nematodes (warm plates must be cooled first). The presence of bacterial growth is essential to retain nematodes on the plate, prevent burrowing, and provide uninterrupted growth. Care should be taken not to gouge the agar surface or spread the bacteria right to the side of the dish.

For simultaneously screening the characteristics of many individual worms, it is convenient to clone individuals in 96- or 24-well microtiter plates (Hirsh and Vanderslice, 1976). For 96-well microtiter plates, 50 μl of a 1% (w/v) solution of bacteria suspended in complete S medium (Rogalski *et al.*, 1988) may be used as the growth medium (see Section VI,A,3 for preparation). For 24-well microtiter plates, 0.5 ml of bacteria solution or 2 ml of NGM agar seeded with OP50 may be used in the larger wells. Care must be taken to avoid worms crawling from well to well. Tissue culture plates having distinctly separate cylindrical wells and having lids fitted with condensation rings are helpful in preventing cross-contamination. Overlaying NGM agar with 2% top agar is helpful in preventing burrowing (Sulston and Hodgkin, 1988).

III. Handling of Nematodes

A. Basic Techniques

A good binocular dissecting microscope is required to work with nematodes. Most work is done at 25× magnification. Magnifications of 50× and 12× are helpful for close observation and scanning a plate, respectively. To transfer individual worms between plates, a wire pick is made by embedding about 1.5 cm of 32-gauge platinum wire in the end of a broken-off Pasteur pipet or in a bacterial inoculating needle equipped with a chuck. Platinum wire cools quickly when flamed. The end of the wire can be cut obliquely with a razor or heavy scissors to fashion a fine point or be flattened and trimmed into a microspatula. An adult worm can easily be scooped up at midbody on the end of the wire. The pick is then held stationary in one hand, while the other hand switches in a new plate under the scope to which the worm is transferred. Any differences in the level of agar between two plates can be accommodated by prefocusing on the plate with the higher level of agar and manually raising the other plate into focus. When the worm to be transferred is lowered to a new plate, a little twist of the pick may help it off onto the plate. With practice, a half dozen or more animals may be transferred at once. Worms are most easily removed from the pick if they are deposited on the bare agar surface of the plate near, rather than in, the bacterial lawn. Picks should be flame-sterilized between transfers, for example, with an alcohol lamp. Accumulated ash debris may be periodically incinerated in a Bunsen burner. Care should be taken to avoid poking holes in the agar or injuring or desiccating animals during transfer. Plates should be labeled on the sides of the dishes and the lids to avoid cross-contamination by accidentally switching lids between plates.

Worms may be transferred from plate to plate in several additional ways. Sterile strips (0.8 × 12 cm) made from charcoal pastel paper or a 3 × 5 index card can be used to scrape masses of worms off one plate and dab them on another. Sterile pointed applicator sticks or flame-sterilized scalpel blades or weighing spatulas allow large numbers of worms to be transferred in agar chunks. Worms may be floated off a plate by gently flooding the plate with M9 buffer (see Section VIII); eggs are preferentially retained. Animals that have burrowed into the agar can be recovered by letting a plate stand with a thin layer of M9 buffer an hour or longer. Larval stage worms, hard to transfer by wire pick, may be individually sucked up in a small volume of buffer using a micropipetter or drawn microcapillary tube. Alternatively, a wad of bacteria can be scooped up on the end of a pick and used as a sticky pad to pick up small worms. Only approximate numbers of worms can be transferred in liquid volume because pipetted worms, particularly adults, settle rapidly.

To grow a large number of adult individuals and larvae, 10 to 20 adult young hermaphrodites should be transferred to a large 9-cm plate spread with OP50. The exact number of parents to use depends on the fecundity of the nematode strain used. After 4 to 5 days at 20°C, 3 days at 25°C, or 6 to 7 days at 16°C, a large plate will contain several thousand adults and tens of thousands of larvae. Proportionally fewer nematodes can be prepared by seeding a 5-cm OP50 cross-hatched plate with three adult hermaphrodites. C. elegans grows so rapidly and reproduces so prolifically that overcrowding and starvation can occur within a day of progeny maturing. Experiments must be well timed. Dauers and young juveniles survive on a starved plate, but a starved plate is useless for most purposes.

B. Mating Nematodes and Maintaining a Male Stock

To mate worms on a large 9-cm plate, 10 to 15 males and a half dozen hermaphrodites are picked to a plate painted with a zigzag of bacteria (a half dozen males and a few hermaphrodites should be used on a 5-cm plate). Mating usually proceeds most efficiently at 20°C. Males tend to crawl off a plate unless a mating plate with a fully grown streak of bacteria is used. To avoid the tedium of having to continually mate males to maintain a male stock, a 9-cm male plate is allowed to starve at 20 or 16°C and may then be kept at 16°C for at least 2 months. By transferring an agar chunk to a fresh plate, males may be grown from the starved stock within 2 days at 20°C. For strains that mate well, an alternative way of having males continuously available is to mate about 12 males and 3 hermaphrodites at 16°C once a week.

C. Storage of Nematode Stocks at 16°C

Worms may be kept several months at 16°C as a special, quiescent third-stage larva, the dauer, that accumulates on starved plates (Figs. 1, 3). Wrapping plates with a strip of stretched Parafilm prevents contamination and prevents evaporation of water. The inclusion of nystatin in stock plates (see Section II, A) helps prevent fungal contamination. Stock plates should be renewed at least every 1 to 2 months by transfer of a chunk of agar to a fresh plate (a paper strip can be used on young plates). To avoid a genetic founder effect in any manipulation involving the transfer of worms, including axenizing and freezing stocks, it is best to propagate scores of worms rather than depend on a few individuals to establish a new stock. Survival is better on a large 9-cm plate but 5-cm plates are adequate and save space. Some mutant strains adventitiously are isolated with secondary mutations that prevent dauer formation, so care must be exercised in holding an unfamiliar strain at 16°C.

IV. Decontamination and Preservation of Nematode Stocks

A. Axenizing Nematode Stocks (Hypochlorite Method)

Because lids are removed from petri plates to manipulate worms and stock plates are stored for months, contamination with mold, yeast, undesirable bacteria, and other microbes can be a serious problem. Mold is the most likely type of contamination to destroy a stock plate and to spread to other plates. Beyond obvious contamination, softening of the agar or failure to clear the bacterial lawn as a plate becomes overcrowded indicates contamination. Although most strains can survive on a contaminated plate, especially if nystatin is included to inhibit fungal growth, stocks must be clean for experimental use and to be reliably frozen. Treatment with alkaline hypochlorite solution (see Section VIII) is the best way to decontaminate nematode stocks. Hypochlorite treatment can also be used to obtain embryos for immunofluorescence analysis (see Chapter 16 in this volume) or *in situ* hybridization (see Chapters 14 and 15 in this volume) and to generate synchronous worm cultures.

In axenizing cultures, it is best to start with a minimally contaminated plate. Serial transfer of a culture by the agar chunk method through several fresh NGM plates can help worms outgrow many contaminants, especially if the agar chunks to be transferred are taken opposite the point of seeding a plate with worms. A plate that contains hundreds of gravid adult worms should be harvested.

In isolating embryos for immunofluorescence or *in situ* hybridization studies, it is best to start with a minimally synchronized culture. Smaller cultures can be started by initially transferring three young adult hermaphrodites to each 5-cm NGM plate seeded with OP50; larger cultures can be started by initially transferring 20 adult hermaphrodites to each 9-cm NGM plate. The worms are harvested after about 3 days of growth at 20°C, or when young gravid adults form the majority of the population.

Adults should be floated off a 9-cm NGM plate in 5 ml of sterile M9 buffer or water and transferred to a sterile disposable 15-ml conical screw-cap centrifuge tube. To avoid removing contamination, no effort should be made to wash off eggs stuck to the plate. Worms are spun down 2 minutes at 1000 rpm (200*g*) in a tabletop clinical centrifuge. The supernatant is removed and the pellet is rinsed by resuspending in fresh buffer or water. The animals are collected again and most of the supernatant is removed. Seven to ten milliliters of alkaline hypochlorite solution (see Section VIII) is added. The solution is allowed to stand 10 to 15 minutes at room temperature with brief and careful vortexing every few minutes to resuspend settled worms (eye protection is advisable) Embryos can die from lack of oxygen or overbleaching so a limited treatment time and frequent agitation are important. For preparing embryos for *in situ* chromosome hybridization, however, a worm pellet should be treated with 1 ml of bleach solution for 7 minutes without agitation. The hypochlorite solution should be made from a bottle of bleach no more than a few months old. Within a few minutes, adult worms should dissolve, leaving a hazy solution of eggs liberated from their carcasses. After hypochlorite treatment, the eggs are collected by centrifugation at 1000 rpm for 2 minutes. The egg pellet is washed twice by resuspension in 10 ml of sterile M9 buffer and collected by centrifugation. The final pellet should be resuspended in a small volume (less than 0.5 ml) for transfer by Pasteur pipet to an NGM plate spread with OP50. The transfer plate will have many newly hatched worms, including some worms hatched and disfigured at the conclusion of the hypochlorite treatment. Repeated treatment of a culture is sometimes necessary to remove all contamination. Spores, especially of some *Bacillus* bacteria, are resistant to hypochlorite treatment. Spreading only half an NGM plate with bacteria and depositing the egg pellet in the bare half of the plate allow the larvae of any mobile strain to crawl away from residual contaminants like spores. The bare agar surface can be excised the next day with sterile applicator stick or flamed weighing spatula. Axenized stocks should be stored wrapped with a single strip of stretched Parafilm to avoid recontamination.

The hypochlorite method may be scaled up to prepare eggs from gram quantities of nematodes. For each volume of worms to be dissolved, 7 to 10 vol of hypochlorite solution should be used. To collect eggs from a large quantity of nematodes, e.g., 50 g, it is helpful to process the worms in several batches and to use a very loose-fitting homogenizer to resuspend the worms rather than rely on vortexing (R. Hecht, personal communication).

B. Freezing Nematode Stocks

Caenorhabditis elegans can be preserved indefinitely at cryogenic temperatures. Successful preservation requires addition of a cryoprotective agent such as glycerol and slow freezing.

A box for freezing worms in an ultralow-temperature freezer can readily be made from an insulated foam box used to ship biological perishables. A suitable box to use should have a rectangular base about 8.5×10 in., be at least 10 in. high without the lid, and have walls 1.5 in. thick. The lid of the box is saved. With a packing knife, the side walls of the box are cut through all around the box 4 in. above the base. A 5.7×7-in. piece of a side wall is saved from the cut off portion of the box to fashion an insert block. Rows of $\frac{3}{8}$ in. holes spaced about $\frac{1}{4}$ in. apart are drilled into the foam insert to provide spaces to hold 80 tubes (best done with a drill press).

Some brands of liquid nitrogen refrigerators provide a foam insert for slow freezing of samples in the neck of the refrigerator. In the experience of the authors in freezing hundreds of mutant strains, freezing above liquid nitrogen yields far fewer survivors and is more unreliable than slow freezing in an ultralow-temperature (-70 to $-100°C$) freezer.

To freeze worms, it is best to use an overgrown plate that has starved for a day or so. The plate should contain thousands of young larvae, as slightly starved L1 and L2 larvae survive freezing best. To prepare four stock vials, including one to be test thawed, the plate is flooded with 3 ml of M9 buffer. The buffer is gently swirled over the agar surface of the plate and removed with a Pasteur pipet by tilting the plate to one side. The worms from each plate are collected in a sterile tube and a roughly equal volume of freezing medium (see Section VIII) is added. The worms are aliquoted out to four 1.8-ml Nunc cryogenic tubes, taking care to resuspend the worms immediately before each transfer. The capped tubes are placed in the foam freezing box and put at $-70°C$. The foam lid is kept only loosely closed. The next day, one of the tubes is test thawed and the remainder of the tubes are stored at $-70°C$ or in liquid nitrogen. We have used regression analysis to analyze data provided by the *Caenorhabditis*

Genetics Center. Survival in liquid nitrogen decreases by only 11% after 11 years of storage (36 to 32%) but survival at −80°C appears to decrease by about 50% (~80 to ~40%) over 10 years regardless of whether the data are fitted by a linear or an exponential decay. Thus, liquid nitrogen appears to offer the surest long-term storage, but worms can be kept safely in an ultralow-temperature freezer for many years. Some mutant strains may survive freezing and recovery much more poorly than the wild type (M. Edgley, pers. comm).

A vial may be thawed by allowing it to stand 15 minutes at room temperature. The contents of a vial are then mixed and poured onto an NGM plate spread with bacteria. Hundreds of worms should survive in a good preparation and many may be seen twitching within minutes of thawing. Freezing many worms in a relatively large volume of liquid (0.5–1.0 ml) seems to favor a good survival rate. Survival of a thawed strain is best judged after overnight growth at 20°C, when possible. One vial of the frozen strain is kept as a permanent master stock never to be thawed except in an emergency. The remaining vials, ideally preserved in a separate freezer, are used as working copies. It is advisable to store at least the master stock in liquid nitrogen to avoid the risk of a mechanical freezer failure (liquid nitrogen suppliers have been known to go on strike, though!).

V. Preparation of Synchronized Cultures and Specific Stages

Synchronously growing animals may be prepared using the same alkaline hypochlorite method employed in axenization. If large numbers of synchronized animals are required, dauer larvae provide a source of worms that will grow to adulthood to lay eggs in approximate synchrony (Wadsworth and Riddle, 1989). Dauer larvae may be prepared by layering 1 ml of 8- to 11-day-old starved liquid culture (see Section VI,A,3) on 2 ml of 15% (w/v) Ficoll 400 (Sigma Chemical Co., No. F4375) in 0.1 M NaCl. After the dauers are allowed to settle for 5 minutes at 1g and the upper layer is removed, dauers may be recovered from the Ficoll layer by several washes with distilled water, pelleting at 2000 rpm. The washed dauers are applied to NGM plates, several thousand per plate. After 48 hours at 25°C, the adults are collected, washed twice with distilled water, and treated with alkaline hypochlorite (Emmons et al., 1979) (see axenization method, Section IV,A). If only small numbers of synchronized animals are needed, eggs may be prepared directly from a plate full of gravid adults rather than starting with dauers. The washed eggs are shaken in M9 buffer for 17 to 22 hours at 25°C. L1 larva, arrested by starvation, resume synchronous growth when reintroduced to bacterial food either on plates or in liquid culture. To avoid the effects of dauer pheromone accumulated during starvation, starved L1s should be washed once with M9 buffer and pelleted by centrifugation before reintroduction to bacteria. The synchrony of hatched postembryonic larva may be monitored by observing pharyngeal beating, which ceases during the molts between larval stages. Synchronously induced dauer larvae may be produced by culture in the presence of dauer pheromone (Golden and Riddle, 1984). Eggs synchronized within the 1- to 30-cell stage may be obtained by hypochlorite treatment of synchronized adults that are just beginning to form eggs (4–6 eggs; Schauer and Wood, 1990; see Table I for development times). Embryos arrested at the 100- to 200-cell stage may be obtained by treatment of parental hermaphrodites with floxuridine (FuDR) (Stroeher *et al.*, 1994).

Care should be exercised in studying the properties of older-stage worms prepared from dauers. The phenotype of some mutants involving the timing of developmental events, for example, *lin-14* (Ambros and Horvitz, 1987), or the formation of cuticle, for example, *sqt-2* (Cox *et al.*, 1980), is known to vary, depending on whether animals pass through the dauer state in maturing.

Adult males may be purified from hermaphrodites by their size and tendency to wriggle through holes (Klass and Hirsh, 1981; Nelson *et al.*, 1982; see Chapter 12 in this volume). A cleaned culture of synchronized young to 1-day-old adults of a *him* strain, such as CB1490 *(him-5),* is first washed on a 35-μm Nitex screen (TETKO, Elmsford, NY) supported on a 13-cm embroidery hoop to separate males from hermaphrodites. Worms from no more than 10 ml of packed culture are allowed to sit undisturbed for 30 minutes. Males in the filtrate may be separated from any young larvae present by layering the filtrate on a 20-μm Nitex screen that is allowed to sit over a petri plate in contact with M9 buffer 30 minutes or longer. The population of worms retained on the filter should be >95% male. The screens, hoops, and glass rod supports for the hoops may be sterilized by soaking in 70% ethanol and drying under a germicidal lamp in a hood for 5 minutes each.

VI. Large-Scale Cultivation of Nematodes

A. Growth of Gram Quantities of Nematodes

Gram quantities of nematodes can be prepared by growth on petri plates or by rotary shaking in a flask at controlled temperatures. Petri plate methods are economical and require no special equipment. Large quantities of nematodes are more easily prepared in fermentor-like devices. Fementors offer the advantage of scalability, minimizing the number of parallel cultures required to grow a large quantity of worms. The yield, cost of expendable materials, and advantages and disadvantages of each method are summarized in Table II.

1. Growth of Nematodes on Enriched Peptone Plates

Gram quantities of nematodes can be grown on enriched peptone plates (see Section VIII) seeded with NA22 bacteria (Schachat *et al.*, 1978) (NA22 is avail-

Table II

Comparison of Culture Methods for Raising Gram Quantities of Nematodes[a]

Method	Size (number of culture vessels)	Yield (g worms)	Cost (dollars/g)	Advantages/disadvantages
NGM plates	9-cm plate (10)	0.47	2.48	High-quality nematodes with no special preparation but low yield
Enriched peptone plates	15-cm plate (10)	3	1.97	High-quality nematodes prepared from readily available ingredients but modest yield
Egg plates	9-cm plate (1)	1	0.14	High yield, inexpensive to prepare but worms may be difficult to purify from egg debris and tend to form dauers from overcrowding
	4-qt dish (1)	10	0.07	
Liquid culture[b]	300 ml in 2800-ml flask (1)[c]	8	0.16	Large quantities prepared in minimal number of culture vessels, but requires special equipment and personnel training; worms grown in liquid appear somewhat starved compared with those grown on NGM plates
	20-liter carboy (1)[c]	200	0.16	
	300-liter fermentor (1)	1500	0.31	

[a] Cost calculations include only expendable materials, not capital equipement or labor. Cost of labor per gram of worms probably decreases going down the table.

[b] May require bacterial fermentor and platform shaker but can be done on modest scale using only compressed house air. Capital cost of equipment can easily range from $4000 to $12,000 according to requirements.

[c] Assumes bacteria prepared using modified SLBH in Labline S.M.S. Hi Density Fermentor.

able from the *Caenorhabditis* Genetics Center, University of Minnesota—St. Paul). Enriched peptone plates are particularly useful for growing moderate quantities of synchronized worms. Enriched peptone plates also provide a better yield per unit weight for some protein preparations, e.g., myosin filaments (Deitiker and Epstein, personal communication), than worms grown in liquid culture. As much as a third of a gram of nematodes can be harvested from a single 15-cm plate seeded with several tens of thousands of L1 larvae.

2. Growth of Nematodes on Egg Plates

As much as a gram of nematodes can be grown on a single 9-cm plate prepared from eggs and up to 10 g of worms may be grown using a 4-qt Pyrex baking dish. Although egg drop medium is inexpensive to prepare and offers an excellent yield, worms may be difficult to purify from egg debris and the worms have a tendency to form dauers at the high density of culture.

The original method described by Baillie and Rosenbluth (personal communication) has been adapted for large-scale nematode culture in 4-qt baking dishes by R. Hecht (pers. comm.). One large egg is added to 50 ml of H broth (see Section VIII) in a sterile 100-ml beaker. The mixture is beaten with a fork sterilized and flamed with 95% ethanol. With a large blunt-ended probe, the mixture is sonicated 5 minutes or until homogeneous. For culturing nematodes on standard NGM plates (9cm), 15 ml of the egg drop mixture is added to each plate. Large Pyrex baking dishes (4 qt) are prepared by autoclaving the empty dish with an aluminum foil cover and then pouring NGM agar to a depth of about 0.6 cm (~250 to 300 ml NGM agar per dish). Eighty milliliters of egg drop mixture is added to the set agar in each 4-qt dish. Each plate or 4-qt dish is inoculated with a stationary culture of OP50 or NA22 (2 to 3 ml of bacteria for a 4-qt dish). The open plates are dried down in a laminar-flow hood by blowing air over them with a small fan. The egg drop medium should be set (still moist) but no longer runny. Egg plates may be stored at 4°C before use (cover 4-qt dishes with plastic wrap). Each dish is inoculated with concentrated worms collected in M9 buffer from overgrown NGM plates (5 plates of worms required for a 4-qt dish).

Worms grown on egg plates must be purified from debris by several rounds of settling. The worms are floated off in M9 buffer and added to the top of a 1-liter graduated cylinder filled with M9 buffer. Worms are allowed to settle at 4°C (30 minutes to an hour). The supernatant is aspirated and the worm pellet is resuspended in M9 buffer and allowed to settle again several more times. The worm pellet may then be further cleaned by flotation on 30% (w/v) sucrose (see Section VI,A,4).

3. Growth of Nematodes on Bacteria in Liquid Culture

Nematodes can readily be grown in large quantity on *E. coli* suspended in S medium, a minimal salts solution (see Section VIII). The bacteria required to grow nematodes can be prepared in bulk quantity and stored at least several weeks at 4°C. Like the nematodes themselves, the bacteria may be grown in a flask or a fermentor, depending on the scale required.

a. Growing Bacteria

Fifteen to twenty grams of bacteria may be prepared per liter of medium by growing bacteria in 2800-ml baffled Fernbach flasks. Yields approaching 30 g of bacteria per liter of medium may be obtained by growing bacteria in Roux bottles with forced aeration, but this method is more prone to contamination.

Bacteria can be grown in high yield in 3XD medium (see Section VIII). The bacteria are freshly streaked out from a frozen permanent stock and a single colony is inoculated into a 10-ml overnight culture made in the same medium. *E. coli* strain NA22 works well, perhaps because it does not form filamentous structures readily. The following day, 5 ml of the overnight culture is inoculated into each of two baffled Fernbach flasks containing 500 ml of 3XD medium. The cultures are grown at 37°C and 250 rpm for a full day. The bacteria are harvested by spinning for 10 minutes at 4000*g* in tared, sterile 500-ml centrifuge bottles with the brake off. The harvested bacteria are weighed. About 25 ml of S medium is then added to each bottle and the bacteria are resuspended in the capped bottles by shaking for 15 minutes to an hour at 250 rpm.

b. Growing Nematodes by Rotary Shaking

By dilution with S complete medium, the bacteria are resuspended at a final density of 30 to 50 g/liter. Unlike bacteria, worms are best grown in an unbaffled 2800-ml Fernbach flask at 20°C shaken at 160 rpm. Bacterial suspension (300–500 ml) is added to each flask to be used. The worm inoculum for each flask should be prepared from a freshly axenized stock that has been allowed to just overgrow a 9-cm plate. Flasks may be covered with commercial closure caps or closures homemade from aluminum foil. A single strip of labeling tape can be used to prevent the closure from riding up on the neck of a flask during days of continuous shaking. If contamination is a problem, plugs made from cotton wrapped in cheese cloth or from silicone sponge (Bellco) can prevent the entry of unfiltered air into a flask. It is helpful to cover flasks fitted with closure plugs loosely with aluminum foil to prevent contamination from settling on the outside of the closure and falling in if the flask is opened for periodical sampling (best not to open before harvesting). An uncontaminated culture will clear of bacteria in 4 to 5 days of growth at 20°C. Freshly cleared cultures should produce a yield of worms equal to about half the weight of the bacteria used. Worms grown in liquid culture will have a longer, thinner look than those grown on plates, and large clumps of eggs may form in liquid culture. The relative numbers of adults and larvae obtained depend on the nematode strain and inoculum used.

In cultures enriched in juvenile worms, some neuronal proteins are a higher percentage of total protein (Lewis *et al.,* 1987). To obtain such cultures, worms may be allowed to continue to grow for several days to a week past the point of clearing. The adults die off, killed by the internal hatching of eggs during starvation. Starved cultures produce a worm yield equal to about a quarter the weight of bacteria used.

c. Growing Nematodes and Bacteria by Forced Aeration

If a rotary shaker is not available, both bacteria and nematodes may be efficiently grown using forced aeration. Cultures of either may be aerated in tall, narrow bottles such as 1-liter Roux bottles (Corning No. 1290-1L) using house-compressed air or a high-capacity fish pump. Up to 500 ml of culture may be grown in an 850-ml bottle. Air should be filtered through sterile cotton. To aerate bacterial cultures, fritted glass dispersion tubes are necessary (12 mm diameter × 250 mm long, Corning No. 3953312EC). Antifoam A concentrate (2 μl, Sigma Chemical Co., No. A 5633) is added to each bottle before aeration is begun. The harvested bacteria are resuspended in complete S medium (see Section VIII), and the culture is inoculated with axenized nemotodes as for growth by rotary shaking. To limit foaming and avoid clogging spargers with worm debris, it is sufficient to aerate the nematode culture with a straight glass tube extending to the bottom of the culture bottle. Bubbling should be vigorous enough to visibly circulate culture medium. Aquarium gang valves are useful in distributing the air among cultures.

4. Cleaning Nematodes

A freshly cleared, uncontaminated culture is easy to clean. In such a culture, the main contaminants are worm cuticles, salt crystals, and a few dead worms and perhaps some residual bacteria. Worms may be collected from large culture volumes by sedimentation overnight at 4°C after chilling on ice. Settling in a large graduated cylinder or a tall, narrow bottle helps concentrate the worms. After the culture medium is aspirated off, the nematodes from a 300-ml culture may be collected in two to four 50-ml centrifuge tubes, using 0.1 M NaCl to wash the worms into a few tubes. Keeping worms cold (0–4°C) helps both in pelleting and in floating worms on sucrose. Worms are pelleted by spinning 2 minutes at 700 rpm (100g) in a tabletop centrifuge with the brake off. Washing worms several times at this step, including settling by gravity, may help remove minor contamination. Flotation of worms on 30% (w/v) sucrose in water is an economical method of cleaning (Sulston and Brenner, 1974), but results in loss of some worms, particularly juveniles, to the bottom of a centrifuge tube by the increased density caused by osmotic shrinkage. For flotation on 30% (w/v) sucrose, worms may be suspended in 0.1 M NaCl and mixed with an equal volume of ice-cold 60% (w/v) sucrose before spinning 5 minutes at 700 rpm (100g). The tubes are spun immediately after mixing, and not too many tubes are spun at once to avoid loss of worms to the bottom of the tube by osmotic shrinkage on standing in 30% sucrose. The floating worms are removed to a fresh tube by sucking them off the wall of the centrifuge tube with a Pasteur pipet. The worms are then washed twice by centrifugation, pelleting them from 0.1 M NaCl by spinning 2 minutes at 700 rpm.

A superior but more expensive method of cleaning moderate quantities of relatively uncontaminated worms is to first sediment the nematodes through 15% (w/v) Ficoll 400 in 0.1 M NaCl and then float the worms on 35% (w/v) Ficoll 400 in 0.1 M NaCl. Ficoll is about 15 times more expensive than sucrose. Some researchers use Renograffin-60, available from Bristol Myers-Squibb or a local pharmacy, as a less expensive, less viscous substitute for Ficoll. Undiluted Renograffin-60 has a density equivalent to that of 75% (w/v) Ficoll. For the sedimentation step, it is helpful to dilute the worm pellet with an equal volume of 0.1 M NaCl before layering it over 15% (w/v) Ficoll to avoid mass transfer of worms into the Ficoll layer. Worms are spun 15 min at 700 rpm (100g). For flotation on 35% (w/v) Ficoll, a small volume of nematodes, no more than a few grams per 50-ml tube, is thoroughly mixed with the flotation medium by inverting the tube. The tube is then spun 15 minutes at 700 rpm. Worms are washed twice with 0.1 M NaCl, spinning 2 minutes at 700 rpm. The pellet may then be homogenized or quick-frozen for storage at −70°C.

Cultures starved for 1 week contain enough debris and dead worms that it is helpful to put the flotation step first to avoid a mass transfer effect in pelleting through Ficoll. Flotation on 30% (w/v) sucrose works best to remove living worms from debris in a starved culture. The worms that float are then washed once with 0.1 M NaCl before pelleting through 15% (w/v) Ficoll 400 in 0.1 M NaCl.

B. Growth of Hundred-Gram Quantities of Nematodes

1. Efficient Large-Scale Growth of Bacteria

Large quantities of the *E. coli* strain NA22 can be grown in a 3-liter Labline S.M.S. Hi-Density Fermentor as follows. The basic SLBH medium (see Section VIII) and the methodology are similar to those described by Sadler *et al.* (1974) with some modifications. To begin fermentation, a 300-ml overnight culture of NA22 grown in modified SLBH medium is inoculated into 3 liters of SLBH medium in the S.M.S. fermentor chamber. The chamber is rotated at 320 rpm at 37°C with an initial oyxgen flow rate of 1 to 2 liters/min. Unlike the method of Sadler and co-workers, all the glycerol needed is present from the start. A hood, if available, is the safest method of exhausting fermentation waste gases. Otherwise, it is helpful to pass the exhaust tube from the fermentor down a drain and up the other side of a trap to avoid unpleasant smells. The drain should be simultaneously flushed with air to avoid O_2 accumulation in the sewer pipes. After 3 or 4 hours fermentation, the O_2 flow rate is turned up to 4 to 5 liters/min for the remainder of the fermentation. Around 4 hours, a slow trickle of cooling water is turned on to keep the temperature of the fermentor at 37°C. After the foam is allowed to settle, bacteria are harvested in eight 500-ml centrifuge bottles with sealing caps. Yields of 250 g bacteria per 3.3 liters of medium can routinely be obtained.

2. Growth of Nematodes in Carboys by Forced Aeration

Large quantities of nematodes can be prepared in the following way. Transparent polycarbonate carboys (20 liter) are fitted with caps that have three holes drilled in their tops. Two holes accommodate $\frac{3}{16} \times \frac{1}{16} \times \frac{5}{16}$-in. Tygon tubing. The tubing to carry incoming air runs through one hole in the cap to the bottom of the carboy and is weighted with a stainless-steel nut held on by a flanged plastic tubing connector. Incoming air is filtered through sterile cotton but not prehumidified. Outlet tubing of the same size begins just inside the lid and is run through the other tubing hole into a hood or sewer pipe. A third hole, $\frac{3}{4}$-in. diameter, is closed with a stopper. Sterile water can be periodically added through the third hole to maintain the liquid level of cultures during vigorous aeration. Carboys are autoclaved with 16 liters of S medium (see Section VIII) and concentrated *E. coli* are added to give a final bacterial concentration of 28 g/liter in a final volume of 18 liters. Before nematodes are inoculated, a carboy is vigorously aerated overnight. Carboys are then inoculated with 50 to 600 ml of a clearing nematode culture grown in flasks by rotary shaking. Aeration should be vigorous enough to form a standing wave 1 to 2 in. high. When the bacteria are exhausted (about 4 days with a 600-ml inoculum), nematodes can be harvested by first chilling the cultures for 2 hours in an ice water-filled sink and then allowing settling to continue overnight at 4°C. Culture medium is removed from the settled worms by aspiration. Worms can be cleaned as described above (see Section V,A,4) by flotation on 30% (w/v) sucrose followed by sedimentation through 15% (w/v) sucrose in 250-ml centrifuge bottles spun in a swinging bucket rotor (Ficoll is expensive for large-scale preps). After two washes with 0.1 *M* NaCl, collected worms are frozen and stored at −80°C. In our experience, nematode proteins are stable for many months in this condition.

About 200 g of nematodes may be obtained from a single carboy if harvested as the bacteria clear, and about 100 g can be obtained if the culture is allowed to starve 1 week for preparation of juveniles.

C. Growth of Kilogram Quantities of Nematodes in Large Fermentors

Kilogram quantities of nematodes can be grown in large fermentors (150–250 liters) by scaling up the same basic recipes for growth of bacteria and nematodes (C. Johnson and A. O. W. Stretton, pers. comm.; Gbewonyo *et al.*, 1994). Bacteria and worm cultures may be harvested by continuous-flow centrifugation or by settling worms in 50-liter separatory funnels after chilling. Worms are purified by filtration through cheesecloth followed by flotation on 30 to 35% (w/v) sucrose and frozen by dribbling into liquid nitrogen. Contamination problems are alleviated by using *E. coli* strain OP50-1, a uracil auxotroph resistant to streptomycin and phage 80 (available from the *Caenorhabditis* Genetics Center, University of Minnesota—St. Paul), and by growing both bacteria and worm cultures in the presence of streptomycin sulfate (50 mg/liter, Sigma No. S 6501) and nystatin (50,000 units or 10 mg/liter, Sigma No. N 3503). More than 1.4 kg of nematodes have been obtained from a fermentor run employing 5 kg of *E. coli*. The final yield of nematodes appears limited only by the efficiency with which *E. coli* can be grown in a large fermentor. Johnson and Stretton found that a 1/1500 dilution of commercial bleach was capable of removing ciliate contamination from a late-stage culture with no apparent effect on nematodes.

Means of homogenizing nematodes and precautions that need to be taken against proteolysis are discussed in Chapter 18 of this volume.

VII. Growth of Radioactively Labeled Worms

Nematodes can be labeled to a high specific radioactivity with ^{35}S, ^{3}H, or ^{32}P by feeding them radioactively labeled bacteria. The nonfeeding dauer stage can be labeled to a lower specific radioactivity by an exchange reaction with $^{14}CO_2$ incorporated into solution as $NaH^{14}CO_3$. Nonradioactive labeling of nematode proteins with biotin offers an alternative to working with large amounts of radio-activity.

A. Labeling *E. coli* with [^{35}S] Sulfate

Nematodes can be labeled with ^{35}S by feeding them *E. coli* that have been labeled with [^{35}S]sulfate or a [^{35}S]methionine/cysteine mix (Epstein *et al.,* 1974; Schachat *et al.,* 1977; Garcea *et al.,* 1978; Cox *et al.,* 1981a; Lewis, unpublished). Care must be taken not to make bacteria so radioactive that nematode growth is inhibited. To prepare nematodes containing more than 10^8 cpm of ^{35}S label, 3 ml of an overnight culture of NA22, a radiation-resistant strain of *E. coli,* is grown in low-sulfate minimal medium (see Section VIII) and inoculated into 300 ml of the same medium containing 1.5 mCi of [^{35}S] sulfate (Dupont NEX-042) or EXPRE$^{35}S^{35}S$ cysteine/methionine protein labeling mix (DuPont NEG-072). For growth on a cysteine/methionine labeling mix, the medium is supple-mented with a 2 $\mu g/ml$ mix of unlabeled cysteine and methionine (1:3 ratio) and the amount of unlabeled sulfate is reduced (see Section VIII). After over-night growth at 37°C, the bacteria are harvested by a 5-minute centrifugation at 4000 rpm in 250-ml centrifuge bottles, being careful not to fill each bottle more than about half-full. The percentage incorporation may be assayed by counting 10 μl of culture fluid before and after pelleting the bacteria. Incorporation should range from 60 to 80% (Bretscher and Smith, 1972; Lewis, unpublished). The bacterial pellet is then resuspended in 45 ml of complete S medium (see Section VIII) in a sterile 500-ml flask covered with a aluminum foil closure and inoculated with several dozen adult worms (30 μl of worm suspension obtained from a 9-cm NGM plate started from 10 wild-type adults and then flooded when clearing with several milliliters of M9 buffer made without magnesium sulfate). The culture is grown by rotary shaking at 20°C at 160 rpm until all bacteria are consumed (about 5 days). The nematodes may be collected and cleaned as described above for the growth of gram quantities of nematodes. To prepare an extract, worms may be broken in a French pressure cell if care is taken to plug the mouth of the collection tube with cotton or a tissue to prevent the escape of a radioactive aerosol. ^{35}S radioactivity incorporated into homogenate fractions may be assayed by trichloroacetic acid precipitation (Garcea *et al.,* 1978). More than 10^9 cpm of radioactivity should be incorporated into the bacteria and the yield of radioactive nematodes should be in excess of 10^8 cpm. About 1 g of radioactively labeled bacteria is obtained from 300 ml of low-sulfate medium, allowing a final yield of about 0.5 g of ^{35}S-labeled worms. A specific radioactivity of about 62.5 Ci/mole sulfur is obtainable. If a larger physical mass of worms is required for preparative work, worms may be grown on ^{35}S-labeled bacteria diluted with unlabeled bacteria in a volume of complete S medium appropriate for the total mass of bacteria (see Section VI,A). For shorter 2-hour pulse-labeling experiments, worms may be fed bacteria labeled to a specific radioactivity of 625 Ci/mole. Label may be incorporated at discrete times in the life cycle by pulse-feeding synchronized L1 larvae or postdauers on ^{35}S-labeled bacteria (Garcea et al., 1978; Cox et al., 1981a) (see Section V for synchrony and staging). If a rotating shaker with temperature control is not available, nematodes may be grown in a thin layer of bacterial solution placed in empty petri dishes or on labeled bacteria placed on plates without peptone (NP plates, see Section VIII). To grow worms in a thin layer of liquid, the bacteria from 100 ml of low-sulfate medium are resuspended in 7.5 ml of complete S medium for one 9-cm dish. To disperse bacteria on NP plates, the pellet from 300 ml of bacterial culture should be resuspended in 10 ml of M9 buffer and 0.5 ml dispensed per NP plate. For short labeling pulses, each plate can support several thousand adults and proportionally greater numbers of juveniles for up to 14 hours at 25°C. The dishes should be sealed with a stretched strip of Parafilm and placed in a tray in a below-ambient-temperature incubator set at the desired growth temperature between 16 and 25°C, with special care taken to avoid spillage. In our experience, it is easiest to efficiently label and recover nematodes from liquid culture.

B. Labeling *E. coli* with [³H]Leucine

When the amount of sulfur in a particular protein is low or unknown, it may be desirable to label proteins more generically with [³H]leucine, a much more common amino acid than cysteine or methionine. ³H decays are detected much less efficiently than ^{35}S decays, but the large amount of radioactivity that can be incorporated compensates for the inefficiency of detection. The same minimal medium used to grow bacteria for ^{35}S labeling is used, except $MgSO_4$ is added to 10 mM. The medium also contains 2 μg/ml unlabeled leucine and 0.5 mCi of [³H]leucine for each 100 ml of bacterial culture to be grown. Allowing for detection efficiency, the same yields of radioactivity incorporated into bacteria and nematodes are obtained with ³H leucine as for ^{35}S labeling.

C. Labeling *E. coli* with [³²P] Orthophosphate

Using ^{32}P-labeled bacteria (1 g, containing 15 mCi ^{32}P), worms from a plate inoculum can be uniformly labeled to a specific radioactivity of 30 Ci/mole by growth over 5 days in low-phosphate medium (Sulston and Brenner, 1974). By pulse labeling with more radioactive bacteria (0.4 g, containing 50 mCi ^{32}P) for 16 hours, an incorporation as high as 200 Ci/mole can be obtained. The culture methods are similar to those described for ^{35}S labeling except low-phosphate medium for bacterial and nematode growth is employed (see Section VIII). As millicurie amounts of ^{32}P are incorporated (0.6 and 14 mCi, respectively) adequate radiation safety measures must be employed.

D. Labeling Dauer Stages Directly with NaH^{14}CO$_3$

During molts, *C. elegans* stops feeding. To label cuticular proteins synthesized during molting, Cox *et al.* (1981b) have employed pulse labeling with NaH^{14}CO$_3$ (40–60 Ci/mole). Several thousand synchronized worms are incubated for 30 to 60 minutes in 0.5 ml of M9 buffer containing 15 to 60 μCi of NaH^{14}CO$_3$. After pulse labeling, the worms are washed 4 to 10 times in chase buffer (667 ml M9 buffer, 8.4 g NaHCO$_3$, water to 1 liter). Harvesting immediately and chasing for more than 1 hour yield similar results. During a 60-minute pulse, 1 to 2% of the label is incorporated into trichloroacetic acid-insoluble macromolecules and at least 50% of the incorporated label comprises amino acids.

E. Nonradioactively Labeling *Caenorhabditis elegans* Proteins with Biotin

Several groups have investigated the nonradioactive labeling of nematode proteins using reactive biotin derivatives. Detection of derivatized proteins by binding of avidin or streptavidin conjugates of alkaline phosphatase or horseradish peroxidase coupled with chemiluminescent detection methodology allows the detection of as little as 10 pg of protein and provides an alternative to the use of the large amounts of radioactivity required for metabolic labeling (see above). The blots can be developed in a day, in contrast to the several days that are required for detection of ^{35}S by fluorography. A potential drawback for some applications is the presence of avidin-binding proteins in *C. elegans* extracts (M. Blaxter, pers. comm.). Detection of specific proteins may be enhanced if a selective fractionation method, such as immunoprecipitation, is used following the biotinylation step. Standard procedures for biotinylation (Hnatowich *et al.,* 1987) and immunoprecipitation (Miyake *et al.,* 1991) can be employed. For immunoprecipitation, care must be taken that the biotinylation reagent is adequately quenched to avoid reaction with the antibody (reaction with 0.1 *M* ethanolamine or glycine, pH 8.0, for 1 hour at 4°C recommended) and that the antigenicity of the targeted protein is not affected by biotinylation.

VIII. Solutions

1. NGM agar (Brenner, 1974): 3 g NaCl, 2.5 g peptone, 17 g agar, 975 ml water. Autoclave. Cool to 55°C, then sterilely add, in order, 1 ml cholesterol

(5 mg/ml in EtOH), 1 ml of 1 M CaCl$_2$, 1 ml of 1 M MgSO$_4$, and 25 ml of 1 M potassium phosphate, pH 6.0 (solution 2). The cholesterol solution need not be sterilized.

2. 1 M Potassium phosphate, pH 6.0: 136 g KH$_2$PO$_4$, add water to 900 ml. Adjust pH to 6.0 with concentrated KOH. Add water to 1 liter. Autoclave.

3. M9 buffer (Brenner, 1974): 6 g Na$_2$HPO$_4$, 3 g KH$_2$PO$_4$, 5 g NaCl, 0.25 g of MgSO$_4$ · 7H$_2$O per liter. Autoclave.

4. Minimal medium for growing OP50 and NA22: To 10 ml sterile M9 buffer (solution 3), add 0.1 ml each of sterile 2 M NH$_4$Cl and 20% (w/v) D-glucose. Add 0.02 ml of sterile 2 mg/ml uracil (may be autoclaved). Growth of OP50 on minimal medium minimizes adventitious contamination in bacterial stock cultures. For maintainence of NA22, omit uracil. Grow cultures overnight at 37°C, shaking at 225 rpm. Store at 4°C. Preserve aliquots of bacterial stock cultures by addition of sterile 80% (w/v) glycerol to a final concentration of 15% (w/v) glycerol and quick-freezing in a cryotube in liquid nitrogen or dry ice/ethanol. Preserve at −70°C or below. Streak out bacteria from ice with flamed wire loop without thawing (or preserve a working aliquot in 50% w/v glycerol at −20°C for months without freezing).

5. Freezing medium (based on Sulston and Brenner, 1974): 20 ml of 1 M NaCl, 10 ml of 1 M KH$_2$PO$_4$, pH 6.0 (solution 2), 60 ml of 100% glycerol, water to 200 ml. Autoclave. Add 0.6 ml of sterile 0.1 M MgSO$_4$.

6. Alkaline hypochlorite solution for axenization and bulk embryo isolation (based on Hecht *et al.*, 1981): 2 ml of fresh Clorox bleach or equivalent (4–6% sodium hypochlorite), 5 ml of 1 N NaOH, to axenize one plate of worms.

7. Enriched peptone plates (based on Schachat *et al.*, 1978): 1.2 g of NaCl, 20 g of peptone, 25 g of agar. Add water to 1 liter. Autoclave. Cool to 55°C. Then sterilely add 1 ml cholesterol (5 mg/ml in EtOH), 1 ml of 1 M MgSO$_4$, and 25 ml of 1 M potassium phosphate, pH 6.0 (solution 2).

8. Hershey broth to prepare egg plates (based on Hershey and Chase, 1952): 8 g nutrient broth (GIBCO, 5 g peptone, 3 g beef extract), 5 g peptone, 5 g NaCl, 1 g dextrose, water to 1 liter. Autoclave.

9. 3XD (Epstein *et al.*, 1974): 10.5 g Na$_2$HPO$_4$, 4.5 g KH$_2$PO$_4$, 0.6 g NH$_4$Cl, 15 g casein hydrolysate (should not be vitamin-free), 24 g glycerol, water to 1 liter. Autoclave. Add 3 ml of 1 M MgSO$_4$. A variation on this recipe suggested by S. Ward, doubling the amounts of NH$_4$Cl and casamino acids, increasing MgSO$_4$ by 2.8 ×, and adding 1 ml of trace metals (solution 13), can increase the bacterial yield by at least 50%.

10. S basal medium (Sulston and Brenner, 1974): 5.9 g of NaCl, 50 ml of 1 M potassium phosphate, pH 6.0 (solution 2), 1 ml of cholesterol (5 mg/ml in EtOH), to 1 liter with water. Autoclave.

11. Complete S medium (Sulston and Brenner, 1974): To each liter of S basal medium (solution 10), add the following sterile components: 10 ml 1 M potassium

citrate, pH 6.0 (solution 12); 10 ml trace metals solutions (solution 13); 3 ml 1 M CaCl$_2$; 3 ml 1 M MgSO$_4$.

12. 1 M potassium citrate, pH 6.0: 268.8 g tripotassium citrate, 26.3 g citric acid monohydrate, water to 900 ml. Adjust pH to 6.0 with concentrated KOH. Add water to 1 liter. Autoclave.

13. Trace metals solution (Sulston and Brenner, 1974): 1.86 g Na$_2$EDTA, 0.69 g FeSO$_4$ · 7H$_2$O, 0.20 g MnCl$_2$ · 4H$_2$O, 0.29 g ZnSO$_4$ · 7H$_2$O, 0.016 g CuSO$_4$, water to 1 liter. Autoclave. Store in the dark.

14. Modified SLBH medium (based on Sadler $et~al.$, 1974): To make 3 liters of SLBH medium, dissolve 67 g of yeast extract (Sigma No. Y 4000), 32 g of casein enzymatic hydrolysate (Sigma No. C 1026), and 87 g of glycerol in 2.7 liters of water. Autoclave. To complete the medium, add 300 ml of 1 M K$_2$HPO$_4$, bringing the pH to about 6.8.

15. Low-sulfate medium for labeling bacteria with ^{35}S (based on Bretscher and Smith, 1972): To make 300 ml for labeling with ^{35}SO$_4$ (DuPont NEX-042), add 30 ml of 10 × M9 buffer made without MgSO$_4$ and 3 ml of 2 M NH$_4$Cl to a 1-liter flask, add water to 300 ml, and autoclave. After cooling, add 1.5 ml of 20% glucose, 0.6 ml of 1 M MgCl$_2$, and 4.8 ml of 5 mM MgSO$_4$. To make 300 ml for labeling with a cysteine/methionine labeling mix (DuPont NEG-072), add only 4.0 ml of 5 mM MgSO$_4$ and supplement the medium with 2 μg/ml mix of unlabeled cysteine and methionine in a 1 : 3 ratio.

16. NP plates without peptone for ^{35}S labeling (Schachat $et~al.$, 1977): 1.2 g of NaCl, 25 g of agar. Add water to 1 liter. Autoclave. Cool to 55°C. Then sterilely add 1 ml cholesterol (5 mg/ml in EtOH), 1 ml of 1 M MgSO$_4$, and 25 ml of 1 M potassium phosphate, pH 6.0 (solution 2).

17. Low-phosphate medium for labeling bacteria with ^{32}P (Sulston and Brenner, 1974): 5 g NaCl, 1.5 g KCl, 1 g NH$_4$Cl, 2 g vitamin-free casamino acids (Difco), 2 g Bacto-Peptone (Difco), 12.1 g Tris base. Add water to 1 liter and adjust pH to 7.4 with HCl. Autoclave.

18. Low-phosphate SLP medium for growing nematodes on ^{32}P-labeled bacteria (Sulston and Brenner, 1974): S medium with only 0.01 M potassium phosphate and the addition of imidazole hydrochloride, pH 6.0, to 0.04 M. Autoclave.

Acknowledgments

The completion of this work was supported in part by Grant GM-08194 from the National Institutes of Health and Grant HRD-92-53024 from the National Science Foundation. Thanks to the many people who generously provided information and advice.

References

Ambros, V., and Horvitz, H. R. (1987). The lin-14 locus of $Caenorhabditis~elegans$ controls the time of expression of specific postembryonic developmental events. $Genes~Dev.$ **1**, 398–414.

Brenner, S. (1974). The genetics of *Caenorhabditis elegans*. *Genetics* **77,** 71–94.

Bretscher, M. S., and Smith, A. E. (1972). Biosynthesis of ³⁵S-L-methionine of very high specific activity. *Anal. Biochem.* **47,** 310–312.

Cox, G. N., Laufer, J. S., Kusch, M., and Edgar, R. S. (1980). Genetic and phenotypic characterization of roller mutants of *Caenorhabditis elegans*. *Genetics* **95,** 317–339.

Cox, G. N., Staprans, S., and Edgar, R. S. (1981a). The cuticle of *Caenorhabditis elegans*. II. State-specific changes in ultrastructure and protein composition during postembryonic development. *Dev. Biol.* **86,** 456–470.

Cox, G. N., Kusch, M., DeNevi, K., and Edgar, R. S. (1981b). Temporal regulation of cuticle synthesis during development of *Caenorhabditis elegans*. *Dev. Biol.* **84,** 277–285.

Emmons, S. W., Klass, M. R., and Hirsh, D. (1979). Analysis of the constancy of DNA sequences during development and evolution of the nematode *Caenorhabditis elegans*. *Proc. Natl. Acad. Sci. U.S.A.* **76,** 1333–1337.

Epstein, H. F., Waterston, R. H., and Brenner, S. (1974). A mutant affecting the heavy chain of myosin in *Caenorhabditis elegans*. *J. Mol. Biol.* **90,** 291–300.

Garcea, R. L., Schachat, F., and Epstein, H. F. (1978). Coordinate synthesis of two myosins in wild-type and mutant nematode muscle during larval development. *Cell* **15,** 421–428.

Gbewonyo, K., Rohner, S. P., Lister, L., Burgess, B., Cully, D., and Buckland, B. (1994). Large scale cultivation of the free living nematode *Caenorhabditis elegans*. *Biotechnology* **12,** 51–54.

Golden, J. W., and Riddle, D. L. (1984). The *Caenorhabditis elegans* dauer larva: Developmental effects of pheromone, food, and temperature. *Dev. Biol.* **102,** 368–378.

Hecht, R. M., Schomer, D. F., Oró, J. A., Bartel, A. H., and Hungerford, E. V., III. (1981). Simple adaptations to extend the range of flow cytometry five orders of magnitude for the DNA analysis of uni- and multicellular systems. *J. Histochem. Cytochem.* **29,** 771–774.

Hershey, A. D., and Chase, M. (1952). Independent functions of viral protein and nucleic acid in growth of bacteriophage. *J. Gen. Physiol.* **36,** 39–56.

Hirsh, D., and Vanderslice, R. (1976). Temperature-sensitive developmental mutants of *Caenorhabditis elegans*. *Dev. Biol.* **49,** 220–235.

Hirsh, D., Oppenheim, D., and Klass, M. (1976). Development of the reproductive system of *Caenorhabditis elegans*. *Dev. Biol.* **49,** 200–219.

Hnatowich, D. J., Virzi, F., and Rusckowski, M. (1987). Investigations of avidin and biotin for imaging applications. *J. Nucl. Med.* **28,** 1294–1302.

Hodgkin, J., Horvitz, H. R., and Brenner, S. (1979). Nondisjunction mutants of the nematode *Caenorhabditis elegans*. *Genetics* **91,** 67–94.

Johnson, T. E., and Wood, W. B. (1982). Genetic analysis of life-span in *Caenorhabditis elegans*. *Proc. Natl. Acad. Sci. U.S.A.* **84,** 6603–6607.

Klass, M., and Hirsh, D. (1981). Sperm isolation and biochemical analysis of the major sperm protein from *Caenorhabditis elegans*. *Dev. Biol.* **84,** 299–312.

Lewis, J. A., Fleming, J. T., McLafferty, S., Murphy, H., and Wu, C. (1987). The levamisole receptor, a cholinergic receptor of the nematode *Caenorhabditis elegans*. *Mol. Pharmacol.* **31,** 185–193.

Miyake, K., Weissman, I. L., Greenberger, J. S., and Kincade, P. W. (1991). Evidence for a role of the integrin VLA-4 lympho-hemopoiesis. *J. Exp. Med.* **173,** 599–607.

Nelson, G. A., Roberts, T. M., and Ward, S. (1982). *Caenorhabditis elegans* spermatozoan locomotion: Amoeboid movement with almost no actin. *J. Cell Biol.* **92,** 121–131.

Riddle, D. L. (1988). The Dauer Larva. In "The Nematode *Caenorhabditis elegans*" (W. B. Wood, ed.), pp. 393–412. Cold Spring Harbor Laboratory, Cold Spring Harbor, New York.

Rogalski, T. M., Bullerjahn, A. M. E., and Riddle, D. L. (1988). Lethal and amanitin-resistance mutations in the *Caenorhabditis elegans* ama-1 and ama-2 genes. *Genetics* **120,** 409–422.

Sadler, J. R., Miwa, J., Maas, P., and Smith, T. (1974). Growth of high density bacterial cultures: A simple device. *Lab. Pract.* **23,** 642–643.

Schachat, F. H., Harris, H. E., and Epstein, H. F. (1977). Two homogenous myosins in body-wall muscle of *Caenorhabditis elegans*. *Cell* **10,** 721–728.

Schachat, F., Garcea, R. L., and Epstein, H. F. (1978). Myosins exist as homodimers of heavy chains: Demonstration with specific antibody purified by nematode mutant myosin affinity chromatography. *Cell* **15,** 405–411.

Schauer, I. E., and Wood, W. B. (1990). Early *C. elegans* embryos are transcriptionally active. *Development* **110,** 1303–1317.

Stroehcr, V. L., Kennedy, B. P., Millen, K. J., Schroeder, D. F., Hawkins, M. G., Goszczynski, B., and McGhee, J. D. (1994). DNA-protein interactions in the *Caenorhabditis elegans* embryo: Oocyte and embryonic factors that bind to the promoter of the gut-specific *ges-1* gene. *Dev. Biol.* **163,** 367–380.

Sulston, J. E., and Brenner, S. (1974). The DNA of *Caenorhabditis elegans*. *Genetics* **77,** 95–104.

Sulston, J., and Hodgkin, J. (1988). Methods. *In* "The Nematode *Caenorhabditis elegans*" (W. B. Wood, ed.), pp. 587–606. Cold Spring Harbor Laboratory, Cold Spring Harbor, New York.

Sulston, J. E., and Horvitz, H. R. (1977). Post-embryonic cell lineages of the nematode, *Caenorhabditis elegans*. *Dev. Biol.* **56,** 110–156.

Wadsworth, W. G., and Riddle, D. L. (1989). Developmental regulation of energy metabolism in *Caenorhabditis elegans*. *Dev. Biol.* **132,** 167–173.

Wood, W. B. (1988). Introduction to *C. elegans* Biology. *In* "The Nematode *Caenorhabditis elegans*" (W. B. Wood, ed.), pp. 1–16. Cold Spring Harbor Laboratory, Cold Spring Harbor, New York.

Wood, W. B., Hecht, R., Carr, S., Vanderslice, R., Wolf, N., and Hirsh, D. (1980). Parental effects and phenotypic characterization of mutations that affect early development in *Caenorhabditis elegans*. *Dev. Biol.* **74,** 446–469.

CHAPTER 2

Mutagenesis

Philip Anderson

Department of Genetics
University of Wisconsin
Madison, Wisconsin 53706

I. Introduction

Mutations are the fuel that drives genetic analysis. Without a plentiful and continuing supply of mutations, the genetic enterprise grinds to a halt. Germ-line mutations occur naturally during growth and reproduction of all strains, but such spontaneous mutations are too infrequent to be generally useful. In most *Caenorhabditis elegans* strains, spontaneous mutations arise at frequencies of about 10^{-6} per gene per generation. Spontaneous mutations are valuable for molecular analyses, but working geneticists need not depend on these rare events for new alleles. A variety of mutagenic agents and treatments are available to assist an investigator in obtaining useful or desired mutations. This chapter summarizes the principles and protocols involved in mutagenesis of *C. elegans*. It is intended as a guide to the choice of mutagens and elaborates basic principles for their rational use. This chapter considers only mutagenesis related to "forward" genetic analysis. "Forward" in this context means the identification of mutant strains following global mutagenesis of the entire genome. "Reverse" genetics and site-directed mutagenesis are considered elsewhere in this volume (see Chapter 3).

The goal of *in vivo* mutagenesis is to increase either the frequency or the variety of mutations contained in a population of animals. The benefit of increasing the frequency of mutations is self-evident; it makes finding the desired mutants easier. This is especially important when methods for phenotypic screening are laborious. The benefit of increasing the variety of mutations may be less obvious, but it is often of great importance. "Variety" in this context means the numbers and types of DNA alterations that cause mutant phenotypes. Correctly interpreting genetic data often relies on explicit or implicit knowledge of the molecular lesion involved. Understanding the mutagenic process can aid these interpretations. More importantly, certain types of mutations can be the key ingredient to subsequent genetic or molecular experiments. For example, having conditional alleles of essential genes simplifies many genetic manipulations. Transposon insertions or other types of gene rearrangement are often key ingredients in successful strategies for cloning genes defined by mutation. An investigator can use knowledge of the mutagenic process to his or her advantage when designing such experiments or interpreting their results.

II. Development of the Germ Line

Only mutations that occur in the germ line are heritable. An understanding of germ-line development (Kimble and Ward, 1988) is therefore necessary to achieve an effective mutagenesis. The adult germ line is descended from a single embryonic stem cell, P4, which is born shortly after fertilization. P4 divides once during embryonic development, yielding two germ-line precursor cells in L1 larvae. Germ-line nuclei proliferate throughout postembryonic development, yielding about 1000 nuclei in hermaphrodites and 500 in males. These numbers increase during adulthood, because in both sexes a population of germ-line descendants continue mitotic division throughout adult growth. Pachytene nuclei, indicating entry of germ-line nuclei into meiosis, are first observed during L3 lethargus in hermaphrodites and during mid-L3 in males. As the developing gonads enlarge during L3 and L4, increasing numbers of nuclei enter meiosis. Primary spermatocytes, indicating gamete differentiation, are first observed during mid-L4 in males and late L4 in hermaphrodites. Oogenesis in hermaphrodites commences shortly after the L4 molts to adulthood. Oogenesis in hermaphrodites and spermatogenesis in males continue throughout the adult reproductive period.

As the goal of a mutagenesis procedure is usually to mutagenize as many gametes as possible, it follows that the most effective development stage for mutagenesis is the late L4 larva or young adult. The number of germ-line nuclei is near its maximum at these stages. Mutagenesis of the appropriate stage can be achieved either by synchronizing a parental population prior to mutagenesis or, more commonly, by picking L4 or young adult animals from a mixed-stage population immediately after they have been mutagenized. Mutagenesis of gravid hermaphrodites is effective, but care must be taken to ensure that eggs contained in gravid adults at the time of mutagenesis are excluded from the offspring population. Eggs are impermeable to most compounds and will, therefore, be unmutagenized.

As germ-line nuclei divide mitotically throughout larval and, to a lesser extent, adult development, a mutation induced in one nucleus can expand into a clone of nuclei that all contain the same mutation. In such cases, recovered mutants often represent repeated isolations of the very same mutational event. The problem is most severe when young larvae, which contain small numbers of rapidly proliferating germ-line nuclei, are mutagenized. Such problems are lessened (but not eliminated) by mutagenizing L4 or young adult animals. Even sexually mature adults maintain a population of mitotic germ nuclei, so the problem persists in all mutagenic protocols. The only way to ensure independence of multiple isolates is to divide mutagenized parents into separate subpopulations before or immediately after mutagenesis and to retain at most a single mutant from each subpopulation.

Either hermaphrodites or males can be mutagenized. Each of the self-fertilized offspring of a mutagenized hermaphrodite contains two sets of mutagenized chromosomes (one sperm, one oocyte). Each of the cross-fertilized offspring of a mutagenized male contains one set of mutagenized chromosomes. These differences must be taken into account if the frequency of mutants is determined among the offspring. Mutant frequencies are most usefully expressed as events per mutagenized gamete (haploid set of chromosomes). Following mutagenesis, the desired mutants are identified based on their phenotype among the F1, F2, or subsequent generations. Provided that late larvae or young adults are mutagenized, mutants identified among the F1 must contain dominant alleles, whereas those identified among the F2 or subsequent generations may contain either dominant or recessive alleles. Hermaphrodite self-fertilization ensures that mutations heterozygous in the F1 are often homozygous in the F2. Maternal effects can cause mutant phenotypes to not be evident until the F3 generation.

III. Mutagen Efficiency versus Mutagen Specificity

Two important, but quite separate, aspects of a mutagen should be considered prior to its use. One is mutagen efficiency. That is, how effective is the mutagen at inducing new mutations? What is the frequency of such events following mutagenesis? The second is mutagen specificity. What types of mutations does a mutagen cause (base substitutions, deletions, etc.)? The goals of a mutagenesis protocol are often conflicting. A very potent mutagen is of little value if it does not increase the frequency of the desired type of lesion. For example, ethyl methanesulfonate is an exceedingly potent mutagen, but almost all of its mutational products are G/C → A/T transitions. Ethyl methanesulfonate is worthless if the goal is to isolate transposon insertions. Conversely, a very specific mutagen may not be helpful if it is inefficient. For example, spontaneous mutations, which in certain strains are often caused by transposon insertion, are quite rare events even in mutator strains (see below). Efficient methods of screening or selection may be needed before spontaneous mutagenesis becomes a realistic strategy. Both the efficiency and specificity of commonly used *C. elegans* mutagens are summarized below.

IV. The Dark Side of the Force

The efficiency with which a mutagen induces new mutations is a two-edged sword. On the one hand, very potent mutagens are advantageous because they increase the frequency of mutations to maximum levels. On the other hand, potent mutagens are disadvantageous because they induce large numbers of extraneous mutations at the same time. *In vivo* mutagenesis procedures are inherently global in nature. The entire genome is mutagenized, and, from a population of mutagenized animals, mutant individuals are identified. Such mutants contain one mutation that causes a phenotype of interest, but they may contain hundreds of additional lesions elsewhere in the genome. Some of these extraneous mutations affect protein coding sequences; others do not. Of those that are in coding regions, some affect function of the gene product; others do not. In cases where extraneous mutations affect phenotype, genetic results can be confusing or misleading. If a mutant exhibits multiple phenotypes, is this due to pleiotropy of a single mutation? Or, is it due to the presence of multiple mutations in the strain? When a DNA sequence change is identified in a particular mutant strain, does that mutation actually cause the phenotype of interest? Or, is the observed lesion extraneous, with another undetected lesion being responsible? These are examples of problems that plague forward genetic analysis. The problems posed by adventitious mutations are most severe when potent mutagens are used. Some startling predictions and cautionary examples of this phenomenon are described below.

Ethyl methanesulfate (EMS) is the most widely used mutagen for *C. elegans*, primarily because it is one of the most potent agents available. The measured frequency of mutations affecting an average-sized gene following EMS mutagenesis (50 m*M,* see below for dose response) is between 1×10^{-4} and 5×10^{-4} per mutagenized gamete (Brenner, 1974; Meneely and Herman, 1979; Greenwald and Horvitz, 1980; Howell and Rose, 1990; Johnsen and Baillie, 1991). Accepting the higher of these figures (a more typical result) implies that a reduction-of-function or loss-of-function allele occurs in one of every 2000 mutagenized gametes. This number (1/2000) represents the frequency of *functionally defective alleles,* not total mutations. Only a small fraction of EMS-induced mutations yield functionally defective gene products (see below). The *C. elegans* genome is estimated to contain 17,800 expressed transcripts (Wilson *et al.,* 1994), of which 2000 to 3500 represent essential genes (Brenner, 1974; Clark *et al.,* 1988; Howell and Rose, 1990; Johnsen and Baillie, 1991). If we assume that the average frequency of loss-of-function alleles of all genes is the same as that of the measured sample, it follows that when a young adult hermaphrodite is mutagenized with EMS and allowed to self-fertilize, every F1 animal is, on average, heterozygous for 18 loss-of-function mutations affecting expressed genes, 2 to 4 of which represent recessive lethal mutations! Clearly, extraneous mutations are a common and serious complication.

The magnitude of the problem is even more apparent when total mutations, not just those that cause functional defects, are considered. As discussed below, almost all EMS-induced mutations are G/C → A/T transitions. The frequency of such mutations following EMS mutagenesis is remarkably high, about 7×10^{-6} per mutagenized G/C base pair. This estimate follows from two observations: (1) The frequency of EMS-induced alleles of the amber suppressors *sup-5* and *sup-7* is about 10^{-5} per mutagenized gamete (Waterston, 1981). (2) For both *sup-5* and *sup-7,* a single C → T transition, in the anticodon of a tRNA^{Trp} gene, is the mutational target for induction of a suppressor allele (Bolten *et al.,* 1984; Kondo *et al.,* 1988; Kondo *et al.,* 1990). Thus, a 2-base-pair (bp) target yields a mutation frequency of 10^{-5} per mutagenized gamete. Similar observations for amber suppressor mutations affecting a different collection of five tRNA^{Trp} genes (Hodgkin, 1985; Kondo *et al.,* 1990) indicate EMS mutation rates of about 8×10^{-6} per mutagenized G/C base pair. Estimates from a larger mutational target are in agreement. The frequency of *unc-54(0)* alleles isolated in an unbiased manner (an F1 clonal screen) is about 1 per 800 mutagenized gametes (Bejsovec and Anderson, 1988; S. Brenner, pers. comm.). Sequencing 18 *unc-54(0)* mutations demonstrates that most of them (16/18) are nonsense alleles (Dibb *et al.,* 1985; Bejsovec and Anderson, 1990). *unc-54* contains 160 G/C base pairs which, if mutated to A/T base pairs, yield a nonsense codon (Karn *et al.,* 1983). Assuming that all such base pairs are mutable, and that all such mutants are genuine *unc-54(0)* alleles, the deduced frequency of mutations is 7×10^{-6} per mutagenized G/C base pair.

The *C. elegans* haploid genome is estimated to be 8×10^7 bp, of which 36% is G/C (Sulston and Brenner, 1974). Assuming the single-base frequency derived above applies to the whole genome, it follows that every mutagenized gamete contains more than 200 G/C → A/T transitions. When hermaphrodites are mutagenized and allowed to self-fertilize, their offspring derive from two mutagenized gametes and, therefore, contain more than 400 such mutations. The genomes of mutagenized animals are replete with unwanted, extraneous mutations.

How are such complications to be avoided? There are several contributing solutions. The first and most important is to thoroughly outcross newly isolated mutants to unmutagenized genetic backgrounds. During the outcross series, Mendelian segregation and crossing over will separate most extraneous mutations from the selected mutation. Linked mutations, however, can be difficult to remove even by repeated outcrossing. For example, an extraneous mutation that is 10 map units away from a gene of interest will be removed by six unselected outcrosses only about half of the time. Forcing deliberate crossovers on both sides of the gene of interest improves the cleansing process. Isolating multiple alleles of a gene can identify the effects of adventitious mutations. Independent alleles each contain a different collection of such mutations. Phenotypes exhibited by several independent mutants are unlikely to be caused by extraneous mutation. Most mutations that affect phenotype are recessive, including those that are extraneous. Examining phenotypes in compound heterozygotes (animals heterozygous for two independent mutations affecting a single gene) reduces the confounding influences of linked or unlinked extraneous mutations.

A corollary of the above discussion is that the frequency of mutants exhibiting any specific phenotype should never be less than about 10^{-5} following EMS mutagenesis. A frequency of about 10^{-5} represents a single-base-pair target. If the frequency is less than this, the phenotypes are probably not single-gene affects, or they are not caused by G/C $\rightarrow$ A/T transitions. For example, resistance to high levels of ivermectin occurs at a frequency of about 10^{-7} per mutagenized gamete following EMS mutagenesis. All of these resistant strains are double mutants. They contain mutations affecting two separate genes, both of which are necessary for high-level resistance (C. D. Johnson, pers. comm.).

V. Chemical Mutagenesis

A. Mutagens

Water-soluble chemical mutagens are among the most potent and easiest to use. EMS is by far the most commonly used mutagen, but chemical mutagens having differing specificities are available as well. Information concerning the efficiency and specificity of a number of chemical mutagens are summarized below. For many mutagens, information concerning their efficiency or specificity in *C. elegans* is limited to one or only a small number of genes. As EMS is the most widely used mutagen, the efficiencies of all other mutagens considered below are compared with its efficiency.

1. Ethyl Methanesulfonate

a. Efficiency

EMS is the most potent and widely used mutagen available for *C. elegans*. As discussed above, the frequency of loss-of-function or reduction-of-function alleles for an average sized gene is about 5×10^{-4} per mutagenized gamete. The frequency of G/C → A/T transitions is about 7×10^{-6} per mutagenized G/C base pair. EMS concentrations of 50 mM are typically used, but lower doses (10–25 mM) can reduce toxicity to the mutagenized parents and mitigate the confounding influences of extraneous mutations. The frequency of induced mutations using 12.5 mM EMS is about half that of 50 mM (Rosenbluth *et al.,* 1983).

b. Specificity

Table I summarizes the sequences of 245 sequenced EMS-induced mutations. Ninety-two percent are G/C → A/T transitions. Because of this extreme specificity, and because stop codons [amber (UAG), ochre (UAA), and opal (UGA)] are rich in A and U residues, EMS is an excellent mutagen for generating nonsense alleles. EMS induces deletions and chromosomal rearrangements also, but the rates of these changes have not been rigorously determined. The data in Table I tend to underestimate the proportion of rearrangements, as alleles chosen for sequencing tend to be point mutations. In cases where a relatively unbiased sample of EMS-induced single-gene, homozygous-viable mutations have been examined by Southern blots or other means for deletions, about 13% (13/102) of EMS-induced mutations are deletions or other rearrangements (Finney *et al.,* 1988; Ruvkun *et al.,* 1989; Bejsovec and Anderson, 1990; Ahringer and Kimble, 1991; Miller *et al.,* 1992; Klein and Meyer, 1993; P. Anderson, unpublished results). Deletions range in size from 4 bp to more than 18 kilobases (kb). EMS-induced deletions appear on average to be small. Of 249 EMS-induced recessive lethals in the *unc-22, sDp2,* or LGV(left) regions, only one is a deficiency by genetic criteria (Clark *et al.,* 1988; Howell and Rose, 1990; Johnsen and Baillie, 1991). This low proportion demonstrates that large deletions are rare among EMS-induced events. EMS may efficiently induce other types of chromosomal rearrangements, however. *sup-3* alleles, which result from duplications and amplifications of the *myo-3* myosin heavy-chain gene (Maruyama *et al.,* 1989), occur following EMS mutagenesis at the remarkably high frequency of 2×10^{-4} per gamete (Riddle and Brenner, 1978). This frequency is only two- to threefold lower than that of EMS single-gene mutation frequencies. It is unclear if this is exceptional or typical for EMS-induced duplications.

2. Nitrosoguanidine

a. Efficiency

The efficiency of mutagenesis by nitrosoguanidine (NTG), EMS, and several other mutagens considered below has been measured using a convenient and easy test system. Loss-of-function alleles of three different genes (*unc-93, sup-9,* and *sup-10*) suppress the uncoordinated and egg-laying defective phenotype of *unc-93 (e1500)* (Greenwald and Horvitz, 1980). Using this system, the single-gene mutation frequency following NTG mutagenesis is about 10-fold lower than that observed with EMS. In other organisms, however, NTG is an exceptionally

Table I
Summary of Sequences of 245 Ethyl Methanesulfonate-Induced Mutations

Gene	Number of alleles	Sequence changes	Reference
unc-54	10	2 G → A[a] 6 C → T 1 A → T[a] 2 deletions	Dibb *et al.*, 1985
unc-54	44	17 G → A 25 C → T 2 deletions	Bejsovec and Anderson, 1990
let-60	25	17 G → A[b] 7 C → T 2 A → T[b]	Beitel *et al.*, 1990 Han and Sternberg, 1991
lin-12	8	4 G → A 4 C → T	Greenwald and Seydoux, 1990
fem-3	9	5 C → T 2 T → C 1 G → T 1 deletion	Ahringer and Kimble, 1991
unc-15	8	4 G → A 3 C → T 1 A → G	Gengyo-Ando and Kagawa, 1991
emb-9	3	3 G → A	Guo *et al.*, 1991
deb-1	2	3 G → A[c] 1 C → T	Barstead and Waterston, 1991
glp-1	15	8 G → A 5 C → T 1 T → A 1 deletion	Kodoyianni *et al.*, 1992
tra-1	8	8 C → T	Zarkower and Hodgkin, 1992
sem-5	6	5 G → A 1 C → T	Clark *et al.*, 1992
dpy-7	4	4 G → A	Johnstone *et al.*, 1992
unc-93	3	2 G → A 1 C → T[d] 1 G → T[d]	Levin and Horvitz, 1992
tra-2	2	1 G → A 1 C → T	Kuwabara *et al.*, 1992
glp-1	17	17 G → A	Lissemore *et al.*, 1993
sdc-3	14	5 G → A 7 C → T 1 C → A 1 deletion	Klein and Meyer, 1993
sqt-1	8	4 G → A 4 C → T	Kramer and Johnson, 1993
ced-3	8	3 G → A 5 C → T	Yuan *et al.*, 1993

continues

Table I

(*continued*)

Gene	Number of alleles	Sequence changes	Reference
rol-6	5	3 G → A 2 C → T	Kramer and Johnson, 1993
dpy-10	3	2 G → A 1 C → T	Levy *et al.*, 1993
dpy-2	2	2 G → A	Levy *et al.*, 1993
unc-17	2	1 G → A 1 G → T	Alfonso *et al.*, 1993
mei-1	14	6 G → A 8 C → T	Clark-Maguire and Mains, 1994
let-23	11	8 G → A 2 C → T 1 C → G	Aroian *et al.*, 1994
mec-4	5	1 G → A 4 C → T	Hong and Driscoll, 1994
ced-9	3	2 C → T 1 T → A	Hengartner and Horvitz, 1994
unc-101	1	1 C → T	Lee *et al.*, 1994
Total:		122 G → A 103 C → T 7 deletions 13 others	

[a] *unc-54(e1152)* contains both a G → A transition and a nearby A → T transversion.
[b] *let-60(s1155)* contains both a G → A transition and a nearby A → T transversion.
[c] *deb-1(st555)* contains three separate G → A transitions.
[d] *unc-93(n200)* contains both a C → T transition and a G → T transversion.

potent mutagen. It seems likely that conditions for optimum NTG mutagenesis of *C. elegans* have not yet been established.

b. Specificity

No information is available.

3. Diethyl Sulfate

a. Efficiency

Using reversion of *unc-93(e1500)* as a measure, the single-gene mutation frequency following diethyl sulfate mutagenesis is about twofold lower than that observed with EMS (Greenwald and Horvitz, 1980).

b. Specificity

Limited information is available. The diethyl sulfate-induced allele *unc-93(n234)* is a G → A transition (Levin and Horvitz, 1992).

4. N-Nitroso–N-ethylurea

a. Efficiency

Using reversion of *unc-93(e1500)* as a measure, the single-gene mutation frequency following *N*-nitroso-*N*-ethylurea (ENU) mutagenesis is about the same as that observed with EMS (D. Stanislaus and B. De Stasio, pers. comm.).

b. Specificity

ENU-induced mutations have not yet been sequenced. Based on results from other organisms, a variety of transitions and transversions are expected (Richardson *et al.*, 1987; Pastink *et al.*, 1989).

5. Formaldehyde

a. Efficiency

The frequency of formaldehyde-induced *unc-22* mutations (2×10^{-4} per mutagenized gamete) is about sevenfold lower than that obtained with EMS (EMS frequency adjusted to reflect 50 mM EMS, Moerman and Baillie, 1981; Rosenbluth *et al.*, 1983). The frequency of formaldehyde-induced recessive lethals balanced by *eT1(III;V)* (1.6% per mutagenized chromosome) is fourfold lower than that obtained with 12.5 mM EMS (Johnsen and Baillie, 1991) and about ninefold less than with 50 mM EMS (Rosenbluth *et al.*, 1983).

b. Specificity

Eleven of thirty-three formaldehyde-induced *unc-22* mutations and 6 of 16 formaldehyde-induced lethals balanced by *eT1(III;V)* are large deficiencies by genetic criteria (Moerman and Baillie, 1981; Rogalski *et al.*, 1982; Johnsen and Baillie, 1988). Such alleles are lethal when homozygous and delete two or more nearby genes. *unc-54(s291)*, a formaldehyde-induced allele, is a small (1275-bp) deletion.

6. Acetaldehyde

a. Efficiency

Using reversion of *unc-93(e1500)* as a measure, the single-gene mutation frequency following acetaldehyde mutagenesis is about 10-fold lower than that observed with EMS (Greenwald and Horvitz, 1980).

b. Specificity

No information is available.

7. Diepoxyoctane

a. Efficiency

The frequency of *unc-54(0)* mutations following diepoxyoctane (DEO) mutagenesis is about two- to threefold lower than that observed with EMS using the same screen (Anderson and Brenner, 1984).

b. Specificity

An estimated 27% of DEO-induced *unc-54* mutations are multigene deletions defined by genetic criteria (Anderson and Brenner, 1984). Such alleles are lethal when homozygous and delete one or more essential genes near *unc-54*. Among 44 homozygous viable DEO-induced *unc-54* alleles, one is a small deletion and one is a 288-bp displaced duplication (Eide and Anderson, 1985c; B. Saari and P. Anderson, unpublished observations). The remainder exhibit no alterations on Southern blots and, therefore, are likely to be point mutations.

8. Diepoxybutane

a. Efficiency

Using reversion of *unc-93(e1500)* as a measure, the single-gene mutation frequency following diepoxybutane (DEB) mutagenesis is about the same as that observed with EMS (Trent *et al.*, 1991).

b. Specificity

Among DEB-induced *unc-54* and *unc-22* alleles, 15% (7/47) are small deletions, ranging in size from 0.5 to 3.5 kb (Trent *et al.*, 1991). This makes DEB very similar to EMS with regard to induction of small deletions. DEB-induced point mutations have not been sequenced.

B. Protocols

All of the mutagens listed below are known or suspected carcinogens. Great care must be exercised in their use. Wear gloves when handling all mutagens and work in a fume hood when using volatile compounds. Use disposable plasticware instead of reusable glass. Dispose of all reagents and contaminated supplies in a safe manner (e.g., a dedicated chemical or radiological disposal procedure). Inactivate mutagens whenever possible before disposal. Consult a qualified chemical safety official for detailed protocols for safe inactivation and/or disposal of these mutagens.

1. Ethyl Methanesulfonate

This procedure is adapted from that of Sulston and Hodgkin (1988). Make a solution of 0.1 *M* EMS (also known as methanesulfonic acid ethyl ester) by adding 0.02 ml (20 μl) of liquid EMS to 2 ml of M9 buffer. Gently agitate until the dense oily liquid has dissolved. Collect nematodes in M9 buffer and wash once with M9. Add 2 ml of the suspension of washed worms to the 2 ml of EMS solution (final concentration 0.05 *M* EMS) in a wide-bore test tube. Incubate for 4 hours at 20°C. Agitate occasionally to increase aeration. After mutagenesis, wash worms once with M9 buffer. Distribute mutagenized worms to NGM plates as desired.

Notes. EMS must be kept anhydrous and solutions made freshly. Store EMS at room temperature. EMS is volatile; work in a fume hood. Solutions containing EMS are inactivated by mixing them with an equal volume of "inactivating solution" (0.1 M NaOH, 20% w/v $Na_2S_2O_3$) for 24 hours. Equipment or accessories contaminated with EMS should be soaked in inactivating solution for 24 hours prior to disposal.

2. Nitrosoguanidine

This procedure is from Greenwald and Horvitz (1980). To 3 ml of washed animals in M9 buffer, add 1 ml of an *N*-methyl-*N'*-nitro-*N*-nitrosoguanidine (Aldrich) solution in M9 buffer, such that the final concentration is 0.5 mg/ml NTG. Incubate for 1 hour at 20°C. Agitate occasionally to increase aeration. Wash the animals two or three times in M9 buffer after mutagenesis. Distribute mutagenized worms to NGM plates as desired.

3. Diethyl Sulfate

This procedure is from Greenwald and Horvitz (1980). To 3 ml of washed animals in M9 buffer, add 1 ml of diethyl sulfate (Aldrich) solution in M9 buffer, such that the final mutagenesis concentration is 1 mM diethyl sulfate. Incubate 2 hours at 20°C. Agitate occasionally to increase aeration. Wash the animals two or three times in M9 buffer after mutagenesis. Distribute mutagenized worms to NGM plates as desired.

Notes. DES is volatile; work in a fume hood.

4. Formaldehyde

This procedure is from Moerman and Baillie (1981). Prepare formaldehyde by warming 5 g of paraformaldehyde (Fisher) in 50 ml of 65°C distilled water. Add NaOH to clear the solution. After clearing, adjust the solution to pH 7.2, dilute to 150 ml with distilled water, and dilute further to 500 ml by adding M9 buffer. This 1% solution is then kept as a stock solution. Collect nematodes in M9 buffer and wash once with M9. To 9 vol of worm suspension, add 1 vol of the formaldehyde stock solution (final concentration 0.1%). Incubate 4 hours at 20°C. Agitate occasionally to increase aeration. After mutagenesis, wash worms once with M9 buffer. Distribute mutagenized worms to NGM plates as desired.

5. Acetaldehyde

This procedure is from Greenwald and Horvitz (1980). To 3 ml of washed animals in M9 buffer, add 1 ml of acetaldehyde (Aldrich) solution in M9 buffer, such that the final mutagenesis concentration is 0.1% acetaldehyde. Incubate 2 hours at 20°C. Agitate occasionally to increase aeration. Wash the animals two or three times in M9 buffer after mutagenesis. Distribute mutagenized worms to NGM plates as desired.

Notes. Acetaldehyde is volatile and flammable; work in a fume hood.

6. Diepoxyoctane

This procedure is from Anderson and Brenner (1984). Make a solution of 40 mM 1,2,7,8-diepoxyoctane by adding 11.4 μl of liquid DEO to 2 ml of M9 buffer. Gently agitate until the light, oily DEO liquid has dissolved. Collect nematodes in M9 buffer and wash once with M9. Add 0.2 ml of 40 mM DEO solution to 3.8 ml of washed worms (final concentration 2 mM). Incubate 3 hours at 20°C. Agitate occasionally to increase aeration. After mutagenesis, wash worms once with M9 buffer. Distribute mutagenized worms to NGM plates as desired.

Notes. DEO should be stored anhydrous. DEO is volatile; work in a fume hood.

7. Diepoxybutane

This procedure is adapted from that of Trent *et al.* (1991). Make a solution of 10 mM 1,2,3,4-diepoxybutane (also known as 1,3-butadiene diepoxide) by adding 2.0 μl of liquid DEB to 2 ml of M9 buffer. Gently agitate until the light, oily DEB liquid has dissolved. Collect nematodes in M9 buffer and wash once with M9. Add 0.04 ml (40 μl) of 10 mM DEB solution to 4.0 ml of washed worms (final concentration 10^{-4} M). Incubate 3 hours at 20°C. Agitate occasionally to increase aeration. After mutagenesis, wash worms three or four times with M9 buffer. Distribute mutagenized worms to NGM plates as desired.

Notes. DEB should be stored anhydrous. DEB is volatile; work in a fume hood.

VI. Radiation Mutagenesis

A. Mutagens

Exposure of *C. elegans* to ultraviolet light, ionizing radiation, or particle bombardment is strongly mutagenic. Radiation mutagenesis is usually performed with the expectation of recovering genome rearrangements. Such rearrangements might be small, intragenic lesions (e.g., small deletions) or large, multigene mutations (e.g., deficiencies and translocations). The efficiency and specificity of commonly used procedures are described below. Where possible, mutagenic efficiencies are compared with that of EMS, the benchmark mutagen. In several cases, mutagenic specificities have been determined using only genetic criteria.

1. Gamma Irradiation

a. Efficiency

Gamma irradiation is a potent mutagen. The frequency of γ-ray-induced recessive lethals balanced by *eT1(III;V)* (4% per mutagenized chromosome: Rosenbluth *et al.,* 1985) is only slightly less than that observed with 12.5 m*M* EMS (6%: Johnsen and Baillie, 1991). If reversion of *unc-93(e1500)* is used as a measure, the single-gene mutation frequency following γ-ray mutagenesis is equal to or slightly higher than that observed with EMS (Greenwald and Horvitz, 1980).

b. Specificity

A large proportion of γ-ray-induced mutations are DNA rearrangements. This is true both for homozygous viable alleles (presumed single-gene mutations) and for alleles isolated in a manner that allows them to be lethal when homozygous. For example, of 16 homozygous viable γ-ray-induced alleles of *unc-93, sdc-3, lin-14,* or *unc-86,* 9 exhibit DNA abnormalities detected on Southern blots (Levin and Horvitz, 1992; Klein and Meyer, 1993; Ruvkun *et al.,* 1989; Finney *et al.,* 1988). Of 29 γ-ray-induced alleles of *unc-93* and LG V(left) (isolated in a manner that recovers lethal alleles), 16 are chromosomal rearrangements (Greenwald and Horvitz, 1980; Rosenbluth *et al.,* 1985). Nine of the sixteen are deficiencies, four are translocations, two are duplications, and one is an uncharacterized crossover suppressor.

2. X Irradiation

a. Efficiency

Like gamma irradiation, X rays are efficient mutagens for generating large deficiencies. Following 7000–8000 rad of X irradiation, LG II and LG X deficiencies occur from 2×10^{-4} to 9×10^{-4} per mutagenized gamete (Meneely and Herman, 1979; Sigurdson *et al.,* 1984). X-ray-induced alleles of *sup-35* and *sup-36,* a screen that demands homozygous viable alleles, occur at frequencies about fivefold lower than those observed with EMS (Schnabel *et al.,* 1991).

b. Specificity

Sixteen of twenty-one X-ray-induced alleles of *unc-105* are large deficiencies by genetic criteria (Sigurdson *et al.,* 1984).

3. Ultraviolet Irradiation

a. Efficiency

Following 120 J/m^2 of UV irradiation, recessive-lethal mutations balanced by *eT1(III;V)* occur at frequencies about half that observed with EMS (Stewart *et al.,* 1991; Johnsen and Baillie, 1991).

b. Specificity

Based on one investigation, UV irradiation appears to generate a large proportion of gene rearrangements among its mutational products. Of 12 recessive lethals balanced by *eT1,* 6 are large deficiencies by genetic criteria, 2 are duplications, 1 is a translocation, and only 3 appear to be single-gene mutations (Stewart *et al.*, 1991). A single sequenced UV-induced allele, *unc-15(su2000)*, is a 3-bp deletion (Gengyo-Ando and Kagawa, 1991).

4. Trimethylpsoralen

a. Efficiency

The frequency of *unc-22* mutations following TMP/UV mutagenesis (Yandell *et al.*, 1994) is about 15-fold lower than that observed with EMS (Moerman and Baillie, 1981).

b. Specificity

The structures of 24 TMP-induced alleles of either *unc-22, pal-1,* or *unc-101* have been reported (Yandell *et al.*, 1994; Lee *et al.*, 1994). Eleven are deletions, one is an insertion, and two are complex rearrangements. This large proportion of deletions makes TMP a particularly attractive mutagen for generating alleles detectable by molecular techniques. Nineteen of twenty-three TMP-induced *unc-22* mutations were viable when homozygous, even though they were isolated initially as heterozygotes (Yandell *et al.*, 1994). Thus, TMP appears to preferentially induce small, rather than large, deletions.

5. ^{32}P Decay

a. Efficiency

The frequency of mutations following ^{32}P decay mutagenesis has not been carefully determined, but it is at least 100-fold higher than the spontaneous frequency (Babu and Brenner, 1981).

b. Specificity

Very little information is available. Three of four ^{32}P-induced *unc-4* alleles are deletions detected with Southern blots. *eT1 (III;V),* a reciprocal translocation, is ^{32}P induced.

6. Ionizing Particles

a. Efficiency

Ionizing particles are very efficient mutagens (Nelson *et al.*, 1989). Low-energy ionized particles (e.g., hydrogen and helium ions) yield mutation rates similar to those observed with 1500-R gamma irradiation, whereas high-energy particles (e.g., argon, iron, and lanthanum ions) yield mutation rates severalfold higher.

b. Specificity

No information is available.

B. Protocols

1. Gamma Irradiation

This procedure is from Rosenbluth *et al.* (1983). Spot washed worms onto a culture plate. Transfer young adults onto a fresh plate. These P_0 animals are mutagenized directly on the plate. Irradiate the worms with a ^{60}Co irradiation source. Depending on the dose rate, vary the time of irradiation such that a total dose of 1500 R is administered. Dose rates between 7.5 and 296 R/s have been reported. Immediately after irradiation, transfer the worms to a fresh plate and allow them to recover for 1 hour before further use. Distribute mutagenized worms to NGM plates as desired.

2. X Irradiation

This procedure is from Meneely and Herman (1979). Follow a procedure similar to that described above for gamma irradiation, substituting an X-ray source in place of ^{60}Co. The standard dose is 7000 to 7500 R, delivered at a dose rate of approximately 650 R/min. As noted for γ-ray mutagenesis (Rosenbluth et al., 1985), lower dose rates, such as 1500 R, may produce fewer complex rearrangements while still providing effective mutagenesis.

3. Ultraviolet Irradiation

This procedure is from Stewart et al. (1991). Worms are irradiated on agar in uncovered petri dishes using a 30-W General Electric UV germicidal lamp. Equilibrate the lamp by turning it on 15 minutes prior to use. Measure the UV dose with a calibrated ultraviolet light meter (Ultraviolet Products, Model J225). Typical irradiations occur at a dose rate of 2 W/m^2/s (about 43-cm distance from source to target). Irradiate for 60 seconds. If differing dose rates are used, irradiate for sufficient time to achieve a total dose of 120 J/m^2 (1 J = 1 W s).

4. Trimethylpsoralen

This procedure is from Yandell et al. (1994) and L. Edgar (pers. comm.). Cut one 15-cm petri dish of slightly starved worms into quarters. Place each quarter on a fresh plate. Incubate at 20°C for 24 hours. Harvest the worms by washing the plates with sterile M9 medium; collect by low-speed centrifugation in conical-bottomed tubes. After washing twice with M9 medium, remove as much liquid as possible. Prepare a 3 mg/ml stock solution of 4,5′,8-trimethylpsoralen (TMP) in dimethyl sulfoxide. For a working solution, dilute this stock with M9 medium to a final TMP concentration of 30 μg/ml. To the concentrated worm suspension add 10 vol of working TMP solution. Wrap the centrifuge tube in foil to screen ambient light. Place on a rocker table and agitate gently for 15 minutes. Pour the treated worms onto a large uncovered petri dish. Irradiate the worms with a UV lamp (Blak-Ray lamp, Model UVL-21) at an intensity of 340 μW/cm^2 for 60 seconds. After irradiation, place the worms on an agar plate spread with *Escherichia coli*. Incubate at 20°C in the dark. After 5 hours, the animals are no longer light sensitive; transfer them onto NGM plates as desired.

Notes. The maximum effective wavelength for irradiation is 360 nm. Use a UV meter to measure and standardize the UV dose. Good mutation rates occur when about 10% of irradiated eggs die. Warm the TMP/dimethyl sulfoxide stock solution to dissolve the crystals. Even at final concentration (30 μg/ml), TMP will crystallize out of solution.

5. ^{32}P Decay

This procedure is from Babu and Brenner (1981). Prepare phosphate-free NGM agar by omitting all phosphate from standard NGM plates. Synchronize a population of worms by collecting only the eggs. Allow the eggs to hatch on phosphate-free NGM plates. After hatching, collect L1 larvae with phosphate-free buffer. Supplement phosphate-free NGM plates with a small amount of cold (unlabeled) phosphate and carrier-free free [^{32}P]phosphate to give a specific activity of about 10 Ci/mole. Grow *E. coli* strain NA22 (a radiation-resistant mutant) on these plates. Place a few hundred of the freshly hatched larvae onto the plates. Incubate the plate at 15°C for 5 days to allow the larvae to grow into adults. These adult worms constitute the mutagenized (P_0) generation. Distribute the animals as desired to cold (unlabeled) NGM plates seeded with *E. coli* strain OP50.

6. High–Energy Ionizing Particles

Investigators with a convenient and plentiful source of cosmic rays or access to a linear accelerator (SuperHILAC) coupled to a synchrotron (Bevatron) should consult Nelson *et al.* (1989) for appropriate protocols.

VII. Spontaneous Mutagenesis

The goals of spontaneous mutagenesis are almost always to isolate transposon insertion alleles. Such alleles are often the key reagents for successful gene cloning strategies. Transposon tagging, first employed in *C. elegans* with *lin-12* and *unc-22* (Greenwald, 1985; Moerman *et al.*, 1986), is a widely used technique. An alternative strategy, positional cloning, is increasingly common as the genome physical map is integrated with the genetic linkage map (Coulson *et al.*, 1986, 1988). With such strategies, alleles that alter a gene's restriction map (revealed with a Southern blot) are especially valuable for pinpointing a gene's location within an otherwise large featureless region (e.g., see Finney *et al.*, 1988). For this purpose, transposon insertions are ideal. They affect gene structure in ways that are almost always detected with Southern blots.

As in most organisms, spontaneous mutations in *C. elegans* are often caused by transposable genetic elements. Care must be exercised, however, in choosing a genetic background for spontaneous mutant hunts. Transposons are active only in certain strains. With one exception (see below), transposon insertions have never been observed in *C. elegans* variety Bristol, the standard laboratory strain. An extensive survey of spontaneous Bristol mutations affecting the *unc-54* myosin heavy-chain gene shows them to be mostly point mutations, with about 20% being small deletions or other gene rearrangements (Eide and Anderson, 1985a). The sobering conclusion from this work is that transposon insertions into *unc-54*, if they occur, do so at frequencies of less than 5×10^{-9} in Bristol.

Six different families of *C. elegans* transposons have been described (Tc1–Tc6). Some characteristics that distinguish these families are shown in Table II. Despite certain similarities in DNA sequence, none of these elements hybridize to each other using typical hybridization conditions. Tc1 is, by far, the element most frequently responsible for insertion mutations, but there are some notable exceptions (see below). It is likely that additional families of elements remain to be discovered. An element related to the *mariner* transposon of *Drosophila* has recently been identified (M. Sedensky, S. Hudson, B. Everson, P. Morgan, pers. comm.). Circumstantial evidence suggests that an as-yet-undiscovered transposon is responsible for at least one spontaneous *smg-3* allele (B. Cali and P. Anderson, unpublished observations).

The frequency of transposon insertion is highly gene dependent. Some genes are good targets for insertions; others are poor targets. For example, in the Bergerac BO strain, the frequencies of Tc1 insertion into *unc-22, lin-12,* and *unc-54* are estimated to be 1×10^{-4}, 3×10^{-5}, and 5×10^{-7}, respectively (Moerman and Waterston, 1984; Greenwald, 1985; Eide and Anderson, 1985b). For some genes, Tc1 insertions have never been recovered, even in strains where Tc1 is known to be active. The reasons for this gene specificity are not understood. A corollary of this is that certain genes appear to be highly transposon specific. Of 51 *unc-22* insertions induced by *mut-2* ("mutator," see below), 43 are caused by Tc1 (Collins and Anderson, 1994). Yet, of nine *unc-86, ced-4, unc-33, unc-116, mec-7,* or *gld-2* insertions induced by *mut-2*, none are caused by Tc1. Two are caused by Tc3, four by Tc4, and two by Tc5 (Finney *et al.*, 1988; Yuan *et al.*, 1991; Li *et al.*, 1992; Patel *et al.*, 1993; C. Savage and M. Chalfie, pers. comm.; A. Jones and T. Schedl, pers. comm.). Collectively, these observations indicate that the frequency of transposon-induced mutations varies greatly from gene to gene and from element to element. Because transposon insertions are often spliced from pre-mRNAs (Rushforth *et al.*, 1993), insertions identified in phenotypic screens may represent only a subset of total insertions that occur.

Insertion of Tc elements within a gene is strongly site specific. Many genes have hotspots that receive a disproportionate number of insertions. The derived "consensus" sequence GA$^{GA}_{TG}$TA$^{TG}_{CC}$T describes the similarities of many Tc1 insertion sites, especially the hotspots (Eide and Anderson, 1988; Mori *et al.*, 1988a). This primary sequence alone, however, does not describe all insertion sites or account for all observed site specificity (van Luenen and Plasterk, 1994).

Transposon insertion alleles are often, but not always, genetically unstable. Depending on the insertion allele, partial or complete revertants can be recovered

Table II
Distinguishing Characteristics of *Caenorhabditis elegans* Transposon Families

| Transposable element | Size (bp) | Element copy number in | | Element termini | Target site duplication | Transposition detected in | | | Reference |
		Bristol	Bergerac BO			Bristol	Bergerac	*mut-2*	
Tc1	1610	30	300–500	54-bp IR[a]	TA	No	Yes	Yes	Rosenzweig et al., 1993 Emmons et al., 1983 Liao et al., 1983
Tc2	2074	6	~20	24-bp IR	TA	No	Yes	Yes	Ruvolo et al., 1992 Levitt and Emmons, 1989
Tc3	2335	15–18	15–18	36-bp IR	TA	No	No	Yes	Collins et al., 1989; D. Schneider et al., unpublished results
Tc4	1605	~20	~20	774-bp IR	TNA	No	No	Yes	Yuan et al., 1991
Tc4v	3483	5	5	130-bp IR	TNA	No	No	Yes	Li and Shaw, 1993
Tc5	3.2 kb	4–6	4–6	~500-bp IR	TNA	No	No	Yes	Collins and Anderson, 1994
Tc6	1603	~24	~24	765-bp IR	?	No	No	No	Dreyfus and Emmons, 1991

[a] IR, inverted repeat.

at high frequency (up to 10^{-3} per chromosome). Revertants arise following precise or, more frequently, imprecise excision of the inserted element (e.g., Eide and Anderson, 1988; Moerman *et al.*, 1991). Tc1, in particular, tends to leave preferred "footprints" behind after excision (Ruan and Emmons, 1987; Eide and Anderson, 1988; Plasterk, 1991). The frequency of reversion is highly allele dependent. Some insertion alleles revert at very high frequency, whereas others have never been seen to revert despite extensive screens. It is likely that genes and proteins tolerant of imprecise excision are those that revert at the highest frequencies (e.g., Eide and Anderson, 1988; Kiff *et al.*, 1988). Reversion is always background dependent. An element-induced mutation will revert only in a genetic background that contains an appropriate mutator allele (see Table II and below). In nonmutator strains (or in inappropriate mutator strains), revertants are not obtained. *mut-4, mut-5,* and *mut-6* activate transposition and excision of Tc1, but these mutators apparently do not activate the other families of transposons (with the possible exception of Tc2). *mut-2* activates transposition and excision of at least Tc1, Tc3, Tc4, and Tc5 (Collins *et al.*, 1987, 1989; Yuan *et al.*, 1991; Collins and Anderson, 1994).

Mutator-dependent reversion of a spontaneous mutation is a strong indication that the allele is caused by transposon insertion. In the case of Tc1, compound heterozygotes harboring both a Tc1-induced and a non-Tc1-induced allele of the same gene can revert at extraordinarily high frequencies (Mori *et al.*, 1990). Such events yield precise, rather than imprecise, excisions and are likely to be the result of double-strand break repair at excision sites (Plasterk and Groenen, 1992). The high-frequency reversion of Tc1 heteroalleles is mutator dependent. *mut-5* and *mut-6* activate heteroallelic excision of Tc1 (Mori *et al.*, 1990), but *mut-2* does not (B. Cali and P. Anderson, unpublished observations; J. Collins, pers. comm.). Because the frequencies of heteroallelic reversion are so high (up to 14% revertants!), this is an excellent method to identify using genetic criteria the Tc1 insertions among a collection of spontaneous alleles.

Transposon insertions are frequently not null alleles. It is now clear that many, if not most, transposons are spliced out of mutant pre-mRNAs in a manner that leaves small in-frame insertions/deletions behind in the mature message. Such mRNA "footprints" have been observed for Tc1 (Rushforth *et al.*, 1993; Benian *et al.*, 1993), Tc3 (M. Mills, J. Glasner, J. Collins, pers. comm.), Tc4 (Li *et al.*, 1992; Li and Shaw, 1993), and Tc5 (C. Parham, K. Butze, J. Beinhorn, J. Collins, pers. comm.). In cases where the encoded protein is tolerant of a mRNA footprint, partial or full gene activity can result (e.g., Moerman and Waterston, 1984; Benian *et al.*, 1993). This causes insertions identified by a mutant phenotype to often be weak (not null) alleles. For insertions identified by reverse genetic means (see Chapter 3 in this volume), such splicing often causes insertion alleles to be fully wild type, even in cases where the affected gene is essential (e.g., Rushforth *et al.*, 1993; A. Rushforth and P. Anderson, unpublished observations). For sequenced genes in which insertion alleles are not null, the methods described by Zwaal *et al.* (1993) can be used to generate intragenic deletions.

VIII. Mutator Strains

A. Choice of Strain

Choosing the correct strain is important for isolating transposon insertions. Transposons have been shown to be active in only four fundamentally different strains of *C. elegans*. These strains and their derivatives are discussed below.

1. Bergerac BO

Tc1 was first discovered in Bergerac BO, hereafter called Bergerac (Emmons *et al.*, 1983; Liao *et al.*, 1983). Tc1 was shown to be genetically active when spontaneous mutations isolated from Bergerac were analyzed molecularly (Eide and Anderson, 1985b; Greenwald, 1985; Moerman *et al.*, 1986). Bergerac, a wild isolate collected in Bergerac, France, sometime before 1949 (Nigon and Dougherty, 1949), contains 300 to 500 copies of Tc1. All transposon insertions isolated to date in Bergerac are Tc1.

Several derivatives of Bergerac are more useful than Bergerac itself for isolating spontaneous mutations. The mutator activity of Bergerac is polygenic, and manipulating its mutator properties by design is not possible. Mori *et al.* (1988b) describe Bristol/Bergerac hybrids in which transposition and excision of Tc1 are dependent on single mutator genes. *mut-4*, which maps near *dpy-14* on LG I, is a natural Bergerac gene that contributes to Bergerac's mutator activity. *mut-5* (near *dpy-10* on LG II) and *mut-6* (near *dpy-13* on LG IV) are apparently transposed derivatives of *mut-4*. *mut-5-* and *mut-6*-containing strains are particularly useful because their Tc1 copy number is about 60, much lower than that of Bergerac. Of these hybrid strains, *mut-6* has the highest levels of activity. Transposition and excision of Tc1 in strain RW7097 (a *mut-6* derivative that is otherwise wild type) is comparable to that found in Bergerac and substantially higher than that observed for *mut-4* or *mut-5* (Mori *et al.*, 1988b).

The highest possible frequencies of transposition and excision are achieved in strains that contain *mut-2(r459)*. *mut-2(r459)* is an EMS-induced mutation that increases the frequency of Tc1 transposition and excision about 40-fold above that seen for Bergerac (Collins *et al.*, 1987). Two *mut-2*-containing strains are particularly useful. Strain TR679 [genotype *mut-2(r459)*] exhibits the highest possible frequency of transposon insertions (about 40-fold above Bergerac). TR679 harbors *mut-2* in a Bristol/Bergerac hybrid (50% Bergerac, 50% Bristol) genetic background. Strain MT3126 [genotype *mut-2(r459), dpy-19(n1347)*] is a descendant of the parent of TR679 in which *mut-2* was crossed 13 times into a Bristol genetic background (Finney, 1987). The *mut-2* activity of MT3126 maps near *unc-13* on LG I. Although the frequency of Tc1 transposition and excision in MT3126 is about 10-fold lower than that of TR679, the frequencies are still severalfold higher than that of Bergerac (J. Collins and P. Anderson, unpublished results). MT3126 contains 60–80 copies of Tc1 (B. Spangler and P. Anderson, unpublished observations).

In addition to its effects on Tc1, *mut-2* activates transposition and excision of Tc3, Tc4, and Tc5 (Collins *et al.*, 1989; Yuan *et al.*, 1991; Collins and Anderson, 1994). Most transposon insertions isolated from *mut-2* are Tc1, but this is highly gene dependent (see above). Significant numbers of Tc3, Tc4, and Tc5 insertions are recovered, with Tc4 probably being the most common non-Tc1 event. Insertions of Tc3, Tc4, and Tc5 have not been recovered in any strain other than a *mut-2*-containing one.

2. DH424

Strain DH424 is a wild isolate collected in California during the 1970s (Liao *et al.*, 1983). It contains several hundred copies of Tc1. At 20°C, transposable element activity is not detected in DH424 (Eide and Anderson, 1985b). At 25°C, however, Tc1 is active in DH424. It is not possible to directly measure Tc1 transposition in DH424 at 25°C, because DH424 cannot be cultivated at elevated temperature. DH424 contains a temperature-sensitive allele of *zyg-12*, just as Bergerac does (Wood *et al.*, 1980). Strain TR1297 is a non-temperature-sensitive derivative of DH424 in which the DH424 *zyg-12* region has been replaced with the corresponding *zyg-12(+)* region of Bristol. In TR1297, Tc1 is inactive at 20°C but active at 25°C (D. Eide and P. Anderson, unpublished observations). TR1297 is useful because it is the only conditional mutator available. The frequencies of Tc1 transposition have not been carefully measured in TR1297 at 25°C.

3. TR403

Strain TR403 is a wild isolate collected in Madison, Wisconsin, in the early 1980s. TR403 has a high copy number of Tc1, and yields *unc-22::Tc1* mutations at a frequency of 2×10^{-5}, severalfold lower than Bergerac (J. Collins and P. Anderson, unpublished observations).

4. KR579

KR579 is a spontaneous mutator derived ultimately from wild-type Bristol (Babity *et al.*, 1990). During cultivation of KR579 or its immediate ancestors, Tc1 was spontaneously activated. Close relatives of KR579 are quiescent. KR579 contains 40 to 60 copies of Tc1 and yields spontaneous *unc-22* alleles at frequencies comparable to those of Bergerac.

B. Growth and Maintenance of Strains

Care must be exercised when propagating mutator strains. Because they exhibit high frequencies of spontaneous mutations, mutator strains accumulate deleterious mutations. If subcultured repeatedly, such mutations can accumulate to the point that most of the animals in a population are visibly sick and reproduce poorly or not at all. Long-term growth tends to select for derivatives that have lower levels of transposon activity. Such "quiescent" derivatives do not accumulate deleterious mutations and, therefore, enjoy a reproductive advantage. Over time, quiescent individuals will become the predominant animals in a population. This problem is most severe with mutator strains that exhibit the highest levels of transposon activity. Because of these problems, mutator strains should never be passaged long term. Rather, fresh strains should be thawed and grown only for the several generations needed to produce populations for screening or selection. When mutator strains are received from other laboratories, a large number of independent vials should be frozen. That way, fresh strains are always available for future use. Mutator strains that have accumulated deleterious mutations and are, therefore, sick or semisterile can be "revived" by outcrossing them. Outcrossing reduces extraneous mutations, because most such mutations segregate independently of the mutator or of other markers in the strain. The difficult part of an outcross is usually identifying descendants that are homozygous for the mutator gene. This can be accomplished either by using mutators that have a well-defined map location (see above) or by crossing markers repeatedly into a fresh mutator background. When new mutants are identified in a mutator strain, they should be quickly outcrossed and the mutations of interest isolated in a nonmutator background. This prevents further accumulation of deleterious mutations.

IX. Summary and Conclusions

Choosing the right mutagen means selecting the right combination of mutagen efficiency and mutagen specificity. For mutagen efficiency, nothing beats EMS. It is extremely potent, it is easy to use, and its mutational specificity is well documented. If mutations other than G/C → A/T transitions are desired, mutagens other than EMS must be used. Based on initial observations, ENU appears to be as efficient as EMS. Work with other organisms predicts that ENU will yield a wider variety of transitions and transversions than EMS. If this proves to be true, ENU will become an important mutagen for routine genetic analysis.

For investigators wanting large multigene deletions, gamma irradiation, UV irradiation, formaldehyde, and DEO are the mutagens of choice. Gamma irradiation yields the highest frequency of events by far, but may also yield more complex rearrangements. Based on limited information, UV irradiation, formaldehyde, and DEO appear to be effective deletion mutagens. Of the three, UV appears to be the most efficient. For investigators wanting small intragenic deletions, TMP appears most effective. TMP is not very potent, but a large proportion of TMP-induced *unc-22* mutations are small deletions. Hopefully this will be true of all genes. For investigators wanting other types of genome rearrangements (e.g., translocations, crossover suppressors), gamma irradiation (or possibly X irradiation) is effective.

For transposon insertions, *mut-2* (especially strain TR679) provides the highest possible frequency of events. Because *mut-2* activates several families of transposons, it yields insertions in genes that are poor targets for Tc1. Manipulating a strain with such high frequencies of spontaneous mutations, however, can be problematical (see above). For Tc1-specific events, *mut-6* (strain RW7097) is the best choice. It provides frequencies comparable to those of Bergerac, but its Tc1 copy number is much lower. A reasonable strategy for spontaneous mutagenesis is to use TR679 only if mutants are not obtained in strains with lower levels of activity (e.g., MT3126 or RW7097).

References

Ahringer, J., and Kimble, J. (1991). Control of the sperm-oocyte switch in *Caenorhabditis elegans* hermaphrodites by the fem-3 3′ untranslated region. *Nature* **349,** 346–348.

Alfonso, A., Grundahl, K., Duerr, J. S., He-Ping, H., and Rand, J. B. (1993). The *Caenorhabditis elegans* unc-17 gene: a putative vesicular acetylcholine transporter. *Science* **261,** 617–619.

Anderson, P., and Brenner, S. (1984). A selection for myosin heavy-chain mutants in the nematode *C. elegans. Proc. Natl. Acad. Sci. U.S.A.* **81,** 4470–4474.

Aroian, R. V., Lesa, G. M., and Sternberg, P. W. (1994). Mutations in the *Caenorhabditis elegans* let-23 EGFR-like gene define elements important for cell-type specificity and function. *EMBO J.* **13,** 360–366.

Babity, J. M., Starr, T. V. B., and Rose, A. M. (1990). Tc1 transposition and mutator activity in a Bristol strain of *Caenorhabditis elegans. Mol. Gen. Genet.* **222,** 65–70.

Babu, P., and Brenner, S. (1981). Spectrum of ^{32}P-induced mutants of *C. elegans. Mutat. Res.* **82,** 269–273.

Barstcad, R. J., and Waterston, R. H. (1991). Vinculin is essential for muscle function in the nematode. *J. Cell Biol.* **114,** 715–724.

Beitel, G. J., Clark, S. G., and Horvitz, H. R. (1990). *Caenorhabditis elegans ras* gene *let*-60 acts as a switch in the pathway of vulval induction. *Nature* **348,** 503–509.

Bejsovec, A., and Anderson, P. (1988). Myosin heavy-chain mutations that disrupt *Caenorhabditis elegans* thick filament assembly. *Genes Dev.* **2,** 1307–1317.

Bejsovec, A., and Anderson, P. (1990). Functions of the myosin ATP and actin binding sites are required for *C. elegans* thick filament assembly. *Cell* **60,** 133–140.

Benian, G. M., L'Hernault, S. W., and Morris, M. E. (1993). Additional sequence complexity in the muscle gene, *unc*-22, and its encoded protein, twitchin, of *Caenorhabditis elegans. Genetics* **134,** 1097–1104.

Bolten, S. L., Powell-Abel, P., Fischhoff, D. A., and Waterston, R. H. (1984). The *sup-7(st5)* X gene of *C. elegans* encodes a tRNATrp-UAG amber suppressor. *Proc. Natl. Acad. Sci. U.S.A.* **81,** 6784–6788.

Brenner, S. (1974). The genetics of *Caenorhabditis elegans. Genetics* **77,** 71–94.

Ciliberto, G., Traboni, C., and Cortese, R. (1982). Relationship between the two components of the split promoter of eukaryotic tRNA genes. *Proc. Natl. Acad. Sci. U.S.A.* **79,** 1921–1925.

Clark, D. V., Rogalski, T. M., Donati, L. M., and Baillie, D. L. (1988). The *unc-22*(IV) region of *Caenorhabditis elegans:* Genetic analysis of lethal mutations. *Genetics* **119,** 345–353.

Clark, S. G., Stern, M. J., and Horvitz, H. R. (1992). *C. elegans* ccll-signalling gene *sem*-5 encodes a protein with SH2 and SH3 domains. *Nature* **356,** 340–344.

Clark-Maguire, S., and Mains, P. E. (1994). *mei*-1, a gene required for meiotic spindle formation in *Caenorhabditis elegans,* is a member of a family of ATPases. *Genetics* **136,** 533–546.

Collins, J. J., and Anderson, P. (1994). The Tc5 family of transposable elements in *Caenorhabditis elegans*. *Genetics* **137**, 771–781.

Collins, J., Forbes, E., and Anderson, P. (1989). The Tc3 family of transposable genetic elements in *Caenorhabditis elegans*. *Genetics* **121**, 47–55.

Collins, J., Saari, B., and Anderson, P. (1987). Activation of a transposable element in the germ line but not the soma of *Caenorhabditis elegans*. *Nature* **328**, 726–728.

Coulson, A., Sulston, J., Brenner, S., and Karn, J. (1986). Toward a physical map of the genome of the nematode *C. elegans*. *Proc. Natl. Acad. Sci. U.S.A.* **83**, 7821–7825.

Coulson, A., Waterston, R., Kiff, J., Sulston, J., and Kohara, Y. (1988). Genome linking with yeast artificial chromosomes. *Nature* **335**, 184–186.

Dibb, N., Brown, D., Karn, J., Moerman, D., Bolten, S., and Waterston, R. (1985). Sequence analysis of mutations that affect the synthesis, assembly and enzymatic activity of *unc*-54 myosin heavy chain of *C. elegans*. *J. Mol. Biol.* **183**, 543–551.

Dreyfus, D. H., and Emmons, S. W. (1991). A transposon-related palindromic repetitive sequence from *C. elegans*. *Nucleic Acids. Res.* **19**, 1871–1877.

Eide, D., and Anderson, P. (1985a). The gene structures of spontaneous mutations affecting a *Caenorhabditis elegans* myosin heavy chain gene. *Genetics* **109**, 67–79.

Eide, D., and Anderson, P. (1985b). Transposition of Tc1 in the nematode *C. elegans*. *Proc. Natl. Acad. Sci. U.S.A.* **82**, 1756–1760.

Eide, D., and Anderson, P. (1985c). Novel insertion mutation in *Caenorhabditis elegans*. *Mol. Cell Biol.* **5**, 1–6.

Eide, D., and Anderson, P. (1988). Insertion and excision of *Caenorhabditis elegans* transposable element Tc1. *Mol. Cell Biol.* **8**, 737–746.

Emmons, S., Yesner, L., Ruan, K., and Katzenberg, D. (1983). Evidence for a transposon in *Caenorhabditis elegans*. *Cell* **32**, 55–65.

Finney, M. (1987). Ph. D. Thesis, Massachusetts Institute of Technology, Cambridge, MA.

Finney, M., Ruvkun, G., and Horvitz, H. R. (1988). The *C. elegans* cell lineage and differentiation gene *unc*-86 encodes a protein with a homeodomain and extended similarity to transcription factors. *Cell* **55**, 757–769.

Gengyo-Ando, K., and Kagawa, H. (1991). Single charge change on the helical surface of the paramyosin rod dramatically disrupts thick filament assembly in *Caenorhabditis elegans*. *J. Mol. Biol.* **219**, 429–441.

Greenwald, I. (1985). *lin*-12, a nematode homeotic gene, is homologous to a set of mammalian proteins that includes epidermal growth factor. *Cell* **43**, 583–590.

Greenwald, I., and Horvitz, H. (1980). *unc*-93(e1500): A behavior mutant of *Caenorhabditis elegans* that defines a gene with a wild-type null phenotype. *Genetics* **96**, 147–164.

Greenwald, I., and Seydoux, G. (1990). Analysis of gain-of-function mutations of the *lin*-12 gene of *Caenorhabditis elegans*. *Nature* **346**, 197–199.

Guo, X. D., Johnson, J. J., and Kramer, J. M. (1991). Embryonic lethality caused by mutations in basement membrane collagen of *C. elegans*. *Nature* **349**, 707–709.

Han, M., and Sternberg, P. W. (1991). Analysis of dominant negative mutations of the *Caenorhabditis elegans let-60 ras* gene. *Genes Dev.* **5**, 2188–2198.

Hengartner, M. O., and Horvitz, H. R. (1994). *C. elegans* cell survival gene *ced*-9 encodes a functional homolog of the mammalian proto-oncogene *bcl*-2. *Cell* **76**, 665–676.

Hodgkin, J. (1985). Novel nematode amber suppressors. *Genetics* **111**, 287–310.

Hong, K., and Driscoll, M. (1994). A transmembrane domain of the putative channel subunit MEC-4 influences mechanotransduction and neurodegeneration in *C. elegans*. *Nature* **367**, 470–473.

Howell, A. M., and Rose, A. M. (1990). Essential genes in the *hDf6* region of chromosome I in *Caenorhabditis elegans*. *Genetics* **126**, 583–592.

Johnsen, R. C., and Baillie, D. L. (1988). Formaldehyde mutagenesis of the *eT1* balanced region in *C. elegans*: Dose-response curve and the analysis of mutational events. *Mutat. Res.* **201**, 137–147.

Johnsen, R. C., and Baillie, D. L. (1991). Genetic analysis of a major segment [LGV(left)] of the genome of *Caenorhabditis elegans*. *Genetics* **129**, 735–752.

Johnstone, I. L., Shafi, Y., and Barry, J. D. (1992). Molecular analysis of mutations in the *Caenorhabditis elegans* collagen gene *dpy-7*. *EMBO J.* **11**, 3857–3863.

Karn, J., Brenner, S., and Barnett, L. (1983). Protein structural domains in the *Caenorhabditis elegans unc-54* myosin heavy chain gene are not separated by introns. *Proc. Natl. Acad. Sci. U.S.A.* **80**, 4253–4257.

Kiff, J., Moerman, D., Schriefer, L., and Waterston, R. (1988). Transposon-induced deletions in *unc-22* of *C. elegans* associated with almost normal gene activity. *Nature* **331**, 631–633.

Kimble, J., and Ward, S. (1988). Germ-line development and fertilization. *In* "The Nematode *Caenorhabditis elegans*" (W. B. Wood, ed.), pp. 191–213. Cold Spring Harbor Laboratory, Cold Spring Harbor, New York.

Klein, R. D., and Meyer, B. J. (1993). Independent domains of the Sdc-3 protein control sex determination and dosage compensation in *C. elegans*. *Cell* **72**, 349–364.

Kodoyianni, V., Maine, E. M., and Kimble, J. (1992). Molecular basis of loss-of-function mutations in the *glp-1* gene of *Caenorhabditis elegans*. *Mol. Biol. Cell* **3**, 1199–1213.

Kondo, K., Hodgkin, J., and Waterston, R. H. (1988). Differential expression of five $tRNA^{Trp}_{UAG}$ amber suppressors in *Caenorhabditis elegans*. *Mol. Cell Biol.* **8**, 3627–3635.

Kondo, K., Makovec, B., Waterston, R. H., and Hodgkin, J. (1990). Genetic and molecular analysis of eight $tRNA^{Trp}$ amber suppressors in *Caenorhabditis elegans*. *J. Mol. Biol.* **215**, 7–19.

Kramer, J. M., and Johnson, J. J. (1993). Analysis of mutations in the *sqt-1* and *rol-6* collagen genes of *Caenorhabditis elegans*. *Genetics* **135**, 1035–1045.

Kuwabara, P. E., Okkema, P. G., and Kimble, J. (1992). *tra-2* encodes a membrane-protein and may mediate cell communication in the *Caenorhabditis elegans* sex determination pathway. *Mol. Biol. Cell* **3**, 461–473.

Lee, J., Jongeward, G. D., and Sternberg, P. W. (1994). *unc-101*, a gene required for many aspects of *Caenorhabditis elegans* development and behavior, encodes a clathrin-associated protein. *Genes Dev.* **8**, 60–73.

Levin, J. Z., and Horvitz, H. R. (1992). The *Caenorhabditis elegans unc-93* gene encodes a putative transmembrane protein that regulates muscle contraction. *J. Cell Biol.* **117**, 143–155.

Levitt, A., and Emmons, S. W. (1989). The Tc2 transposon in *Caenorhabditis elegans*. *Proc. Natl. Acad. Sci. U.S.A.* **86**, 3232–3236.

Levy, A. D., Yang, J., and Kramer, J. M. (1993). Molecular and genetic analyses of the *Caenorhabditis elegans dpy-2* and *dpy-10* collagen genes: A variety of molecular alterations affect organismal morphology. *Mol. Biol. Cell* **4**, 803–817.

Li, W., Herman, R. K., and Shaw, J. E. (1992). Analysis of the *Caenorhabditis elegans* axonal guidance and outgrowth gene *unc-33*. *Genetics* **132**, 675–689.

Li, W., and Shaw, J. E. (1993). A variant Tc4 transposable element in the nematode. *C. elegans* could encode a novel protein. *Nucleic Acids Res.* **21**, 59–67.

Liao, L., Rosenzweig, B., and Hirsh, D. (1983). Analysis of a transposable element in *Caenorhabditis elegans*. *Proc. Natl. Acad. Sci. U.S.A.* **80**, 3585–3589.

Lissemore, J. L., Currie, P. D., Turk, C. M., and Maine, E. M. (1993). Intragenic dominant suppressors of *glp-1*, a gene essential for cell-signaling in *Caenorhabditis elegans*, support a role for *cdc10/ SW16*/ankyrin motifs in GLP-1 function. *Genetics* **135**, 1023–1034.

Maruyama, I. N., Miller, D. M., and Brenner, S. (1989). Myosin heavy chain gene amplification as a suppressor mutation in *Caenorhabditis elegans*. *Mol. Gen. Genet.* **219**, 113–118.

Meneely, P., and Herman, R. (1979). Lethals, steriles and deficiencies in a region of the X chromosome of *C. elegans*. *Genetics* **92**, 99–115.

Miller, D. M., Shen, M. M., Shamu, C. E., Burglin, T. R., Ruvkun, G., Dubois, M. L., Ghee, M., and Wilson, L. (1992). *C. elegans unc-4* gene encodes a homeodomain protein that determines the pattern of synaptic input to specific motor neurons. *Nature* **355**, 841–845.

Moerman, D., and Baillie, D. (1981). Formaldehyde mutagenesis in the nematode *C. elegans*. *Mutat. Res.* **80**, 273–279.

Moerman, D., Benian, G., and Waterston, R. (1986). Molecular cloning of the muscle gene *unc-22* in *Caenorhabditis elegans* by Tc1 transposon tagging. *Proc. Natl. Acad. Sci. U.S.A.* **83**, 2579–2583.

Moerman, D., and Waterston, R. (1984). Spontaneous unstable *unc-22IV* mutations in *C. elegans* var. Bergerac. *Genetics* **108**, 859–877.

Moerman, D. G., Kiff, J. E., and Waterston, R. H. (1991). Germline excision of the transposable element Tc1 in *C. elegans*. *Nucleic Acids Res.* **19**, 5669–5672.

Mori, I., Benian, G., Moerman, D., and Waterston, R. (1988a). Transposable element Tc1 of *Caenorhabditis elegans* recognizes specific target sequences for integration. *Proc. Natl. Acad. Sci. U.S.A.* **85**, 861–864.

Mori, I., Moerman, D. G., and Waterston, R. H. (1988b). Analysis of a mutator activity necessary for germline transposition and excision of Tc1 transposable elements in *Caenorhabditis elegans*. *Genetics* **120**, 397–407.

Mori, I., Moerman, D. G., and Waterston, R. H. (1990). Interstrain crosses enhance excision of Tc1 transposable elements in *Caenorhabditis elegans*. *Mol. Gen. Genet.* **220**, 251–255.

Nelson, G. A., Schubert, W. W., Marshall, T. M., Benton, E. R., and Benton, E. V. (1989). Radiation effects in *Caenorhabditis elegans*. Mutagenesis by high and low LET ionizing radiation. *Mutat. Res.* **212**, 181–192.

Nigon, V., and Dougherty, E. (1949). Reproductive patterns and attempts at reciprocal crossing of *Rhabditis elegans* Maupas 1900, and *Rhabditis briggsae* Dougherty and Nigon, 1949 (Nematoda: Rhabditidae). *J. Exp. Zool.* **112**, 485–503.

Pastink, A., Vreeken, C., Nivard, M. J. M., Searles, L. L., and Vogel, E. W. (1989). Sequence analysis of N-ethyl-N-nitrosourea-induced *vermillion* mutations in Drosophila melanogaster. *Genetics* **123**, 123–129.

Patel, N., Thierry-Mieg, D., and Mancillas, J. R. (1993). Cloning by insertional mutagenesis of a cDNA encoding *Caenorhabditis elegans* kinesin heavy chain. *Proc. Natl. Acad. Sci. U.S.A.* **90**, 9181–9185.

Plasterk, R. H. A. (1991). The origin of footprints of the Tc1 transposon of *Caenorhabditis elegans*. *EMBO J.* **10**, 1919–1925.

Plasterk, R. H. A., and Groenen, J. T. M. (1992). Targeted alterations of the *Caenorhabditis elegans* genome by transgene instructed DNA double strand break repair following Tc1 excision. *EMBO J.* **11**, 287–290.

Richardson, K. K., Richardson, F. C., Crosby, R. M., Swenberg, J. A., and Skopk, T. R. (1987). DNA base changes and alkylation following in vivo exposure of Escherichia coli to N-methyl-N-nitrosourea or N-ethyl-N-nitrosourea. *Proc. Natl. Acad. Sci. U.S.A.* **84**, 344–348.

Riddle, D., and Brenner, S. (1978). Indirect suppression in *C. elegans*. *Genetics* **89**, 299–314.

Rogalski, T., Moerman, D., and Baillie, D. (1982). Essential genes and deficiencies in the *unc-22 IV* region of *C. elegans*. *Genetics* **102**, 725–736.

Rosenbluth, R., Cuddeford, C., and Baillie, D. (1983). Mutagenesis in *C. elegans*. I. A rapid eukaryotic mutagen test system using the reciprocal translocation *eT1(III V)*. *Mutat. Res.* **110**, 39–48.

Rosenbluth, R., Cuddeford, C., and Baillie, D. (1985). Mutagenesis in *C. elegans*. II. A spectrum of mutational events induced with 1500 R of gamma-radiation. *Genetics* **109**, 493–511.

Rosenzweig, B., Liao, L., and Hirsh, D. (1983). Sequence of the *C. elegans* transposable element Tc1. *Nucleic Acids Res.* **11**, 4201–4209.

Ruan, K., and Emmons, S. (1987). Precise and imprecise somatic excision of the transposon Tc1 in the nematode *C. elegans*. *Nucleic Acids Res.* **15**, 6875–6881.

Rushforth, A. M., Saari, B., and Anderson, P. (1993). Site-selected insertion of the transposon Tc1 into a *Caenorhabditis elegans* myosin light chain gene. *Mol. Cell Biol.* **13**, 902–910.

Ruvkun, G., Ambros, V., Coulson, A., Waterston, R., Sulston, J., and Horvitz, H. R. (1989). Molecular genetics of the *Caenorhabditis elegans* heterochronic gene *lin-14*. *Genetics* **121**, 501–516.

Ruvolo, V., Hill, J. E., and Levitt, A. (1992). The Tc2 transposon of *Caenorhabditis elegans* has the structure of a self-regulated element. *DNA Cell Biol.* **11**, 111–122.

Schnabel, H., Bauer, G., and Schnabel, R. (1991). Suppressors of the organ-specific differentiation gene *pha-1* of *Caenorhabditis elegans*. *Genetics* **129**, 69–77.

Sigurdson, D., Spanier, G., and Herman, R. (1984). *Caenorhabditis elegans* deficiency mapping. *Genetics* **108**, 331–345.

Stewart, H. I., Rosenbluth, R. E., and Baillie, D. L. (1991). Most ultraviolet irradiation induced mutations in the nematode *Caenorhabditis elegans* are chromosomal rearrangements. *Mutat. Res.* **249,** 37–54.

Sulston, J., and Brenner, S. (1974). The DNA of *C. elegans. Genetics* **77,** 95–104.

Sulston, J., and Hodgkin, J. (1988). Methods. *In* "The Nematode *Caenorhabditis elegans*" (W. B. Wood, ed.), pp. 587–606. Cold Spring Laboratory Press, Cold Spring Harbor, New York.

Trent, C., Purnell, B., Gavinski, S., Hageman, J., Chamblin, C., and Wood, W. B. (1991). Sex-specific transcriptional regulation of the *C. elegans* sex-determining gene *her-1. Mech. Dev.* **34,** 43–56.

van Luenen, H. G., and Plasterk, R. H. (1994). Target site choice of the related transposable elements Tc1 and Tc3 of *Caenorhabditis elegans. Nucleic Acids Res.* **22,** 262–269.

Waterston, R. (1981). A second informational suppressor, *sup-7X,* in *C. elegans. Genetics* **97,** 307–325.

Wilson, R., Ainscough, R., Anderson, K., Baynes, C., Berks, M., Bonfield, J., Burton, J., Connell, M., Copsey, T., Cooper, J., Coulson, A., Craxton, M., Dear, S., Du, A., Durbin, R., Favello, A., Fraser, A., Fulton, L., Gardner, A., Green, P., Hawkins, T., Hillier, L., Joer, M., Johnston, L., Jones, M., Kershaw, J., Kirsten, J., Laisster, N., Latreille, P., Lightning, J., Lloyd, C., Mortimore, B., O'Callaghan, M., Parsons, J., Percy, C., Rifken, L., Roopra, A., Saunders, D., Shownkeen, R., Simms, M., Smaldon, N., Smith, A., Smith, M., Sonnhammer, E., Staden, R., Sulston, J., Thierry-Mieg, J., Thomas, K., Vaudin, M., Vaughan, K., Waterston, R., Watson, A., Weinstock, L., Wilkinson-Sproat, J., and Wohldman, P. (1994). 2.2 Mb of contiguous nucleotide sequence from chromosome III of *C. elegans. Nature* **368,** 32–38.

Wood, W., Hecht, R., Carr, S., Vanderslice, R., Wolf, N., and Hirsh, D. (1980). Parental effects and phenotypic characterization of mutations that affect early development in *C. elegans. Dev. Biol.* **74,** 446–469.

Yandell, M. D., Edgar, L. G., and Wood, W. B. (1994). Trimethylpsoralen induces small deletion mutations in *Caenorhabditis elegans. Proc. Natl. Acad. Sci. U.S.A.* **91,** 1381–1385.

Yuan, J., Finney, M., Tsung, N., and Horvitz, H. R. (1991). Tc4, a *Caenorhabditis elegans* transposable element with an unusual fold-back structure. *Proc. Natl. Acad. Sci. U.S.A.* **88,** 3334–3338.

Yuan, J., Shaham, S., Ledoux, S., Ellis, H. M., and Horvitz, H. R. (1993). The *C. elegans* cell death gene *ced-3* encodes a protein similar to mammalian interleukin-1β-converting enzyme. *Cell* **75,** 641–652.

Zarkowcr, D., and Hodgkin, J. (1992). Molecular analysis of the *C. elegans* sex-determining gene *tra-1:* A gene encoding 2 zinc finger proteins. *Cell* **70,** 237–249.

Zwaal, R. R., Broeks, A., van Meurs, J., Groenen, J. T., and Plasterk, R. H. (1993). Target-selected gene inactivation in *Caenorhabditis elegans* by using a frozen transposon insertion mutant bank. *Proc. Natl. Acad. Sci. U.S.A.* **90,** 7431–7435.

CHAPTER 3

Reverse Genetics: From Gene Sequence to Mutant Worm

Ronald H. A. Plasterk

Division of Molecular Biology
Netherlands Cancer Institute
1066 CX Amsterdam, The Netherlands

I. Introduction

I. A. Reverse Genetics

Caenorhabditis elegans is in all likelihood the first metazoan animal whose entire genome sequence will be determined (Wilson *et al.,* 1994). In addition, a very detailed description of the animal's morphology, development, and physiology is available (see elsewhere in this book, and Wood, 1988.) Thus, the complete phenotype and genotype of an animal will be known. What is not known is how genotype determines phenotype; to study this, one needs to establish connections between genome sequence and phenotype.

Much has been done by classic or forward genetics: mutagenesis experiments have identified loci involved in a specific trait. Many of these loci have already been defined at the molecular level, and the genome sequence will certainly aid in the identification of many more. The opposite approach, reverse genetics, becomes naturally more important when more of the genome sequence is determined: Given the sequence of a gene of which nothing else is known, how can the function of that gene be determined?

Reverse genetics is more than targeted inactivation. One can study a gene's function by several approaches:

1. Comparison of the gene sequence with those of other genes can indicate possible functions. A clear overall similarity to a gene of known function can identify a gene as a member of a gene family (e.g., a transcription factor), but even without that one can obtain hints about the possible mechanistic role of a putative protein by recognition of specific domains or motifs (e.g., a membrane spanning domain, a GTP-binding domain).

2. The tissue- and stage-specific expression pattern can give a hint of the gene's function (also see Chapters 14 and 21). It can at least exclude a function in those cells and those stages in which no expression is found.

3. In some cases, one can design dominant negative mutants that can be introduced as a transgene (see Chapter 19), or one can direct expression levels, times, or tissue by fusion to foreign promoters. The phenotypes of such recombinant nematodes may indicate a function of the gene, although it should be interpreted with care: overproduction of, for example, a kinase may result in aberrant phosphorylation of nonphysiological targets and thus result in phenotypes unrelated to the physiological role of that kinase.

4. Sometimes one can use prior knowledge to set up specific biochemical assays for recombinant proteins based on the gene sequence. For example, one can recognize a sequence of a glycosyltransferase and study the precise nature of it by overproduction and purification of the protein and determination of the specificity of the transferase *in vitro*.

5. Finally one can alter the endogenous gene and study the effect on phenotype. The alteration can be complete inactivation, partial inactivation (e.g., compare Greenstein *et al.*, 1994), or a more specific change. These types of experiments could be referred to as reverse genetics in a stricter sense, and points 1 to 4 as reverse genetics in a wider sense. This chapter further addresses the former.

I. B. Notes for Nematode Novices

The purpose of all genetic analysis is to understand phenotype in terms of genotype. The *C. elegans* genome project removes the bottleneck of gene mapping, cloning, and sequencing, and, as discussed in this chapter and elsewhere in this book, the bottlenecks of transgenesis and target-selected gene inactivation are largely removed as well. This attracts people to this experimental model who were not previously studying it; researchers interested in a specific class of genes find that sequenced members of that class are known in *C. elegans* and consider studying them. That is probably a good decision, but the following should be kept in mind: inactivation of a gene is not a goal in itself, but a means to study gene function, and one should be prepared that the phenotype of a knockout is not always directly informative and that much detailed study of *C. elegans* biology may be necessary to interpret mutant phenotypes. One should realize that the most likely outcome of a gene inactivation experiment is that the homozygous mutant is either lethal or shows no obvious defects. As someone said, "death is a boring phenotype," and experimentally it may indeed require very much effort and detailed study of nematode development or physiology to draw interesting conclusions from it. The absence of an obvious phenotype forces one into a detailed analysis as well.

The purpose of genetics is to understand the complexity of life in terms of the complexity of the genome, and one encounters that complexity inevitably. Forward genetic studies start with a clean and well-defined phenotype and end with genes of diverse mechanistic roles, so that difficult choices have to be made about which genes to study. Reverse genetics, on the other hand, starts with a well-defined set of genes, and the difficult choice to be made is which of the many aspects of phenotype will be studied once a mutant animal is obtained. Especially when no phenotype is apparent, one can continue indefinitely testing diverse phenotypes such as periodic defecation (Thomas, 1990), thermotaxis (I. Mori, pers. comm.), and response to diverse odorants (Bargmann, 1993), to name a few.

Another point to keep in mind is that the biological meaning of function can be different at different levels. If a gene knockout results in loss of the ability to form dauer larvae, then one can call that ability the gene's function. If that gene encodes a kinase, then one can also say that the phosphorylation of one or a few targets is the gene's function. As most genes seem to have homologs in diverse species, one is well advised to consider at which level one wishes to study gene function. If the goal is a biochemical analysis of an intracellular signalling pathway, then one may be better off studying that in a unicellular organism such as *Dictyostelium*, because that would allow analysis of homogeneous cell populations, addition of radiolabeled precursors, and so on. Similarly one may choose to study the regulation of the cell cycle in yeast. In general, one will probably choose well-differentiated animals such as the nematode and fruit fly primarily when the genes studied are probably involved in aspects of multicellular life: cell differentiation, cell–cell communication, and so on.

These cautionary remarks are not intended to frighten anybody away from reverse genetics of *C. elegans*. The combination of having a complete genome sequence and having a complete description of the cell lineage, the entire wiring of the nervous system, and many mutants in behavior and development should be a gold mine for everyone interested in the molecular biology of development and physiology. It is hoped the remainder of this chapter will serve as a guide on one of the many paths into the mine.

II. Strategies

II. A. Alternative Strategies for Gene Inactivation

This chapter aims to describe a method that can be used to obtain nematodes that have a gene of interest inactivated. Use of the transposon Tc1 for that purpose is discussed, because since at present it is the only method that works in practice. Alternative strategies are only briefly mentioned here, and the reader is referred to the literature for discussion of their potential application and their limitations.

1. The strategy of targeted gene interruption by homologous recombination with transgenic DNA has been tried, but has never worked satisfactorily. The common way to introduce DNA into the germ line of a large number of worms is microinjection into the gonads (Fire, 1986; Mello *et al.*, 1992). It is possible that the frequency with which naked microinjected DNA integrates homologously into the nematode genome is not very different from that in other species, but the absolute number of progeny that have been exposed to the transgenic DNA is limited by the number of injections one can perform. Nevertheless, a few cases of success have been reported, using either plasmid DNA or oligonucleotides (Broverman *et al.*, 1993; C. C. Mello, pers. comm.).

2. An alternative that has clear use is antisense RNA. It has been shown that one can largely inactivate the function of a gene by introduction of a transgene that carries a gene segment in inverted orientation with respect to the promoter (Fire *et al.*, 1991). An advantage of this approach is that one can in principle aim to inactivate gene function in a subset of cells only, by the choice of a specific promoter. Two limitations should also be considered: it is possible that gene inactivation is lethal, which would result in inability to generate the transgenic line (with a knockout one can always make the mutants first, as heterozygote, and test the phenotype of the homozygote subsequently). A more important limitation is that the absence of a phenotype does not mean much: either it could be the real effect of loss of gene function, or it could reflect insufficient effect of the transgene. An advantage of the strategy lies in this same effect: in cases

where total loss of gene function is lethal, an antisense strategy may result in less severe phenotypes, thus allowing selection of extragenic suppressors.

3. A third strategy is not detailed here, as it is not strictly reverse genetics: one can make an assumption about phenotype (e.g., that a gene is essential for viability) and use that to search for mutants among a mutagenized population (see Barstead and Waterston, 1991). For example, one can precomplement with an extrachromosomal transgene that contains the gene of interest in many copies, mutagenize the strain, and look for progeny that have become obligatory transgenics (and die when the transgene is lost).

II. B. Target–Selected Mutagenesis

The subtlety in the title of this subsection is that the gene interruption per se is not targeted, but that one mutagenizes randomly and selectively searches for animals that have a gene of known sequence mutated. The mutagen can be of several kinds, but because the search is based on the gene sequence, one needs a mutagen that induces major recognizable changes in the gene sequence. One possibility is a mutagen that induces deletions, so that one can search with polymerase chain reaction (PCR) primers that correspond to sequences so far apart that no visible PCR product is obtained from wild-type DNA; one can then visualize genomes that have lost DNA between these sites (Yandell *et al.,* 1994).

The remainder of this chapter discusses interruption with the transposon Tc1 (Rushforth *et al.,* 1993; Zwaal *et al.,* 1993), combined with the generation of a frozen mutant library. A discussion of several aspects of this approach, including an overview of previous literature, is presented elsewhere (Plasterk, 1992) and will not be repeated here.

III. Isolation of Tc1 Alleles from a Mutant Library

What follows is a description of the method currently used in the author's laboratory. Obviously not all alternatives have been analyzed systematically, and the revelance of all parameters has not been tested, but the method has been used for 3 years and has been altered and improved as a result. Not every step is motivated explicitly, and readers wishing to know if a certain step is essential or arbitrary can contact the author.

Every natural isolate of *C. elegans* contains several copies of the Tc1 transposon; the element is mobile in several strains (reviewed in Moerman and Waterston, 1989, and most recently in Plasterk, 1994). Insertion of Tc1 into a gene can interrupt that gene and therefore inactivate it. As will be discussed below, insertion into introns may leave gene function intact. Such insertions that do not result in loss of gene function may nevertheless be used as a first step toward gene inactivation, as progeny may be selected in which the transposon plus (part of) the interrupted gene sequences have been lost (see Section V).

Over the last year we have isolated many Tc1 insertion alleles for colleagues elsewhere, taking advantage of the fact that we had already invested the time to generate a mutant library and that we have gained some experience with the technique. This chapter should allow laboratories that expect to interrupt many genes to set up their own library. That is not very difficult and, compared with many common genetic techniques, not so very much work.

The method is derived from a method that has found some use in the fruit fly (Ballinger and Benzer, 1989; Kaiser and Goodwin, 1990; Littleton *et al.,* 1993), although its application there has thus far been limited by the logistics of the procedure and the strong regional preferences for P transposon insertion. A strain that contains several copies of the Tc1 transposon and is permissive for Tc1 transposition is taken as a source of new "spontaneous" insertion alleles. The insertions are recognized by PCR, using one primer specific for the Tc1 element and one for the gene of interest (Rushforth *et al.,* 1993; Zwaal et al., 1993). This mutagenesis and detection protocol has been combined with the establishment of a library of thousands of frozen worm cultures, so that many of the laborious steps (worm culturing, DNA isolation) have to be performed only once, and can be used for almost indefinite series of mutant hunts.

III. A. Outline of the Strategy

The reader is advised to read the publication describing the strategy (Zwaal *et al.,* 1993) before going into details described below. A typical library consists of three sets of 960 cultures of worms and a corresponding set of crude lysates. These lysates are inspected by PCR in such a way that insertions of Tc1 into a gene of interest are visualized. The PCR employs two sets of primers: one specific for Tc1, the other one specific for the gene of interest. Products are obtained only if Tc1 sequences are properly juxtaposed to the sequences of the gene of interest. In theory one could perform 3×960 PCRs to screen the library, but the workload can be very much reduced by ordered pooling of the crude lysates before DNA is purified.

The library is analyzed by blocks of 960 cultures: 10 racks of 12×8 (see Fig. 1a). The standard nomenclature for positions within each rack is as follows: 8 rows A–H, and 12 columns 1–12. The first screen determines in which of the 8 rows an address can be found ("first-dimension address"): for that purpose we pool some material of all of the 120 lysates of row A, of row B, and so on. Thus 960 samples are reduced initially to 8 DNA pools.

The method has to contend with a background caused by DNA that has Tc1 insertions that occured in somatic cells. In practice, the signal-to-background ratio is barely sufficient to recognize addresses. We solve this by doing the screening in fourfold. We dilute the DNA samples so far that most of the samples that do not correspond to an address contain not a single amplifiable mutant

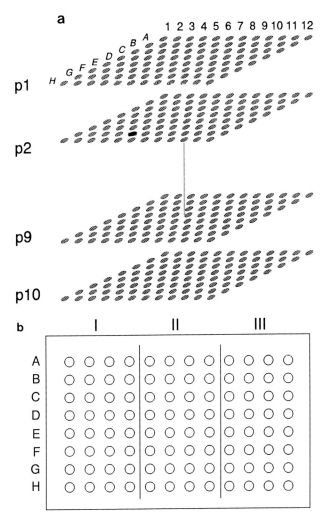

Fig. 1 (a) Pooling strategy for one set of 960 cultures. (b) Layout of PCR for initial screening. Compare with the gel shown in Fig. 2.

DNA. The PCR is aimed at reaching a plateau, so that one gets clear bands on an ethidium bromide-stained gel independent of the number of molecules at the start. If an address is real, then each sample of the corresponding DNA preparation will yield the same PCR product; on the other hand, the DNA of a nonaddress will yield either no products or incidental products of variable length. A positive sample contains mutant molecules, but note that we have diluted so far that weak but real addresses contribute mutant DNA to only a fraction of the samples; in other words we amplify four samples from the same DNA pool, and finding that three of the four result in the same PCR product is taken to indicate an address. Figure 2a illustrates the point. Note that one makes judgment calls that need to be confirmed by repetition (see Section III,C,2).

If no address is observed, one does not need to bother further. Once the bottleneck of finding a first-dimension address is passed, and we know that in one of the tubes (e.g., in row B) there is a mutant, we use that information in the next step. Thus we do not screen the 10 racks for all rows, but only for row B. This requires that an extra set of 80 DNA preparations is available for every 960 lysates which correspond to 10 DNA preparations for each row. The signal-to-background ratio is reduced by a factor of 12 in the screening in the second dimension, as compared with the first dimension. So once we know that row B has a potential mutant, we screen 10 DNA samples: rack 1B, rack 2B, rack 3B, and so on. This is done in triplicate (which is a bit overkill, but we find that it is much more work to repeat a series of reactions than it is to analyze more samples). Finding a second-dimension address (rack 4, row B) is an additional verification of the first-dimension address (see Fig. 2b). The final address is determined by analyzing which of the 12 samples in rack 4, row B has the mutant (Fig. 2c); we go back to the original lysates, take a bit of it, and because the signal-to-background ratio is again higher and the absolute concentration of mutant molecules in the crude lysate is high, one does not need to purify the DNA before PCR. We remove excess sodium dodecyl sulfate by a

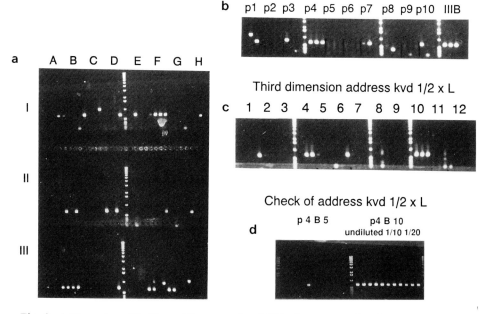

Fig. 2 (a) Screening of the library. Three sets of each 960 cultures are analyzed. The interpretation of the data is discussed in the text. (b) Second-dimension address. (c) Final address. (d) Confirmation of final address.

single alcohol precipitation, resuspend the pellet, and take a small fraction of the solution into PCR. The PCR for the last dimension is again done in triplicate. A real address should now be positive in triplicate, whereas most of the other lysates produce no product.

III. A. 1. Generation of a Mutant Library

The screening procedure described below is chosen because it fits nicely within the dimensions of the necessary equipment, and analyzes 3×960 (approximately 3000) cultures. That is the size of a library that we screen, usually with success, to isolate mutants and we therefore think it is initally not necessary to make the library larger than this.

III. A. 2. Culturing of Worms

For our library we used the strain MT3126 (Finney, 1987). It contains the *mut-2* mutation, as a result of which it is permissive for jumping of Tc1 (and probably Tc3). Even though we have no evidence that the mutator phenotype can be lost in time, we go back to glycerol stocks every now and then. Ten-centimeter NGM plates are prepared as described (Wood, 1988), but twice the amount of peptone is added, and they are seeded with *Escherichia coli* OP50. This is done in a sterile hood. After 1 or 2 days the plates are inoculated with 5 to 10 MT3126 worms of mixed age, as follows: a suspension of MT3126 is prepared in M9 in a dish, and a micropipetter with yellow tip is used to transfer each time 5 μl from the dish onto a plate. The first plates are inspected to count the number of worms. The petri dishes are put back into the cardboard boxes in which they were delivered, and the box is loosely closed. The box is incubated at 20°C (we found that incubation at 25°C was not a good idea, as our version of the MT3126 strain seems slightly thermosensitive). When the bacterial lawn is consumed and the worms have burrowed in the agar (usually starting on day 11 or 12 after, a bit longer than two generation times of the worm), 4 ml of M9 buffer is pipetted onto a plate, and the plates are put again in a cardboard box and shaken overnight at 18 to 20°C. This serves two purposes: all burrowed worms go into the supernatant, and they are further starved.

III. A. 3. Storage of Worms

Micronic racks and tubes are used (Micronic, The Netherlands; Costar seems to supply similar material). Racks are filled with 96 tubes, three racks of 96 are prepared per 96 worm cultures. The racks are autoclaved and are marked clearly on front, side, and top. It is important that the marking be large and clear, as one will later need to recognize it when the racks are in the −80°C freezer. Care is taken that the orientation of the plate later will not be mistaken. The tubes are not further marked, and their identification thus depends solely on the position within the racks. A complete address is defined by plate, letter of row (A–H), and number of column (1–12).

The shaken worm plates and marked racks are transferred to the sterile hood. Each plate is taken, tilted to let the M9 plus worms flow to one side, and gently moved so that the worms are fully suspended. Note that the volume of M9 will be diminished, due to absorption into the plate and evaporation. Then using a 1-ml blue tip and a micropipetter, we transfer 400 μl to each corresponding position of the first two racks and the remainder of the suspension into the third rack. Because of differences in the dryness and thickness of plates, the remaining M9 volume may differ; if less than 1 ml is on a plate (estimated by eye), then a few extra drops of fresh M9 are added before the worms are aliquoted.

The first two racks are meant to be frozen for survival. Once the rack is full, using a multiwell micropipetter we add 400 μl of freezing solution to each tube (30% glycerol, 25 mM KPO$_4$, pH 6.6, 50 mM NaCl, 2.5 μg/ml cholesterol), and close the tubes with sterile caps (8 caps on a strip, Micronic). A lid is put on the plates, and the plates are inverted a few times to mix the freezing solution with the M9. The racks are wrapped in cotton wool and then in two towels and are slowly frozen overnight in a −80°C Revco freezer. Then the racks are unwrapped and stored at −80°C. The duplicate should ideally be stored in a separate freezer, and both freezers equipped with a temperature alarm.

While the first two racks are being packed, the third rack is left, so that the worms have sedimented. These are used for DNA analysis and can be taken out of the sterile hood. Using a Pasteur pipet we remove the M9 supernatant. The worm pellets (plus a bit of remaining M9, which does not interfere with subsequent steps) can either be stored frozen or lysed directly.

To each wet pellet we add 200 μl of lysis solution (0.2 M NaCl, 0.1 M Tris–HCl, pH 8.5, 50 mM EDTA, 0.5% sodium dodecyl sulfate, freshly added 100 μg/ml protease K). The tubes are capped, and the lid is put on the rack. The rack is left in a stove at 65°C for minimally 2 hours and occasionally inverted to resuspend the debris. Then the lysates can be stored at −20 or −80°C, apparently indefinitely. The lysates are used for two purposes: ordered pooling, followed by extensive DNA purification (to obtain DNA later used to search for addresses), or (for the last step in determination of an address) partial purification by an alcohol precipitation.

An alternative that can be considered, but has not been tried by us, is to lyse the worms with a milder detergent ("single-worm lysis buffer", see Section III,D,2). After pooling, one could still add a stronger detergent to the pooled materials before the DNA is extracted. The advantage is that in the last step one can test the crude lysate immediately (as the mild detergent, diluted into PCR buffer, does not inactivate Taq polymerase).

III. B. Preparation of DNA for Screening of the Library

Using a multiwell pipetter we pool 20 μl of each of 12 lysates in a row into a Micronic tube. This results in eight pools per rack (A–H). Then the pooled lysates are vortexed, and 180 μl from the A tube of each of 10 plates is pooled and DNA is purified as described previously (Wood, 1988: a phenol extraction, a phenol/chloroform extraction, a chloroform extraction, and an alcohol precipitation). The DNA is resuspended in 100 μl TE (10 mM Tris-HCl, 1 mM EDTA, pH 7.6) and stored in a $-20°C$ freezer. This stock can be used for many searches, as it can be diluted far. The optimal dilution is best determined empirically; we usually dilute 10 to 50 times. The diluted DNA is stored in capped Micronic tubes in a Micronic rack; the microtiter format allows later dispension into microtiter format PCR plates.

The remainder of the lysates of eight pools per plate is also purified by phenol extractions and ethanol precipitation and resuspended in 200 μl TE or water, and the 80 purified DNA samples per 960 cultures are stored in a Micronic rack. These DNAs are used to determine second-dimension addresses. Once a second-dimension address is obtained, we only need to determine which of the 12 cultures in a row contains the mutants. Therefore, we go back to the original lysates, take a minimal volume that can be taken out using a multiwell pipetter (e.g., 5 μl), and add 100 μl of a mixture of 6.25 ml 96% ethanol, 1.25 ml H_2O, and 250 μl of 3 M Na acetate, pH 4.8, at room temperature. The mixture is centrifuged 20 minutes at room temperature. We have had success with precipitations that were done using a Falcon flat-bottom microtiter plate, which has the advantage that one can process lysates for several putative addresses at the same time, and use a multiwell pipetter to dispense DNA for the PCR.

III. C. Determination of the Presence of a Mutant

III. C. 1. PCR with Nested Primers

III. C. 1. a. Tc1-Specific Primers

We visualize insertions in genes of interest by PCR, using a primer specific for the transposon end and one for the gene. To make the reaction more specific and more sensitive we perform two rounds of PCR, using nested primers in the second round. The L1 and R1 primers are used for the first PCR (each for one orientation of Tc1), L2 and R2 for the second. The sequence of Tc1 specific primers is the following:

L1: 5′ CGTGGGTATTCCTTGTTCGAAGCCAGCTAC 3′

L2: 5′ TCAAGTCAAATGGATGCTTGAG 3′

R1: 5′ TCACAAGCTGATCGACTCGATGCCACGTCG 3′

R2: 5′ GATTTTGTGAACACTGTGGTGAAG 3′

Note that we chose the first primers somewhat removed from the transposon termini. This probably explains why the method works at all. In a genome that contains 50 copies of Tc1 (M. Finney, pers. comm.), the chances of obtaining Tc1 insertion near a Tc1 element are on average 50 times larger than those of obtaining one in a single-copy gene of interest. Thus one would expect that some selection step is required to remove the PCR products that result from amplification of the region between two Tc1 elements. This, however, is not the case (see results in Fig. 2a): the likely explanation is that Tc1–Tc1 amplicons generated during the first PCR round have long inverted repeats at their ends that extend from the L1 or R1 prime site in one Tc1 element to the L1 or R1 site in the neighboring element. This inverted repeat of a few hundred base pairs folds back immediately during the cooling after denaturation, and prevents priming by oligonucleotide primers.

III. C. 1. b. Gene-Specific Primers

The choice of gene-specific primers is based on a few general guidelines; we have chosen to keep the PCR conditions identical for all screens. This is made possible by the high specificity of nested PCR; we probably use annealing values that are a bit lower than optimal for most primers, which could lead to artifactual products, but these are cleaned up completely by the additional specificity of the second PCR.

Two sets of nested primers are chosen, each at one end of a region of 3 kb, pointing inward. This is the maximum area that can be screened; if a gene is much larger than this, one can choose to use more primer pairs, although in practice one may not need to. The distance is chosen also with the purpose that once an insertion is obtained, the same primer pairs can be used for isolation of deletion derivatives (see Section V). We find that primers that follow the following rules of thumb work well in more than 90% of the cases. We have not compared performance of primers chosen by these criteria with that of primers chosen by computer algorithms. The guidelines are based on those for collaborators who have sent us oligonucleotides. If they seem unnecessarily detailed, it is because we have found that to be necessary in some cases.

1. The primers of a pair are chosen close together, preferably within 200 bp.

2. Primers are approximately 50% GC, are 21 to 23 nucleotides long, have no funny sequences (palindromes, repeats, blocks of identical nucleotides), and have a somewhat balanced composition of all four nucleotides and a G or C at the 3' end.

3. Primers are all stored in stock solutions of 100 μM in TE or water; 100 μl is plenty.

4. We use simple names for the primers, Jon 1, Jon 2, Jon 3, Jon 4, and choose them such that Jon 2 is the nested primer for Jon 1, and Jon 4 is the nested primer for Jon 3. (Note that this is easily mixed up, as the primer sites within a gene will thus be in the order Jon 1,2,4,3 from left to right).

5. Some Ph.D.'s in biochemistry need to be reminded that not all marker pens hold on plastic and that stickers may come loose if tubes get wet. A second labeling of the top of the tube can be convenient.

c. PCR Protocol

PCR is performed in Perkin-Elmer 9600 machines. These take plates in a microtiter format, so that large series of reactions are easily prepared, because the DNA is stored in this format (see above) and because reagents can be dispensed over 96 PCR tubes using a multiwell pipetter. Another advantage is that one can perform reactions in small volumes (usually 10 μl per reaction), which saves reagents (particularly Taq polymerase). A final advantage is that reactions can be done without an oil overlay, which facilitates gel loading, etc. The PCR program can be quick, according to the suppliers, but because we are searching insertions of unknown size and unpredictable nucleotide composition we have not tried to minimize incubation times during PCR, and probably use too long programs. An important consideration in this stage is formed by the costs of the PCR. We have used Perkin Elmer tubes, and rubber Perkin Elmer overlays instead of caps. The overlays are much cheaper than new caps for every reaction, and they can be used indefinitely. We have never cleaned them or tried to remove traces of DNA. One might expect contaminations due to products of previous PCRs, but we do not find them. The contamination problem is probably somewhat exaggerated in general; in our case it helps that we never use the same primer sets for long, as we switch to new gene-specific primers for every search.

The only disposables are thus the PCR tubes, as the racks are also used indefinitely. Some suppliers have recently come up with cheaper versions of the tubes (Biozym) and with single plates, which we have not yet tried but expect to perform equally well. We compared several Taq polymerases in a blinded experiment and found several to perform well. Taking into account the price as well, we decided to use BRL Gibco Taq polymerase (5 U/μl).

The PCR conditions have been tested to some extent. We found the following to work well:

2 μl	DNA
1 μl	dNTP ($10\times$ = 2 mM for each dNTP)
1 μl	reaction buffer ($10\times$ = 0.5 M KCl, 0.1 M Tris–HCl, pH 8.3, 15 mM MgCl$_2$, 200 μg/ml gelatin)
1 μl	L1 or R1 primer ($10\times$ = 2 μM)
1 μl	gene primer 1 ($10\times$ = 2 μM)
4 μl	water (doubly distilled)
0.05 μl	Taq polymerase (5 U/μl)
10 μl	

The DNA is always dispensed first, and the other reagents are added after they have been mixed. For example, to do a "first-dimension screen," with the same primers on 96 DNA samples, we make a reaction mixture for 120 reactions, distribute them over 12 Micronic tubes in a rack, and use a multiwell pipetter to dispense 8 × 9 μl. Note that we always make a bit more reagent than is required. The layout of the PCR tray is of course arbitrary, but we have chosen the size of the library (3 × 960 samples) and the pooling strategy (8 samples per 960, to be checked in quadruplicate) such that the layout as shown in Fig. 1b is certainly convenient. As every primer pair can be checked with L and R primers, one can screen the complete series of 3×960 cultures for insertions in the vicinity of one primer pair by doing two parallel sets of two PCRs.

The PCR program is

3′	94°C
35×	1′ 94 C, 1′ 55°C, 2′ 72°C
3′	70°C
(indef)	10°C or room temperature

The second PCR can be prepared shortly before the first PCR is finished. A mixture is made similar to the one described above, but now primer L2 or R2 is used, as is gene primer 2. No DNA is added (see below), and the volume is compensated with extra water. After the mixture is dispensed, we do the following: with a multichannel pipetter we add 100 μl water to each tube of the first PCR. Then we stick a 96-pin stainless-steel "hedgehog" into the diluted PCR samples, pull it out, and stick it into the second PCR mixture. This small inoculum is sufficient. The homemade hedgehog is kept in a small iron tray containing ethanol and, before and after use, is pulled through a flame. This "sterilization" removes all DNA, as judged by the fact that all our work is done using a single hedgehog, and we see no contaminations.

III. C. 2. Gel Electrophoresis: Interpretation of the Gel Pattern

After the second PCR we add loading dye for agarose gel electrophoresis, again with a multichannel pipetter. The samples are analyzed by electrophoresis on horizontal 1% agarose gels. Note that it is not necessary to change tips or flush the tips with buffer after loading a sample, as one is only interested to see strong bands in the gel and is therefore not worried by slight carryover. This very much speeds up gel loading. The layout of the gel should be such that:

1. All quadruplicates are loaded next to each other, so that potential hits are easily recognized.

2. The lanes can be easily identified. We do this by loading DNA size markers between small series of samples.

3. Many samples can be separated on one gel. All potential addresses will be checked anyway, so one does not require optimal separation. As shown in Fig. 2a, we run up to three (sometimes even six) rows of samples on one 30-cm gel. In principle, one can thus analyze 120 (or 240) samples per gel (including markers), but following the PCR format (see above) we analyze a series of 96 samples plus the markers. We load A, B, C, and D of the first 960 cultures (I), then a size marker, then E, F, G, and H, and another size marker. The next row on the gel has the same pattern for the second 960 (II), and the third for the last 960 (III).

Figure 2 shows a gel that is typical. Several important considerations can be illustrated by interpretation of the gel in this figure.

1. The size marker helps to count off the sets of four lanes.

2. We look only at the strong bands.

3. If all bands were at the same position one might be suspicious of the result, but we see bands at many different positions, the normal spread expected for Tc1 insertions. The maximal size of products that we see in these experiments is approximately 2 kb, but these are rarer than products of up to 1 kb. Note that there seem to be "favorite" positions in the gel, reflecting hot sites for Tc1 insertion (see Van Luenen and Plasterk, 1994).

4. We now look for bands at the same position in four lanes from one sample (I F, III B). We also sometimes see cases of two or three out of four. Quite often these are found to be real addresses on repetition. The normal rules of statistics apply: a doublet or triplet at a position that is "hot" in the whole gel has more of a chance of being the result of chance than a doublet at a unique position.

III. D. Isolation of a Mutant

III. D. 1. Determination of the Address of a Mutant

The analysis described in Section III,C indicates sets of cultures that may contain a Tc1 insertion mutant. We usually store the information from screens with different sets of primers until, for example, 16 putative addresses have been obtained. Then each putative address is checked six times. We try to choose an even number of putative addresses per primer combination, so that two series of six reactions can fill a row of 12 tubes on a microtiter plate. After this control experiment one can usually conclude with reasonable certainty whether a first-dimension address is real. It should be noted that the subsequent analysis implicitly reconfirms this conclusion; in the rare case that no second-dimension address is obtained for a PCR product of the expected size, then one has to conclude that the bands observed in the more complex mixtures of the first dimension resulted from an unfortunate coincidence (or experimental error, such as contamination).

The experimental procedures for analysis of the second and third dimension of the address are the same as for the first dimension, except that usually it is not necessary to repeat the series of reactions after a putative second-dimension address is obtained (as the complexity of the DNA is lower, and thus the signal-to-background ratio is higher). If we have identified the lysate of the culture that contains the mutant, we perform one more PCR series on dilutions of that DNA and of a neighboring sample as a negative control (Fig. 2d).

III. D. 2. Isolation of a Mutant Line from a Positive Culture

Once an address has been determined one of the two corresponding stocks is thawed: the tube is taken from the $-80°C$ freezer, and thawed quickly, by warming between thumb and fingers. As soon as the tube is thawed completely, we remove most of the supernatant and transfer the remaining 40–50 μl containing the sedimented worms to a 10-cm seeded NGM plate. Occasionally we find that the frozen culture contains contaminating bacteria of unknown species, in which case we seed the duplicate cultures on plates that contain antibiotics (note that these plates are seeded with a thicker *E. coli* OP50 bacterial lawn, as these bacteria hardly grow on them). In most cases hundreds of larvae are found to have survived the procedure; it is important to keep an eye on the number of survivors, as it is not useful to screen a number of progeny worms much larger than the number of survivors.

The cultures were oligoclonal from the start, and thus we do not know what fraction of the survivors contains the mutation of interest. Our screening procedure is sensitive enough to detect mutants that constitute significantly less than 1% of a culture. This poses a dilemma: screening unnecessarily large numbers of single survivors is a lot of work if one in five turns out to be mutant, whereas screening too small numbers may not identify the mutant. We particularly want to avoid having to set up new cultures of worms after an initial screen was found to be negative. The following compromise results in relatively little work and no chance of missing mutants:

Two to three days after thawing a culture we pick 100 to 150 young adults individually onto small seeded NGM plates (Costar 12-well Cluster dishes, No. 3512), and at the same time seed oligoclonal cultures of rising complexity: 10 plates of 10 worms, 5 of 20 worms, 5 of 50 worms, 5 of 100 worms, and a plate of the rest. Two to four days later, 96 parental worms that have laid viable eggs are picked into 2.5 μl of "single-worm lysis buffer" (50 mM KCl, 10mM Tris–HCl, pH 8.3, 2.5 mM MgCl$_2$, 0.45% Nonidet P-40, 0.45% Tween 20, 0.01% gelatin, freshly added 60 μg/ml proteinase K). A culture of the mutator strain MT3126 always contains sterile individuals, and this seems even more so after thawing of a frozen culture. This is why we seed 100 to 150 individuals; the number 96 is obviously chosen by the PCR format. A quick way to analyze 96 single worms is the following: fill 96 tubes of a Perkin Elmer 9600 plate with 2.5 μl of single-worm lysis buffer, and pick and transfer single worms into the tube using a platinum wire (we check each transfer with a dissecting microscope). Add 5 μl paraffin oil to each tube. The oil is to prevent evaporation during the lysis step; the Perkin Elmer 9600 machine uses heating of the top of the tubes to prevent evaporation, but this requires minimally 5 to 10 μl of fluid. The subsequent PCR requires sufficient dilution of the lysis buffer. Lysis is for 60 minutes at 65°C in the 9600 PCR apparatus, followed by 10 minutes at 95°C for inactivation of proteases. We perform PCR in a total volume of 25 μl, using the outer PCR primers. As a control, we do the same reaction on a microliter of the original DNA sample of the positive culture. In this case we take samples of the first PCR and analyze these on gel; in principle, a mutant allele should result in a clear product of the expected size. The second PCR (using nested primers) is also performed and serves as control. In rare cases we see that the first PCR does not result in a clear PCR product, and the second one does, and subsequent analyses have indicated that the allele was indeed present.

Usually the mutant is found in this series, in which case we check some progeny of the mutant line again by single-worm PCR (and of a negative neighbor as control). If this is positive, then the other cultures are discarded. If, on the other hand, the series of single worms did not yield a mutant, then the cultures of rising complexity are analyzed. The worm pellets are lysed in 100 μl of single-worm lysis buffer (now with 200 μl/ml proteinase K), and 2 μl is analyzed by PCR. The most complex culture is in principle a replica of the culture that was indicated as positive in the screen, and it should again show the mutation. We take the culture of lowest complexity that is positive in the PCR, pick single worms out of these onto plates, and test them one generation later. If the only positive culture is of high complexity (more than 100), then it is advisable to go through one more step of sib selection, and plate, for example 50 cultures of 10 worms.

IV. Analysis of Mutants

IV. A. Initial Analysis of Tc1 Insertion Mutants

It is important to investigate whether a mutant is homozygous. A first impression can be obtained by PCR on, for example, 12 or 24 progeny worms, using the Tc1 and gene-specific primers. If all progeny contain the mutation, then one may conclude that probably the parent was homozygous, unless of course the wild-type allele is fortuitously coupled to an unrelated lethal mutation. If this experiment indicates that the strain is probably homozygous, one can do Southern blot analysis to confirm this. Most lines that we find are homozygous: if there is no selective pressure against homozygosity (so if the homozygous allele is normally viable and fertile) then chances are that the strain is homozygous as a result of inbreeding during the few generations before and after the thawing. And, indeed, most alleles that we find are apparently without clear phenotype for the homozygote. In addition, the requirement for a TA sequence at the Tc1 integration site, in combination with the A/T richness of introns, results in a bias toward intron insertions, so that even for essential genes we often pull out homozygous intron insertion alleles.

If the line is found to be heterozygous, then based on the arguments above, one may suspect that the homozygote has selective disadvantage or is lethal, and one should not grow the strain for too long without cloning and checking by PCR. One can then attempt to stabilize the strain by crossing in a balancer (see Chapter 7), or cross the allele into a strain that contains a transgene with the entire wild-type gene and attempt to obtain a homozygous mutant in this background (see below).

Once homozygous (or balanced), the strain is best frozen in multiple copies so that it will not be lost. The strain gets a new strain and allele number (see Appendix).

IV. B. Determination of the Insertion Site Sequence

The size of the PCR fragment can give a reasonable indication of the insertion site. The amplified DNA region runs from a known position near the Tc1 ends to a known position in the gene of interest and, therefore, contains the junction between the two sequences. One can determine the precise sequence of the insertion site quite easily, using one of the many protocols available for sequencing PCR products, using the L2 or R2 PCR primer as sequencing primer. Note that the sequence can be determined even before the clonal mutant line is obtained or before the address is thawed. This may be useful if multiple addresses are obtained, and one has reasons to prefer insertions in certain areas. Most insertions are in noncoding regions and, therefore, probably not used for phenotypic analysis anyway, but only for isolation of deletion derivatives (see below). One might argue that for this reason it is not important to know the precise insertion site, as the approximate site, derived from the size of the PCR product, is sufficient to choose primers for subsequent detection of deletion derivatives. We think there are good reasons to sequence the insertions nevertheless; in some cases the insertion allele may have interesting phenotypic properties (and then one wants to define the allele at the molecular level), determination of the sequence is proof that the PCR product is indeed the result of an insertion into the gene of interest, and the insertion site is the best way to document the allele. The entire genome sequence is becoming available through networked computer databases (see Chapter 23), and provides an infrastructure for sharing information about genotype and phenotype. The resolution of the genetic analysis of *C. elegans* will soon be at the level of the nucleotide, and it seems perferable to define transposon insertion alleles at this level too, so that they can be introduced into the "DNA sequence" window option of the ACeDB database (see Chapter 25).

V. Isolation of Deletion Derivatives

Tc1 alleles are not guaranteed null alleles: insertions in introns are removed from mature RNA together with the rest of the intron by normal splicing, and even insertions in exons can be removed by an aberrant splicing process that seems to be rather good at removing Tc1 sequences (perhaps as a result of the terminal inverted repeats that can form a stem-loop in RNA; Rushforth *et al.*, 1993). Zwaal *et al.* (1993) demonstrated that Tc1 insertion allels can be used as a starting point for isolation of deletion derivatives and can be selected in a strictly reverse genetic strategy (i.e., based on knowledge of the DNA sequence only). PCR is used to visualize deletions: the primers are chosen 3 kb apart in the genomic DNA, which implies that the amplicon is too large to be efficiently amplified, and thus one selectively visualizes rare deletion derivatives in a culture. A second PCR with nested primers is used to make the reaction more specific.

We usually choose the primers used for isolation of an insertion allele 3 kb apart (see Section III,C1,b), so that the same primers can be used for isolation of deletions. Note that the primers bias the search for deletions; a deletion can be visualized only if it has removed a large enough DNA segment yet is fully contained between the prime sites.

The mechanism of Tc1-induced deletion formation is not known with certainty, but because it has been shown that Tc1 (and the related element Tc3) transposes after excision of the element (Plasterk, 1992; Plasterk and Groenen, 1992; Vos *et al.*, 1993; Van Luenen *et al.*, 1995), it is reasonable to assume that the deletions result from the repair of the double-strand DNA break that is left after Tc1 excision. This is important because it implies that one can only find germ-line deletions using a strain that shows excision of Tc1 in the germ line. That means that the original strain in which the Tc1 insertion was isolated should not be outcrossed with, for example, the standard laboratory strain Bristol N2, because that would result in loss of the "mutator" gene that directs Tc1 jumping. Either the strain should not be outcrossed at all, or one may consider using a strain that carries markers on chromosome I (DR102 *dpy-5 unc-29*), as this is where the *mut-2* gene, which is thought to be responsible for Tc1 jumping, maps. The presence of small direct repeats at many deletion endpoints indicates that the process of deletion formation is not fully sequence independent, and this may be why not all Tc1 alleles seem to generate deletions at similar frequencies. If one encounters no deletions at reasonable frequency, it may be better to use a different set of primers to alter the area where deletions are sought.

We usually start approximately 100 cultures on small NGM plates and initiate each culture with not too many worms (5–10) of mixed age. After the plates are full grown, half of the worms are lysed in 50 to 100 μl "single-worm lysis buffer" by incubation for 2 to 3 hours at 65°C. Proteinase K is inactivated by heating the samples to 95°C for 15 minutes, and 1 μl of each lysate is analyzed in a 20-μl PCR. The sensitivity of the PCR protocol is such that one often sees false positives, which may result from deletions in somatic cells, or deletions that occurred very late during the culturing. Therefore, positive preparations are analyzed again by performing a convenient number (e.g., 6 or 12) of PCRs, using the same lysate. Preferably a deletion should be visible in one round of PCR. Once it has been established that a culture indeed contains a deletion allele, subcultures of different complexities are started (see above).

The lysis and PCR are repeated, and the culture of lowest complexity that contains a mutant allele is analyzed further as described above (either direct single-worm analysis or more sib selection steps).

Once a deletion derivative is obtained, one can again analyze whether it is homozygous, and if the homozygote is lethal one can introduce a balancer or a transgene with the wild-type gene (see Section IV,A). We have had good experience with the following approach: a transgene of the cloned gene is made in the strain Bristol N2. The transgene contains an extrachromosomal mixed array of the gene of interest (in our case *gpb-1*: R. Zwaal and RHAP, unpublished) and the visible marker gene $rol-6^D(su1006)$. The resulting strain is a Rol that segregates wild-type animals at approximately 50% as a result of spontaneous loss of the extrachromosomal transgene. Then we cross males with the heterozygous deletion mutant, and pick F1 males (50% of these will contain the deletion allele) and cross these with transgenic Rol hermaphrodites. Progeny Rol hermaphrodites are picked onto separate plates, and after they have laid eggs they are inspected by PCR for the presence of the deletion allele. From positive cultures we pick single Rol animals and culture these. Some are found to have 100% Rol progeny (plus, on closer inspection, dead larvae). Analysis of their DNA indicates that these strains are homozygous for the deletion allele, and this explains why they had become dependent on the presence of the transgene for survival. These obligatory transgenic animals are a good source of homozygous mutants for further study. Note that the rescue is formal proof that the lethal phenotype is the result of the deletion mutation, and not of another linked defect.

VI. Concluding Remarks

This chapter introduces some thoughts behind target-selected gene inactivation and some simple protocols. Genetic analysis obviously does not end with description of a mutant phenotype. One can assay whether expression in one type of cells is sufficient to perform certain functions by introducing the gene fused to a foreign promoter into a null mutant. Having a null mutant with a defined phenotype and rescue by the cloned gene, one has in principle an assay for site-directed point mutants of the gene; each mutant can be tested for its ability to rescue the null mutant. Epistatic interaction between null alleles and alleles of other genes can be studied. And, finally, mutants with a clear phenotype [Tc1 insertion mutants, or deletion derivatives, or transgenic lines where the phenotype is (partially) rescued] can be used for the isolation of extragenic suppressor mutants, which may help to unravel pathways of interacting gene products.

Acknowledgments

Work in author's laboratory is supported by a Pionier grant of the Dutch organization for Scientific Research (NWO) and recently by NIH/NCRR grant RR 10082-01. I am grateful to members of my laboratory for very stimulating discussion, to Sandra Pennington, Rik Korswagen, Richard Zwaal, Annegien Broeks, and Marianne de Vroomen for critical reading of the manuscript, and to José Groenen, Joyce van Meurs, and Marianne de Vroomen for technical assistance.

References

Ballinger, D. G., and Benzer, S. (1989). Targeted gene mutations in *Drosophila*. *Proc. Natl. Acad. Sci. U.S.A.* **86,** 9402–9406.
Bargmann, C. I. (1993). Odorant-selective genes and neurons mediate olfaction in *C. elegans. Cell* **74,** 515–527.

Barstead, R. J., and Waterston, R. H. (1991). Vinculin is essential for muscle function in the nematode. *J. Cell. Biol.* **114,** 715–724.

Broverman, S. A., MacMorris, M. M., and Blumenthal, T. (1993). Alteration of *Caenorhabditis elegans* gene expression by targeted transformation. *Proc. Natl. Acad. Sci. U.S.A.* **90,** 4359–4363.

Finney, M. (1987). The genetics and molecular biology of unc-86, a *C. elegans* cell lineage gene. Ph.D. Thesis. Massachusetts Institute of Technology, Cambridge, MA.

Fire, A. (1986). Integrative transformation of *C. elegans. EMBO J.* **5,** 2673–2680.

Fire, A., Albertson, D. G., Harrison, S. W., and Moerman, D. G. (1991). Production of antisense RNA leads to effective and specific inhibition of gene expression in *C. elegans* muscle. *Development* **113,** 503–514.

Greenstein, D., Hird, S., Plasterk, R. H. A., Andachi, Y., Kohara, Y., Wang, B., Finney, M., and Ruvkun, G. (1994). Targeted mutations in the *Caenorhabditis elegans* POU homeo box gene *ceh-18* cause defects in oocyte cell cycle arrest, gonad migration, and epidermal differentiation. *Genes Dev.* **8,** 1935–1948.

Kaiser, K., and Goodwin, S. F. (1990). "Site-selected" transposon mutagenesis of *Drosophila. Proc. Natl. Acad. Sci. U.S.A.* **87,** 1686–1690.

Littleton, J. T., Stern, M., Schulze, K., Perin, M., and Bellen, H. J. (1993). Mutational analysis of *Drosophila synaptotagmin* demonstrates its essential role in Ca^{2+}-activated neurotransmitter release. *Cell* **74,** 1125–1134.

Mello, C. C., Kramer, J. M., Stinchcomb, D. T., and Ambros, V. (1992). Efficient gene transfer in *C. elegans:* Extrachromosomal maintenance and integration of transforming sequences. *EMBO J.* **10,** 3959–3970.

Moerman, D. G., and Waterston, R. H. (1989). Mobile elements in *Caenorhabditis elegans* and other nematodes. *In* "Mobile DNA" (D. E. Berg and M. M. Howe, eds.), pp. 537–556. American Society for Microbiology, Washington, D.C.

Plasterk, R. H. A. (1992). Reverse genetics of *Caenorhabditis elegans. Bioessays* **14,** 629–633.

Plasterk, R. H. A., and Groenen, J. T. M. (1992). Targeted alterations of the *Caenorhabditis elegans* genome by transgene instructed DNA double strand break repair following Tc1 excision. *EMBO J.* **11,** 287–290.

Plasterk, R. H. A. (1994). The Tc1/*mariner* transposon family. *In* "Transposable Elements" (H. Saedler and A. Gierl, eds.), Springer Verlag, Heidelberg, in press.

Rushforth, A. M., Saari, B., and Anderson, P. (1993). Site-selected insertion of the transposon Tc1 into a *Caenorhabditis elegans* myosin light chain gene. *Mol. Cell. Biol.* **13,** 902–910.

Thomas, J. H. (1990). Genetic analysis of defecation in *C. elegans. Genetics* **124,** 855–872.

Van Luenen, H. G. A. M., Colloms, S. D., and Plasterk, R. H. A. (1993). Mobilization of quiet, endogenous Tc3 transposons of *Caenorhabditis elegans* by forced expression of Tc3 transposase. *EMBO J.* **12,** 2513–2520.

Van Luenen, H. G. A. M., and Plasterk, R. H. A. (1994). Target site choice of the related transposable elements Tc1 and Tc3 of *Caenorhabditis elegans. Nucleic Acids Res.* **22,** 262–269.

Van Luenen, H. G. A. M., Colloms, S. D., and Plasterk, R. H. A. (1995). The mechanism of transposition of Tc3 in *C. elegans. Cell* **79,** 293–301.

Vos, J. C., Van Luenen, H. G. A. M., and Plasterk, R. H. A. (1993). Characterization of the *Caenorhabditis elegans* Tc1 transposon *in vivo* and *in vitro. Genes Dev.* **7,** 1244–1253.

Wilson, R., Ainscough, R., Anderson, K., Baynes, C., Berks, M., Bonfield, J., Burton, J., Connell, M., Cooper, J., Copsey, T., Coulson, A., Craxton, M., Dear, S., Du, Z., Durbin, R., Favello, A., Fraser, A., Fulton, L., Gardner, A., Green, P., Hawkins, T., Hillier, L., Jier, M., Johnston, L., Jones, M., Kershaw, J., Kirsten, J., Laisster, N., Latreille, P., Lightning, J., Lloyd, C., Mortimore, B., O-Callaghan, M., Parsons, J., Percy, C., Rifken, L., Roopra, A., Saunders, D., Shownkeen, R., Sims, M., Smaldon, N., Smith, A., Smith, M., Sonnhammer, E., Staden, R., Sulston, J., Thierry-Mieg, J., Thomas, K., Vaudin, M., Vaughan, K., Waterston, R., Watson, A., Weinstock, L.,

Wilkinson-Sproat, J., and Wohldman, P. (1994). 2.2 Mb of contiguous nucleotide sequence from chromosome III of *C. elegans. Nature* **368,** 32–38.

Wood, W. B., (ed.) (1988). "The Nematode *C. elegans*" Cold Spring Harbor Laboratory Press, New York.

Yandell, M. D., Edgar, L. G., and Wood, W. B. (1994). Trimethylpsoralen induces small deletion mutations in *Caenorhabditis elegans. Proc. Natl. Acad. Sci. U.S.A.* **91,** 1381–1385.

Zwaal, R. R., Broeks, A., Van Meurs, J., Groenen, J. T. M., and Plasterk, R. H. A. (1993). Target-selected gene inactivation in *Caenorhabditis elegans,* using a frozen transposon insertion mutant bank. *Proc. Natl. Acad. Sci. U.S.A.* **90,** 7431–7345.

CHAPTER 4

Genetic Mapping with Polymorphic Sequence-Tagged Sites

Benjamin D. Williams

Department of Genetics
Washington University School of Medicine
St. Louis, Missouri 63110

I. Introduction

The number of easily distinguishable mutant phenotypes in *Caenorhabditis elegans* is relatively small, and this constrains the number of factors that can be followed in standard genetic crosses. Consequently, a new mutation is mapped, first to a chromosome using two-factor data from one or more crosses, and then to a chromosomal subregion by successive three-factor crosses (see Sulston and Hodgkin, 1988, for description of standard mapping methods).

Mapping would be more efficient if it were possible to score a large number of well-distributed markers in a single cross. The advent of the polymerase chain reaction (Saiki *et al.*, 1988) makes this approach feasible by allowing polymorphic genomic regions to serve as genetic markers that are easily scored in DNA released from individual animals. The only "phenotype" is a band on a gel, so the segregation of many of these markers can be followed in a single cross. Following the terminology proposed by Olsen *et al.* (1989), we refer to polymorphisms that can be scored by appropriately designed polymerase chain reaction (PCR) assays as polymorphic sequence-tagged sites (STSs).

In *C. elegans*, copies of the transposable element Tc1 are a source of easily identified and well-distributed polymorphisms. Tc1s are present at approximately 500 loci dispersed throughout the genome of the Bergerac strain, but absent from most of these positions in the Bristol strain (Emmons *et al.*, 1983; Liao *et al.*, 1983). Identification and genetic mapping of Tc1 polymorphisms near genes of interest (Ruvkun *et al.*, 1989) have been used to facilitate the isolation of these genes from the physical map of the *C. elegans* genome (Coulson *et al.*, 1986, 1988, 1991). Conversely, Tc1 polymorphisms have been used as genetic markers to place cloned genes on the linkage map (Files *et al.*, 1983). Tc1 polymorphisms have also been used to clone genes by transposon tagging (Moerman *et al.*, 1986).

To develop a set of polymorphic STS markers useful for a genomewide, genetic mapping strategy, 200 Tc1-containing clones from a random library of Bergerac genomic DNA were positioned on the *C. elegans* genomic physical map (Williams *et al.*, 1992). From the 73 independent sites identified, 40 were developed into STS markers that would effectively cover most of the genome. Each Tc1 polymorphism is scored by a unique PCR assay that amplifies a product only when the Tc1 is present, thus distinguishing between the Tc1(+) (Bergerac DNA) and Tc1(−) (Bristol DNA) polymorphic states. By combining several such assays in a single reaction, multiple STSs can be scored simultaneously in DNA released from an individual animal. This permits a very efficient mapping strategy that requires only a single interstrain cross and analysis of a small number of progeny.

The absence of a visible phenotype associated with STS markers, and the ability to score them in DNA released from single embryos as well as adults, provides advantages beyond simply reducing the number of crosses necessary to map a new mutation. For example, the first of these features simplifies the mapping of X-linked mutation by allowing X-linked STS markers to be introduced directly through males (*C. elegans* males are hemizygous for X, and males carrying standard X-linked recessive marker mutations, causing a dumpy or uncoordinated phenotype, for example, are often ineffective maters). The second feature simplifies the mapping of recessive lethal mutations by allowing developmentally arrested embryos to be scored directly for STS markers. In contrast, standard marker mutations usually cannot be scored in these embryos, so a less sensitive linkage test must be used that requires an additional generation. Several additional advantages of the STS markers are described below.

A more detailed description of the polymorphic STS mapping technique has been published previously (Williams *et al.*, 1992).

II. Polymorphic Sequence–Tagged Site Markers

Each STS assay includes a primer that anneals to a unique region flanking a particular Tc1 insertion site and a primer that anneals to the Tc1 (Table I). Together the primers amplify a DNA fragment from the Bergerac Tc1 (+) "filled" site, but not from the Bristol Tc1 (−) "empty" site. Because the fragment is amplified from DNA of a Tc1 (+)/Tc1(−) heterozygote, each Tc1 behaves as a dominant genetic marker.

The genetic and physical map positions of the current set of 40 polymorphic STS markers are shown in Fig. 1. Precise physical map positions for these markers are available within the ACeDB/CEMAP database (see Chapter 25 of this volume). The STS genetic map positions were initially deduced directly from physical map position of the Tc1-containing clones, relying on the extensive correspondence that has been established between the *C. elegans* physical and genetic maps. To detect any obvious errors in these deduced map positions, which, for example, might reflect an error in physical mapping of a particular Tc1, each polymorphic STS has also been mapped genetically to the appropriate chromosomal subregion in crosses with standard marker mutations (Williams *et al.*, 1992).

To map efficiently, groups of STS assays have been designed to work together within a single reaction that can detect from three to nine different STSs simultaneously. In each of these "multiplex" reactions, a common Tc1 primer works in combination with several different STS-specific flanking primers. The product amplified from a particular STS is a characteristic size that is easily distinguishable from other STS products by standard nondenaturing acrylamide gel electrophoresis. The standard multiplex reactions are shown in Fig. 2. Useful assay sets include a chromosome assignment reaction, which detects centrally placed markers on each autosome, and chromosome-specific reactions, each detecting multiple markers distributed along individual chromosomes. Two reactions are shown for chromosome V, one designed for mapping on the left side of this chromosome and one for the right side. Two reactions are also shown for chromosome III, one detecting an additional Tc1 present in only one of the two Bergerac strains used for mapping.

III. Summary of Mapping Strategy

The mapping strategy is diagrammed in Fig. 3. Mutations generated in the Bristol background are mapped by constructing a mutant heterozygote that is a Bristol/Bergerac hybrid. Heterozygous F1 hermaphrodites are allowed to self-

Table I
Primer Sequences for STS Assays[a]

Primer	Polymorphism	Band size (bp)	Sequence (5′ → 3′)							
618[b]			GAA	CAC	TGT	GGT	GAA	GTT	TC	
Chromosome I										
093	stP124	115	GAC	GCA	GAC	AGA	CGA	AGT	G	
734	hP4	130	CGG	AAA	TAT	TAT	CAG	CAC	AGC	
437	TCbn2	150	GCA	TAA	AAA	GCC	TCC	AAG	TCA	
Chromosome II										
543	stP196	133	CCA	AAA	GTT	TAA	AGG	AAA	TGA	AGC
363	stP100	198	GGA	AAC	CAA	GAA	CAT	TGG	ACG	
133	stP101	118	CGC	CTG	ATT	TTT	CCA	GGT	GC	
816	stP50	180	TCC	AGA	TAT	CAT	ATA	GCT	TGT	TC
886	stP36	153	CAC	TGT	CTT	GTC	GAT	ACC		
437	stP98	269	AAG	TAG	AAA	AAT	TGC	CTT	GCG	
723	maP1	234	CCA	ATT	TTC	CGG	AAG	TTT	TCG	
Chromosome III										
570	eP64	137	TAA	TAA	TTT	GTC	AGG	AAA	CGA	G
845	stP19	216	ACA	AGC	GGG	TCT	ACT	GAA	CC	
587	mgP21	165	GGA	ACA	AAA	GTG	CCT	TGG	G	
401	stP127	233	GCA	TCG	ATA	CAA	GTG	GAA	GC	
548	stP120	149	AAT	AAT	CAG	TGA	AGC	CTC	ATG	
800	stP17	183	CTC	GAT	GTG	TCT	CAA	TAG	TTC	C
Chromosome IV										
815	stP13	236	CCC	ACA	ACC	TTT	TGC	TAC	AAC	
056	stP51	281	GTT	CGT	TTT	TAC	TGG	GAA	GG	
931	stP44	209	CCA	TCG	TTT	GTG	TCT	AGA	GTC	
653	sP4	179	TTT	CTG	TTT	TGT	GCT	TAG	ACG	
510	stP5	261	GGA	TTA	TTA	CCG	TCT	TAC	GCA	
536	stP35	149	GCA	GTC	TCT	AAT	AGA	GCT	GC	
Chromosome V										
813	stP3	153	GTC	GCA	TTT	CCA	TTC	ATG	CAG	
440	stP192	290	GCA	CGC	TGA	GAG	TAA	GTG	C	
997	stP23	135	TTG	TCA	ACT	ATT	TTA	CAG	CGA	G
736	bP1	119	AAC	ACA	TTT	AGG	TAA	TGT	AGC	AC
998	stP6	170	TCA	CAA	TCG	ATG	ACT	AAG	TAC	TGG
862	stP18	203	TTG	AAC	TTC	TCC	CAC	TCC	TC	
438	stP108	135	AAA	GAT	AAA	CGC	GCT	TTT	TGG	
439	stP105	152	GGG	TAG	TTG	TTC	ATG	TCT	CG	
652	stP128	200	GCA	ACG	CTT	TGT	GGA	TCT	G	
Chromosome X										
930	stP41	193	TGT	CTA	CTT	ACC	TTA	ACT	TAC	C
888	stP40	229	GTA	TGA	GCT	AAT	TGT	ACC	CTC	
449	stP156	143	TGG	AGG	ATT	CGG	GCG	ATT	G	
112	stP33	260	CGT	CTA	GTC	GTG	TGT	TTC	C	
453	stP103	209	GAC	GAA	AAG	AGG	TAC	ACG	AG	
454	stP129	160	CCA	CTT	ATT	GCC	ACT	TTT	TGG	
450	stP61	176	GAA	TTG	GTG	TCC	GGA	ACA	C	
452	stP72	112	CTT	GAA	AAT	ACC	ATG	GCA	TAC	
887	stP2	127	CAA	AAC	GGT	ATA	CTC	TGG	TG	

[a] Reprinted with permission from Williams *et al.* (1992).
[b] Common Tc1 primer used in every STS assay.

fertilize, and then individual F2 mutant homozygotes are assayed for specific Tc1s in two successive mapping steps. The first step (Fig. 3A) establishes linkage to an autosome, and the second (Fig. 3B) refines map position to a chromosomal subregion. X linkage is determined earlier during the generation of the Bristol/Bergerac hybrid (see below).

In the first step, 20 to 30 F2 mutants are tested individually with the chromosome assignment reaction. Each unlinked Tc1 should be detected in three-fourths of these animals, as expected for dominant genetic markers. In contrast, the linked Tc1 will be detected in significantly fewer animals because this requires recombination between the mutation and the Tc1 (see Fig. 3A). Tight linkage will be detected easily because the linked Tc1 will be inherited by few, if any, of the F2 mutants. Loose linkage may be detected only after additional F2 mutants are scored and a statistically significant reduction from three-fourths inheritance is observed for one of the Tc1s.

Once the mutation has been mapped to a chromosome, additional F2 mutant homozygotes are tested with the appropriate chromosome-specific reaction. Recombination events can be positioned along the chromosome based on the inheritance of the linked Tc1s, allowing the mutation to be mapped to a chromosomal subregion as in standard multifactor analysis (see Fig. 3B).

IV. Results

We mapped the recessive lethal mutation *deb-1(st385)* to test the method. Mutant *deb-1(st385)* homozygotes arrest during late embryogenesis, sometimes hatching as misshapen L1 larvae (Barstead and Waterston, 1991). Figure 4A shows the results of the first mapping step. The unlinked Tc1s marking chromosomes, I, II, III, and V were detected in approximately three-fourths of the 25 F2 mutants that were scored. In contrast, the Tc1 marking chromosome IV was detected in none of the mutants, placing *deb-1(st385)* on chromosome IV, close to STS *sP4*.

The second mapping step is shown in Fig. 4B. Thirty-three additional F2 mutants were scored with the chromosome IV reaction, and 10 were positive for one or more STSs. The five different types of recombinants are illustrated by the representative reactions shown in lanes A to E. An interpretation of the corresponding crossover events between the Bristol and Bergerac chromosomes is shown in Fig. 4C. These data position *deb-1(st385)* between *stP51* and *sP4*, but do not order it with respect to the closely linked polymorphism *stP44*.

Additional mapping experiments using this technique, including mapping of X-linked mutations, have been published previously (Williams *et al.*, 1992). The sensitivity of the linkage test is illustrated by mapping an *unc-52* mutation. The *unc-52* locus is approximately 20 map units from STS *maP1*, which marks chromosome II in the chromosome assignment reaction. Linkage was demonstrated by scoring 39 F2 mutants (Williams *et al.*, 1992).

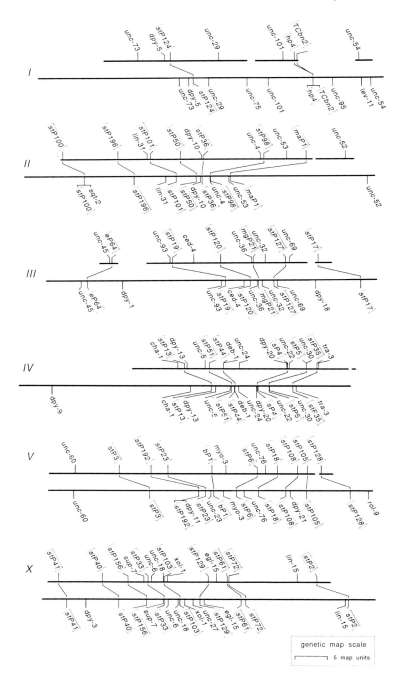

====== **V. How to Use the Method**

A. Strains

The mapping method is appropriate for mutations generated in the Bristol N2 background, and Bristol N2 males are used in most of the crosses described below. For the generation of Bristol/Bergerac hybrids, two Bergerac strains can be used, RW7000 (see in Section V,G) and the derivative strain DP13. DP13 contains an additional Tc1 on chromosome III, *eP64*, but lacks one Tc1 chromosome V, *stP128* (see Fig. 2).

B. Genetic Crosses

Bergerac males of strain RW7000 or DP13 do not mate effectively. Consequently, crosses to generate Bristol/Bergerac hybrids are started with Bristol males. This contraint results in different procedures for autosomal and X-linked mutations.

For autosomal mutations, Bristol hermaphrodites homozygous or heterozygous (recessive lethal or sterile mutations) for the unmapped mutation are crossed with Bristol males. Ten to fifteen male progeny from this cross are mated with 20 to 30 Bergerac hermaphrodites. Because RW7000 and DP13 are homozygous for an uncharacterized recessive mutation causing sluggish movement, outcross F1 animals can often be identified as well-moving animals. Approximately 40 well-moving F1 animals are picked to seperate plates (fewer are needed if the male parents were generated in a cross with a mutant homozygote). F1s heterozygous for the unmapped mutation are recognized when they produce homozygous mutant F2 self progeny. Approximately 70 F2 mutant worms or, for recessive lethal mutations, 70 F2 developmentally arrested embryos are picked individually into separate microfuge tubes containing lysis buffer and stored for later scoring.

This STS-based mapping strategy can also be adapted for maternal effect mutations. Because expression of the mutant phenotype is dependent not on the

---

Fig. 1 Physical (top line) and genetic (bottom line) maps of chromosomes I, II, III, IV, V, and X, showing the positions of polymorphic STSs (boxes) and other loci to provide orientation. STS genetic map positions are based on their physical map positions and genetic mapping data published previously (Williams *et al.,* 1992). This figure was modified from Fig. 1 of Williams *et al.* (1992), and incorporates an updated version of the physical map. The positions of several markers have changed. On chromosome I, STSs *hP4* and *TCbn2* have been moved to the right of *unc*-101, based on the current physical map positions of these markers. On chromosome V, STS *stP108* has been moved to the left of *dpy-21,* based on unpublished genetic mapping data (Kim Ferguson, pers. comm.). The physical maps are scaled to chromosome size; estimated sizes are 15 megabases (Mb) (I), 18 Mb (II), 13 Mb (III), 18 Mb (IV), 25 Mb (V), and 21 Mb (X).

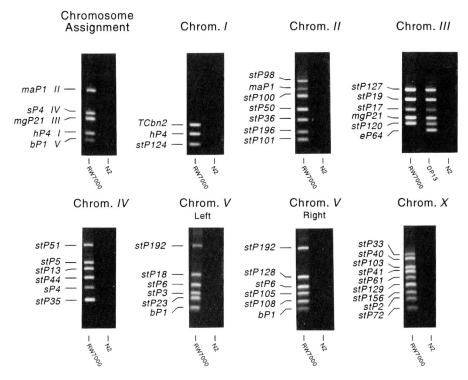

Fig. 2 Polymerase chain reaction performed on DNA released from single Bergerac (RW7000, DP13) and Bristol (N2) animals, as negative controls, illustrates the chromosome assignment reaction and each of the chromosome-specific reactions. Tc1 *eP64* is present only in DP13 (see chromosome III). Tc1 *stP128* is present in RW7000 (see chromosome V, right), but absent from DP13 (not shown). Reprinted with permission from Williams *et al.* (1992).

genotype of the zygote, but rather the genotype of its hermaphrodite parent, in the mapping scheme presented here, F2 mutant homozygotes will appear wild type. They are recognized, however, by cloning individual F2 animals to separate plates and allowing them to self. F2 mutant homozygotes will segregate progeny with the mutant phenotype, and then these F2 parents can then be picked into separate tubes of lysis buffer for later scoring.

X-linked mutations are first recognized during the initial crosses of the mapping scheme, because *C. elegans* males are hemizygous for the X chromosome. Some of the males produced in the first cross will be hemizygous for the unmapped mutation and will display the mutant phenotype. If the unmapped mutation is lethal, the XO zygotes will be inviable (and, therefore, indistinguishable from lethal homozygotes produced by self-fertilization), so X-linkage is first indicated by the failure to introduce the lethal mutation into the F1 hybrid strain through

A

Segregation of linked and
unlinked STS's in F2
mutant homozygotes

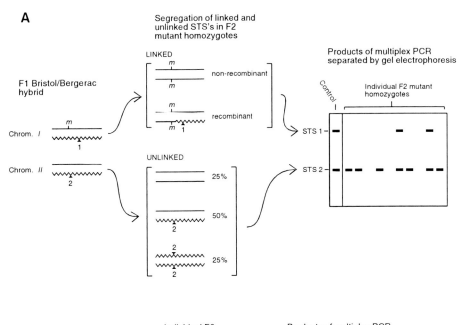

B

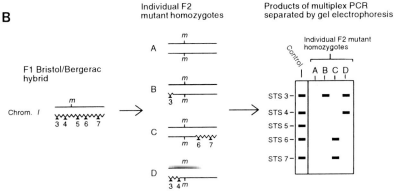

Fig. 3 Two-step polymorphic STS mapping strategy. (A) Step 1, mapping to an autosome. A Bristol/
Bergerac F1 hybrid (Bristol DNA = straight lines, Bergerac DNA = jagged lines, Tc1s = numbered
triangles) that is heterozygous for new mutation *m* is allowed to self, and individual F2 mutant
homozygotes are assayed by multiplex PCR for STSs marking each autosome, STSs 1 and 2 in this
example. The unlinked STSs (exemplified by STS 2) are detected in 75% of the animals, whereas
the linked STS (STS 1) is partially or completely "excluded" from the mutant homozygotes, as it
is inherited only when there is a crossover between it and the mutation. A diagram of an acrylamide
gel displaying the PCR products is shown on the right. Each lane represents a single reaction with
DNA of an individual F2 mutant homozygote. Unlinked STS 2 is detected in 7 of 10 animals assayed,
whereas linked STS 1 is detected in only 2 of 10 animals. The control lane shows a reaction with
Bergerac DNA. (B) Step 2, mapping to a chromosomal subregion. Additional F2 mutant homozygotes
from the same F1 parental strain are assayed for several STSs on the appropriate chromosome,
again by multiplex PCR. Several expected F2 mutant genotypes are illustrated (A–D) along with
the corresponding PCR results. In this example, the PCR data can be used to infer the positions of
crossovers between the Bristol and Bergerac chromosomes and place *m* between STSs 4 and 6, but
do not order it with respect to STS 5. Alternative positions for *m* would require more complex
patterns of recombination. Modified from Williams *et al.* (1992).

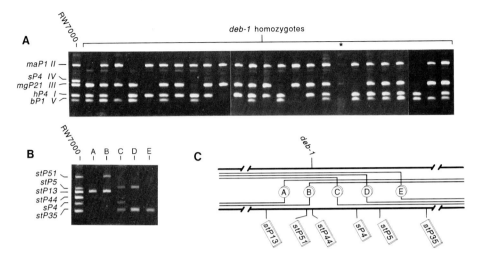

Fig. 4 Test mapping of lethal mutation *deb-1(st385)*. (A) Mapping *deb-1* to chromosome IV. Control reaction with RW7000 DNA shows the positions of bands corresponding to STSs marking chromosomes I, II, III, IV, and V. Additional lanes show 25 separate reactions, each performed with DNA from an individual *deb-1* F2 homozygote produced by self-fertilization of a Bristol/ Bergerac hybrid. Each STS was detected in approximately 75% of the animals with the exception of *sP4*, marking chromosome IV, which was detected in none of them. The asterisk indicates a failed PCR reaction. (B) Mapping *deb-1* to a chromosome IV subregion. A control reaction with RW7000 DNA shows the bands corresponding to STSs arrayed along chromosome IV. Lanes A–E show representative reactions for each type of *deb-1* homozygote that was positive for one or more chromosome IV STSs. Class A (*n* = 4), class B (*n* = 1), class C (*n* = 1), class D (*n* = 3), class E (*n* = 1); the remaining 23 mutants tested negative for all of the chromosome IV STSs. (C) For classes A–E, diagram of the proposed recombination events between the Bristol (top line) and Bergerac (bottom line) chromosomes of the F1 hybrid. This interpretation places *deb-1* between *stP51* and *stP5*, which corresponds to its previously established genetic and physical map positions. Reprinted with permission from Williams *et al.* (1992).

a male parent. In either case a hybrid strain for further mapping is constructed as follows. Hybrid males containing a Bergerac X chromosome are produced by crossing Bergerac hermaphrodites with Bristol males. These hybrid males are then mated to Bristol hermaphrodite mutant homozygotes or heterozygotes (lethal or sterile mutations). Approximately 30 individual F1 progeny (fewer if the hermaphrodite parent is homozygous) are then cloned to separate plates and allowed to self. Plates with F2 mutant homozygotes are retained, and 30 to 50 F2 mutants are scored individually with the X chromosome reaction. It should be noted that when using a heterozygous Bristol parent in this scheme, nonhybrid Bristol F1 mutant heterozygotes can be produced by self-fertilization. These animals are recognized by testing each F1 with the X chromosome reaction before F2 progeny are used for mapping. F1s that test negative are assumed to be nonhybrids, and these plates are discarded.

C. Complications Due to Spontaneous Mutations and Tc1 Excision

1. Spontaneous Mutations

Spontaneous mutations occur at a relatively high rate in the Bergerac mutator background (Moerman and Waterston, 1984) and can occasionally cause problems. For example, a spontaneous mutation can cause an F1 Bergerac nonhybrid (produced by self-fertilization of the Bergerac parent) to be mistaken for an F1 hybrid that is heterozygous for the unmapped mutation. This has happened, although infrequently, while we were mapping lethal mutations. In each instance all of the mutant F2s from a particular F1 tested positive for every STS in the chromosome assignment reaction. The F1 was a Bergerac animal that had apparently acquired a spontaneous lethal mutation. This kind of artifact is easily recognized if F2 mutants are scored as groups of siblings. If F2s from several different F1s are picked and then scored in random order, however, the artifact may go unnoticed during the first mapping step, and could lead to an overestimation of the map distance between the mutation and the linked marker.

2. Tc1 Excision

Tc1 excision can cause the loss of an STS marker from the parental Bergerac strain. Consequently, the parental strain should be tested with the relevant multiplex reaction as a positive control in each mapping experiment. In the course of several years of mapping, we have only once detected the loss of an STS marker from our RW7000 strain. Those plates were discarded and the strain reinitiated from frozen stocks. To reduce the chances of losing a Tc1 marker during propagation, the Bergerac strains are not maintained by transferring an individual hermaphrodite to a fresh plate. Instead, fresh plates are seeded with many animals.

Tc1 excision in the germ line of the Bristol/Bergerac F1 hybrid (Mori et al., 1988, 1990) is another potential problem. We have detected apparent spontaneous excision of several different STS Tc1s in the hybrid germ line (Williams et al., 1992). These events occured with low enough frequency that they should not significantly affect the assignment of a new mutation to linkage group. Misinterpretation of an excision event as the loss of a Tc1 due to recombination could, however, lead to errors in subsequent mapping to a chromosomal subregion. Our experience to date suggests that enough redundant information is generated when mapping with STSs that an infrequent excision event should be recognized and, therefore, should not lead to mapping errors.

D. Recipes

1. Lysis buffer: 50 mM KCl, 10 mM Tris (pH 8.3), 2.5 mM MgCl$_2$, 0.45% Nonidet P-40, 0.45% Tween 20, 0.01% (w/v) gelatin. Autoclave and then store in aliquots at $-20°C$; just before use add proteinase K to 60 μg/ml.

2. Proteinase K stock: 10 mg/ml proteinase K (Boehringer-Mannheim) in water. Store in aliquots at $-20°C$.

3. Chitinase solution: 20 mg/ml chitinase (Sigma No. c-6137) in 50 mM NaCl, 70 mM KCl, 2.5 mM MgCl$_2$, 2.5 mM CaCl$_2$. Store in aliquots at $-20°C$.

4. 10× Taq buffer: 100 mM Tris (pH 8.3), 500 mM KCl, 15 mM MgCl$_2$, 0.01% (w/v) gelatin. Autoclave and store in aliquots at $-20°C$.

5. PCR cocktail: 1.1× Taq buffer, 5 nmole each dNTP per reaction, 25 pmole Tc1 primer 618 per reaction, 25 pmole each STS-specific primer per reaction (see Table I for primer sequences, see below for alternative primer concentrations), 0.6 unit Taq DNA polymerase (Perkin Elmer Cetus) per reaction. Final amplification reaction should be 1× Taq buffer; PCR cocktail is freshly made just before use.

E. DNA Preparation

Methods for DNA preparation and "single-worm" PCR were adapted with slight modification from Barstead *et al.* (1991). A single worm is transferred using a standard platinum wire "worm picker" directly from the culture plate to a 2.5-μl drop of lysis buffer in the cap of a 0.5-ml tube suitable for thermocycling (tube still attached). Care is taken to avoid transferring a large amount of bacteria with each worm, usually by picking the worm up from a region of the plate where there is no bacterial lawn. After the worm is observed within the drop of lysis buffer, the tube is closed, centrifuged briefly to move the drop to the bottom of the tube, and frozen at $-70°C$ for 10 minutes. Samples can be stored at $-70°C$ for weeks. After a drop of mineral oil is added as an overlay, the tube is heated to 60°C for 1 hour, followed by 95°C for 15 minutes, and then kept at 4°C until the PCR cocktail is added.

When lethal mutations are mapped, eggs containing arrested embryos are handled essentially the same as single worms, except that they are treated briefly with chitinase. Eggs are picked up using a 5-μl capillary tube pulled to an approximate 100-μm inner diameter and filled with chitinase solution. Particular care should be taken to observe directly the successful transfer of the egg to the lysis buffer, and only a small volume of chitinase solution should be transferred with each egg. The same capillary can be used for multiple transfers without cross-contamination of samples.

We have only used embryos arrested near the end of development. It remains to be determined if mutants arresting earlier, before many cell divisions have been completed, will yield enough DNA to give reproducible results.

F. Polymerase Chain Reaction Conditions

PCR cocktail (22.5 μl) is added on top of the mineral oil overlay that covers the DNA sample. When all the samples are ready, the tubes are centrifuged for a few seconds to move the PCR cocktail through the oil, mixing it with the

2.5 μl DNA sample to bring the reaction volume to 25 μl. The tubes are immediately transferred to the thermocycler and cycled 30 times with the following conditions: 94°C for 30 seconds, 58°C for 1 minute, and 72°C for 1 minute. Ten microliters of each reaction is run on a 6% acrylamide minigel (Mighty Small II, Hoeffer Scientific Instruments) buffered with 1× TBE (90 mM Tris-borate, 2 mM EDTA) and stopped when the bromphenol blue dye front reaches the bottom. Conditions for gel electrophoresis and staining are as described for nondenaturing DNA gels in Sambrook *et al.* (1989).

Each experiment should include several reactions scoring single animals from the Bergerac parental strain. These serve as a positive controls and as STS standards for interpreting the gels. Several animals from the Bristol parental strain should also be assayed as negative controls.

The protocol described here uses an equimolar mixture of primers in each reaction. A more economical alternative is to keep the Tc1 primer 618 at 25 pmole per reaction, and reduce the STS-specific primers to 5 pmole per reaction (J. Kramer, pers. comm.). In some instances this may reduce the intensity of the STS bands, however.

G. Troubleshooting

If control reactions with Bergerac DNA are not working well, i.e., they give faint bands, the problem might be solved by titrating the level of Taq DNA polymerase. The protocol described here uses 0.6 unit of Taq polymerase (Perkin Elmer) per reaction, and this is the low end of an acceptable range. Doubling the amount of Taq polymerase does not cause any problems, and may give better results. We have not needed to retitrate Taq levels with different lots of Taq polymerase, but anticipate that this might be necessary depending on the source of the enzyme.

In our experience, the PCR reactions work well most of the time, with a failure rate of approximately 1 in 20 when mapping with individual embryos. Based on many control reactions with DNA from single Bergerac animals, when reactions fail, they fail completely. We have not seen reactions in which only one or a subset of STSs failed to amplify, while others have worked well. The complete failure of a reaction should not lead to mapping errors using the mapping approach described here.

Although we have not encountered the partial failure of a multiplex reaction, i.e., the failure of a subset of STS assays while others work well, this could produce inconsistent results when mapping a new mutation to a chromosomal subregion. We, however, anticipate that this problem will occur infrequently and would be easily recognized due to the amount of redundant information generated by the STS mapping method. If partial failure of a multiplex reaction becomes a problem in a particular mapping experiment, one approach would be to routinely clone the F2 mutant homozygotes to separate plates and allow them to produce F3 self progeny before preparing the F2s for PCR. If data from a particular F2 were in question, 10 of its progeny could be retested with the same chromosome-specific reaction. Artifactual failure to amplify an STS in F2 DNA would be recognized by its detection in DNA from one or more of the F3s.

One additional complication that should be considered are non-STS background bands that are sometimes amplified in the reactions. Extra bands are not surprising considering the number of primers in the reactions and the high Tc1 copy number in the F2 animals. In our experience, faint background bands migrating near the position of STS bands rarely interfere with interpretation of the data and, in most experiments, are not visible at all. The procedure described above appears to reduce the intensity of background bands by minimizing the time that the mixed reactions spend before they are denatured in the first amplification cycle. If background bands do become a problem, however, one approach is to simplify the reaction mix by omitting several STSs. Alternatively, similar to the approach described just above, F2 mutant homozygotes can be cloned to separate plates and allowed to self before they are scored. If data from a particular F2 animal is ambiguous, several of its progeny can be tested for the STS in question using a simplified reaction.

Finally, in several instances other laboratories using this procedure have encountered difficulty due to use of a misidentified strain from the *Caenorhabditis* Genetics Center. Strains distributed as RW7000 prior to 1992 may not be correct. In mapping experiments conducted with the misidentified strain, none of the STSs included in the chromosome assignment reaction were detected (the strain has not been tested for other STSs). The *Caenorhabditis* Genetics Center is now distributing the correct RW7000 strain.

VI. Conclusions and Prospects

This mapping method offers a number of advantages over standard procedures. (1) It is rapid and requires only a single interstrain cross rather than a succession of crosses involving many different strains and requiring an elapsed time of several weeks. (2) STSs behave as dominant markers, permitting efficient and sensitive mapping strategies. In contrast, most conventional mapping in *C. elegans* uses recessive visible markers and less efficient strategies to detect linkage. (3) STSs can be scored in embryos. This permits efficient mapping of lethal mutations because the markers can be scored in lethal homozygotes that have arrested during embryonic development. With standard methods lethal mutations must be mapped using a less sensitive linkage test that requires an additional generation. (4) X-linked STS markers can be easily introduced into a mapping strain through males. In contrast, mapping on X with visible markers is often complicated by ineffective mating of hemizygous mutant males, and may require the construction of XX *tra-1* (Hodgkin and Brenner, 1977) males. (5) Only one mutant phenotype is scored, avoiding complications that may arise when scoring the phenotype of an unmapped mutation in a background of one or more visible marker phenotypes. (6) Each STS is a landmark connecting the genetic and physical maps, potentially useful if a goal of genetic mapping is the isolation of corresponding clones from the physical map. Although generally useful, many of these characteristics make the STS mapping method particularly desirable for mutations that present special difficulties when using standard methods. These include lethal, sterile, maternal effect, suppressor, and X-linked mutations.

It should also be noted that this mapping technique may permit new kinds of genetic analysis in *C. elegans*. One example is the mapping of multiple factors that contribute to quantitative traits (Lander and Botstein, 1989). This has not been possible using standard mapping methods but, with the ability to follow many markers in a single cross, may now be feasible.

Acknowledgments

The STS mapping method was developed in collaboration with Bertold Schrank and Chau Huynh while the author was a postdoctoral fellow in Robert H. Waterston's laboratory. I thank R. H. Waterston for many insightful discussions and for providing a superb research environment. I thank R. H. Waterston, J. Waddle, and J. McCarter for helpful comments on the manuscript. This work was supported by National Institutes of Health Grants GM-23883 and HG-00375 to R. H. Waterston. B.D.W. was supported by Postdoctoral Fellowship GM-12625.

References

Barstead, R. J., and Waterston, R. H. (1991). Vinculin is essential for muscle function in the nematode. *J. Cell Biol.* **114,** 715–724.

Barstead, R. J., Kleiman, L., and Waterston, R. H. (1991). Cloning, sequencing and mapping of an α-actinin gene from the nematode *Caenorhabditis elegans. Cell Motil. Cytoskel.* **20,** 69–78.

Coulson, A., Sulston, J., Brenner, S., and Karn, J. (1986). Toward a physical map of the genome of the nematode *Caenorhabditis elegans. Proc. Natl. Acad. Sci. U.S.A.* **83,** 7821–7825.

Coulson, A., Waterston, R., Kiff, J., Sulston, J., and Kohara, Y. (1988). Genome linking with yeast artificial chromosomes. *Nature (London)* **335,** 184–186.

Coulson, A., Kozono, Y., Lutterbach, B., Shownkeen, R., Sulston, J., Waterston, R. (1991). YACs and *C. elegans* genome. *Bioessays* **13,** 413–417.

Emmons, S. W., Yesner, L., Ruan, K.-S., and Katzenberg, D. (1983). Evidence for a transposon in *Caenorhabditis elegans. Cell* **32,** 55–65.

Files, J. G., Carr, S., and Hirsh, D. (1983). Actin gene family of *Caenorhabditis elegans. J. Mol. Biol.* **164,** 355–375.

Hodgkin, J. A., and Brenner, S. (1977). Mutations causing transformation of sexual phenotype in the nematode *Caenorhabditis elegans. Genetics* **86,** 275–287.

Lander, E. S., and Botstein, D. (1989). Mapping Mendelian factors underlying quantitative traits using RFLP linkage maps. *Genetics* **121,** 185–199.

Liao, L. W., Rosenzweig, B., and Hirsh, D. (1983). Analysis of a transposable element in *Caenorhabditis elegans. Proc. Natl. Acad. Sci. U.S.A.* **80,** 3585–3589.

Moerman, D. G., and Waterston, R. H. (1984). Spontaneous unstable *unc-22 IV* mutations in *Caenorhabditis elegans* var. Bergerac. *Genetics* **108,** 859–877.

Moerman, D. G., Benian, G. M., and Waterston, R. H. (1986). Molecular cloning of the muscle gene *unc-22* in *Caenorhabditis elegans* by Tc1 transposon tagging. *Proc. Natl. Acad. Sci. U.S.A.* **83,** 2579–2583.

Mori, I., Moerman, D. G., and Waterston, R. H. (1988). Analysis of a mutator activity necessary for germline transposition and excision of Tc1 transposable elements in *Caenorhabditis elegans*. *Genetics* **120,** 397–407.

Mori, I., Moerman, D. G., and Waterston, R. H. (1990). Interstrain crosses enhance excision of Tc1 transposable elements in *Caenorhabditis elegans*. *Mol. Gen. Genet.* **220,** 251–255.

Olson, M., Hood, L., Cantor, C., and Botstein, D. (1989). A common language for physical mapping of the human genome. *Science* **245,** 1434–1435.

Ruvkun, G., Ambrose, V., Coulson, A., Waterston, R., Sulston, J., and Horvitz, H. R. (1989). Molecular genetics of the *Caenorhabditis elegans* heterochronic gene *lin-14*. *Genetics* **121,** 501–516.

Saiki, R. K., Gelfand, D. H., Stoffel, S., Scharf, S. J., Higuchi, R., Horn, G. T., Mullis, K. B., and Erlich, H. A. (1988). Primer-directed enzymatic amplification of DNA with a thermostable DNA polymerase. *Science* **239,** 487–491.

Sambrook, J., Fritsch, E. F., and Maniatis, T. (1989). "Molecular Cloning" Cold Spring Harbor Laboratory Press, Cold Spring Harbor, New York.

Sulston, J., and Hodgkin (1988). Methods, In *The Nematode Caenorhabditis elegans,* W. B. Wood, ed., pp. 587–606. Cold Spring Harbor, New York: Cold Spring Harbor Laboratory.

Williams, B. D., Schrank, B., Huynh, C., Shownkeen, R., and Waterston, R. H. (1992). A genetic mapping system in *Caenorhabditis elegans* based on polymorphic sequence-tagged sites. *Genetics* **131,** 609–624.

CHAPTER 5

Genetic Dissection of Developmental Pathways

Linda S. Huang and Paul W. Sternberg

Howard Hughes Medical Institute and Division of Biology 156-29
California Institute of Technology
Pasadena, California 91125

A major tool of developmental geneticists is the ordering of genes in functional pathways. In this chapter, we explain the logic behind constructing pathways, starting from the knowledge of the relevant phenotypes associated with the genes of interest, assuming that careful analysis of the phenotype has been carried out. We discuss the construction and interpretation of phenotypes of double mutants, screening for and analysis of extragenic suppressors, as well as issues regarding complex pathways and genetic redundancy. Avery and Wasserman (1992) have provided a brief theoretical discussion of epistasis analysis; here we explain the more practical aspects of how models of developmental pathways are built in *Caenorhabditis elegans*.

I. Epistasis Analysis

Epistasis is the masking of the phenotype of one mutant by the phenotype of a mutant in another locus. Hence, epistasis analysis can be used to determine a functional order of action of two genes, regardless of the directness of the interaction. Epistasis analysis is most informative, however, when the genes analyzed control a common process. Thus, it is important to determine the relationships between the mutations of interest before embarking on the construction of a formal genetic pathway.

Two different kinds of pathways exist (Fig. 1). Historically, these have been distinguished as regulatory pathways and assembly or metabolic pathways. As both types of these pathways require "regulation," for the purpose of this chapter we refer to the classic regulatory pathway as a switch regulation pathway and the classic assembly pathway as a substrate-dependent pathway. The switch regulation pathway involves genes or gene products that can be turned "on" or "off"; these different states of the genes (or their products) involved determine the outcome of the pathway. Mutations in genes involved in this type of pathway have two distinct and opposite phenotypes and also have the ability to bypass the requirement for upstream genes. The second type of pathway involves a substrate, where an obligate series of sequential steps are required to generate the final outcome; classic examples of this second type of pathway include metabolic pathways and bacteriophage morphogenesis. Mutations in genes involved in the substrate-dependent pathway have phenotypes that suggest a progression of events. Sometimes, determining which of the two types of pathways the genes of interest are involved in requires extensive phenotypic analysis of the relevant mutations.

Consider, for example, vulval differentiation in *C. elegans*. In wild-type animals, three of six multipotent vulval precursor cells differentiate to form the vulva. These six precursor cells are a subset of the 12 "Pn.p" cells (the posterior daughters of the 12 ectoblasts, P1 through P12). Although loss-of-function mutants in *lin-26* (*lin* = *lin*eage abnormal), *lin-39,* and *let-23* (*let* = *let*hal) are all vulvaless and have the same phenotype when examined under a dissecting microscope, these genes are involved in very different aspects of vulval differentiation. *lin-26* is involved in the formation of the Pn.p cells, *lin-39* is involved in determining which of the Pn.p cells become potential vulval precursor cells, and *let-23* is involved in the fate decision regarding which Pn.p cells will actually differentiate into vulval tissue. Phenotypic analysis under higher-magnification Nomarski optics demonstrates that the vulvaless phenotype of animals mutant in *lin-26* is due to the absence of Pn.p cells; in *lin-39* mutants, the vulval precursor cells are not generated; and in *let-23* mutants, the vulval precursor cells are not differentiating.

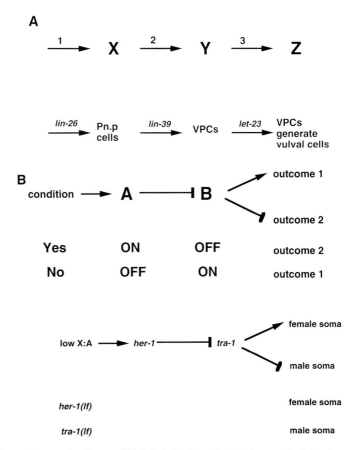

Fig. 1 General types of pathways. (A) Substrate-dependent pathway: vulval development. A series of genes (1, 2, and 3) are necessary to produce a series of outcomes (X, Y, and Z). *lin-26* is necessary for the development of Pn.p cells. *lin-39* is necessary to select a subset of Pn.p cells to become vulval precursor cells (VPCs). *let-23* is necessary for the VPCs to generate vulval cells. (B) Switch regulation pathway: somatic sex determination. A formal regulatory pathway is shown with conditions regulating which of two outcomes (1 or 2) will occur. If the condition is met (e.g., presence of a signal, particular environmental conditions, chromosome constitution), outcome 1 occurs. A specific example is shown at the bottom. A low ratio of X chromosomes to autosome sets results in the activation of *her-1* via a series of other genes. *her-1* activity inactivates *tra-1* via a series of other genes. *tra-1* activity results in female somatic differention; *tra-1* inactivity leads to male somatic differentaion. *lf*, loss-of-function mutation. Arrows represent positive regulation; bars represent negative regulation.

In this example, the Pn.p cells are the substrate; *lin-26, lin-39*, and *let-23* act to change the state of this cell. A mutation in each of these genes represents a step in the pathway that provides the appropriate context or substrate for the next step. Here, arrows are used to show a progression of events from one step to the next (Fig. 1A). Epistasis analysis of substrate-dependent pathways will confirm the order of events seen by phenotypic analysis.

On the other hand, mutations involved in a switch regulation pathway should all have the same phenotype or the direct opposite phenotype (Fig. 1B). In effect, the mutations will represent one of two states of an event, either ON or OFF. An example of this type of pathway in *C. elegans* involves the *tra-1* (*tra* = *tra*nsforming) and *her-1* (*her* = *her*maphroditization) genes, which are needed for proper sex determination (reviewed by Villeneuve and Meyer, 1990). These genes are part of a negative regulatory pathway and thus bars are used instead of arrowheads to symbolize the relationship between them. In *C. elegans*, the sex of the animals is determined by the number of X chromosomes in an animal; an XX animal is hermaphroditic, whereas an XO animal is male. The *her-1* loss-of-function mutation causes feminization of XO animals without affecting XX animals. The *tra-1* loss-of-function mutation causes the opposite phenotype, masculinization of XX animals, without affecting XO animals. These genes are involved in a switch regulation pathway because XO animals can be either one of two states, male or hermaphrodite; the same is true for XX animals.

The definition of a switch regulation pathway versus a substrate-dependent pathway depends on the phenotype studied or the event assayed. In the study of the pathway containing the receptor tyrosine kinase encoded by *let-23*, its effects on the decision of the vulval precursor cells to take on vulval versus nonvulval fates constitutes a switch regulatory pathway. Synthesis of the LET-23 receptor would, however, constitute a substrate-dependent pathway; one event would lead to another and the presence of LET-23 is required. Biochemical experiments do not necessarily define a substrate-dependent pathway. Studies on how ligand activation of LET-23 leads to a phosphorylation cascade of downstream targets would be a switch regulation pathway; two distinct states are being analyzed, for example, phosphorylated and nonphosphorylated. Further, an obligate substrate is not needed in this pathway, as activation of a downstream target can bypass the need for LET-23 (e.g., a gain-of-function mutation in the *let-60 ras* gene will activate the pathway even in the absence of LET-23). It is imperative to distinguish whether the mutations of interest affect a switch regulation versus a substrate-dependent pathway, as the logic used to order the genes involved is different and thus the resultant pathway constructed can be very different. The ordering of genes in a substrate-dependent pathway can be determined through an examination of the state of the substrate (i.e., the state of the Pn.p cell given above); epistasis analysis serves to confirm what is inferred from the phenotypic analysis or to imply the sequence of events. In the next section of this chapter, we consider the logic behind constructing a switch regulation pathway, where pure phenotypic analysis will not allow gene ordering.

II. Epistasis Analysis of Switch Regulation Pathways

A. Double-Mutant Construction

Once it is determined that the mutations of interest might constitute a switch regulation pathway, double mutants can be constructed to determine the epistatic relationships between the two mutations. The *epistatic* mutation is the one whose phenotype is displayed in the doubly mutant animal; the mutation whose phenotype is not displayed is *hypostatic* to the other. Thus, an epistasis test can only be performed on two mutations in different loci and with opposite phenotypes; epistasis relationships cannot be determined using mutations with the same phenotypes. Genes with mutations of the same phenotype, however, can be ordered by epistasis analysis using a mutation in a gene that functions between the two and that causes the opposite phenotype.

We outline three basic strategies for constructing double mutants in Fig. 2. The first method is the simplest (Fig. 2A), as it involves taking animals carrying the single mutations and using them directly to make the double mutants. Epistasis is determined by the self progeny of the F2 animals. If animals of phenotype A produce progeny of phenotypes A and B while animals of phenotype B only produce progeny of phenotype B, gene B is epistatic to gene A. Gene A would be epistatic to gene B if the opposite were true. Furthermore, the animals of phenotype B from parents of phenotype A will be the desired double mutant; these animals can be cultured to maintain the doubly mutant strain. Although this method is the simplest, it cannot be used if gene A and gene B are tightly linked on the same chromosome.

The second method used for construction involves using a closely linked marker in *cis* to (on the same chromosome as) each gene of interest (Fig. 2B). The construction then involves making the strain carrying both marked chromosomes. The advantage of this method is that the strain can be constructed by simply following the mutations used as markers without regard to the phenotypes of interest. Once the doubly marked animal is obtained, the phenotype of interest can be determined. If the doubly marked animal has phenotype A, gene A is epistatic to gene B and vice versa. A control experiment must be done, however, to construct double mutants with just the two markers, to make sure there is no effect on the phenotype of interest. Sometimes this method cannot be used because the markers will occlude scoring the phenotypes of interest.

The best method for determining epistatic relationships involves using linked markers in *trans* to (on the homologous chromosome as) the mutations of interest (Fig. 2C). This eliminates nonspecific marker effects, while ensuring that the double mutation of the two genes of interest is actually being constructed. The markers should be close to the gene of interest to reduce the possibility of recombination. These markers can be either mutations in an unrelated gene or, better yet, balancer chromosomes (see Chapter 7 in this volume for an explanation of how to use balancers). This construction is similar to the first construction described, except that doubly mutant animals can be ascertained by the methods described above and also by their failure to segregate the *trans* markers.

A combination of methods can also be used. No matter which method is used to construct the double mutant, it is important to demonstrate that the presumptive doubly mutant animal actually carries both mutations of interest. One way that this can be done is by allowing males to mate with the doubly

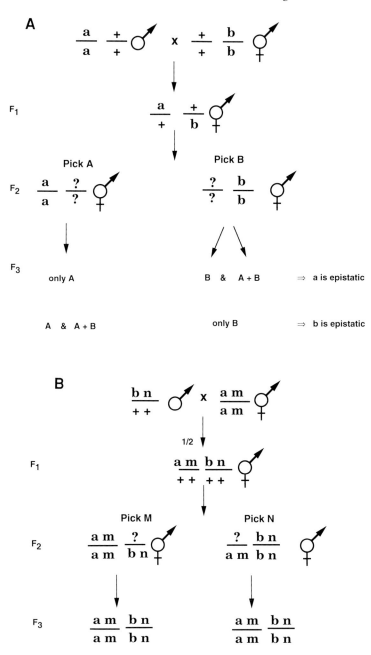

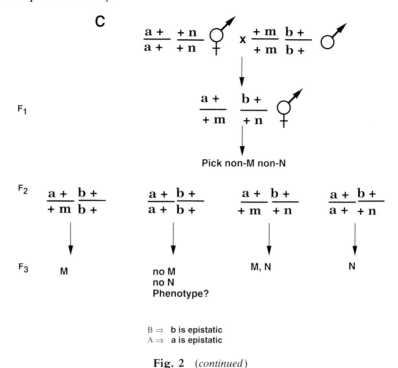

Fig. 2 (*continued*)

Fig. 2 Construction of double-mutant strains. (A) No markers. Animals carrying mutations in one gene of interest (gene A) with phenotype A are mated with animals carrying mutations in the other gene of interest (gene B) with phenotype B. The F1 heterozygote (gene $a/+$, gene $b/+$) will produce progeny of both phenotype A and phenotype B. Next, F2 animals of phenotype A and phenotype B are individually cultured and their F3 progeny examined to determine whether animals of phenotype A produce progeny of phenotype B or vice versa. By analyzing both classes, one can ensure that the desired strain will be constructed, even if one's assumption about the double-mutant phenotype is incorrect. "?" indicates that the allele at a given locus in a particular animal is not inferable from its phenotype or the genotype of its parents. (B) Linked markers in *cis*. The second method used for epistasis analysis involves using markers linked in *cis* to (on the same chromosome as) the genes of interest. The markers linked to the two genes should be different, closely linked to the gene of interest to avoid recombinants, not have any epistatic relationships to each other, not have any interactions with the genes of interest, and be easily scored as a double mutant. Males carrying mutation *b* with linked marker *n* are mated to hermaphrodites homozygous for mutation *a* and linked recessive marker *m*. Cross-progeny are non-M and heterozygous for *a* and *b*. Cross-progeny that do not produce N progeny are discarded, as they did not receive the *bn* chromosome from their father. From this heterozygote, hermaphrodites with phenotype M or N are picked, and the double mutant *MN* (also homozygous for *a* and *b*) is easily recognized. (C) Linked markers in *trans*. The best method for determining epistatic relationships involves using markers (*m, n*) linked in *trans* to (on the homologous chromosome as) the genes of interest. This eliminates nonspecific marker effects while ensuring that the double mutation of the two genes of interest is actually being constructed. Once again, the markers should be fairly close to the gene of interest to reduce the possibility of recombination. This construction is similar to that in part A, except that doubly mutant animals can be ascertained by the method described above and also by their failure to produce progeny carrying the markers linked in *trans*.

mutant hermaphrodites and picking F1 heterozygous animals. Animals of both phenotype A and phenotype B should be produced by the heterozygous animals, demonstrating that both mutations were present in the putative doubly mutant animal. Also, F1 heterozygous males can be picked and outcrossed to test whether each carries the A and B mutations.

B. Interpretation of Epistasis

In a switch regulation pathway, the epistatic gene is the downstream gene because these genes are negatively regulating each other. This rule can be derived from analysis of the single- and double-mutant phenotypes, as illustrated in the analysis of two genes involved in sex determination, *tra-1* and *her-1*. As mentioned above, the *tra-1* mutation transforms XX animals into males, whereas the *her-1* mutation transforms XO animals into hermaphrodites. The *tra-1; her-1* double mutant has the *tra-1* phenotype; XX animals are males. *tra-1* is epistatic to *her-1* and thus downstream of *her-1*. *tra-1* cannot be upstream of *her-1* because the wild-type activity of *tra-1* is to activate the hermaphrodite program of development, whereas the wild-type activity of *her-1* is to activate the male program of development. If *tra-1* were upstream of *her-1*, inactivation of *tra-1* would eliminate the repression of *her-1*, activating the male program of development. Inactivation of *her-1* would lead to the inability to activate the male program of development, resulting in the hermaphrodite program of development. Removal of both *tra-1* and *her-1* would make *tra-1* unable to repress *her-1* (which does not matter because *her-1* is inactivated by mutation) and *her-1* unable to activate the male program of development. This would result in the double mutant exhibiting the *her-1* phenotype. The experimental evidence says this is not true, so *tra-1* is downstream of *her-1*; that is, inactivation of *tra-1* obviates the need for *her-1*.

Comprehensive double-mutant analysis with genes involved in a common process allows the construction of a pathway (see Fig. 3). For example, during vulval induction, three of six vulval precursor cells (VPCs) normally adopt vulval fates while the other three adopt nonvulval epidermal fates. By removing the inductive signal through ablation of the signaling cell, the three VPCs that normally become vulva now adopt nonvulval epidermal fates. Mutations that mimic the signaling-cell ablation phenotype [all six VPCs adopt nonvulval epidermal fates, also known as vulvaless (Vul) mutations] include *let-23*, *lin-3*, *let-60*, and *lin-45*. Mutations also exist that have the opposite phenotype [all six VPCs adopt vulval fates, also known as multivulva (Muv) mutations]; these include *lin-15* and *lin-1*. Double-mutation construction using Muv and Vul mutations yield the following results:

lin-1 is epistatic to *let-23*	*let-23* is epistatic to *lin15*
lin-1 is epistatic to *lin-3*	*lin-15* is epistatic to *lin-3*
lin-1 is epistatic to *let-60*	*let-60* is epistatic to *lin-15*
lin-1 is epistatic to *lin-45*	*lin-45* is epistatic to *lin-15*

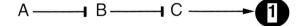

	Genotype			Phenotype		Inferred Pathway
				transformation	duplication/ deletion	
i	$\frac{+}{+}$	$\frac{+}{+}$	$\frac{+}{+}$	none (both 1 and 2)	none	
ii	$\frac{a}{a}$	$\frac{+}{+}$	$\frac{+}{+}$	$1 \to 2$	missing 1	A ➝ ●
iii	$\frac{+}{+}$	$\frac{b}{b}$	$\frac{+}{+}$	$2 \to 1$	extra 1	B —●
iv	$\frac{+}{+}$	$\frac{+}{+}$	$\frac{c}{c}$	$1 \to 2$	missing 1	C ➝ ●
v	$\frac{+}{+}$	$\frac{b}{b}$	$\frac{c}{c}$	$1 \to 2$	missing 1	B — C ➝ ●
vi	$\frac{a}{a}$	$\frac{b}{b}$	$\frac{+}{+}$	$2 \to 1$	extra 1	A — B —●

Fig. 3 Epistasis analysis. The phenotypes of a set of genotypes and the inferences are shown. The inferred pathway leading to outcome 1 (black oval) is shown at the top. The default outcome is 2. Phenotypes are described in two ways in this figure: as transformations from 1 to 2 or 2 to 1, or as missing and extra structures, states, or parameters. The inference from the phenotype of each genotype is shown. For example, in (ii), the absence of A leads to no 1; thus, A promotes outcome 1. In (iii), however, the absence of B leads to extra 1; thus, B inhibits outcome 1.

As two states are being assayed, the ability of the VPCs to adopt vulval fates versus their ability to adopt nonvulval fates, the following pathway can be constructed, using the rule of the epistatic gene being the downstream gene:

$$lin\text{-}3 \frown\!\!\!\searrow lin\text{-}15 \frown\!\!\!\searrow \genfrac{}{}{0pt}{}{let\text{-}60}{lin\text{-}45}{let\text{-}23} \frown\!\!\!\searrow lin\text{-}1 \frown\!\!\!\searrow vulval\ fates$$

C. Importance of Using Null Alleles

The examples of epistasis given above result from double-mutant analyses using severe-loss-of-function recessive alleles. Epistasis analysis is based on the assumption that the mutations in the genes involved remove the function of that gene in the cell, tissue, or process being analyzed. Thus, it is important to determine by dosage analysis whether the alleles involved are hypermorphs (increased function), hypomorphs (reduction of function), amorphs ("null," complete loss of function), or neomorphs (novel function) [see Muller (1932) for details; see Sternberg (1990) and Greenwald and Horvitz (1980) for a discussion regarding the determination of a gene's null phenotype].

Null mutations are important for epistasis because the logic behind epistasis analysis is valid only if the two mutations used can be presumed to have no assayable activity. For example, consider two genes, A and B, in a regulatory pathway where there exists a null mutation in gene A but there exists no null mutations in gene B, only a hypomorphic mutation. If A is epistatic to B, this would not be as critical, because the normal function of B is to negatively regulate A. In this case, A is downstream of B. So, even if B has residual activity, the double-mutant animals do not have functional A activity so the residual B activity cannot regulate A activity.

On the other hand, if B is downstream of A, the double-mutant animal may display a misleading phenotype because the B mutation used contains residual activity and the doubly mutant animal has no A activity to regulate this residual activity. As B and A have opposite phenotype, having some wild-type B activity will lead to some expression of the A mutant phenotype, depending on how much activity the hypomorphic B mutation retains. Therefore, the outcome of an epistasis experiment where one or both of the mutations used are not null alleles could be coexpression, where both A and B phenotypes are expressed, or a misleading double-mutant phenotype, where the animal displays the A phenotype.

A practical example of this phenomenon can be found in Ferguson *et al.* (1987). Epistasis analysis using the *lin-15* allele, *n309,* and the *let-23* allele, *n1045,* resulted in *let-23(n1045); lin-15(n309)* doubly mutant animals expressing either the Muv or the Vul phenotype. It is now known that *let-23(n1045)* makes some wild-type product (Aroian *et al.,* 1994) and that *lin-15(n309)* is not a complete deletion of the locus (Huang *et al.,* 1994; Clark *et al.,* 1994). It is not possible to use a complete null allele of *let-23* to analyze its phenotype in late larval development (without mosaic analysis) because, as the name implies, a *let-23* null is lethal and would not survive to make the vulva. The *sy97* allele of *let-23,* however, is a severe loss-of-function allele with respect to the vulva, such that vulval differentiation is essentially not seen (see Aroian and Sternberg, 1991, for an example of tissue-specific activities of a genetic locus). Molecular analysis also identified a *lin-15* allele, *e1763,* whose lesion removes more coding sequence than *n309.* When epistasis analysis is performed using *let-23(sy97)* and *lin-15(e1763),* all the doubly mutant animals display a Vul phenotype (Huang *et al.,* 1994). Of course, the *let-23(sy97)* allele did not exist in 1987 and the molecular nature of the *lin-15* alleles was not known, so the analysis was performed using the best of what existed and was known at the time.

D. Use of Dominant Mutations

As mentioned above, epistasis analysis cannot be performed using mutations that display the same phenotype. This can lead to subsets of the pathway where the order of some genes is not known. Sometimes these genes can be ordered through the use of gain-of-function alleles, which will display the opposite phenotype of the loss-of-function mutations. In these cases, it is important to know that the gain-of-function mutation in the gene of interest increases the normal activity of the gene and does not confer a novel activity.

In the example of the pathway regulating vulval differentiation given above, the genes *let-60, let-23,* and *lin-45* cannot be separated by epistasis using hypomorphic alleles, as all display the Vul phenotype. There exists, however, a gain-of-function allele of *let-60;* animals carrying this allele display the Muv phenotype. Double-mutant construction using the *let-60* gain-of-function allele and the *lin-45* and *let-23* hypomorphic alleles gives the following results:

Genotype	Phenotype
lin-45; let-60(gf)	Vul
let-23; let-60(gf)	Muv

Therefore, the *let-60* gain-of-function allele can be used to split the order of action of *let-23* and *lin-45*. These results imply the order

$$let\text{-}23 \longrightarrow let\text{-}60 \longrightarrow lin\text{-}45.$$

Arrows are used because the wild-type function of the genes is to positively regulate each other. The gain-of-function phenotype of *let-60* results in the opposite phenotype of hypomorphic *let-60* alleles and allows the ordering of these genes using the logic used for epistasis for switch regulation pathways.

E. Complex Pathways

Epistasis analysis does not always result in simple interpretations of gene order. Sometimes this is because the mutations used are not null alleles; the consequences of this are discussed above. Sometimes this is because the mutations used are not part of a switch regulation pathway but, instead, are part of a complex pathway that combines both switch regulation processes and substrate-dependent processes. In fact, complex pathways are more often the rule than the exception. Development proceeds through a series of steps; often, a set of decisions about a fate leads to an execution of a particular fate, which may then lead to decisions about another fate. Development can be viewed as a set of substrate-dependent pathways leading to switch regulation pathways, which lead to more substrate-dependent pathways, and so on.

Because the logic of epistasis differs for switch regulation and substrate-dependent pathways, it is important to determine if the mutations involved in a complex pathway are all involved in the same step of the pathway being studied. This is not always obvious and may require careful phenotypic analysis. For example, animals carrying the mutation *n300* are Vul when examined under a dissecting microscope. Because animals carrying the *lin-15* mutation are Muv and, superficially, Muv and Vul are opposite phenotypes, the epistasis analysis of these two genes seems simple. The doubly mutant animal of genotype *n300; lin-15* is Vul (Ferguson *et al.*, 1987); the simple interpretation is that *n300* is downstream of *lin-15*. This, however, is not the case. Careful examination of the *n300* phenotype reveals its involvement in the generation of the VPCs; *n300* animals are Vul because the VPCs are not there and thus cannot make a vulva. The correct interpretation is *n300* is upstream of *lin-15*, operating in the pathway required to generate the VPCs and not in the regulation of VPC fate, as *lin-15* does.

The process of programmed cell death is an excellent example of a complex pathway (reviewed in Ellis *et al.*, 1991a) (Fig. 4). In *C. elegans,* 131 of the 1030 cells generated during development of the adult hermaphrodite undergo programmed cell death. Programmed cell death is a complex process, involving first the specification of whether or not a cell will die, followed by the process of killing the cell, and finishing with the engulfment and degradation of cell corpses. Mutations have been found in genes affecting each of these processes. For example, the genes *ced-3* (*ced* = *c*ell death abnormal), *ced-4,* and *ced-9* are involved in the killing process (Ellis *et al.*, 1991b; Hengartner *et al.*, 1992). Genes involved in the engulfment of cell corpses include *ced-1, ced-2, ced-5, ced-6, ced-7, ced-8,* and *ced-10;* mutations in these genes causes cell corpses to persist. The process of cell death thus consists of

specification of death ⟶ killing of cells ⟶ engulfment of cell corpses.

Epistasis can only be interpreted using the logic discussed for switch regulation pathways for genes involved in a common process; *ced-3* and *ced-1* are involved in different processes and thus phenotypic analysis elucidates their order relative to each other.

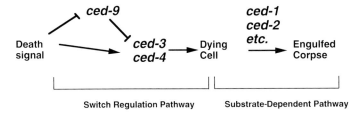

Fig. 4 Mixed switch regulation and substrate-dependent pathway: programmed cell death. An example of a mixed pathway. Some signal controls activities of either *ced-9* or *ced-3* and *ced-4,* resulting in activation of a pathway by which cells die. Inactivation of *ced-9* results in extra cells dying. Inactivation of either *ced-3* or *ced-4* results in the survival of cells that would otherwise die. Inactivation of *ced-1, ced-2,* etc., results in cells that die, but whose corpses are not engulfed by surrounding tissue.

ced-3, ced-4, and ced-9 are involved in regulating the killing of cells. In animals without ced-3 or ced-4 function, cells survive that normally die by programmed cell death. Animals without ced-9 function die. When ced-9 mutant animals also lack either ced-3 or ced-4, they live, suggesting that functional ced-3 or ced-4 is necessary for the ced-9 gene product to function. This interpretation is consistent with the gain-of-function phenotype of ced-9, which results in the survival of cells that normally die by programmed cell death (this is the same phenotype as loss-of-function of ced-3 and ced-4). These results imply the gene order of

$$ced\text{-}9 \diagdown\kern-1.2em\diagup \searrow ced\text{-}3,\ ced\text{-}4.$$

When double mutants are made using mutations in ced-3 and ced-1, a gene involved in the engulfment of cell corpses, the doubly mutant animal displays the ced-3 phenotype; however, ced-1 and ced-3 are part of the same substrate-dependent pathway but not part of the same switch regulation pathway. For one, ced-3 and ced-1 do not have opposite phenotypes. Phenotypic analysis would suggest that the cell must first be specified to die by ced-3 before its corpse can be engulfed through the activity of ced-1. Also, the engulfment pathway that ced-1 regulates is not necessary for causing cell death like ced-3, because mutations that prevent engulfment do not prevent most cell deaths (Hedgecock et al., 1983; Ellis et al., 1991a). The action of ced-3 leads to the action of ced-1. Thus, the pathway should be drawn as

$$\text{specification of death} \longrightarrow ced\text{-}9 \diagdown\kern-1.2em\diagup \searrow ced\text{-}3,\ ced\text{-}4 \longrightarrow ced\text{-}1.$$

These examples regarding n300 and lin-15 in the vulval differentiation pathway and the genes in the programmed cell death pathway illustrate the importance of detailed phenotypic characterization of the singly mutant animals in preventing misinterpretation of double-mutant phenotypes. Once it is determined that two genes are in a switch regulation pathway, the rule that the epistatic gene resides downstream of the hypostatic gene can be simply applied. In contrast, if two genes are involved in a substrate-dependent pathway, double-mutant analysis again confirms the order of events that have been visualized, although in this case, the epistatic gene is the upstream gene. Whether two genes are involved in a switch regulation process or a substrate-dependent process can be determined only by careful analysis of the phenotypes of the mutations involved.

F. Genetic Redundancy

Another factor that can complicate the interpretation of epistatic relationships is genetic redundancy. Discussions on the theoretical implications of genetic redundancy can be found in Thomas (1993) and Tautz (1992); these issues are beyond the scope of this chapter. In practice, genetic redundancy can be discovered in three ways, by backcrossing newly isolated mutants of interest, by undertaking a screen for redundant genes, or by constructing double mutants with two different genes (Fig. 5).

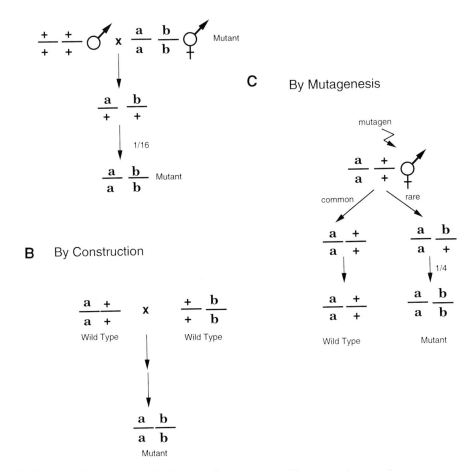

Fig. 5 Synthetic phenotypes. (A) Discovery by backcrossing. If two recessive mutations are responsible for the phenotype, then 1 of 16 progeny of the double heterozygote will display the phenotype. (B) Discovery by construction. (C) Discovery by mutagenesis.

Discovering genetic redundancy by backcross involves examination of the frequency of segregation of the mutation involved from a heterozygous animal (Fig. 5A). This method is most often used during the analysis of a new mutation following mutagenesis (e.g., see Ferguson and Horvitz, 1989). A recessive phenotype caused by a single gene trait will usually segregate from a heterozygote animal at a frequency of 1/4. If, however, two genes are required to cause the phenotype, animals expressing this phenotype will segregate from a heterozygous parent at a frequency of 1/16, assuming they are unlinked from each other. Once it is determined that two genes cause the phenotype of interest, the phenotype of each mutation alone should be determined. If these two mutations are genetically redundant, they will cause the phenotype of interest only in combination with each other and should display either a reduced phenotype or possibly even no phenotype alone.

Another method for discovering genetic redundancy involves constructing double-mutant animals using existing mutations (Fig. 5B). This is usually done when mutations are recovered that display an incomplete phenotype or that display no phenotype with respect to the phenotype of interest (i.e., a silent mutation). This method was extremely informative in the discovery of the two sets of genes involved in the engulfment process during programmed cell death (Ellis *et al.*, 1991a) and the redundancy seen in the dauer formation pathway (Thomas *et al.*, 1993).

A third method for discovering genetic redundancy involves screening for new mutations that synergize with the original mutation to cause the phenotype of interest (Fig. 5C) (also see Ferguson and Horvitz, 1989). This technique is especially useful if it is already known that redundancy exists in the system, using molecular information or by the discovery of genetic redundancy through other methods, as described above.

The formal interpretation of genetic redundancy is that the redundant genes are involved in parallel pathways, regulating the process of interest. For two redundant genes, A and B, that negatively regulate gene C that negatively regulates gene D, the pathway would look like

In this case, the animal carrying mutations in both gene A and gene B would display the phenotype opposite that of animals mutant in gene C and would display the same phenotype as animals mutant in gene D. Thus, when epistasis analysis is done with genetically redundant genes, both redundant genes should be eliminated because only then is the phenotype of interest seen. In this case, because gene A only partially negatively regulates gene C, even doing epistasis with a null allele of gene A will not completely eliminate the function of that particular step; both gene A function and gene B function need to be completely eliminated to create the phenotype that represents a lack of function at that step. Thus, the triply mutant animal lacking gene A, gene B, and gene C must be constructed for epistasis analysis.

G. Limits of Epistasis

The ordering of genes in pathways using genetic epistasis is a powerful tool; however, it merely provides a working model for more phenotypic studies or molecular analysis and should not be taken as the "answer." One limitation of epistasis is that it assumes a linearity of events. This is not always the case; sometimes pathways are branched or contain multiple inputs. Also, some pathways use tissue-specific regulators that are not necessarily used in other developmental processes that use a subset of these same genes. Ultimately, these issues can be resolved by careful phenotypic analysis of the genes involved in the pathway, although where to look may not be initially obvious.

One example of a branched pathway in *C. elegans* is the sex determination pathway (Fig. 6). A high X chromosome-to-autosome ratio (X : A) negatively regulates the *fem-1*, *fem-2*, and *fem-3* genes, which negatively regulate the *tra-1* gene. *tra-1* functions to activate the developmental program for the female soma while repressing the developmental program for the male soma. The role of the *fem-1*, *fem-2*, and *fem-3* gene products, however, is not just to regulate *tra-1*; these genes are also responsible for promoting male germ-line development and negatively regulating female germ-line development. In the case of a high X : A ratio, inactive *fem-1*, *fem-2*, and *fem-3* would lead to female germ-line development. By recognizing the branch point at *fem-1*, *fem-2*, and *fem-3* and realizing that germ-line development is regulated differently than somatic development, the intersex phenotype of animals carrying the *tra-1* mutation can be interpreted. XX *tra-1* mutant animals have a male soma because they have no functional *tra-1* to repress male somatic development; these XX animals also have a female germ-line because *fem-1*, *fem-2*, and *fem-3* are repressed by the high X : A ratio.

This example also illustrates the existence of tissue-specific regulators of a particular pathway. Although *tra-1* is downstream of *fem-1* in somatic development, it is not so in germ-line development. Thus, the order of gene action should be determined by epistasis analysis with the genes involved for the particular developmental process of interest, looking at their action in the tissue of interest. Another example of this is the use of the heterochronic genes *lin-4*, *lin-14*, *lin-28*, and *lin-29* (Ambros and Moss, 1994). Animals carrying loss-of-function mutations in *lin-4* and *lin-14* have widespread defects in temporal control. By examining their effects in the temporal control of the hypodermal seam cells, a regulatory pathway was constructed with the more specifically used heterochronic genes, *lin-28*, and *lin-29*. A complete description of the construction of this

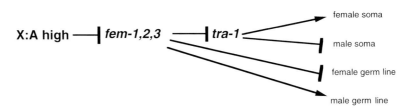

Fig. 6 Branched pathway: somatic and germ-line sex determination. The ratio of X to autosomes determines sexual phenotype (see Villeneuve and Meyer, 1990, for a review). A high ratio of X chromosomes to autosomes results in repression of activity of the *fem* genes. For somatic sexual determination, the *fem* genes negatively regulate *tra-1* activity. For germ-line sex determination, the *fem* genes control sexual identity independently of *tra-1*.

pathway is found in Ambros (1989); this paper also contains an excellent explanation of how the logic of epistasis analysis was used to construct the pathway.

Another variation on branched pathways are pathways with more than one input (Fig. 7). An example of this is the *C. elegans* vulval differentiation pathway. The pathway given in previous sections consists of

$$lin\text{-}3 \longrightarrow lin\text{-}15 \longrightarrow let\text{-}23 \longrightarrow let\text{-}60$$
$$lin\text{-}45 \longrightarrow lin\text{-}1 \longrightarrow \text{vulval fates.}$$

Molecular identification of the *lin-3* gene product as a growth factor/ligand-like molecule and the *let-23* gene product as a receptor tyrosine kinase, however, suggests that *lin-3* encodes the ligand for *let-23* (reviewed by Sternberg, 1993). Furthermore, previous phenotypic characterization of *lin-15* demonstrated that although *lin-15* mutant animals exhibit the mutant Muv phenotype, even in the absence of the inductive tissue, their VPCs are still capable of responding to the signal. Thus, *lin-15* does not belong directly downstream of the *lin-3* signal, but instead, as a second input on *let-23:*

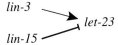

The examples of the vulval differentiation pathway and the sex determination pathway given above underscore the importance of careful phenotypic analysis in the construction of developmental regulatory pathways. This is not to say that epistasis analysis should not be performed until an exhaustive understanding of

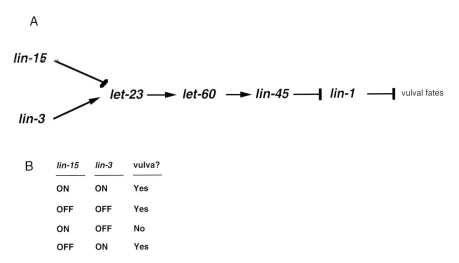

Fig. 7 Multiple inputs: vulval induction. (A) Abbreviated pathway of vulval induction (see Sternberg, 1993, for a review). (B) A "truth table" schema for the combined action of *lin-15* and *lin-3* to control vulval differentiation.

the mutant phenotype exists; however, pathways constructed through epistasis analysis should be considered models that can change over time, given new information from further phenotypic or molecular analysis.

H. Extension to Other Perturbations

The logic presented in this chapter can be extended to other nongenetic interactions, such as cell–cell interactions that can be dissected using cell ablations. Rather than remove the function of a gene by mutation, a cell can be removed by laser ablation (see Chapter 10 in this volume) or by a pharmacological agent (see Chapter 8). One example of using cell ablations instead of mutation for epistasis is the analysis of cell signaling during male spicule development (Chamberlin and Sternberg, 1993). B_γ and $B\delta$ are two different cell fates adopted by certain progeny of the B cell, a male-specific blast cell involved in spicule development. Ablation of the nearby Y.p cell (the posterior daughter of the male-specific blast cell, Y) leads to a defect in the $B\delta$ lineage; ablation of the pa cells (the two cells B.alpa and B.arpa, great-great granddaughters of the blast cell, B; sisters of B_γ and $B\delta$) leads to a defect in B_γ. As B_γ and $B\delta$ are alternative cell fates, ablation of the Y.p cell can be considered to cause phenotypes opposite from that caused by ablation of the pa cells. The double ablation of both Y.p and pa cells has a defect similar to ablation of the Y.p cell alone. Using the logic of epistasis, the role of the pa cells might be to negatively regulate the effect of Y.p.

III. Extragenic Suppressors

To further analyze a pathway, it is often desirable to identify additional genes. One method for doing this involves starting with a wild-type animal and screening for additional mutations with the phenotypes of interest. Another method involves isolating extragenic suppressor mutations of a previously identified mutant gene in the pathway (see Chapter 2 in this volume for information regarding the different mutagens available). Suppression screens can be better than direct screens because the presence of the starting mutation might suppress the lethality of the suppressor mutation, and thus allow the mutation to be recovered. Screens for mutations that enhance a partial mutant phenotype can also identify new genes.

A. Screens for Extragenic Suppressors

Screens for extragenic suppressors seem deceptively simple; a mutation in the pathway is chosen and a screen is performed to look for new mutations that no longer express the mutant phenotype, either in the F1 generation (for dominant suppressors) or in the F2 generation (for recessive suppressors) (Fig. 8). Although the screening process is straightforward, the key to the success of an extragenic suppressor screen involves choosing the most appropriate starting mutation for the purpose of the screen, as the choice of a starting strain affects the suppressor mutations isolated.

One consideration when choosing a starting mutation is to decide what type of mutation to suppress: a null mutation, a loss-of-function mutation, or a gain-of-function mutation. Suppression of a null mutation (X) will allow recovery of new mutations that allow bypass of the gene of interest. These will be either gain-of-function (gf) mutations of downstream genes in the same substrate-dependent pathway (Y) or loss-of-function (lf) mutations of downstream negative regulators (W). Suppression of a null mutation, however, will not allow recovery of mutations in genes that directly interact with the starting gene's product.

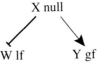

On the other hand, suppression of a reduction-of-function mutation (X) will allow recovery of mutations in genes that interact with the gene of interest. A

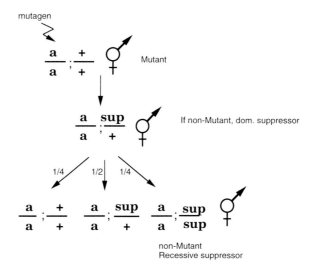

Fig. 8 Suppressor screens. From mutant parents that have been mutagenized, the F1 progeny and F2 grandprogeny are examined for phenotypic revertants, that is, animals that do not display the mutant phenotype. Each F1 examined screens two mutagenized gametes, as either the sperm or the ova could carry a mutation. If the F2 are examined, the number of mutagenized gametes is also two per F1. m, starting mutation; sup, suppressor mutation.

mutation in an interacting gene will be recovered if it removes the negative regulation of an upstream interacting gene (V). Mutations that allow bypass of the gene of interest will also be recovered (W and Y), as with using the null. Upstream genes that, when mutated, increase the activity of the loss-of-function mutation used will also be recovered (Z).

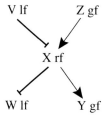

Suppression of a gain-of-function mutation can allow the subsequent recovery of the opposite spectrum of alleles as suppression of a loss-of-function mutation. For example, loss-of-function mutations of downstream genes will be recovered (Y) as will gain-of-function mutations of downstream negatively regulated genes (W). These screens can be very powerful [e.g., see Wu and Han (1994) and Lackner *et al.* (1994) regarding suppression of the gain-of-function *let-60 ras* mutations; Riddle (1977) for suppression of dauer defective mutants; and Hodgkin (1986) for suppression of sex determination mutations]. It is important, however, to know that the starting mutation (X) increases normal gene activity.

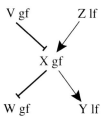

Besides choosing a starting mutation for a suppression screen based on the nature of the mutation, the more information known about a particular mutation, the better the choice that can be made. For example, screens using an amber suppressible allele will not only yield suppressors of interest, but can also yield mutations in amber suppressor tRNAs. If the suppressors of interest occur at a very low frequency, the other more nonspecific mutations may overwhelm the recovery of the desired mutations. Similarly, screens using alleles that are splice site mutations may yield mutations in splicing components as well as the suppressors of interest. Of course, it is not always possible to begin with knowledge of the exact defect of the mutation of interest; nonetheless, one can test by construction whether a starting mutation is suppressed by known informational suppressors, for example, *sup-7* and *smg-1* (see below for further details).

B. Analysis and Interpretation of Suppressors

Analysis of suppressor mutations involves separating the suppressors of interest from intragenic revertants and informational suppressors, testing dominance, checking for phenotypes in an otherwise wild-type background, mapping the suppressor locus, and determining the spectrum of suppression. When a suppressor mutation is isolated, its only known phenotype is that it suppresses the original mutation. Thus, no assumptions can be made about the phenotype of the suppressor on its own; it could have an unexpected phenotype, be lethal, or be silent. Because of this, strains for the analysis of suppressor mutations must carry the starting mutation to allow scoring of the suppressor phenotype. In essence, the strain with the starting mutation is the background strain for further analysis. Besides this, analysis of suppressor mutations proceeds as for any other mutation. For example, to establish linkage with a recessive suppressor mutation, *mut/mut; sup/sup* animals can be crossed to *mut; marker* strains to construct a *mut/mut; marker/+; sup/+* heterozygote, and linkage of *sup* and *marker* observed among the progeny (*mut* = starting mutation, *sup* = suppressor mutation,

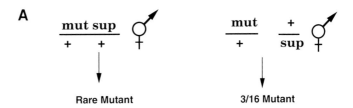

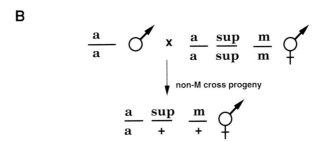

Fig. 9 Analysis of suppressor mutations. (A) Linked versus unlinked suppressors. Assuming complete penetrance and recessivity of the *sup* mutation, only *mut +/mut sup* recombinants will be detected among the progeny of animals heterozygous for *mut* and *sup*. These occur at a frequency of $2p/4 = p/2$, where p is the map distance (see Sulston and Hodgkin, 1988). (B) Test for dominance. Animals heterozygous for the *sup* mutation and homozygous for the starting mutation, *a*, are constructed to determine the phenotype.

marker = any unrelated marker) (Fig. 9A). Dominance can be tested by crossing *mut; sup* males to *mut; marker* hermaphrodites and examining the phenotype of the nonmarker cross-progeny (Fig. 9B). Similarly, complementation of recessive suppressor mutations can be tested by crossing *sup-1; mut* males to *sup-2; mut; marker* hermaphrodites.

Intragenic revertants will be linked; extragenic linked suppressors can be separated by recombination. For analysis of intragenic revertants see Greenwald and Horvitz (1980). Such revertants can be informative with respect to the structure, function, or expression of a particular gene, but are not helpful in defining a pathway.

It is important to determine the spectrum of suppression of a suppressor mutation: Does it suppress other alleles of the starting gene? If not, it might suggest informational suppression (see below) or a protein–protein interaction, depending on the nature of the alleles. Does it suppress hypomorphic or null alleles? If it only suppresses hypomorphic alleles, the suppressor might act upstream in a pathway or act in branch of the pathway. Does it suppress other phenotypes of the starting mutation? This would tell you if it acts in all pathways in which your starting mutation functions. Does it suppress mutations in other genes in the pathway, and if so, does it only suppress mutations that lie upstream? Not only can these types of data reveal whether a suppressor is informational, but they also indicate the specificity of the suppressor gene defined. Whether specific or generally acting suppressors are of greater interest is a matter of personal taste.

One class of extragenic suppressors are informational suppressors (reviewed by Hodgkin *et al.,* 1987). Formally, informational suppressors are allele specific, gene nonspecific, and thus act on particular types of mutations, rather than particular types of gene products. The classic informational suppressor is an amber suppressor, for example, *sup-7* in *C. elegans.* A new class of informational suppressors, the *smg* genes, were found by reversion of three independent phenotypes; the *smg* genes affect mRNA stability (Pulak and Anderson, 1993). The informational nature of their suppression was discovered by the realization that three different genetic screens for unrelated pathways identified the same set of suppressor mutations (Hodgkin *et al.,* 1989).

C. Silent Suppressors

Once the map position of a suppressor mutation is determined, markers can be used in *trans* to separate the suppressor from the original mutation so that the phenotype of the suppressor alone can be determined. The simplest suppressor mutations to interpret are those that confer a phenotype opposite that of the starting mutation, with suppression by virtue of epistasis [e.g., suppression of *lin-15* multivulva by *let-60* vulvaless (Han *et al.,* 1990); suppression of *tra-3* masculinization by *fem-1, fem-2,* or *fem-3* feminization (Hodgkin, 1986); suppression of dauer constitutive by dauer defective (Riddle *et al.*, 1981)]. Many suppressor mutations, however, have an unrelated phenotype or no phenotype other than suppression of the starting mutation; these are silent suppressors as they have no effect with respect to the phenotype of interest. There are various types of experiments one can carry out but no generalizable formula is available to determine what will be the most informative types of silent suppressor mutations. Note that silent suppressors can identify genes that would otherwise not have been identified.

Some suppressor mutations enhance other mutations that have the phenotype opposite that of the starting mutation, suggesting that they indeed control activity of the pathway of interest. Some suppressor mutations have synthetic phenotypes; that is, the double-mutant animal carrying two suppressor mutations displays a phenotype opposite that of the starting mutation; this is due to the redundant action of the genes defined by the suppressor mutations. The synthetic phenotype can then be used in epistasis tests. If there is clear epistasis of the suppressor double mutant with mutations in the pathway, the redundant suppressors most likely act in a parallel subset of the otherwise linear pathway, with redundant genes A and B defined by suppressors of X (see Thomas *et al.*, 1993, for an example). This pathway would look like

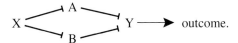

If suppressor mutations suppress hypomorphic alleles but not null alleles, then they are more likely to be a side branch of the main pathway. These mutations are in a side branch because they are unable to bypass the null allele and, thus, do not define a downstream component regulated by an upstream gene (see Lee *et al.*, 1994, for an example). Silent suppressors that do not show synthetic phenotypes cannot be placed in a pathway using epistasis, but the spectrum of suppression of mutations in the pathway of interest can suggest their role.

IV. Prospects: Use of New Technologies for Pathway Analysis

Transgenes add to the arsenal of tools for pathway analysis: they can be used for suppression and epistasis. For example, the high copy number of *lin-3* provided by a transgene results in a multivulva phenotype; this phenotype is hypostatic to the *let-23* vulvaless phenotype, consistent with *lin-3* acting upstream of *let-23* (Hill and Sternberg, 1992). A powerful technique in the future will be reversion of the dominant effects of transgenes. One potential problem may be a high degree of intragenic revertants, that is, deletions, of the integrated transgenes. In one case, this did not happen; rather, reversion of integrated *lin-3* transgene using ethyl methanesulfonate (EMS) as the mutagen yielded suppressor mutations in expected genes such as *let-23*, but not deletions of the transgene (J. Liu and P. Sternberg, unpublished observations).

In *Saccharomyces cerevisiae,* high-copy suppression using plasmid libraries is a powerful tool for finding interacting or related genes. In *C. elegans,* similar analysis will be more difficult, but still possible. Because of the larger genome size compared with yeast, testing on the order of 500 transgenic lines, each with multiple copies of five cosmids (assuming good representation of the genome with 2500 cosmids), would be required. The ability to create mutations in genes of interest will be a powerful tool. As genetically defined genes are cloned and homologies are seen, other molecularly defined components that may lie in the pathway of interest can be cloned through reverse genetics and engineered into a genetic mutation (see Chapter 3 for further details) for further analysis. Finally, from a geneticist's perspective, the Genome Project makes it more attractive to pursue the characterization of silent suppressor mutations because the molecular cloning will be increasingly facile.

V. Conclusion

The determination of the functional order of genes in a developmental pathway provides a working model for the design of additional experiments. New genes can be added to the pathway once they are found, either at a branchpoint or directly in the pathway. The gene order can be refined on receipt of more information about the phenotype of the mutations involved, the isolation of new mutations that allow more epistasis analysis to be performed, as well as more information about the molecular and biochemical nature of the pathway of interest. Eventually, individual pathways will be connected to other pathways, evolving into a network of gene interactions for developmental processes.

Acknowledgments

The authors thank Paul Garrity, Wendy Katz, Ralf Sommer, John DeModena, Marie-Anne Félix, Yvonne Hadju-Cronin, Howard Lipshitz, Katharine Liu, Anna Newman, and the editors for critical comments. Research in our laboratory discussed here was supported by the U.S. Public Health Service, the March of Dimes Birth Defects Foundation, and the Howard Hughes Medical Institute, with which P.W.S. is an Investigator.

References

Ambros, V. (1989). A hierarchy of regulatory genes controls a larval to adult developmental switch in *C. elegans. Cell* **57,** 49–57.

Ambros, V., and Moss, E. G. (1994). Heterochronic genes and the temporal control of *C. elegans* development. *Trends Genet.* **10,** 123–127.

Aroian, R. V., and Sternberg, P. W. (1991). Multiple functions of *let-23,* a *C. elegans* receptor tyrosine kinase gene required for vulval induction. *Genetics* **128,** 215–267.

Aroian, R. V., Lesa, G. M., and Sternberg, P. W. (1994). Mutations in the *Caenorhabditis elegans let-23* EGFR-like gene define elements important for cell-type specificity and function. EMBO J. **13,** 360–366.

Avery, L., and Wasserman, S. (1992). Ordering gene function: The interpretation of epistasis in regulatory hierarchies. *Trends Genet.* **8,** 312–316.

Chamberlin, H. M., and Sternberg, P. W. (1993). Multiple cell interactions are required for fate specification during male spicule development in *Caenorhabditis elegans. Development* **118,** 297–323.

Clark, S. G., Lu X., and Horvitz, H. R. (1994). The *C. elegans* locus *lin-15,* a negative regulator of a tyrosine kinase signaling pathway, encodes two different proteins. *Genetics* **137,** 987–997.

Ellis, R. E., Jacobson, D. M., and Horvitz, H. R. (1991a). Genes required for the engulfment of cell corpses during programmed cell death in *Caenorhabditis elegans. Genetics* **129,** 79–94.

Ellis, R. E., Yuan, J., and Horvitz, H. R. (1991b). Mechanisms and functions of cell death. *Annu. Rev. Cell. Biol.* **7,** 663–698.

Ferguson, E., and Horvitz, H. R. (1989). The multivulva phenotype of certain *C. elegans* mutants results from defects in two functionally-redundant pathways. *Genetics* **123,** 109–121.

Ferguson, E. L., Sternberg, P. W., and Horvitz, H. R. (1987). A genetic pathway for the specification of the vulval cell lineages of *Caenorhabditis elegans. Nautre* **326,** 259–267.

Greenwald, I. S., and Horvitz, H. R. (1980). *unc-93(e1500)*: A behavioral mutant of *Caenorhabditis elegans* that defines a gene with a wild-type null phenotype. *Genetics* **96,** 147–164.

Han, M., Aroian, R., and Sternberg, P. W. (1990). The *let-60* locus controls the switch between vulval and non-vulval cell types in *C. elegans. Genetics* **126,** 899–913.

Hedgecock, E. M., Sulston, J. E., and Thomson, J. N. (1983). Mutations affecting programmed cell deaths in the nematode *Caenorhabditis elgans. Science* **220,** 1277–1279.

Hengartner, M. O., Ellis, R. E., and Horvitz, H. R. (1992). *Caenorhabditis elegans* gene *ced-9* protects cells from programmed cell death. *Nature* **356,** 494–499.

Hill, R. J., and Sternberg, P. W. (1992). The *lin-3* gene encodes an inductive signal for vulval development in *C. elegans. Nature* **358,** 470–476.

Hodgkin, J. (1986). Sex determination in the nematode *Caenorhabditis elegans*: Analysis if *tra-3* suppressors and characterization of *fem* genes. *Genetics* **114,** 15–52.

Hodgkin, J., Kondo, K., and Waterston, R. H. (1987). Suppression in the nematode *Caenorhabditis elegans. Trends Genet.* **3,** 325–329.

Hodgkin, J., Papp, A., Pulak, R., Ambros, V., and Anderson, P. (1989). A new kind of informational suppression in the nematode *Caenorhabditis elegans. Genetics* **123,** 301–313.

Huang, L. S., Tzou, P., and Sternberg, P. W. (1994). The *lin-15* locus encodes two negative regulators of *C. elegans* vulval development. *Mol. Biol. Cell* **5,** 395–412.

Lackner, M. R., Kornfeld, K., Miller, L. M., Horvitz, H. R., and Kim, S. K. (1994). A MAP kinase homolog, *mpk-1,* is involved in *ras*-mediated induction of vulval cell fates in *Caenorhabditis elegans. Genes Dev.* **8,** 160–173.

Lee, J., Jongeward, G. D., and Sternberg, P. W. (1994). *unc-101,* a gene required for many aspects of *C. elegans* development and behavior, encodes a clathrin-associated protein. *Genes Dev.* **8,** 60–73.

Muller, H. J. (1932). Further studies on the nature and causes of gene mutations. Int. Congr. Genet. **6,** 213–255.

Pulak, R., and Anderson, P. (1993). mRNA surveillance by the *Caenorhabditis elegans smg* genes. *Genes Dev.* **7,** 1885–1897.

Riddle, D. L. (1977). A genetic pathway for dauer larva formation in *Caenorhabditis elegans. Stadler Genet. Symp.* **9,** 101–120.

Riddle, D. L., Swanson, M. M., and Albert, P. S. (1981). Interacting genes in nematode dauer larva formation. *Nature* **290,** 668–671.

Sternberg, P. W. (1990). Genetic control of cell type and pattern formation in *C. elegans. Adv. Genet.* **27,** 63–115.

Sternberg, P. W. (1993). Intercellular signaling and signal transduction in *C. elegans. Annu. Rev. Genet.* **27,** 497–521.

Sulston, J., and Hodgkin, J. (1988). Methods. *In* "The Nematode *Caenorhabditis elegans*" (W. B. Wood, ed.), pp. 587–606. Cold Spring Harbor Laboratory, Cold Spring Harbor, New York.

Tautz, D. (1992). Redundancies, development and the flow of information. *BioEssays* **14,** 263–268.

Thomas, J. H. (1993). Thinking about genetic reduncancy. *Trends Genet.* **9,** 395–399.

Thomas, J. H., Birnby, D. A., and Vowels, J. J. (1993). Evidence for parallel processing of sensory information controlling dauer formation in *Caenorhabditis elegans. Genetics* **134,** 1105–1117.

Villeneuve, A. M., and Meyer, B. J. (1990). The regulatory hierarchy controlling sex determination and dosage compensation in *Caenorhabditis elegans. Adv. Genet.* **27,** 117–188.

Wu, Y., and Han, M. (1994). Suppression of activated Let-60 Ras protein defines a role of *C. elegans* Sur-1 MAP kinase in vulval differentiation. *Genes Dev.* **8,** 147–159.

CHAPTER 6

Mosaic Analysis

Robert K. Herman

Department of Genetics and Cell Biology
University of Minnesota
St. Paul, Minnesota 55108

I. Questions Addressed by Mosaic Analysis

Geneticists like to point out that the ultimate test of a proposed function for a gene and its encoded product (or products) in a living organism involves making a mutant and analyzing its phenotype. This is the goal of reverse genetics: a gene is cloned and sequenced, its transcripts and protein coding sequence are analyzed, and a function may be proposed; one must then introduce a mutation in the gene in a living organism to see what the functional consequences are. The analysis of genetic mosaics takes this philosophy a step further. In mosaics, some cells of an individual are genotypically mutant and other cells are genotypically wild type. One then asks what the phenotypic consequences are for the living organism. This is not the same as asking what cells transcribe the gene or in what cells the protein product of the gene is to be found, but rather it is asking in what cells the wild-type gene is needed for a given function.

One does not undertake a mosaic analysis of a gene until one knows something about the phenotype of the completely mutant organism. If the description of the mutant phenotype is fairly general, such as "uncoordination" in the case of *Caenorhabditis elegans,* and has not progressed to a description of cellular abnormalities, then one can generate mosaics and ask what cells, for example, body muscle or motor neurons, must carry the wild-type gene for the animal to exhibit wild-type coordination: The animal displays the wild-type phenotype if and only if the responsible cells carry the wild-type gene regardless of the genotypes of all other cells. In this way, one can, in principle at least, determine the anatomical focus of a gene's action (Fig. 1).

When a description of the mutant phenotype has progressed to the identification of specific cellular abnormalities, the experimentalist can use genetic mosaics to ask whether the abnormalities are cell autonomous (Fig. 2). This is equivalent to asking if the appearance of the cellular abnormality depends solely on the genotype of the affected cell and not on the genotype of any other cells in the body. When the action of a mutation is cell *non*autonomous, it means that the genotype of one or more other cells is important and that the abnormal cell is made abnormal by interaction with another cell or cells. Mosaic analysis may then be used to try to identify the responsible interacting cell or cells.

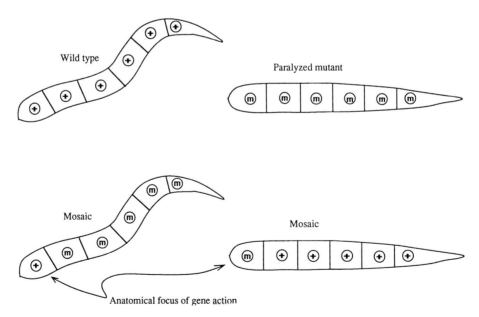

Fig. 1 Mythical six-celled wild-type worm, a paralyzed mutant, and two mosaics. The behavioral phenotype is determined in this example by the genotype of the animal's most anterior cell.

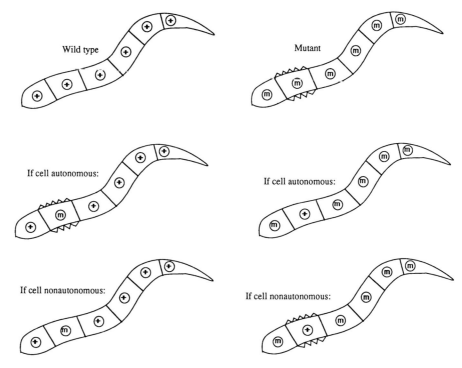

Fig. 2 Mythical six-celled wild-type worm, a mutant with a discernible abnormality in one cell, and four mosaic animals indicative of cell autonomous or cell nonautonomous gene action. Cell nonautonomous gene action means that the cellular abnormality is caused by interaction with one or more other cells. An interacting cell might be a neighbor that interacts structurally, for example, or it might secrete an important component of extracellular matrix or a specific signaling ligand such as a growth factor. The affected cell may also contribute to an extracellular component but not provide enough by itself to lead to a completely wild-type phenotype.

Genetic procedures for generating genetic mosaics, as opposed to methods involving cell or tissue transplants (the products of which are often called chimeras rather than mosaics), generally involve the loss of a wild-type gene from a progenitor cell during development, which then leads to the generation of a mutant clone. It should be remembered for such methods, however, that wild-type product synthesized in the progenitor cell or its ancestral cells prior to gene loss might persist and be transmitted to descendant cells even though they lack the gene; this is referred to as *perdurance* (Garcia-Bellido and Merriam, 1971). The effect of perdurance would be to prevent the appearance of or to weaken the expected mutant phenotype. The complications of perdurance for the interpretation of mosaic results are discussed further in Section II,E,4.

One form of perdurance that is very important developmentally is usually referred to as a maternal effect. The simplest demonstration of a maternal effect is provided by those situations where the homozygous mutant progeny of heterozygous mutant mothers are less severely mutant than the progeny of a homozygous mutant mother (Fig. 3). This simple assay for a maternal effect is impossible when the homozygous mutant animals are inviable or infertile, but a maternal effect may nonetheless be demonstrated by making use of mosaic mothers. The most important type of mosaic mother would be a germ-line mosaic, in which the soma of the hermaphrodite parent is heterozygous and the germ line is homozygous mutant (Fig. 3). Germ-line mosaics have been analyzed extensively by *Drosophila* developmental geneticists (Lawrence, 1991; Wilkins, 1993), but they have so far received rather little attention from *C. elegans* researchers. One example is provided by an analysis of the *C. elegans* recessive mutation *rh59:* it causes an early larval arrest among the self progeny of heterozygous hermaphrodite parents and early embryonic arrest, prior to morphogenesis,

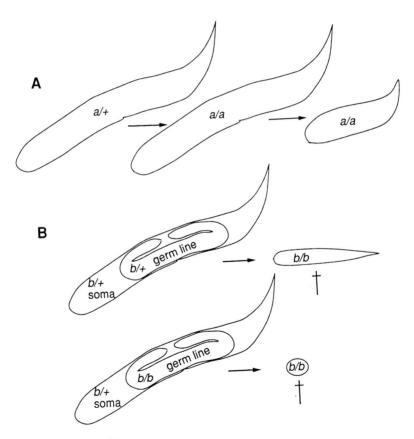

Fig. 3 Maternal effects. (A) The mutant phenotype of an *a/a* animal is more severe if its mother is *a/a* rather than *a/+*. (B) The lethal phenotype of the *b/b* animal is more severe (earlier lethal arrest) if its mother has a *b/b* germ line.

among the self progeny of heterozygous parents that have homozygous mutant germ lines (E. Hedgecock and R. Herman, unpublished results), from which it has been concluded that maternal germ-line expression of the wild-type allele of *rh59* is important for embryogenesis.

Maternal effects are not invariably the result of germ-line expression. Some maternal effect genes in *Drosophila,* for example, have been shown to exert their effects in the mesodermal follicle cells, which surround the developing oocyte (Wilkins, 1993). The *C. elegans vit* genes, which encode vitellogenins, are expressed most strongly in the hermaphrodite intestine (Kimble and Sharrock, 1983; Sharrock, 1984; Blumenthal *et al.,* 1984; Spieth and Blumenthal, 1985); the yolk protein products must then be transported to the developing oocytes. Analysis of hermaphrodites mosaic for the sex determination gene *tra-1* has suggested that *vit* gene expression in the intestine of the hermaphrodite parent is essential for embryogenesis (Hunter and Wood, 1990).

II. Generation of Mosaics by Spontaneous Mitotic Loss of Free Duplications

Most genetic mosaics that have been analyzed in *C. elegans* were generated by the spontaneous somatic loss of free chromosome fragments (Herman, 1984; for review, see Herman, 1989), called *free duplications*. The normal chromosomes in every case were homozygous for a recessive allele of the gene to be analyzed, and the free duplication carried a dominant (almost always wild-type) allele. *C. elegans* chromosomes are holocentric (Albertson and Thomson, 1982), which means that the mitotic and meiotic (Albertson and Thomson, 1993) spindle fibers attach over large extents of the metaphase chromosomes rather than at specific localized sites. Because the chromosomes do not have localized centromeres, the problem of unstable acentric fragments does not arise, and many free duplications of many different regions of the genome, each present in one copy per cell, segregate fairly regularly at mitosis. On the other hand, free duplications are subject to spontaneous mitotic loss, the frequency of loss depending on the specific duplication and other factors discussed below. Albertson and Thomson (1982) observed, by light microscopy, free duplications lying at the outer edge of the metaphase plate or lagging behind normal chromosomes at anaphase and suggested that free duplications may occasionally missegregate owing to an insufficient number of attached microtubules to pull them to the spindle poles. According to this view, duplications smaller than some minimum size may be too unstable to be maintained in stock.

Some somatic duplication losses involve nondisjunction. E. Hedgecock and R. Herman (unpublished results) analyzed 80 mosaic animals in which the duplications *sDp3(III,f)* was lost by the cell AB, one of the daughters of the first embryonic cleavage (Sulston *et al.,* 1983). Two independent methods were used to estimate duplication copy number in the descendants of P_1, the sister of AB

(Fig. 4). Both assay methods made use of the fact that P_1 is a progenitor of the germ line. In one set of experiments, oocytes were stained with diamidino-phenolindole (DAPI) (Sulston and Hodgkin, 1988) and screened for the presence of two stained free duplications; in the other set of experiments, self progeny ratios were used to estimate duplication copy number in the germ line. The two methods were in good agreement and led to the conclusion that about 60% of the losses of *sDp3* at AB involved a nondisjunction event in which P_1 received two copies of the duplication. It is not known why the free duplication seems prone to nondisjunction. The mechanism of simple duplication loss (not involving nondisjunction) is also unknown. It is possible that a lagging duplication at anaphase is sometimes omitted from the newly formed nucleus. Failure to replicate a duplication is another possibility.

Whatever the mechanism by which a duplication is lost, the loss leads to the generation of a homozygous recessive clone in a background of duplication-bearing cells. Duplication loss is best scored by making use of a cell autonomous genetic marker carried by the duplication in addition to the gene under study. Because the cell lineage is rigidly specified, it is frequently possible by scoring a few well-chosen cells to pinpoint precisely the position in the lineage where the duplication must have been lost, in which case the genotypes of virtually all cells in the mosaic animal can be deduced. From the analysis of a series of mosaic animals, the goal is to correlate the unmasking of a gene's recessive phenotype with the loss of the free duplication from a particular cell or set of cells, which then define the anatomical focus of action of the gene. The requirement for

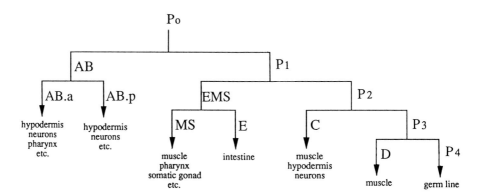

Fig. 4 Early embryonic cell divisions and lineal derivations of general cell types (Sulston *et al.*, 1983). AB.a and AB.p are anterior and posterior daughters, respectively, of AB. Several genes affecting coordinated movement, including *unc-3, unc-7, unc-26, unc-30,* and *unc-36,* exert their effects at least primarily among the descendants of AB.p (see text for references), which is the progenitor of nearly all the motor neurons of the ventral and dorsal nerve cords (Sulston *et al.*, 1983). Genes whose foci appear to be in body muscle, which is generated almost entirely from descendants of P_1(MS, C, and D), are *ace-1, sup-10,* and *unc-29* (see text for references). Genes whose action seems to be hypodermis, which derives from AB.a, AB.p, and C, include *dpy-1, dpy-4, dpy-17, dpy-18,* and *lin-15.*

conducting the mosaic analysis of a gene by this technique, then, is a free duplication that is subject to mitotic loss and that carries both the gene of interest and a cell autonomous marker. As will be discussed below, additional genetic markers on the duplication can be useful for picking out potential mosaics under the dissecting microscope.

A. Sources of Free Duplications

Roughly half of the genome is currently covered by free duplications; methods for generating new free duplications will be described. Some of the available free duplications are very stable mitotically, making the occurrence of mosaicism rare; methods will be described for reducing the sizes of duplications, with the purpose of generating less stable derivatives.

Any stock carrying a free duplication will segregate self progeny that lack the duplication simply as a consequence of meiotic segregation. It is therefore important that the duplication carry a dominant allele (almost always the wild-type allele) of a visible marker for which the normal chromosomes are homozygous recessive; this makes it easy to identify duplication-bearing progeny under the dissecting microscope, as they are the animals in which the duplication complements the visible mutation.

1. Methods for Generating New Free Duplications

Some methods are specific for the recovery of duplications of X chromosomal regions. *C. elegans* hermaphrodites have two X chromosomes (XX) and five pairs of autosomes; males differ only in having a single X chromosome (XO). In one scheme (Herman *et al.*, 1976, 1979), wild-type males are exposed to ionizing radiation, 1500 to 7000 roentgens, and then mated with X-linked visible mutant hermaphrodites, genotype *gen-1/gen-1*, where *gen-1* refers to a hypothetical recessive mutation in the *gen-1* gene conferring the phenotype Gen-1. (A guide to *C. elegans* nomenclature used in this chapter is given in Table I.) The progeny are screened for exceptional wild-type (non-Gen-1) males of putative genotype *gen-1/0; Dp[gen-1(+)]*, which are then backcrossed to *gen-1/gen-1* hermaphrodites. The issuance of wild-type males from the latter cross signifies the transmission of an unlinked X duplication (or a suppressor of the visible mutation), as cross-progeny males normally inherit their one X chromosome from their hermaphrodite parent. Duplications may be either translocated or free; translocated duplications will acquire linkage to chromosomal markers. The presence of a free duplication should be confirmed by chromosome staining, say with 4', 6-diamidino-2-phenylindole dihydrochloride (DAPI) (Sulston and Hodgkin, 1988).

The above isolation scheme requires that the partial diploidy for the X chromosome not preclude male development and fertility. This is usually a useful requirement in that duplications that cannot be transmitted by males are much more

Table I
A Brief Guide to *Caenorhabditis elegans* Nomenclature[a]

Examples of terminology	Explanation
rh59 or *e1551*	Mutation names; consist of a one- or two-letter italicized prefix, which refers to the laboratory of isolation (registered with the *Caenorhabditis* Genetics Center), and an italicized Arabic number
dpy-1 or *unc-36*	Gene names; consist of three italicized letters (referring to the mutant phenotype such as *dumpy* or *uncoordinated*), a hyphen, and an italicized Arabic number
him-10(e1551)	Refers to the mutation *e1551* and indicates that it is an allele of the *him-10* gene
dpy-17 III; unc-42 V	Genotype of a double mutant; mutations in *dpy-17*, which is on linkage group *III*, and *unc-42*, which is on linkage group *V*, are understood even though the mutation (allele) names are not specified
dpy-1(+)	Refers to the wild-type allele of *dpy-1*
sDp3(III;f)[dpy-1(+)]	Duplication name; consists of the same italicized prefix as is used for mutation names (referring to the laboratory of isolation), *Dp* for duplication, and an italicized Arabic number; included in (optional) parentheses in this example are the affected linkage group, *III*, and *f* for free duplication; the genotype of the duplication, such as *dpy-1*(+) in this example, may be specified in brackets
Dpy or Unc or non-Unc	Phenotypic abbreviations; not italic, non-Unc refers to a wild-type phenotype with regard to uncoordination

[a] Based on Horvitz *et al.* (1979).

difficult to manipulate genetically. On the other hand, usually only a small percentage of wild-type male candidates (which are themselves rare) sire progeny, and the duplication of one or more X regions in males may lead to inviability owing to defects in dosage compensation (Hodgkin *et al.*, 1994; Akerib and Meyer, 1994). In an alternative scheme that does not require duplication-bearing males to be fertile, wild-type males are irradiated as before and mated with, for example, *him-8 IV; dpy-3 unc-6X* hermaphrodites. The progeny are screened for Dpy non-Unc or Unc non-Dpy hermaphrodites, which may be produced by the fusion of a duplication-bearing sperm carrying either *dpy-3*(+) or *unc-6*(+) and a diplo-X ovum; the generation of the latter is promoted by *him-8*, which results in high-frequency X chromosome nondisjunction (and a *high incidence of male* self progeny).

Autosomal duplications have been identified by a variety of methods. In one scheme (Herman *et al.*, 1979; Hunter and Wood, 1992), males that were *trans* heterozygous for two closely linked markers, genotype *gen-1 gen-2*(+)/*gen-1*(+) *gen-2*, were irradiated and mated with homozygous double-mutant hermaphrodites, genotype *gen-1 gen-1/gen-1 gen-2*. The progeny were screened for wild-type animals, some of which were either *Dp[gen-1(+)]/gen-1 gen-2(+)/gen-1 gen-2* or *Dp[gen-2(+)]/gen-1(+) gen-2/gen-1 gen-2*, where *Dp[gen-1(+)]* refers to a duplication carrying *gen-1*(+). Other wild-type candidates might have carried a wild-type recombinant chromosome from the male parent or might have been trisomic, having received two homologous chromosomes from the male parent. The various possibilities were distinguished by progeny testing. In another scheme (Rosenbluth *et al.*, 1985; Stewart *et al.*, 1991), *gen-1 gen-2(+)/gen-1(+) gen-2* hermaphrodites were irradiated (with ionizing radiation or ultraviolet light), wild-type self progeny were picked, and their broods were screened for the absence of either Gen-1 (or Gen-2) animals; among those animals giving no Gen-1 progeny were those that were *gen-2/gen-2/Dp[gen-2(+)]*. In a third scheme (Rogalski and Riddle, 1988), irradiated wild-type males were crossed to hermaphrodites homozygous for a semidominant marker in the region to be duplicated (*dpy-13 IV*); most cross-progeny, genotype *dpy-13(+)/dpy-13*, were semi-Dpy, but duplication-bearing animals, genotype *dpy-13(+)/dpy-13; Dp[dpy-13(+)]*, were found among rare non-Dpy cross progeny. Finally, duplications were identified after crossing irradiated wild-type males with autosomally marked hermaphrodites, picking wild-type progeny and recognizing aberrant patterns of segregation among their broods (Rose *et al.*, 1984).

Free duplications have also been generated from translocations, either by recovery of half translocations as duplications (Herman *et al.*, 1982; McKim *et al.*, 1988, 1993) or by recovery of a breakdown product of a translocation as a duplication (DeLong *et al.*, 1987). It is possible that duplications of chromosome ends, which may require a single break, are more easily recovered than duplications of internal regions, which presumably require at least two breaks. If so, it might make sense first to generate a large free duplication that carries a normal chromosome end and then to make smaller derivatives of it; methods for pruning free duplications are described in the next section.

Most free duplications recombine little if at all with the homologous regions of the normal chromosomes (see Chapter 7 in this volume). There are, however, specific regions, where recombination between a free duplication and the chromosome appears to be frequent: the right end of linkage group (LG) I (Rose *et al.*, 1984), the left of end of LG IV (Rogalski and Riddle, 1988), and the left end of the X (Herman and Kari, 1989). Frequent recombination between duplication and chromosome complicates the maintainance of the duplication and renders mosaic analysis of such regions by the method of mitotic duplication loss extremely difficult.

2. Pruning Existing Free Duplications to Enhance the Frequency of Mitotic Loss

Many investigators (Herman, 1984; Austin and Kimble, 1987; McKim and Rose, 1990; Hunter and Wood, 1990; Yuan and Horvitz, 1990; McKim *et al.*, 1993) have generated shortened duplications, and the method is straightforward. A stock of genotype *gen-1 gen-2/gen-1 gen-2;Dp[gen-1(+) gen-2(+)]* is constructed. One then identifies and picks Gen-1 non-Gen-2 or Gen-2 non-Gen-1 self progeny. Such animals can be generated as a consequence of mosaicism (see below for further discussion), but a Gen-1 non-Gen-2 animal carrying a duplication that has lost *gen-1(+)*, for example, will segregate Gen-1 non-Gen-2 (duplication-bearing: *gen-1 gen-2/gen-1 gen-2*; *Dp[gen-2(+)]*) and Gen-1 Gen-2 (nulloduplication: *gen-1 gen-2/gen-1 gen-2*) self progeny. A duplication lacking *gen-1(+)* can arise as a consequence of recombination with the homologous chromosome rather than from deletion formation; however, it is frequently found that additional, closely linked markers have also been lost, which presumably occurs through duplication shortening. Many duplications have been shown to suffer deletions spontaneously, at as high a frequency as 1/500 per generation (Herman, 1984), but the frequency of deletion formation can be enhanced further by exposure to ionizing radiation (McKim and Rose, 1990).

B. Cell Markers for Tracking Duplication Loss

The best cell autonomous genetic marker known for tracking a duplication is *ncl-1*. Mutation in *ncl-1* (the original allele was identified by E. Hedgecock, unpublished; a second allele was identified by C. Kenyon, unpublished) results in enlarged nucleoli, as observed in living animals by Nomarski differential interference contrast microscopy at all stages of development. The nucleoli of nearly all cells, including neurons, hypodermis, and muscle, are markedly enlarged. Intestinal and germ-line nucleoli, however, which are quite large in wild-type animals, are not noticeably larger in *ncl-1* animals. Each of the *ncl-1* mutations is recessive to *ncl-1(+)*. E. Hedgecock (unpublished) identified *ncl-1* mosaics generated from *dpy-1 ncl-1*; *sDp3(III;f)[dpy-1(+) ncl-1(+)]* zygotes. The results established that the patterns of mosaicism of the Ncl phenotype can be explained as the consequence of somatic duplication loss and the cell autonomous action of *ncl-1*. In hypodermal syncytial cells containing a mixture of *ncl-1(+)*-containing and *ncl-1* mutant nuclei, all nucleoli appear wild-type in size; it is presumed that *ncl-1(+)* gene product synthesized in the common cytoplasm represses nucleolar enlargement in both mutant and nonmutant nuclei.

E. Hedgecock and R. Herman (unpublished results) characterized 100 *ncl-1* clones that arose through mitotic duplication loss in the lineages leading to six neurons. Each of the six neurons is produced in 10 or 11 embryonic cell divisions from the zygote. It was concluded that the probability of duplication loss was approximately the same for all of these divisions. [This may not be a property of all free duplications, although Herman (1984) concluded that it was at least approximately true for *mnDp2(X;f)*.] It was also found that losses that occurred at the last division or next-to-last division (losses at these divisions were not distinguishable because the sisters of the six neurons suffer programmed cell death and therefore could not be scored) resulted in *ncl-1* neurons with completely enlarged nucleoli; that is, the *ncl-1(+)* gene showed no sign of perdurance.

In summary, *ncl-1* is cell autonomous, shows no perdurance, and can be readily scored in nearly every cell of a living animal. These features make it an ideal marker for mosaic analysis. Indeed, it has been used in the mosaic analysis of *glp-1* (Austin and Kimble, 1987), *lin-12* (Seydoux and Greenwald, 1989; Seydoux *et al.,* 1990), *tra-1* and *her-1* (Hunter and Wood, 1990, 1992), *pal-1* (Waring and Kenyon, 1991), various lethal mutations (Bucher and Greenwald, 1991), *unc-5* (Leung-Hagesteijn *et al.,* 1992), and *mpk-1* (Lackner *et al.,* 1994). Some effort has been devoted to exploiting the utility of *ncl-1* as a cell marker in the mosaic analysis of genes that are not closely linked to *ncl-1 III.* One approach is to fuse a duplication carrying the gene to be analyzed with a *ncl-1*(+)-bearing duplication (see Section III). A second approach is to fuse an extrachromosomal array carrying the gene of interest to a free duplication carrying *ncl-1*(+) (see Section IV). And a third approach is to generate an extrachromosomal array carrying *ncl-1*(+) in addition to the gene of interest and, perhaps, an additional marker to aid in the maintenance of the array or in the enrichment for classes of potential mosaics (see Section V).

Other cell markers have been used for mosaic analysis. Two markers that appear to be cell autonomous and that affect many cells over much of the lineage are *ced-3* and *ced-4* (Yuan and Horvitz, 1990). These genes are involved in the pathway of programmed cell death. Programmed cell deaths can be scored in living animals by Nomarski differential interference contrast microscopy (Sulston and Horvitz, 1977). Mutations in 25 other genes affect the ability of a set of chemosensory neurons to fill with fluorescent dye. When living wild-type animals are exposed to a solution containing a dye such as fluorescein isothiocyanate, the cell bodies and processes of 12 chemosensory neurons in the head and four neurons in the tail fill with dye and can be readily visualized by fluorescence microscopy (Hedgecock *et al.,* 1985). Mutations that reduce or abolish dye filling map to all six linkage groups (Perkins *et al.,* 1986; T. Starich *et al.,* 1995) and could be useful as cell markers for tracking duplication loss. Two of the genes have so far been used in this way: *osm-1* appears to behave cell autonomously, and the focus of action of *daf-6* has been mapped to four nonneuronal support cells that surround distinct sets of the neurons that fill with dye (Herman, 1987).

Although no germ-line cell markers are known, one can identify germ-line mosaics simply from the consequence that the duplication is transmitted to none of the self progeny. The germ line descends exclusively as a clone derived from P_4 (Fig. 4), which is four cell divisions removed from the zygote (Sulston *et al,* 1983). Thus, germ-line mosaics will be generated by duplication loss at P_1–P_4 (Fig. 4). It should, however, be noted that a mitotic duplication loss occurring in a descendant of P_4 may not eliminate all of the maternal dowry, even for those oocytes whose nuclei lack the duplication. This is because syncytial germ-line nuclei appear to be involved in the formation of the cytoplasm of each oocyte (for review, see Kimble and Ward, 1988).

For some mosaic analyses, an additional cell marker for tracking duplication loss is unnecesary. When the gene of interest itself affects the microscopic appearance of several cells, then the patterns of mosaicism that are found may by themselves provide compelling evidence for cell autonomy, based on the known cell lineage (Sulston *et al.,* 1983). Because most tissues and sensilla in *C. elegans* are not clonally generated, many cells that occupy neighboring positions in the animal are distantly related by ancestry. This means that the cells constituting a mutant clone are often situated among wild-type cells, and this makes the case for cell autonomy very convincing. Examples of genes that have given excellent cell autonomous mosaic patterns are *mab-5* (Kenyon, 1986) and *tra-1* (Hunter and Wood, 1990).

C. Use of Visible Markers to Identify Potential Mosaics

If the duplication carries two dominant visible markers with different anatomical foci of action, then one can screen self progeny of duplication-bearing hermaphrodite parents under the microscope for phenotypic recombinants, which are likely to be generated as a consequence of duplication loss at specific points in the lineage. Consider as an example animals of genotype *dpy-1 ncl-1 unc-36*; *sDp3(III;f)*[*dpy-1*(+) *ncl-1*(+) *unc-36*(+)]. The focus of action of *dpy-1* with respect to the overall Dpy phenotype has been assigned to hyp7, a large syncytial hypodermis that covers much of the body (E. Hedgecock, pers. comm.). The cells that form hyp7 derive from both AB and its sister P_1, which means that duplication loss by either of these cells does not result in a completely mutant hyp7 or a Dpy animal (Fig. 4). The focus of *unc-36*, however, is among the descendants of both daughters of AB.p (Kenyon, 1986), which means that duplication loss by AB or AB.p gives an Unc animal. Therefore, if an embryo of genotype *dpy-1 ncl-1 unc-36*; *sDp3* suffers duplication loss at AB or AB.p, it will become Unc but non-Dpy, a phenotype that is easy to pick out. The precise nature of the putative mosaic can then be confirmed by scoring a cell-specific marker, *ncl-1* in this example, by higher-resolution microscopy.

The approach of screening for rare phenotypic recombinants as potential mosaics can be a great time saver. Other visible markers whose foci have been localized primarily among descendants of AB.p include *unc-3* (Herman, 1984, 1987), *unc-7* (Starich *et al.*, 1993), *unc-26* (Yuan and Horvitz, 1990), and *unc-30* (Yuan and Horvitz, 1990). For some of these genes, animals with a semi-Unc phenotype were identified; such animals were generally mosaic, having suffered duplication loss among one or more early descendants of AB.p (Fig. 4). Visible loci whose foci of action have been localized among descendants of P_1 (probably body muscle) include *ace-1* (Herman and Kari, 1985; Johnson *et al.*, 1988), *unc-29* (Lackner *et al.*, 1994), and *sup-10* (Herman, 1984; Villeneuve and Meyer, 1990). Three other *dpy* genes have been analyzed in mosaics; the focus of all three (along with *dpy-1*, as already noted) may be in hypodermis, but the descendants of P_1 appear to be most important for *dpy-17* (Kenyon, 1986) and *dpy-18* (Hunter and Wood, 1990) function, whereas AB descendants seem more important for *dpy-4* (Yuan and Horvitz, 1990). When a new region of the genome is analyzed by mosaic methods, information about the foci of action of visibles in the region can be obtained, which can then make further mosaic analysis in the region easier.

D. Frequencies of Mitotic Duplication Loss

Different duplications exhibit different frequencies of spontaneous mitotic loss. Figure 5 shows frequencies of duplication loss per cell division for various free duplications. One apparent factor affecting the frequency of somatic duplication loss is duplication size. Duplications derived from larger duplications by pruning (see Section II,A,2) frequently exhibit higher frequencies of duplication loss than their larger progenitors. Examples include *qDp3* (Austin and Kimble, 1987) and *ctDp6* (Hunter and Wood, 1990), which were derived from *mnDp37*; *ctDp2* (Hunter and Wood, 1990), which was derived from *eDp6*; *nDp3* (Yuan and Horvitz, 1990), which was derived from *yDp1*; and *mnDp84*, *mnDp86*, and *mnDp90*, which were derived from *sDp3*. Factors other than size seem also to be important, however. The frequencies of loss of *sDp3(III;f)* and *qDp3(III;f)* have been compared in identical genetic backgrounds; the frequency of loss of *qDp3* was only about 5% that of *sDp3* (Fig. 5) despite the fact that the DNA content of *qDp3* appears to be less than that of *sDp3* (D. Albertson, pers. comm.).

Growth temperature has only a mild effect on the frequency of mitotic loss of *sDp3(III;f)*: the frequency of loss for animals reared at 24°C was about 50%

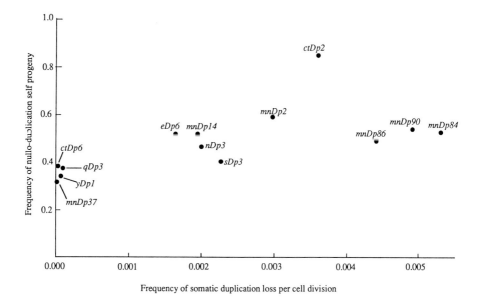

Frequency of somatic duplication loss per cell division

Fig. 5 Frequency of somatic duplication loss per cell division (abscissa) versus frequency of nulloduplication self progeny (ordinate) for each of 13 free duplications. The data for *ctDp2(III;f)*, *ctDp6(III;f)*, *eDp6(III;f)*, and *mnDp37(III;f)* are from Hunter and Wood (1990); *yDp1(IV,V;f)* and *nDp3(IV,V;f)* from Yuan and Horvitz (1990); *mnDp2(X;f)* from Herman (1984); *mnDp14(X;f)* from Herman and Kari (1985); *sDp3(III;f)* from Kenyon (1986); and *mnDp84(III;f)*, *mnDp86(III;f)*, *mnDp90(III;f)*, *qDp3(III;f)*, and *sDp3(III;f)* from R. K. Herman (unpublished).

higher than for those reared at 16°C. A chromosomal mutation that affects mitotic chromosome segregation (A. Villeneuve, pers. comm.), *him-10(e1551ts) III*, has been shown to increase the frequencies of somatic loss of several free duplications by factors of 4 to 6 in animals reared at 20°C (R. Herman, unpublished). The *him-10* mutation is temperature sensitive with respect to its effects both on increasing the incidence of male self progeny (Hodgkin *et al.*, 1979) and on fertility, and it was only about half as effective at 16°C as at 20°C in promoting mitotic duplication loss of *mnDp84*. Clearly, *him-10* may be very useful in raising frequencies of mitotic loss of duplications that are otherwise lost rarely.

Measuring the frequency of somatic duplication loss can be difficult if something is not already known about the focus of action of genes carried by the duplication, and it can be tedious in any case. One, however, can usually get some idea what the frequency of mitotic duplication loss will be simply by measuring the frequency at which the duplication is transmitted to self progeny. Figure 5 shows the relationship for a number of free duplications between the frequency of somatic duplication loss and the frequency of self progeny that fail to inherit the duplication. There seems to be a general but rather imprecise correlation between these two measures of duplication stability. The frequency of transmission of a duplication to self progeny depends on its premeiotic germ-line stability and its meiotic stability in both sperm and oocyte lines; it should perhaps not be surprising that the frequency of transmission of a duplication to self progeny is only a rough predictor of the duplication's somatic stability.

E. Potential Problems and Complications

1. Duplication Breakdown

Free duplications can become altered, either by recombination with the chromosome or by spontaneous mutation. Recombination appears to be very rare except for a few specific regions, as already noted. Spontaneous deletion formation, on the other hand, can occur at high frequency compared with chromosomal mutation rates (Herman, 1984; McKim and Rose, 1990; Villeneuve and Meyer, 1990). An animal that inherits an altered duplication, regardless of how the alteration occurred, can be mistakenly classified as a potential mosaic by virtue of exhibiting a recombinant phenotype (see Section II,C). It is thus important to confirm the mosaic nature of phenotypic recombinants by additional criteria, such as by showing with a cell-specific marker that some cells are mutant and others are wild type. The presence of an altered duplication will also be revealed by the phenotypes of a hermaphrodite's self progeny.

All altered duplications that have been studied were transmissable from parent to progeny and were therefore altered in the germ line. Recombination between duplication and homologous chromosome is presumably restricted, at least primarily, to meiosis, but it is not known if deletion formation in duplications is similarly restricted. If not, it is possible that duplications could suffer deletions in somatic cells, which could lead to incorrect conclusions about gene activity in mosaics. If, for example, a cell autonomous marker but not the gene being analyzed were deleted somatically to produce a clone, then one might conclude wrongly that the gene under study is cell nonautonomous. No clear example of this phenomenon has been demonstrated; one would need two cell autonomous markers on the same duplication and then need to show that loss of one marker could give rise to a mutant clone without simultaneously affecting expression of the other marker in the same cells. This experiment has not been done rigorously, but there have been several examples of mosaics in which two or more genes appeared to be invariably lost simultaneously from the descendants of a somatic cell; for example, Unc non-Dpy progeny of *dpy-1 ncl-1 unc-36; sDp3* hermaphrodites are expected to lack *unc-36*(+) from descendants of AB.p, and among 150 such animals, none was found in which *ncl-1*(+) was not missing from most if not all AB.p descendants (R. Herman, unpublished).

If duplications can suffer deletions somatically, we would in any case expect the frequency to be rare compared with the frequency of duplication loss: if a specific locus has a probability of deletion 1/500 per generation in the germ line, then the frequency of loss per cell division would be estimated at less than one-tenth this value when one takes into account the number of germ-line divisions occurring per generation. Finally, it was noted earlier that many putative duplication losses are associated with mitotic nondisjunction of the duplication; it seems unlikely that these events generate deleted duplications.

2. Consecutive Mosaics

In his analysis of *ncl-1* mosaics arising from *dpy-1 ncl-1; sDp3* animals, E. Hedgecock found animals in which *sDp3* was lost at two or three consecutive cell divisions. The frequency of such "consecutive mosaics" (Fig. 6) was rare compared with "simple mosaics" but higher than expected by chance. We do not know the mechanism of duplication loss in these cases; it might involve an error in replication or segregation of the duplication but seems unlikely to involve nondisjunction. In any case, we suppose that consecutive mosaics arise when an error at one cell division remains uncorrected at one or more succeeding cell

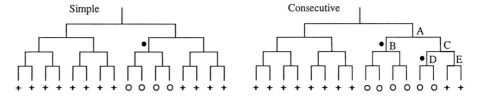

Fig. 6 Illustrations of simple and consecutive mosaics. The trees represent cell lineages. The terminally differentiated cells in the lineage have been scored for a cell autonomous marker carried by the free duplication; + indicates that the duplication is present and o indicates that it is absent. The heavy dots mark the presumed points of duplication loss within the cell lineages.

divisions. Consecutive mosaics have the potential for leading to mistakes in interpretation of mosaic results. Consider the consecutive mosaic illustrated in Fig. 6. Duplication losses occurred at cells B and D, daughter and granddaughter, respectively, of cell A. The experimentalist might see that descendants of both B and C, daughters of A, are mutant and conclude incorrectly that duplication loss occurred at A; that is, it would be wrongly concluded that the descendants of E also lack the duplication. This problem is avoided by scoring more cells in an animal for mosaicism; descendants of all four granddaughters of the cell in which duplication loss occurred should be mutant. If only a few cells can be scored, one should at least base conclusions on more than a very few mosaic animals.

3. Limitations Introduced by the Cell Lineage

The kinds of possible mosaic animals that can be generated by a single somatic duplication loss are obviously determined by the nature of the cell lineage, which is essentially invariant. This is usually not a serious problem when a gene is shown to act cell autonomously because fairly small mutant clones presumably can be identified, and small clones permit one to exclude from consideration as possible interacting cells all but perhaps the most closely related cells, which, because of the nature of the lineage, are often not very plausible candidates for interaction. Thus, in the mosaic analyses of *glp-1* (Austin and Kimble, 1991), *lin-12* (Seydoux and Greenwald, 1989), and *pal-1* (Waring and Kenyon, 1991), each of which had already been implicated in cell–cell signaling, the interacting cells that were analyzed were not closely related, and appropriate clones were found that showed that each gene acts not in the signaling cells but in the receiving cells. The cell lineage can become a serious limitation, however, when a gene's focus of action with respect to a particular phenotype is diffuse and distributed among cells of disparate lineage. In this case, the fully mutant phenotype may be apparent only in mosaic animals in which the duplication is lost by a progenitor of all or nearly all of the responsible cells; the examples of *unc-3* and *unc-36*, in which a fully uncoordinated phenotype requires that descendants of both AB.pl and AB.pr (the left and right daughters of AB.p) be mutant, have already been noted. The fact that AB.pl(−) (symbolizing duplication loss at AB.pl) and AB.pr (−) mosaics exhibit a semi-Unc-3 phenotype is consistent with the view that the focus of *unc-3* action is distributed among descendants of both AB.pl and AB.pr. Both of these cells generate many cell types, primarily neurons and hypodermis; a focus among motor neurons of the ventral and dorsal nerve cords was suggested for *unc-3*, primarily because duplication loss by AB.prp (posterior daughter of AB.pr) or AB.plp (posterior daughter of AB.pl), which generate cord motor neurons but do not contribute to the midhypodermis, led to semi-uncoordinated phenotypes (Herman, 1987).

Several hypodermal cells, including hyp7, which is a single cell covering much of the body, are syncytial, formed by the fusion of mononucleate cells, and the cells that fuse typically arise from distantly related parts of the lineage. Hyp7 is formed by cells that descend from both AB and P_1, the products of the very first embryonic cleavage; therefore, no simple mosaic can generate a completely mutant hyp7. The focus of *lin-15* action in promoting the formation of ectopic pseudovulvas (the Muv or multivulva phenotype; Ferguson and Horvitz, 1985) has been proposed to be in hyp7 (Herman and Hedgecock, 1990). In this case, duplication loss by AB.pl, AB.pr, or P_1 resulted in a variable and partial Muv phenotype, as if the level of *lin-15*(+) expression within the hyp7 syncytium was variably reduced below a critical level in these mosaic animals. The nature of the cell lineage makes it very difficult to conduct a finer-grained mosaic analysis of hyp7.

Mosaic analysis is usually undertaken with the purpose of testing a specific hypothesis or deciding between two alternative hypotheses. For some genes it may be enough to determine the phenotypes of a few very specific mosaics; for example, AB(−) mosaics and P_1(−) mosaics should distinguish between a neuronal and body muscle focus: all body muscles but one descend from P_1, and all nonpharyngeal neurons but one descend from AB (Sulston *et al.*, 1983).

4. Perdurance

Perdurance, the persistence of gene product after the gene has been lost, is clearly not a problem when a homozygous mutant clone results in a recessive mutant phenotype. When, however, a mutant clone does not result in a mutant phenotype, the possibility of perdurance must be considered. For example, in a mosaic analysis of *sdc-1,* a gene involved in both sex determination and dosage compensation, neither AB(−) nor P_1(−) mosaics exhibited any of the sexual transformations in cell fate that *sdc-1* causes in completely mutant animals. One possible interpretation (among others) of this result was that *sdc-1*(+) is transcribed in the one- or two-cell embryo and that this early transcription results in sufficient perdurance of *sdc-1*(+) product to produce a wild-type phenotype in the mosaics (Villeneuve and Meyer, 1990).

III. Fusing Two Unlinked Free Duplications

A duplication carrying the wild-type allele of a gene that one wants to analyze in mosaics may be available, but the duplication may not carry a cell autonomous marker for tracking its somatic loss. One possible solution to this problem is to fuse the duplication carrying the gene to be analyzed with a *ncl-1*(+)-bearing duplication. This approach was used successfully by Hunter and Wood (1992), who fused *ctDp8(V;f)[her-1(+)]* and *sDp3(III;f)[ncl-1(+)]* and then showed, using *ncl-1* on the fused duplication, that *her-1* behaves cell nonautonomously in its effect on sex determination. To fuse two unlinked duplications, one must first create a stock carrying both duplications in a suitable genetic background, in the above example, a strain of genotype (in part; only genes relevant to this discussion are given) *dpy-17 III; sDp3(III;f)* [*dpy-17(+) ncl-1(+)*]; *unc-42 V; ctDp8(V;f)*[*unc-42(+)her-1(+)*]. The two unlinked duplications segregated independently at meiosis, yielding the recombinant classes, Dpy non-Unc and Unc non-Dpy animals, as well as wild-type and Dpy Unc animals. After exposing hermaphrodites of this genotype to 3800 rad of gamma irradiation, wild-type progeny were picked to separate plates. Self progeny broods were then inspected for the presence of wild-type and Dpy Unc animals only, which would be the consequence of the fusion of the two duplications. One fused-duplication-bearing strain was found among 201 animals screened. In experiments of identical design, five fused duplications carrying *ncl-1(+)* and *unc-3(+)* were identified among 414 fertile F_1 progeny of γ-irradiated *sDp3(III;f)–mnDp14(X;f)*-bearing hermaphrodites, and one fused duplication carrying *ncl-1(+)* and *unc-6(+)* was identified among 538 *sDp3–mnDp30*-bearing hermaphrodites (R. Herman and C. Kari, unpublished). A potential difficulty with this approach is that the fused duplication is generally more stable than either of the constituent duplications, perhaps because of its larger size. The frequency of somatic duplication loss can then be stimulated by putting the fused duplication in a *him-10(e1551ts)* genetic background (as noted in Section II,D). The *him-10* gene maps near *ncl-1* and is carried by *sDp3*, but *mnDp90(III;f)*[*dpy-1(+) ncl-1(+) unc-36(+)*] has been derived from *sDp3* in such a way that it lacks the *him-10(+)* gene; it is therefore suggested that *mnDp90* is a good *ncl-1(+)*-bearing duplication to use for duplication fusions.

IV. Fusing a Free Duplication and an Extrachromosomal Transgenic Array

If a gene to be analyzed in mosaics has been cloned and if the cloned gene is capable of transforming mutant animals, then a synthetic duplication of the gene can be constructed. This approach was used by Leung-Hagesteijn *et al.* (1992) in their mosaic analysis of *unc-5*. These authors injected a cosmid clone containing *unc-5(+)* into the germ line of *unc-5* hermaphrodites and recovered transformed animals carrying a transgenic extrachromosomal array (see Chapter 19 in this volume) called *eEx15*. Such extrachromosomal arrays are transmitted during mitosis and meosis much like a free duplication, generally as a single copy per cell (Stinchcomb *et al.*, 1985). Next, animals of genotype *unc-5(e53); eEx15*[*unc-5(+)*]; *dpy-1 ncl-1; sDp3*[*dpy-1(+) ncl-1(+)*] were constructed. The extrachromosomal array and free duplication assorted independently, to give four classes of self progeny: non-Unc non-Dpy, non-Unc Dpy, Unc non-Dpy, and Unc Dpy. After irradiation with 3600 rad from a ^{137}Cs γ-ray source, non-Unc non-Dpy progeny were cultured individually. About 1% of the broods yielded only non-Unc non-Dpy and Unc Dpy self progeny, suggesting a linkage of the array and the free duplication. In three of nine such strains, the linked *unc 5(+)* and *dpy-1(+)* genes remained mitotically unstable, and one of these synthetic duplications, called *evEx8*, was shown to carry *ncl-1*(+) as well as *unc-5*(+) and *dpy-1*(+) and was used for mosaic analysis. The *unc-5* mosaics showed that *unc-5* acts cell autonomously in migrating cells and pioneering neurons, a result that supports the proposal that *unc-5* protein is a transmembrane receptor expressed on the surface of motile cells and growth cones to guide dorsalward movements (Leung-Hagesteijn *et al.*, 1992).

V. Using Extrachromosomal Arrays for Mosaic Analysis

If the gene one wants to analyze by mosaic analysis has been cloned, it is now possible to dispense entirely with free duplications for mosaic analysis, by generating an extrachromosomal array carrying both *ncl-1*(+) and the gene of interest (Lackner *et al.*, 1994; L. Miller, D. Waring and S. Kim, pers. comm.). One uses germ-line injection of DNA (see Chapter 19) containing the gene of interest, the cosmid C33C3 [which carries *ncl-1*(+)] and at least one additional gene that complements a visible marker to follow the transmission of the array from parent to progeny. The injected clones tend to form an extrachromosomal multicopy array (Stinchcomb *et al.*, 1985; Fire, 1986; Mello *et al.*, 1991; Chapter 19 in this volume); *in situ* hybridization has shown that such extrachromosomal arrays are subject to somatic loss (Stinchcomb *et al.*, 1985). The array used for mosaic analysis is maintained in a strain that is otherwise homozygous mutant for *ncl-1*, the gene of interest, and the visible marker, and the Ncl phenotype of individual cells is scored to track somatic loss of the extrachromosomal array. This approach was used by Lackner *et al.* (1994) to show that *mpk-1*, which encodes a mitogen-activated protein kinase affecting vulval development, acts cell autonomously in the vulval precursor cells. In addition, L. Miller and S. Kim (pers. comm.) have shown that *lin-31*, which is an HNF-3/*fork head* transcription factor homolog, also affects vulval cell fate determination cell autonomously.

This is potentially a powerful approach for mosaic analysis. The technique is new, however, and it will be important to confirm that the patterns of mosaic expression are generally due to loss of the array rather than to spotty expression. As discussed by Mello and Fire in Chapter 19, the expression of individual transgenes has frequently been shown to vary from animal to animal, and the variability seems not to be attributable solely to somatic duplication loss. This is most obvious in transgenic lines in which the DNA is integrated; these lines may also exhibit variable expression. Factors affecting mosaic expression, such as copy number of the transforming DNA, are discussed by Mello and Fire (in Chapter 19). The overall pattern of transgene expression is generally deduced from the average pattern obtained from several animals (see, for example, Krause *et al.*, 1994), but this approach may not be easy to apply to the analysis of genetic mosaics.

There are other potential problems with using extrachromosomal arrays for mosaic analysis. In some cases, for example, transgenes are expressed in inappropriate tissues, apparently as a consequence of being driven by inappropriate promoters or of lacking negative regulatory sequences (see Chapter 19). Extra-chromosomal arrays may also introduce unexpected dominant effects, which apparently can result from a variety of causes (see Chapter 19). Finally, it is possible that overexpression from a transgenic array may magnify perdurance effects. All of these potential problems are array specific, which means that they should be assessed for each extrachromosomal array used in mosaic analysis.

VI. Other Methods for Generating Mosaics

A. Transposon Excision

The *C. elegans* transposable element Tc1 is subject to somatic excision at high frequency (for review, see Moerman and Waterston, 1989). The excision events tend to be imprecise, but some of the excisions may restore, at least partially, a wild-type phenotype. Among animals carrying Tc1 inserted in *unc-54*, a structural gene for myosin heavy chain, Eide and Anderson (1985) found animals showing patches of partially revertant body wall muscle, as revealed by polarized light microscopy. Similarly, Moerman *et al.* (1988) identified mosaics in which Tc1 had excised somatically from the *unc-22* gene, which encodes a large muscle protein. Revertant muscle cells were shown to react with antibody to the *unc-22* protein, whereas contiguous nonrevertant cells did not. It was concluded from this result that *unc-22* acts cell autonomously within body muscle cells. This method of generating mosaics does not allow one to use a separate genetic marker for assessing cellular genotypes of the mosaic animals.

B. Targeted Single-Cell Induction of Gene Products

Stringham and Candido (1993) have described a novel scheme for inducing gene expression within selected *C. elegans* cells. They constructed transgenic strains carrying a heat shock gene promoter fused to *lacZ* (see Chapter 19 in this volume) and then used a laser microbeam to induce a sublethal heat shock to individual cells. It was found that the cells so treated, whether of endodermal, mesodermal, or ectodermal origin, were induced to synthesize β-galactosidase. This technique may thus allow one to express a cloned gene in whatever cells one wants at whatever time one wants; this method might be particularly useful for looking at the consequences of selected ectopic expression of a cloned gene.

VII. Conclusions

Important information is likely to be obtained from the mosaic analysis of many more genes in *C. elegans*. The methods described here are likely to be refined; as more and more genes are cloned, the technique that makes use of extrachromosomal arrays containing $ncl-1(+)$ as a cell marker is likely to become increasingly popular.

Good candidates for mosaic analysis are genes that affect patterns of cell lineage, cell migration, or neuron process outgrowth; it is often not clear at the outset that these genes will behave cell autonomously. When molecular analysis has shown that a gene is expressed specifically in the same cells that are affected phenotypically by mutation in the gene, the inference may seem strong that the gene is behaving cell autonomously, in which case the impetus to conduct a mosaic analysis is lessened. On the other hand, a gene may be expressed in many cells, most neurons for example, and only be required functionally in a subset; mosaic analysis may be required to demonstrate this. It is also possible that eliminating gene expression in some cells (in mosaic animals) will lead to a novel or intermediate phenotype, which may be informative.

A few mosaic studies of lethals have been performed (Park and Horvitz, 1986; Johnson *et al.*, 1988; Bucher and Greenwald, 1991), and it seems likely that essential genes will be good subjects for future mosaic work; without mosaics, only the lethal arrest phenotype may be available for study. Two broad questions about lethals may be addressed. First, what is the lethal focus of the gene? That is, what kinds of mosaics are viable and what kinds are inviable? And second, what are the cellular and behavioral phenotypes of various mosaics in which different sets of cells are genotypically mutant?

Acknowledgment

I acknowledge support from National Institutes of Health Grant GM-22387.

References

Akerib, C. C., and Meyer, B. J. (1994). Identification of X chromosome regions in *Caenorhabditis elegans* that contain sex determination signal elements. *Genetics* **138**, 1105–1125.

Albertson, D. G., and Thomson, J. N. (1982). The kinetochores of *Caenorhabditis elegans. Chromosoma* **86**, 409–428.

Albertson, D. G., and Thomson, J. N. (1993). Segregation of holocentric chromosomes at meiosis in the nematode, *Caenorhabditis elegans. Chromos. Res.* **1**, 15–26.

Austin, J., and Kimble, J. (1987). *glp-1* is required in the germ line for regulation of the decision between mitosis and meiosis in C. elegans. *Cell* **51**, 589–599.

Blumenthal, T., Squire, M., Kirtland, S., Cane, J., Donegan, M., Spieth, J., and Sharrock, W. (1984). Cloning of a yolk protein gene family from *Caenorhabditis elegans. J. Mol. Biol.* **174**, 1–18.

Bucher, E. A., and Greenwald, I. (1991). A genetic mosaic screen of essential zygotic genes in *Caenorhabditis elegans. Genetics* **128**, 281–292.

DeLong, L., Casson, L. P., and Meyer, B. J. (1987). Assessment of X chromosome dosage compensation in *Caenorhabditis elegans* by phenotypic analysis of *lin-14. Genetics* **117**, 657–670.

Eide, D., and Anderson, P. (1985). Transposition of Tc1 in the nematode *Caenorhabditis elegans. Proc. Natl. Acad. Sci. U.S.A.* **82**, 1756–1760.

Ferguson, E. L., and Horvitz, H. R. (1985). Identification and characterization of 22 genes that affect the vulval cell lineages of the nematode *Caenorhabditis elegans. Genetics* **110**, 17–72.

Fire, A. (1986). Integrative transformation of *Caenorhabditis elegans*. *EMBO J.* **5,** 2673–2680.

Garcia-Bellido, A., and Merriam, J. R. (1971). Genetic analysis of cell heredity in imaginal discs of *Drosophila melanogaster*. *Proc. Natl. Acad. Sci. U.S.A.* **68,** 2222–2226.

Hedgecock, E. M., Culotti, J. G., Thomson, J. N., and Perkins, L. A. (1985). Axonal guidance mutants of *Caenorhabditis elegans* identified by filling sensory neurons with fluorescein dyes. *Dev. Biol.* **111,** 158–170.

Herman, R. K. (1984). Analysis of genetic mosaics of the nematode *Caenorhabditis elegans*. *Genetics* **106,** 165–180.

Herman, R. K. (1987). Mosaic analysis of two genes that affect nervous system structure in *Caenorhabditis elegans*. *Genetics* **116,** 377–388.

Herman, R. K. (1989). Mosaic analysis in the nematode *Caenorhabditis elegans*. *J. Neurogenet.* **5,** 1–24.

Herman, R. K., and Hedgecock, E. M. (1990). Limitation of the size of the vulval primordium of *Caenorhabditis elegans* by *lin-15* expression in surrounding hypodermis. *Nature* **348,** 169–171.

Herman, R. K., and Kari, C. K. (1985). Muscle-specific expression of a gene affecting actylcholinesterase in the nematode *Caenorhabditis elegans*. *Cell* **40,** 509–514.

Herman, R. K., and Kari, C. K. (1989). Recombination between small X chromosomal duplications and the X chromosome in *Caenorhabditis elegans*. *Genetics* **21,** 723–737.

Herman, R. K., Albertson, D. G., and Brenner, S. (1976). Chromosome rearrangements in *Caenorhabditis elegans*. *Genetics* **83,** 91–105.

Herman, R. K., Madl, J. E., and Kari, C. K. (1979). Duplications in *Caenorhabditis elegans*. *Genetics* **92,** 419–435.

Herman, R. K., Kari, C. K., and Hartman, P. S. (1982). Dominant X-chromosome nondisjunction mutants of *Caenorhabditis elegans*. *Genetics* **102,** 379–400.

Hodgkin, J., Horvitz, H. R., and Brenner, S. (1979). Nondisjunction mutants of the nematode *Caenorhabditis elegans*. *Genetics* **91,** 67–94.

Hodgkin, J., Zellan, J. D., and Albertson, D. G. (1994). Identification of a candidate primary sex determination locus, *fox-1*, on the *X* chromosome of *Caenorhabditis elegans*. *Development* **120,** 3681–3689.

Horvitz, H. R., Brenner, S., Hodgkin, J., and Herman, R. K. (1979). A uniform genetic nomenclature for the nematode *Caenorhabditis elegans*. *Mol. Gen. Genet.* **175,** 129–133.

Hunter, C. P., and Wood, W. B. (1990). The *tra-1* gene determines sexual phenotype cell-autonomously in C. elegans. *Cell* **63,** 1193–1204.

Hunter, C. P., and Woods, W. B. (1992). Evidence from mosaic analysis of the masculinizing gene *her-1* for cell interactions in C. elegans sex determination. *Nature* **355,** 551–555.

Johnson, C. D., Rand, J. B., Herman, R. K., Stern, B. D., and Russell, R. L. (1988). The acetylcholinesterase genes of *Caenorhabditis elegans:* Identification of a third gene (*ace-3*) and mosaic mapping of a synthetic lethal phenotype. *Neuron* **1,** 165–173.

Kenyon, C. (1986). A gene involved in the development of the posterior body region of C. elegans. *Cell* **46,** 477–481.

Kimble, J. E., and Sharrock, W. J. (1983). Tissue-specific synthesis of yolk proteins in *Caenorhabditis elegans*. *Dev. Biol.* **96,** 189–196.

Kimble, J., and Ward, S. (1988). Germ-line development and fertilization. *In* "The Nematode *Caenorhabditis elegans*" (W. B. Wood, ed.), pp. 191–213. Cold Spring Harbor Laboratory, Cold Spring Harbor, New York.

Krause, M., Harrison, S. W., Xu, S.-Q., Chen, L., and Fire, A. (1994). Elements regulating cell- and stage-specific expression of the C. elegans MyoD family homolog *hlh-1*. *Dev. Biol.* **166,** 133–148.

Lackner, M. R., Kornfeld, K., Miller, L. M., Horvitz, H. R., and Kim, S. K. (1994). A MAP kinase homolog, *mpk-1*, is involved in *ras*-mediated induction of vulval cell fates in *Caenorhabditis elegans*. *Genes Dev.* **8,** 160–173.

Lawrence, P. A. (1992). "The Making of a Fly" Blackwell, Oxford.

Leung-Hagesteijn, C., Spence, A. M., Stern, B. D., Zhou, Y., Su, M.-W., Hedgecock, E. M., and Culotti, J. G. (1992). UNC-5, a transmembrane protein with immunoglobulin and thrombospondin type 1 domains, guides cell and pioneer axon migrations in C. elegans. *Cell* **71,** 289–299.

McKim, K. S., and Rose, A. M. (1990). Chromosome *I* duplications in *Caenorhabditis elegans*. *Genetics* **124,** 115–132.

McKim, K. S., Howell, A. M., and Rose, A. M. (1988). The effects of translocations on recombination frequency in *Caenorhabditis elegans*. *Genetics* **120,** 987–1001.

McKim, K. S., Peters, K., and Rose, A. M. (1993). Two types of sites required for meiotic chromosome pairing in *Caenorhabditis elegans*. *Genetics* **134,** 749–768.

Mello, C, C., Kramer, J. M., Stinchcomb, D., and Ambros, V. (1991). Efficient gene transfer in *C. elegans:* Extrachromosomal maintenance and integration of transforming sequences. *EMBO J.* **10,** 3959–3970.

Moerman, D. G., and Waterston, R. H. (1989). Mobile elements in *Caenorhabditis elegans* and other nematodes. *In* "Mobile DNA" (D. E. Berg and M. H. Howe, eds.), pp. 537–556. American Society for Microbiology, Washington, D.C.

Moerman, D. G., Benian, G. M., Barstead, R. J., Schriefer, L. A., and Waterston, R. H. (1988). Identification and intracellular localization of the *unc-22* gene product of *Caenorhabditis elegans*. *Genes Dev.* **2,** 93–105.

Park, E.-C., and Horvitz, H. R. (1986). *C. elegans unc-105* mutations affect muscle and are suppressed by other mutations that affect muscle. *Genetics* **113,** 853–867.

Perkins, L. A., Hedgecock, E. M., Thomson, J. N., and Culotti, J. G. (1986). Mutant sensory cilia in the nematode *Caenorhabditis elegans*. *Dev. Biol.* **117,** 456–487.

Rogalski, T. M., and Riddle, D. L. (1988). A *Caenorhabditis elegans* RNA polymerase II gene, *ama-1 IV,* and nearby essential genes. *Genetics* **118,** 61–74.

Rose, A. M., Baillie, D. L., and Curran, J. (1984). Meiotic pairing behavior of two free duplications of linkage group *I* in *Caenorhabditis elegans*. *Mol. Gen. Genet.* **195,** 52–56.

Rosenbluth, R. E., Cuddeford, C., and Baillie, D. L. (1985). Mutagenesis in *Caenorhabditis elegans*. II. A spectrum of mutational events induced with 1500 R of γ-irradiation. *Genetics* **109,** 493–511.

Seydoux, G., and Greenwald, I. (1989). Cell autonomy of *lin-12* function in a cell fate decision in C. elegans. *Cell* **57,** 1237–1245.

Seydoux, G., Schedl, T., and Greenwald, I. (1990). Cell-cell interactions prevent a potential inductive interaction between soma and germline in C. elegans. *Cell* **61,** 939–951.

Sharrock, W. J. (1984). Cleavage of two yolk proteins from a precursor in *Caenorhabditis elegans*. *J. Mol. Biol.* **174,** 419–431.

Spieth, J,, and Blumenthal, T. (1985). The *Caenorhabditis elegans* vitellogenin gene family includes a gene encoding a distantly related protein *Mol. Cell. Biol.* **5,** 2495–2501.

Starich, T. A., Herman, R. K., and Shaw, J. E. (1993). Molecular and genetic analysis of *unc-7,* a *Caenorhabditis elegans* gene required for coordinated locomotion. *Genetics* **133,** 527–541.

Starich, T. A., Herman, R. K., Kari, C. K., Yeh, W.-H., Schackwitz, W. S., Schuyler, M. W., Collet, J., Thomas, J. H., and Riddle, D. L. (1995). Mutations affecting chemosensory neurons of *Caenorhabditis elegans*. *Genetics* **139,** 171–188.

Stewart, H. I., Rosenbluth, R. E., and Baillie, D. L. (1991). Most ultraviolet irradiation induced mutations in the nematode *Caenorhabditis elegans* are chromosomal rearrangements. *Mutat. Res.* **249,** 37–54.

Stinchcomb, D. T., Shaw, J. E., Carr, S. H., and Hirsh, D. (1985). Extrachromosomal DNA transformation of *Caenorhabditis elegans*. *Mol. Cell. Biol.* **5,** 3484–3496.

Stringham, E. G., and Candido, E. P. M. (1993). Targeted single-cell induction of gene products in *Caenorhabditis elegans:* A new tool for developmental studies. *J. Exp. Zool.* **266,** 227–233.

Sulston, J., and Hodgkin, J. (1988). Methods. *In* "The Nematode *Caenorhabditis elegans*" (W. B. Wood, ed.), pp. 587–606. Cold Spring Harbor Laboratory, Cold Spring Harbor, New York.

Sulston, J. E., and Horvitz, H. R. (1977). Postembryonic cell lineages of the nematode *Caenorhabditis elegans*. *Dev. Biol.* **56,** 110–156.

Sulston, J. E., Schierenberg, E., White, J. G., and Thomson, J. N. (1983). The embryonic cell lineage of the nematode *Caenorhabditis elegans*. *Dev. Biol.* **100,** 64–119.

Villeneuve, A. M., and Meyer, B. J. (1990). The role of *sdc-1* in the sex determination and dosage compensation decisions in *Caenorhabditis elegans*. *Genetics* **124,** 91–114.

Waring, D. A., and Kenyon, C. (1991). Regulation of cellular responsiveness to inductive signals in the developing *C. elegans* nervous system. *Nature* **350,** 712–715.

Wilkins, A. S. (1993). "Genetics of Animal Development" 2d ed. Wiley-Liss, New York.

Yuan, J. Y., and Horvitz, H. R. (1990). The *Caenorhabditis elegans* genes *ced-3* and *ced-4* act cell autonomously to cause programmed cell death. *Dev. Biol.* **138,** 33–41.

CHAPTER 7

Genetic Balancers

Mark L. Edgley, * **David L. Baillie,** † **Donald L. Riddle,** ‡ **and Ann M. Rose** *

* Department of Medical Genetics
University of British Columbia
Vancouver, British Columbia
Canada V6T 1Z3
† Institute of Molecular Biology and Biochemistry
Simon Fraser University
Burnaby, British Columbia
Canada V5A 1S6
‡ Division of Biological Sciences
University of Missouri
Columbia, Missouri 65211

I. Introduction

Genetic balancers are genetic constructs or chromosomal rearrangements that allow lethal or sterile mutations to be stably maintained in heterozygotes. In this chapter we use the term *balancer* primarily to refer to chromosomal duplications or rearrangements that suppress crossing over. In addition, we define *lethal* as any mutation that blocks survival or reproduction. Phenotypes associated with lethal mutations in *Caenorhabditis elegans* range from egg or larval lethality to adult sterility and maternal effect lethality, and can include conditional effects such as temperature sensitivity. The number of essential genes in *C. elegans* (those identified by lethal mutations) may range as high as 7000 according to genetic estimates (Clark *et al.*, 1988; Howell and Rose, 1990; Johnsen and Baillie, 1991). Thus, lethal mutations constitute a rich source of information about basic biological processes in this nematode.

This chapter assumes the reader is somewhat familiar with *C. elegans* genetic nomenclature. A few basic definitions are given here,[1] but for full reference see Horvitz *et al.*, (1979).

Maintenance of mutations is an important aspect of *C. elegans* genetics. Genetic strains carrying nonconditional recessive lethal mutations, at present the largest class of lethals, cannot be kept as homozygotes, and in heterozygotes the mutations can be lost easily through segregation unless there is a means to identify the heterozygotes that carry them. Maintainance of the heterozygous genotype from one generation to the next requires selection of heterozygous individuals, a task that becomes burdensome if more than a few strains must be maintained. For example, the self progeny of an unmarked recessive lethal heterozygote (*let-x*/+) are either arrested *let-x* homozygotes (*let-x*/*let-x*), *let-x* heterozygotes (*let-x*/+), or wild-type animals (+/+) that cannot be distinguished phenotypically from heterozygotes. Many phenotypically wild-type animals must be selected each generation to ensure the propagation of heterozygotes, and the presence of the lethal mutation must be confirmed through direct observation of *let-x*

---

[1] Gene names are italicized and consist of three lowercase letters, followed by a hyphen and isolation number for individual genes. The name is usually a mnemonic referring to the nature of mutations in the gene. For example, the name *dpy* refers to a class of mutation characterized by a short, fat body, and stands for *dumpy*. The name *dpy-18* refers to a particular *dpy* gene. Some other names used throughout the chapter are *let* (lethal), *unc* (uncoordinated), *lon* (long), *rol* (roller), and *bli* (blistered). Phenotypes are represented by nonitalicized gene names with the first letter capitalized. For example, the general phenotype for all *dpy* mutations is written Dpy, and the phenotype for *dpy-18* mutations is written Dpy-18. Rearrangement names are italicized and consist of a lowercase laboratory allele prefix followed by a capitalized abbreviation indicating the type of rearrangement, an isolation number, and optional chromosomal origin and location information in parentheses. For example, the name *sDp2(I;f)* represents the second chromosomal duplication isolated in the Baillie laboratory (allele prefix "s"). The "I;f" indicates that it is a duplication of part of LG I and that it is "free" (not attached to another chromosome). For translocations, the parenthetical information indicates the chromosomes involved. For example, *eT1(III;V)* indicates a translocation between LG III and LG V. The rearrangement abbreviations used here are *C* (dominant crossover supressor), *Df* (deficiency), *Dp* (duplication), *In* (inversion), and *T* (translocation).

homozygotes. If the normal homolog carries a morphological marker, *in trans* to the lethal mutation, heterozygotes can be reliably identified; however, loss of the lethal can still occur through recombination and subsequent segregation. For example, in a *let +/+ dpy* heterozygote, a crossover between the *let* and *dpy* loci produces two recombinant chromosomes, one that carries both mutations and one that is completely wild type. A zygote carrying the wild-type recombinant chromosome and a parental *dpy* chromosome (*+/dpy*) will have a wild-type phenotype, and will produce wild-type and Dpy progeny just as the original heterozygote, but the desired lethal will no longer be present in the strain. Thus, the presence of the lethal in each generation still must be confirmed through direct observation or be deduced through the ratio of wild-type to Dpy progeny, which is very tedious (about 2 : 1 in *let +/+ dpy* heterozygotes and 3 : 1 in *+/dpy* heterozygotes).

Clearly, any sort of large-scale isolation and analysis of lethal mutations requires more effective methods to prevent their loss. The investigator must have an easy way to distinguish between progeny heterozygous for a lethal-bearing chromosome and those homozygous for the nonlethal homolog and, further, must be able either to detect directly when recombination has occured between the lethal mutation and marker mutations or to reduce the incidence of recombination to a negligible level. A balancer provides these functions.

Many different genetic constructs (genotypes) have been used to balance lethal mutations, but they have the same basic characteristics: (1) heterozygotes possess a unique phenotype (wild type or mutant) so that they can be selected reliably; (2) progeny phenotypes allow the investigator to tell when recombination has occurred; (3) close proximity of markers increases the degree of balancing by decreasing the frequency of recombination between lethals and markers; and (4) in the majority of cases, common visible markers linked to the lethals ease all phases of analysis.

Linking lethals to morphological markers is especially helpful for analysis, as it is much easier to score for the absence of a particular morphological phenotype than to score arrested progeny. Furthermore, linked markers facilitate two-factor mapping, and markers common to an entire set of lethals allow rapid *inter se* complementation tests. For example, recombination frequency can be measured between a lethal mutation and a linked marker mutation by scoring viable marker homozygotes among the progeny segregated from a heterozygote. Complementation between two lethal mutations can be assayed by performing a cross to construct animals heterozygous for both lethals and the same marker mutation, and scoring for marker homozygotes. Presence of these homozygotes indicates complementation, and absence indicates failure to complement.

Three examples of the use of simple genotypes to balance lethal mutations follow. To maintain newly generated deficiencies on linkage group (LG) III that were lethal as homozygotes, Greenwald and Horvitz (1980) kept them as heterozygotes over an *unc-93 dpy-17* chromosome. These animals were Unc-93 in phenotype because the deficiencies deleted *unc-93*, and they segregated Unc-

93, Unc-93 Dpy-17, and lethal (deficiency homozygote) progeny. The deficiencies could be maintained by picking Unc animals, as the recombination frequency between *dpy-17* and the deficiency endpoints was low. In a second example, Moerman and Baillie (1979) isolated lethals linked to a conditionally dominant *unc-22* mutation, which causes dominant twitching in the presence of 1% nicotine. Conditional dominance results in a unique heterozygous phenotype. In screens for new mutations, worms heterozygous for *unc-22* were screened for the absence or near absence of fertile adult Unc-22 progeny. Once obtained, these lethals could be maintained by picking animals that moved normally but were induced to twitch in 1% nicotine. Crossing over between a lethal and *unc-22* was easily detected by scoring the rare Unc-22 progeny in the absence of nicotine. The closer the lethal was to *unc-22*, the less often recombinational loss occurred. In a third example, Rose and Baillie (1980) mutagenized a phenotypically wild-type strain of genotype + *unc-15* +/*dpy-14* + *unc-13* and screened for lethal mutations linked to the *dpy-14 unc-13 I* chromosome. The new lethals were maintained simply by picking wild-type animals (heterozygotes) and checking to see that they gave wild-type and Unc-15 progeny but no Dpy-14 Unc-13 progeny. Lethals were balanced because of the short genetic distances. In all cases, recombination was easily detected by the presence of Dpy, Unc, or DpyUnc recombinant animals among the self progeny of a heterozygote. The types and numbers of recombinant progeny gave distance and gene order relative to the markers.

A drawback of these methods is that they are not easily adapted for the isolation of large numbers of lethal mutations over large genetic regions. They may require many different sets of appropriate marker mutations, which either may be too difficult to score or may not exist. A more sophisticated approach makes use of heterozygous chromosomal rearrangements adapted for use as balancers. There are two types of balancing rearrangements: (1) those that reduce or eliminate recombination between a lethal-bearing chromosome and a homolog carrying a wild-type allele of the locus, and (2) those that provide an extrachromosomal or integrated wild-type allele that complements a homozygous lethal mutation. As balancers, these rearrangements have several advantages over simple marked chromosomes. They can balance large genomic regions, and the choice of markers to which lethals can be linked is much broader, requiring only that the markers lie in the balanced region. By virtue of their effects on recombination, they can be heritably stable vehicles for the maintenance of large numbers of lethal mutations. Finally, genetic variants of the rearrangements themselves can be generated to aid in strain construction, mutant screens, and analysis of balancer structure.

Rearrangements as balancers are the focus of this chapter. We describe the features and behavior of each class of balancer currently used in *C. elegans*, using a well-characterized member of the class; present a discussion of the practical aspects of day-to-day balancer use; give an overview of the state of balancing for each chromosome; and lay out in guidebook form information for understanding and maintaining the most commonly used *C. elegans* balancers and their genetic variants. A great deal of detailed analysis beyond the scope of this chapter has been accumulated on balancers (see citations for individual rearrangements), and we encourage the reader to seek out the published works for a more complete understanding of the behavior of particular balancers. Information contained in the cited work is especially helpful when designing mutant screens and carrying out complementation and mapping protocols.

II. Types of Balancers

In *C. elegans*, Herman *et al.* (1976) first characterized duplications with the intention of using them to recover recessive lethal mutations on the X chromosome. Subsequent work by many different groups has resulted in the isolation and characterization of an array of rearrangement types that together balance approximately 65% of the *C. elegans* genome. These rearrangements, including translocations, duplications, and inversions, constitute a powerful set of tools for investigators. In addition, other dominant crossover suppressors and transgenes have been adapted for use as balancers. The physical structures of several balancers have been deduced through genetic analysis. Recent work using fluorescence *in situ* hybridization (FISH) analysis (see Chapter 15 in this volume) shows the potential for determining balancer structure through molecular means. The following discussion gives an overview of the different classes of balancer.

A. Translocations

Translocations are chromosomal rearrangements in which parts of nonhomologous chromosomes are exchanged (Fig 1). Translocations in *C. elegans* have been

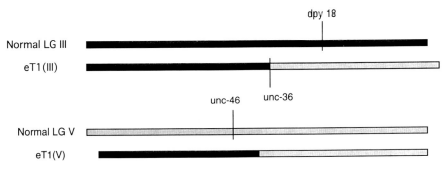

Fig. 1 Diagram of reciprocal translocation *eT1*, showing mutations present in the reference heterozygous strain. The *dpy-18* and *unc-46* mutations are carried on the normal chromosomes, and the *unc-36* mutation is caused by the breakpoint of the translocation on LG III. Recombination is suppressed in the region to the right of *unc-36* on LG III, balancing *dpy-18*, and in the region to the left of *unc-42* on LG V (not shown, see Fig. 7), balancing *unc-46*. *eT1(III)* recombines with the normal LG III in the region to the left of *unc-36*. *eT1(V)* recombines with the normal LG V in the region to the right of *unc-23* (not shown, see Fig. 7).

recovered in specific screens for X-chromosome nondisjunction (Herman *et al.*, 1982), suppression of recombination between widely spaced linked markers (Herman, 1978; Fodor and Deak, 1985), linked lethals (Rosenbluth *et al.*, 1985; McKim *et al.*, 1993), and pseudolinkage of normally unlinked marker mutations (McKim *et al.*, 1988, 1993). A number of existing translocations have been characterized genetically, and several have proven to be reliable balancers for lethal mutant screens (*eT1*: Rosenbluth and Baillie, 1981; Rosenbluth *et al.*, 1983; *nT1*: Clark *et al.*, 1988; *hT1*: Howell and Rose, 1990). They balance large genomic regions, and they are easily manipulated in genetic crosses.

The first *C. elegans* translocation for which reciprocal exchange of chromosomal segments was demonstrated is *eT1(III;V)* (Rosenbluth and Baillie, 1981), which is viable as a homozygote and was originally called *unc-72* (Brenner, 1974). Marker mutations crossed onto or induced on *eT1* were employed to show linkage between appropriate normally unlinked markers on both half-translocations. Several other translocations have since been shown to be reciprocal using similar protocols, for example, *mnT2* and *mnT10* (Herman *et al.*, 1982); *szT1* and *hT1* (McKim *et al.*, 1988); and *hT2* (McKim *et al.*, 1993). Segregation data for *nT1* (Ferguson and Horvitz, 1985; Clark *et al.*, 1988) and *hT3* (McKim *et al.*, 1993) are consistent with their being reciprocal translocations, but rigorous proof is lacking.

In the case of *eT1*, the left portion of LG V is translocated to the left portion of LG III, and the right portion of III is translocated to the right portion of V (Fig. 1). In heterozygotes, the half-translocation carrying the left portion of III [referred to as *eT1(III)*] recombines with the normal III in the region to the left of *unc-36*, and the half-translocation carrying the right portion of V [*eT1(V)*] recombines with the normal V in the region to the right of *unc-23* (refer to Fig. 7 for position of markers). The regions that recombine segregate from each other during meiosis (Rosenbluth and Baillie, 1981; McKim *et al.*, 1988, 1993). Thus, *eT1(III)* segregates from the normal III, and *eT1(V)* segregates from the normal LG V. Recombination is suppressed along the length of the translocated portion of each chromosome, from *unc-36* to the right end of LG III, and from between *unc-23* and *unc-42* to the left end of LG V. The boundaries of crossover suppression thus correspond to the translocation breakpoints. Recombination is not suppressed in the regions that segregate from their normal homologs, from *unc-36* to the left end of LG III, and from between *unc-23* and *unc-42* to the right end of LG V; nor is it suppressed in *eT1* homozygotes. These observations have led to the proposal that these regions do not recombine in heterozygotes due to their inability to pair with normal homologs (Rosenbluth and Baillie, 1981). To maintain the translocation as a heterozygote, the normal homologs are marked with morphological mutations in the recombination-suppressed region [in the case of *eT1*, the most frequently used strain carries *dpy-18(III)* and *unc-46(V)*]. In this way, heterozygotes (which have a wild-type phenotype) can be distinguished from normal homolog homozygotes. Self progeny of *eT1* heterozygotes are wild-type heterozygotes; *eT1* homozygotes (which have an Unc-36 phenotype because the translocation breakpoint lies in the *unc-36* gene on LG III); Dpy-18 Unc-46 homozygotes; and a large percentage of aneuploid progeny (10/16) that arrest development (Fig. 2) as embryos or early larvae (Turner and Baillie, unpublished results; Adames and Rose, unpublished results). Aneuploid progeny are those with an abnormal complement of chromosomes. Figure 2 illustrates how they arise. The *unc-46* and *dpy-18* mutations appear to be linked (they are pseudolinked) because all singly mutant homozygotes are aneuploid, and this arrangement cannot break down in the absence of recombination. If a strain carries a recessive lethal mutation in the recombination-suppressed region

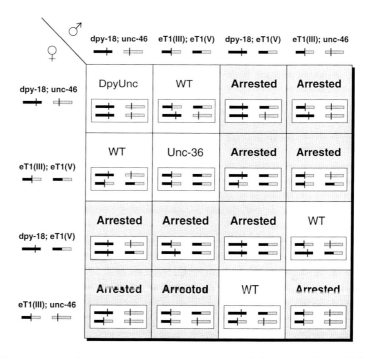

Fig. 2 Punnett square showing normal progeny genotypes and phenotypes that result from selfing a *dpy-18/eT1 III; unc-46/eT1 V* heterozygote. Phenotypes are indicated for each progeny class. Genotypes for gametes and zygotes are given in gene and rearrangement names according to standard nomenclature, and in drawings representing normal and translocation chromosomes with genetic markers in place. The normal LG III is shown as a black bar, with a vertical line indicating the position of the *dpy-18* mutation. The normal LG V is shown as a shaded bar, with a vertical line indicating the position of the *unc-46* mutation. The half-translocation *eT1(III)* is shown as a half-black, half-shaded bar with a vertical line indicating the position of the *unc-36* mutation caused by the translocation breakpoint on LG III. The half-translocation *eT1(V)* is shown as a half-black, half-shaded bar with no vertical line. Boxes of the square representing viable progeny are unshaded. Boxes representing aneuploid progeny, all of which arrest during development, are shaded. All wild-type progeny are heterozygous for the translocation chromosomes and the normal chromosomes. Unc-36 progeny are *eT1* homozygotes, and Dpy Unc progeny are *dpy-18; unc-46* homozygotes. Aneuploid progeny account for 10/16ths of the total.

of either normal homolog, all of the homozygous DpyUnc progeny will die. To characterize these arrested animals, they must not be confused with aneuploid progeny segregated by translocation heterozygotes (See section III,F,6 for more detailed discussion).

B. Duplications

Duplications are chromosomal segments that are present in the nucleus in addition to a full complement of normal chromosomes (Fig. 3). Duplications have been generated by mutagenesis with ionizing radiation or UV light, and recovered as genetic elements that rescue the phenotypic expression of particular mutations (Herman *et al.*, 1976, 1979, 1982; Hodgkin, 1980; Greenwald *et al.*, 1983; Herman, 1984, 1987; Meneely and Wood, 1984; Rose *et al.*, 1984; Rosenbluth *et al.*, 1985, 1988; Austin and Kimble, 1989; DeLong *et al.*, 1987; Meneely and Nordstrom, 1988; Rogalski and Riddle, 1988; Herman and Kari, 1989; Howell and Rose, 1990; Hunter and Wood, 1990; McKim and Rose, 1990; Yuan and Horvitz, 1990; Stewart *et al.*, 1991; Marra and Baillie, 1994). They have also been recovered as exceptional segregants from translocation strains (*mnDp11*: Herman *et al.*, 1982; *szDp1*: McKim *et al.*, 1988; *hDp133, hDp134, hDp135*: McKim *et al.*,

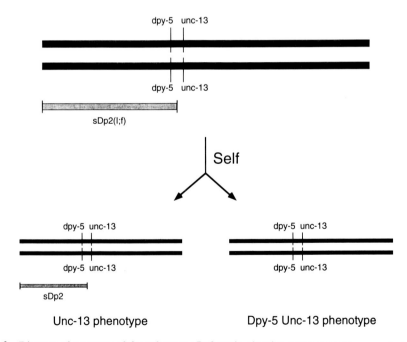

Fig. 3 Diagram of genotype of the reference *sDp2* strain, showing progeny genotypes and phenotypes that result from selfing. The strain is homozygous for *dpy-5* and *unc-13* mutations, and carries one copy of *sDp2*. Animals of this genotype are Unc-13 in phenotype. Progeny not carrying the duplication are Dpy-5 Unc-13.

1993), and as products of a rare recombination event in an inversion strain (Zetka and Rose, 1992). Most duplications in *C. elegans* are "free" elements that segregate in a non-Mendelian fashion. They have been described as extrachromosomal fragments of genetic material, and they can be lost both mitotically and meiotically during gametogenesis (Herman *et al.,* 1976). Mitotic chromosomes exhibit multiple spindle attachment points (Albertson and Thomson, 1982), whereas meiotic chromosomes exhibit a localized spindle attachment point (Albertson and Thomson, 1993). Hence, mitotic segregation of chromosome fragments is more easily understood than is meiotic segregation. The mechanism of free duplication transmission during meiosis is unknown. Each duplication has a characteristic frequency of transmission to gametes. Generally, the larger the duplication, the more stable it is in the germ line (McKim and Rose, 1990). Mitotic loss of certain free duplications from somatic cells during development has made possible mosaic analysis of the gene function (see Chapter 6 in this volume). A small percentage of duplications exist as integrants into otherwise normal chromosomes, in which case segregation becomes Mendelian. Many duplications have been used as balancers (e.g., *mnDp1*: Meneely and Herman, 1979; *sDp2*: Howell *et al.,* 1987; *qDp3*: Bucher and Greenwald, 1991; *sDp3*: Stewart and Baillie, unpublished results).

There are two basic classes of duplication, those that do not recombine with the normal homologs and those that do. Discussion of the significance of this observation can be found in Herman *et al.* (1979) and Rose *et al.* (1984). Members of the nonrecombining class can be used as effective balancers (Rose *et al.,* 1984; Stewart and Baillie, unpublished results). For example, *sDp2* has been used extensively in screens for lethal mutations, and it has been shown to permit identification of the same range of essential genes as does a translocation (*hT1*) that balances the same region (McKim *et al.,* 1988). Rarely, free duplications have been observed to shorten spontaneously, which reduces the extent of the balanced region (McKim and Rose, 1990).

Free duplications generally exist as a single copy, but strains carrying two copies have been documented in some cases (Herman *et al.,* 1979; Rogalski and Riddle, 1988). The reference strain carrying *sDp2* is homozygous for mutant alleles of *dpy-5* and *unc-13* and, in addition, has a single copy of *sDp2* (Fig. 3). The strain has an Unc-13 phenotype, as the duplication carries a wild-type allele of *dpy-5* but not of *unc-13*. It segregates Unc-13 progeny (carrying the duplication) and Dpy-5 Unc-13 homozygotes. The possibility of losing either marker is eliminated by the homozygous state of the marked chromosomes and lack of recombination with the duplication. If a strain is also homozygous for a lethal mutation on the same chromosome in the duplicated region, then the Dpy Unc progeny class will die and the only viable progeny will be those carrying the duplication. The lethal mutation is thus effectively balanced.

C. Transgenes

A transgene is a segment of cloned DNA containing the complete coding element and control elements of a gene, present in the nucleus in addition to a complete complement of normal chromosomes. Direct transformation of mutant strains using cloned DNA is performed in *C. elegans* by germ-line microinjection (Fire, 1986; Chapter 19 in this volume). The microinjected molecules (containing one or more transgenes) assemble into tandem arrays that can be maintained extrachromosomally. Expression of wild-type transgenes in the array can complement, or "rescue," a mutant phenotype. An important advance in these procedures involved coinjecting the DNA to be tested for rescue along with clones of a selectable marker mutation, such as the dominant *rol-6* mutation (Mello *et al.*, 1991), which causes animals carrying it to roll along their long axes. Transgenic progeny displaying the marker phenotype were scored for rescue of the strain's mutant phenotype.

Germ-line microinjection becomes laborious if one wishes to assay the rescuing ability of a group of cosmids in a set of mutants. A more general approach takes advantage of the ability to manipulate transgenes genetically, as if they were free duplications. McKay, McDowall, and Rose (unpublished results) have used transgenes as genetic elements in large-scale experiments to rescue lethal mutations in the *dpy-5* and *dpy-14* regions of chromosome I. Copies of a marker plasmid containing *rol-6(su1006)* were coinjected with sets of two or three overlapping cosmids from the genomic region of interest into wild-type animals or animals homozygous for a morphological mutation. Tranformants were selected on the basis of their Rol-6 phenotype, and individual lines were established that exhibit a high frequency of transmission of the transgene. Standard duplication complementation tests were then used to assay for rescue of a mutation. Rescue was confirmed by establishment of a nonmutant line from the complementation test that exhibited the Rol-6 phenotype, with the transgene as an effective balancer, and that segregated nonrolling progeny (not carrying the transgenic array) that were not rescued. As cosmid contigs cover nearly all the *C. elegans* genome (Coulson *et al.*, 1986), this method can be used with virtually any mutation.

Complementation tests with extrachromosomal arrays containing more than one cosmid increase the efficiency of the analysis, as every mutation does not have to be tested separately against every cosmid. If the transgenic arrays are properly designed, a small number of crosses can establish exactly which individual cosmid is responsible for the rescue. Arrays containing single rescuing cosmids can then be generated to confirm the result.

Transgenic arrays have also been used as balancers in screens for new mutations. Labouesse and Horvitz (pers. comm.) used a transgenic strain carrying a cosmid that rescues *lin-26* in a noncomplementation screen for new mutations mapping to the region balanced by the cosmid. A wild-type clone of *dpy-10* was coinjected with the cosmid into a *dpy-10* mutant strain as a marker to identify transformants. The resulting non-Dpy transgenic animals were mutagenized, and their F2 progeny screened for the presence of new *lin-26* mutations or other mutations balanced by the cosmid. These were identified in the Dpy segregants that had spontaneously lost the transgenes. One new mutation, in the gene *let-253*, was recovered among the progeny of 2727 F1's. This technique allows balancers to be used in tightly focused screens for mutations in very small genomic regions. Plasterk (Chapter 3 in this volume) also used such arrays to screen for lethal transposon-induced deficiencies.

D. Inversions

Inversions are chromosome segments that break from the intact chromosome and rejoin it in the original location but in opposite orientation. The only proven example of an inversion is *hIn1* (Fig. 4), in which a portion of the right half of LG I, from about *unc-75* to about *unc-54*, is inverted (Zetka and Rose, 1992). The mapping of mutations in *hIn1* homozygotes revealed the inverted gene order relative to wild type. It was recovered in a screen for rearrangements that suppress crossing over specifically in this previously unbalanced region. Recombination between the breakpoints is almost completely suppressed in *hIn1* heterozygotes, presumably because of a lack of DNA alignment or interruption of sites required for pairing. The inversion is viable as a homozygote, with normal brood sizes, and in the homozygous state exhibits normal levels of recombination in the inverted interval. It has been used in screens for lethal mutations on LG I to the right of *unc-75* (Ho and Rose, unpublished results).

The original *hIn1* was generated on a wild-type chromosome, making it impossible to distinguish between inversion heterozygotes and homozygotes. To circumvent this difficulty and to make the balancer more useful for mutant screens, new *unc-75* (two lethal alleles), *unc-54*, and *unc-101* mutations were induced on *hIn1* (Lee *et al.*, 1994; Zetka and Rose, 1992). The reference strain is a phenotypically wild-type heterozygote in which an *hIn1*[*unc-54*] chromosome balances *unc-75 unc-101*. Selfing the strain produces wild-type heterozygotes, balancer homozygotes (Unc-54 phenotype), and *unc-75 unc-101* homozygotes. If the normal homolog carries a lethal mutation in addition to *unc-75* and *unc-101*, and it lies within the genetic extents of the inversion, it will also be balanced and the *unc-75 unc-101* homozygotes will be arrested in development. *hIn1* may not

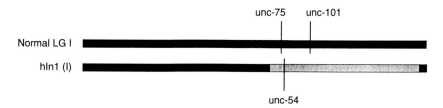

Fig. 4 Diagram of genotype of reference *hIn1* inversion strain. The *unc-75* and *unc-101* mutations are carried on the normal LG I. The *unc-54* mutation was induced secondarily on the inversion chromosome. Recombination is suppressed along the length of the inverted segment in heterozygotes (boundaries of suppression correspond to breakpoints). Terminal sequences are most likely not included in the inverted interval, as a deficiency of the ribosomal gene cluster (*eDf24*) to the right of *unc-54* on normal LG I is apparently not balanced.

include the physical end of the chromosome, as *eDf24* (a deletion of part of the ribosomal gene cluster that lies to the right of *unc-54*) apparently is not balanced by the inversion (M. Zetka, pers. comm.).

E. Other Crossover Suppressors

Several chromosomal rearrangements exist in *C. elegans* that dominantly suppress crossing over but that remain uncharacterized with regard to their structures. Two examples are *mnC1* (Herman, 1978), which balances the right half of LG II from *dpy-10* to around *unc-52*, and *sC1* (Stewart and Baillie, unpublished results), which balances an approximately 15-map-unit segment of the left half of LG III, from around *unc-45* to the region left of *dpy-17*. Crossover suppression in these two cases is presumably restricted to a single chromosome, in contrast to translocations. Pattern of crossover suppression, meiotic properties, brood size, and progeny phenotypes are consistent with their being inversions, but proof is lacking. Both have been used successfully in screens for lethal mutations in the regions they balance. *mnC1*, marked with *dpy-10* and *unc-52* mutations, has been especially useful in isolating and maintaining a high-resolution set of deficiencies (Sigurdson *et al.*, 1984). It is phenotypically wild type as a heterozygote, gives broods of relatively normal size, and is viable as a DpyUnc homozygote but with very small broods. *sC1* was generated on a wild-type chromosome, is viable as a homozygote, and morphologically marked variants have been generated to facilitate its use (Stewart and Baillie, unpublished results).

F. Deficiencies

Deficiencies are segments of chromosomes entirely missing from the genome. Deficiencies are detected after mutagenesis by various methods (e.g., Riddle and Brenner, 1978; Sigurdson *et al.*, 1984; Moerman and Baillie, 1981; Greenwald and Horvitz, 1980; Rosenbluth *et al.*, 1985; Yandell *et al.*, 1994). They are useful as genetic mapping tools, but some deficiencies dominantly reduce recombination frequency in particular genetic regions. Several of the latter class were described by Rosenbluth *et al.*, (1990). A chromosome carrying a small deficiency in the gene cluster of LG I, *hDf8*, was also associated with reduced recombination frequency, from around *dpy-14* to around the left end of the chromosome (McKim *et al.*, 1992).

III. Practical Considerations of Balancer Use

A. Characteristics of Good Balancers

Balancers are used for a variety of tasks, including balancing existing mutations, facilitating strain construction, and screening for new mutations. At a minimum, a balancer should have the properties already described: heterozygotes must have a phenotype distinguishable from that of each homozygote; recombination should be virtually eliminated; progeny phenotypes must allow ready detection of rare recombination; and the construct should be stable (balanced mutations should not spontaneously become unbalanced). It is also helpful if the balancer can be manipulated easily in genetic crosses, particularly if it can be passed through male sperm, and if morphologically marked or lethal variants exist.

Balancing existing mutations is probably the least demanding of these tasks, requiring only that a suitable balancer exists and that the mutation/balancer heterozygote is viable. A minor degree of instability in the heterozygote is acceptable, as long as the investigator checks the strain routinely. Strain construction can be aided by particular qualities of a few balancers, and often requires balancers marked with particular mutations (see Section III,C).

By far the most stringent test of a balancer is to use it to screen for lethal mutations. The major additional requirement imposed on the balancer is that the apparent spontaneous mutation frequency should be low (no higher than in the reference wild-type strain, N2). Studies using two different reciprocal translocations (eT1 and szT1) illustrate this point.

1. eT1(III;V)

This translocation is an extremely stable balancer that has been used extensively for lethal screens. The size of the balanced region was about 40 map units (mu). Rosenbluth et al. (1983) conducted a dose–response study for balanced lethal mutations using ethyl methanesulfonate (EMS) and gamma irradiation, and determined the spontaneous mutation frequency for lethal mutations. A strain of genotype dpy-18/eT1 III; unc-46/eT1 V was used to screen for new lethal mutations linked to either dpy-18 or unc-46. Lethals were recovered at reasonable frequency with both mutagens (6.6% at 12 mM EMS, and 4.3% at 1500 R gamma). The frequency of accumulation of spontaneous mutations was very low. Two control experiments, involving 3198 F1 heterozygous progeny of two P_0 animals, resulted in a total of two balanced lethal mutations for a frequency of 0.06%. In addition, eT1 seems to be completely stable. It has been used to screen many thousands of mutagenized chromosomes, is currently used to balance hundreds of lethal mutations, and it has never been observed to break down.

2. szT1(I;X)

This translocation is very stable, and it has been useful in strain constructions and for balancing existing mutations. It has been used to a limited extent to recover new lethal mutations. Experiments to determine the spontaneous lethal mutation frequency in the region balanced by szT1 gave results different from those obtained with eT1. McKim et al. (1988) detected unusual segregants among the progeny of a strain of genotype dpy-5 unc-13/szT1[lon-2] I; unc-3/szT X.

This strain has a wild-type phenotype and normally segregates wild types, Dpy-5 Unc-13 Unc-3 homozygotes, a few Lon-2 males (as a result of meiotic nondisjunction of the X chromosome), and aneuploids that arrest as embryos or young larvae. From among the progeny of 1104 unmutagenized wild-type heterozygotes, 34 animals were recovered that did not give Dpy Unc-13 Unc-3 progeny and thus appeared to carry a new lethal in one of the balanced regions. These animals, however, did not give progeny appropriate for an *szT1* heterozygote and, on further analysis, appeared to carry a compound chromosome consisting of *szT1(X)* fused to the normal X carrying the *unc-3* mutation. These types of spontaneous rearrangements reduce the utility of *szT1* as a balancer for lethal screens, although it has been used successfully after mutagenesis to recover lethals linked to *dpy-5* (McKim *et al.,* 1988).

B. Genetically Marked Balancers

In properly designed strains, animals heterozygous for a balancer and a balanced mutation (and marker mutations), or homozygous for the mutations and carrying a balancing duplication, possess a unique phenotype. These strains can be maintained by selecting animals with this phenotype and checking their progeny to be sure that appropriate phenotypic classes are segregated. The genetic details vary among individual balancers, and a good understanding of these details is required to maintain a given strain. Specific information on normal progeny genotypes and phenotypes for each class of balancer can be found in Section II, and information on homozygous balancer phenotypes and standard marker mutations for particular balancers can be found in Section V.

The original isolates of some balancers carry mutations that were in the genetic background of the strains from which the balancers were generated (e.g., *dpy-10* and *unc-52* in the case of *mnC1*) or carry mutations in genes interrupted by rearrangement breakpoints (e.g., *unc-36* in *eT1*). In addition, existing balancers have been specially marked with lethal or morphological mutations for particular tasks. These variants can be useful for strain construction (Rosenbluth and Baillie, 1981), maintenance of balanced mutations (Johnsen and Baillie, unpublished results), and analysis of mutations and balancer structure (Rosenbluth and Baillie, 1981). They can be generated by different means, including spontaneous mutation (Rogalski *et al.,* 1988), mutagenesis or recombination (Rosenbluth and Baillie, 1981), and DNA fusion (Hunter and Wood, 1990). The new mutations they carry may be recessive or dominant and may be conditional or nonconditional.

Lethal variants of homozygous viable balancers can be used when it is desirable to remove balancer homozygotes from a population, leaving heterozygotes as the only viable class of progeny. For example, Johnsen and Baillie (unpublished results) used a lethal derivative of *eT1* to maintain lethal mutations in strains in which balancer homozygotes were the most vigorous progeny class. Lethal variants are useful to keep balancer homozygotes from overgrowing a population under any conditions in which heterozygotes cannot be selected routinely, such as large-scale preparations for biochemical analysis or DNA extraction.

Morphologically marked balancer variants are used when a homozygous viable balancer does not already have a unique phenotype, when its phenotype is similar to that of one of the progeny classes, or when a second scorable phenotype is needed in addition to the balancer's native homozygous phenotype. For example, Rosenbluth and Baillie (1981) induced new mutations on *eT1* to determine the segregation patterns of the half-translocations. Zetka and Rose (1992) induced a new *unc-54* mutation on the inversion *hIn1,* which originally had a wild-type homozygous phenotype, to distinguish homozygotes from heterozygotes.

Most of the lethal or morphological balancer variants in common use were generated by mutagenesis with EMS and are thus not very likely to be structurally altered. That is, they may generally be expected to balance the same regions as their parent balancers. On the other hand, balancers subjected to mutagenesis with ionizing radiation could be expected to carry new rearrangements (Rosenbluth *et al.,* 1985; McKim and Rose, 1990; McKim *et al.,* 1993). Thus, it may be necessary to test the extent of balancing for particular variants.

C. Crossing Schemes

Crosses to move mutations into or out of different genetic backgrounds are basic to genetic analysis. For example, crosses are necessary to genetically map mutations; to complement them against deficiencies, duplications, or other mutations; to study the effects of different mutations on each other; and to remove unwanted deleterious mutations after mutagenesis. If one wishes to cross a balanced mutation into another genetic background, males that carry the mutation and are able to mate may be needed. Three methods can be employed to accomplish this. First, a mixed population of heterozygous males, half of which carry the balancer and half of which carry the balanced mutation, can be made by crossing heterozygous hermaphrodites with wild-type males. Second, males can arise in balanced strains by spontaneous X-chromosome nondisjunction, the frequency of which can be increased by a *him* mutation in the genetic background (Hodgkin *et al.,* 1979) or by heat stock (Sulston and Hodgkin, 1988), and these males can be used to propagate balanced male stocks. Third, and most desirable, balanced phenotypically unique males can be made from each balanced strain on demand by crossing to a standard male balancer strain.

The first method complicates analysis by requiring F2 progeny testing to ensure that the correct marker has been transferred. The second method may or may not require progeny testing, depending on whether the desired F2 cross-progeny have a unique phenotype; however, it requires that a male stock be maintained for each balanced mutation. Strain construction and complementation tests are made much simpler if the genotypes and corresponding phenotypes resulting from crosses are unique, and if the required males can be generated as needed.

The following discussion presents a few examples of useful crossing protocols of the latter class for particular balancers. The original published works, or the investigators themselves, are still the best source for specific detail and advice.

1. *hIn1(I)*

Ho and Rose (unpublished results) devised a simple scheme to facilitate the complementation testing of a set of lethal mutations induced using the inversion *hIn1* as a balancer. A single cross for each balanced lethal generated wild-type males of a single genotype that could be used in complementation tests against deficiencies and other lethal mutations. For example, males of a standard balancer strain, of genotype *hIn1[unc-54]/unc-75 unc-101,* were crossed to *hIn1[unc-54 unc-75]/unc-101 lev-11 let-x* hermaphrodites (Fig. 5). The only phenotypically wild-type male progeny, of genotype *hIn1[unc-54]/unc-101 lev-11 let-x,* were then crossed to other identically balanced lethals in complementation tests (e.g., *hIn1[unc-54]/unc-101 lev-11 let-y*). In this case, complementation of *let-x* by *let-y* was indicated by the presence of viable, fertile Unc-101 Lev-11 progeny (*unc-*

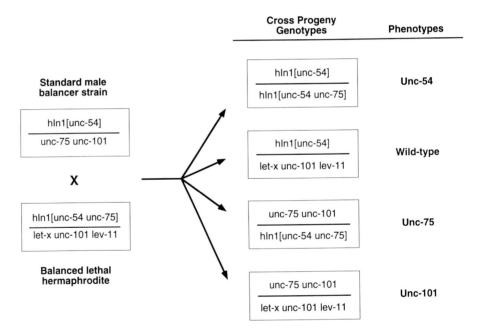

Fig. 5 Example of a crossing scheme using *hIn1* to generate genotypically and phenotypically unique balanced males carrying a desired lethal mutation. The standard male balancer strain and a sample balanced lethal strain are represented by genotypes in the boxes on the left. The genotypes and phenotypes of the four classes of cross-progeny resulting are shown on the right. Both male and hermaphrodite cross-progeny will be present. This example illustrates a basic principle of marker manipulation, which can be adapted for other balancers and markers.

101 lev-11 let-x/unc-101 lev-11 let-y). Failure to complement was indicated by the absence of this progeny class. The same scheme was used to map the lethals against deficiencies that deleted both *lev-11* and *unc-54* (such as *eDf3*). In these cases, complementation or its failure was indicated by the presence or absence of Lev-11 progeny, as none of the deficiencies deleted *unc-101*.

2. *szT1(I;X)*

An advantage of *szT1* in crossing protocols is its spontaneous segregation of fertile males that have a distinct Lon-2 phenotype and are hemizygous for the translocation. These males have been used effectively for strain construction and complementation tests (McKim and Rose, 1990) and elucidation of the structure of the translocation (McKim *et al.*, 1988). The translocation was induced in a strain carrying *lon-2(e678)*, and this mutation is thus present on one half-translocation (Fodor and Deak, 1985). Males from *szT1* strains carrying *lon-2* must have a Lon-2 phenotype, as they are hemizygous for the X chromosome. These males carry both half-translocations and one copy of a normal LG I. As males arise spontaneously in *szT1* strains at a frequency of approximately 10% (Fodor and Deak, 1985; McKim and Rose, 1990), it is not necessary to make males that carry either the half-translocations or the balanced LG I markers by crossing balanced hermaphrodites with wild-type males.

The three basic uses of the Lon males depend on their exclusive transfer of the normal LG I to all viable male progeny and of the translocation chromosomes to all viable hermaphrodite progeny (Fig. 6). First, the males can be used to balance existing mutations. For example, *dpy-5* could be balanced with *szT1* simply by crossing Lon-2 males to a *dpy-5* homozygote. As all wild-type hermaphrodite progeny resulting from the cross must be heterozygous for both *szT1* and *dpy-5*, the mutation is balanced in a single step. Second, the males can be used to generate wild-type males heterozygous for *szT1* balanced lethal mutations for use in complementation tests against other *szT1*-balanced lethals, assuming the lethals have a morphological marker in common and assuming that failure to complement can be scored reliably in male progeny. Third, they can be used for purposes that require F3 hermaphrodite progeny carrying two copies of the normal LG I. For example, McKim and Rose (1990) used *unc-11 dpy-14/szT1(I); szT1(X)/0* males to generate wild-type males of genotype *unc-11 dpy-14/dpy-5 let-x unc-13*. These were then crossed to other strains to test for complementation of *let-x* by a set of duplications. Presence of the *unc-11 dpy-14* chromosome allowed them to select progeny of the desired genotype without progeny testing.

3. *mnDp1(X;V)*

This duplication of part of the right end of LG X is translocated to LG V. It is sterile as a homozygote, but heterozygous males are fertile (Herman *et al.*, 1976). Normally, analysis of X-linked mutations is complicated because males

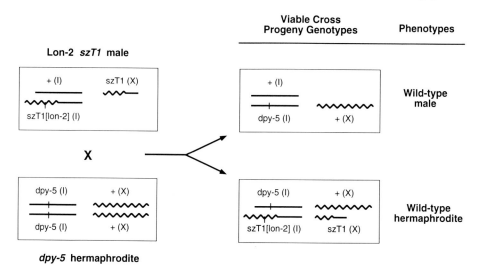

Fig. 6 Example of a crossing scheme using spontaneous Lon-2 males from an *szT1* strain to balance a *dpy-5* mutation. The male and hermaphrodite parents are represented by genotypes in the boxes on the left. The genotypes and phenotypes of the two classes of viable cross-progeny are shown on the right. Male parents are hemizygous for LG X and, because of the *lon-2* mutation carried on *szT1*, must have a Lon phenotype. All wild-type male progeny will be heterozygous for *dpy-5* and will not carry the translocation. All wild-type hermaphrodite progeny will be heterozygous for both *dpy-5* and the translocation. All other cross-progeny are aneuploid, and arrest during development.

are hemizygous for the X chromosome and thus express the mutant phenotype. For example, males resulting from crossing wild-type males to a homozygous mutant *unc-3* (LG X) hermaphrodite would have the genotype *unc-3/0 (X)*. These would have an Unc-3 phenotype and be unable to mate. The use of *mnDp1* (and similar duplications for other parts of the X chromosome) solves this problem. A hermaphrodite strain carrying two mutant copies of *unc-3* and one copy of *mnDp1* has a wild-type phenotype, as the duplication provides a wild-type copy of the *unc-3* gene. Males resulting from crossing wild-type males with this strain have one of two genotypes and correspondingly unique phenotypes. Half will have the genotype *+/+ V; unc-3/0* and be Unc-3, and half will have the genotype *mnDp1/+ V; unc-3/0* and a wild-type phenotype. The latter are able to mate and transfer both the duplication and the *unc-3* mutation in crosses. Meneely and Herman (1979) used these properties of *mnDp1* to analyze recessive lethal mutations balanced by *mnDp1* that are either linked to or delete *unc-3*. Wild-type males of genotype *mnDp1/+ V; unc-3 let-x/0* were used to transfer the two X mutations into different genetic backgrounds for two- and three-factor mapping and for complementation tests with other balanced lethals.

D. Accumulation of Spontaneous Mutations

Rosenbluth *et al.* (1983) measured the spontaneous lethal mutation frequency in the 40-mu region balanced by *eT1* and found it to be 0.06%. Extrapolated to the whole genome, approximately 1 in every 119 selfed hermaphrodites may be expected to be heterozygous for a new lethal mutation. These mutations would quickly be lost by segregation if they appeared in strains that carried no balancer and were maintained in culture. If, however, the mutations occur in a balanced region, segregational and recombinational loss will be eliminated. Indeed, spontaneous mutations of all types (not only lethal) tend to accumulate in balancer strains. Great care must therefore be taken by the investigator to confirm that a given balanced strain has not acquired any additional mutations subsequent to the original mutagenesis. It is preferable to keep strains frozen if they are not actually being used in experiments, and strains that have been passaged should be checked closely. The effects of an additional lethal mutation in a strain that already carries a lethal can be especially subtle. For example, if the original mutation results in arrest at a midlarval developmental stage, an additional mutation that causes the animal to arrest slightly earlier may not be noticed. New mutations causing later developmental arrest are phenotypically undetectable in a lethal that arrests as an embryo. These unrecognized secondary mutations may confound analyses.

E. Exceptional Segregants and Balancer Breakdown

The value of a balancer is reduced if balanced mutations spontaneously become unbalanced, or if balancer strains appear to acquire new mutations at high frequency. The point at which a balancer is no longer considered a balancer is when it cannot be used successfully for its intended purpose. This is the decision of the particular investigator. Although it is possible for any balancer to undergo recombination that results in loss of balanced mutations, it is important to distinguish between exceptional progeny that result from recombination and those that may result from chromosome nondisjunction, as described below. The determination of the nature of a putative breakdown event must always be documented through recovery and analysis of diagnostic progeny.

Exceptional segregants may lead the investigator to believe that recombination has occurred in a balancer strain. For example, the normal progeny of a strain carrying *dpy-5 I* and *unc-3 X* mutations balanced by *szT1 (dpy-5/szT1 [lon-2] I; unc-3/szT1 X)* are wild-type heterozygotes, Dpy-5 Unc-3 homozygotes, Lon-2 males, lethal *szT1* homozygotes, and lethal aneuploid progeny. Dpy non-Unc and Unc non-Dpy progeny are not usually produced because the markers are pseudolinked. Rare Unc-3 progeny do arise (McKim and Rose, 1990), which at first glance could be the product of a recombination event between the normal LG I and *szT1(X)* that resulted in loss of *dpy-5* from the normal LG I. Careful analysis of one such event, however, revealed that no recombination had occurred. Instead, one of the half-translocations, *szT1(X)*, carrying a portion of LG I, was present as a duplication in addition to two normal copies of LG I (marked with *dpy-5*) and two normal copies of LG X (marked with *unc-3*). As this duplication, named *szDp1,* carried a wild-type copy of *dpy-5* but not of *unc-3*, the strain had an Unc-3 phenotype. Analogous exceptional segregants have been recovered from a number of translocation strains, for example, *mnDp11* from *mnT2* (Herman *et al.,* 1982), *hDp133* from *hT1, hDp134* from *hT2,* and *hDp135* from *hT3* (McKim *et al.,* 1993). Thus, the investigator must be aware of the possibility that a translocation heterozygote will give rise to apparent recombinant progeny and must analyze the exceptional progeny before concluding that a crossover has occurred. Physical breakdown of a few balancers has been documented. For example, some duplications of LG I have been observed to shorten spontaneously, resulting in exposure of previously balanced mutations (McKim and Rose, 1990). Also, Zetka and Rose (1992) documented two rare recombination events in *hIn1* heterozygotes that resulted in deficiencies. In all these cases, the fact that physical rearrangement had occured was documented through the recovery and analysis of exceptional progeny.

F. Use of Balancers in Mutant Screens

Balancers have been used in mutant screens most commonly for recovery of lethal mutations, but they can also be used to recover nonlethal mutations. For example, they can be used in noncomplementation screens for new alleles of existing morphological mutations. The work summarized below is concerned mostly with lethal mutations, but it provides practical information for anyone contemplating a mutant screen. The following information will not substitute for a thorough knowledge of balancer genetics and the published works, but the points are good guides for avoiding unnecessary work and confusion.

1. Mutagenizing Balancer Strains

Ideally, nonbalancer strains are mutagenized and the new mutations are captured in crosses to balancers, to prevent inducing mutations on the balancer itself. Such crosses also replace approximately half the mutagenized genome with unmutagenized chromosomes, helping to remove unwanted second-site mutations. For large screens, however, routine backcrossing is not practical, and it is much more efficient to mutagenize balancer strains directly. Genetic mapping and *inter se* complementation of the new mutations can be accomplished rapidly with strains that are already balanced and appropriately marked, but that have not been backcrossed, as discussed previously. The problem of second-site mutations can be minimized by the use of low mutagen doses (see below). Before more extensive characterization is undertaken for particular mutations, backcrossing can be done using schemes similar to those presented in Section III,C.

2. Mutagen Dose

Screens should be done at low mutagen doses for all mutagens to decrease the incidence of multiple mutational events. Studies undertaken by Rosenbluth *et al.* (1983, 1985) demonstrated the utility of low doses of EMS and gamma irradiation, and characterized a number of rearrangements generated in these experiments. Based on these studies, we recommend doses in the range 1500 to 3000 R for gamma irradiation and 6 to 18 mM for EMS. It is tempting to use higher doses to increase the efficiency of recovery, but the benefits are more than outweighed by the increased complication of analysis. At the very least, the use of lower doses can help keep the amount of work down by reducing the need for extensive backcrossing prior to analysis. Rare multiple events are usually spotted in the process of mapping, although this is not always the case (see also Chapter 2 in this volume).

3. Mutation Types

Mutagenesis of balancer strains has yielded point mutations, deficiencies, duplications, and translocations. Some of these can be very complicated to analyze. The investigator should be conversant with all the published work involving a prospective balancer before using it to recover lethals, and should also be conversant with the detailed study by Rosenbluth *et al.* (1985) of the types and frequency of mutations recovered in screens with *eT1*.

4. Chromosomal Location of Balanced Lethals

Screens using reciprocal translocations will recover lethals in the two genomic regions balanced by the two half-translocations. Figuring out on which chromosome they reside requires linkage tests or mapping (e.g., with deficiencies). Linkage mapping is fairly trivial if the original balanced strain carries morphological markers on both balanced chromosomes. For example, refer to Fig. 2. Mapping to chromosome can be done by outcrossing to remove the translocation and examining segregating progeny for reduced numbers of either Dpy-18 (indicating a lethal on LG III) or Unc-46 (indicating a lethal on LG V). Subsequent higher-resolution positioning can be accomplished using recombination mapping and complementation tests with deficiencies or duplications.

5. Mutations Outside the Balanced Region

Translocation and inversion screens can yield lethal mutations that are balanced because they are close to the rearrangement breakpoints, but they lie outside the rearrangement and may be lost through recombination. Duplications have a precise recovery boundary, as they balance by complementation of the lethal (presence of a wild-type allele). A duplication screen will only yield lethals that lie inside the genetic extents of the duplication. Deficiencies spanning the duplication endpoint will not be recovered if they delete any essential genes outside the endpoint.

6. Linked Markers

The presence of morphological mutations linked to lethals in balancer strains has several benefits. First among these is the ease of recovery of the lethals. It is much easier to screen for the absence of a particular morphological mutant class than it is to screen for arrested embryos or larvae. The second major advantage is that presence of the markers eases genetic mapping, complementation analysis, and arrest-stage determination of the lethals. A disadvantage is that the investigator may encounter marker effects. The presence of particular markers may result in a lethal arresting at a different developmental stage than it would without the markers, or a given mutation may be lethal in the presence of a marker but completely viable in its absence. For example, *dpy-14* exhibits a synthetic lethal phenotype in doubly mutant constructs involving a number of muscle mutants, such as *unc-15* and *unc-54* (Rose and Baillie, 1980). It is best to remove the markers prior to phenotypic analysis.

7. Selecting Lethal Homozygotes

Care must be taken when selecting homozygous progeny for further developmental or molecular characterization to understand the correspondence of phenotypes and genotypes segregated from a balanced lethal heterozygote. For example, translocation strains segregate a large proportion of aneuploid progeny (Fig. 2) that arrest as embryos or early larvae, but these are not the lethal homozygotes of interest. To be certain that the arrested embryos or animals are of the correct genotype, the lethal-bearing chromosome must be crossed to a nonbalanced genetic background and resegregated as a homozygote (Johnsen and Baillie, 1991).

G. Screens for Transposon-Induced Mutations

The advantages of balancers for lethal mutant screens seem ideal for extension to screens conducted in mutator genetic backgrounds that exhibit a high frequency of Tc1 transposition (Moerman and Waterston, 1989; Chapter 2 in this volume). The ease of maintenance and crossing is especially attractive given the necessity of removing the mutator from the background once a mutation has been induced. Although these screens may produce desired mutations, they may not be as generally useful as are screens using other mutagens. Using *mut-4(st7000)I*, Clark *et al.* (1990) analyzed 28 spontaneous lethal mutations (probably Tc1-induced) in the 49-mu region balanced by *nT1*. The distribution of these mutations was skewed: 86% of them mapped to LG V, as compared with 43%

of EMS-induced lethal mutations recovered over *nT1*. Furthermore, the types of mutations obtained were different from those obtained using EMS, formaldehyde, or gamma irradiation. Two were new mutations in previously unidentified genes, six were mutations in *lin-40,* and seven were deficiencies. All of the latter deleted the left end of the chromosome, and five of them had right endpoints in or near *lin-40.*

The distribution of transposon-induced mutations is changing with identification methods that do not require that an insertion result in a scorable phenotype (see Chapter 3 in this volume). Also, analysis of secondary deletion mutants derived from strains carrying transposon insertions is resulting in information about the null phenotypes of these genes. Balancers may prove useful in such schemes for maintaining heterozygosity of induced mutations and identifying animals homozygous for the insertions or their spontaneous derivatives.

IV. The Balancer Map

Over half the *C. elgans* genome is covered by reliable, tested balancers (Fig. 7). Well-balanced regions include virtually all of LG I, the right half of LG II, all of LG III, the right half of LG IV, the left 66% of LG V, and the right 80% of LG X (based on genetic, not physical, extents of each chromosome). Incompletely balanced regions include most of the remaining areas. Balancers may or may not include the physical ends of chromosomes. When drawn or referred to as including the end, it means only that the most distal genetic marker appears to be balanced.

Certain chromosomal regions not covered by translocations have proven somewhat resistant to efforts to obtain effective balancers. For example, several balancers for the right arm of LG V have been recovered, but all to date have exhibited unacceptable levels of crossing over and thus are of limited value for lethal screens (Stewart and Baillie, unpublished results). Such incomplete balancers may still provide a useful degree of balancing for existing mutations, and their use should be evaluated case by case.

V. A Field Guide to Balancers

This guide presents alphabetically the most fully characterized and commonly used *C. elegans* balancers. It is by no means an exhaustive list. The "field guide" format is an attempt to present information critical for the use of each balancer in a brief and consistent manner. Standardized descriptors help compare and contrast the choices for a particular genetic region.

Most of the balancers listed here, and some of the derivatives and marked variants, are available from the Caenorhabditis Genetics Center (CGC). Those

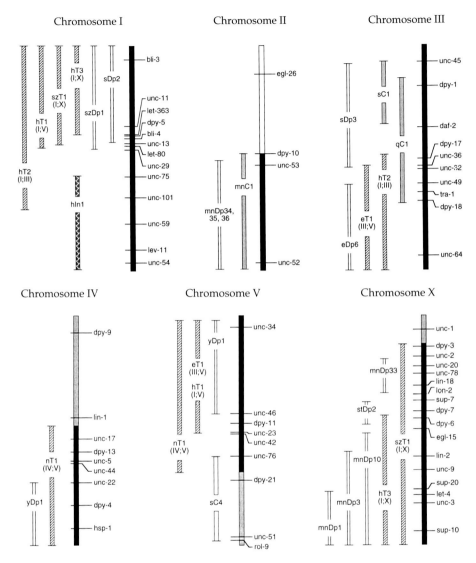

Fig. 7 Map of the balanced regions of *C. elegans* chromosomes. Each chromosome is represented by a vertical bar with cross lines indicating genetic positions of a subset of identified genes (some genes defining the endpoints of minor balancers are not shown where space is limited). By convention, the top end of each vertically drawn chromosome corresponds to the left end when drawn horizontally, and the bottom of each corresponds to the right end. Shading of the chromosomes indicates the degree of balancing. Black represents well-balanced regions, crosshatching represents regions balanced by unstable or uncharacterized rearrangements, and no shading represents regions for which no balancers exist. Approximately 65% of the genome is well balanced. Balancers are drawn to the left of each chromosome as double-line bars (duplications) or bars with different shading patterns (other balancers). Endpoint lines on each balancer indicate its genetic extents. Some rearrangements that provide balancing of limited reliability are not shown. Also not shown are duplications that balance small intervals.

variants not stocked by the CGC generally have not been the subject of wide interest, but they may prove useful for certain screens or strain constructions. For more information about whether a particular variant is available, the investigator should contact the originating laboratory.

A. Explanation of Descriptors

Most of the descriptors are self-explanatory, but a few require more detail. For translocations, inversions, and other crossover suppressors, *stability* refers generally to the frequency at which unusual progeny may be segregated. Measures of stability are necessarily subjective, as very few data have been accumulated on the frequency of such progeny and the nature of the events that produced them. The stability descriptor therefore represents a consensus opinion based on published information and the experiences of the authors' laboratories. *Extremely stable* means that neither recombination nor unusual segregants have been documented. *Very stable* means that rare unusual segregants have been recovered, but the utility of the balancer is not generally affected. *Stable* means that unusual segregants have been recovered at somewhat higher frequency, and utility of the balancer is potentially compromised. Details are given where the nature of unusual segregants has been deduced through further analysis.

For all balancers, *Recommended use* is broken down into four categories, presented in increasing order of characteristics required in the balancer. *General balancing* means that it is useful for small-scale use. *Strain construction* is listed only for balancers known to be especially useful in crossing protocols because of specific characteristics or the existence of marked variants. By definition, males carrying these balancers must be able to mate. *Strain maintenance* means that a balancer is stable enough for large-scale use, although it may be unsuitable for mutant screens. *Mutant screens* means that a balancer has been proven reliable in screens for lethal mutations.

B. The Balancers

1. *eDp6(III;f)*

Summary: Free duplication, moderately well characterized, not observed to recombine with normal homologs. Very effective balancer for right portion of LG III from right end through *tra-1* and *vab-7*.

Origin: Acetaldehyde mutagenesis.

Recommended use: General balancing, strain maintenance.

Reference strain: CB1517, *eDf2 III; eDp6(III;f)*.

Phenotype: Unc-119.

Segregants: Unc-119.

Handling: Unc phenotype of reference strain is characteristic of the combination of two copies of *eDf2* and one copy of *eDp6*. This is due to deletion of the *unc-119* locus by *eDf2* and incomplete complementation of the deletion by the duplication (D. Pilgrim and M. Maduro, pers. comm.).

References: Hodgkin, 1980, 1987; Hunter and Wood, 1990).

2. *eT1(III;V)*

Summary: Reciprocal translocation, well characterized, extremely stable. Very effective balancer for left portion of LG V from left end through *unc-23*, and right portion of LG III from right end to *unc-36*. *eT1(III)* is LG V (left) translocated to LG III (left), disjoins from normal LG III. *eT1(V)* is LG III (right) translocated to LG V (right), disjoins from normal LG V.

Origin: ^{32}P mutagenesis of N2.

Recommended use: General balancing, strain construction, strain maintenance, mutant screens.

Reference strain: BC2200, *dpy-18(e364)/eT1 III; unc-46(e177)/eT1 V.*

Phenotype: Wild type.

Segregants: Wild type, Unc-36 *eT1* homozygotes, Dpy-18 Unc-46, and large numbers of arrested aneuploid progeny.

Growth characteristics: Original isolate homozygous viable with Unc-36 phenotype caused by the translocation breakpoint. Brood size in heterozygotes ~100, in homozygotes ~160. *eT1* homozygotes can overgrow a population, especially in balanced strains carrying certain lethal mutations or deficiencies.

Handling: Easy to manipulate. Heterozygous male stocks mate well.

Marked variants: Morphological: *eT1[bli-5(s277)]*, *eT1[dpy-11(s287)]*, *eT1[sma-2(s262)]*, *eT1[sma-3(e491)]*, *eT1[unc-42(e270)]*. Lethal: *eT1[let-500(s2165)]*.

References: Rosenbluth and Baillie, 1981; Rosenbluth *et al.*, 1983, 1985; McKim *et al.*, 1988; Nelson *et al.*, 1989).

3. *hIn1(I)*

Summary: Inversion, well characterized, very stable. Very effective balancer for right portion of LG I from *unc-75* through *unc-54*. Extreme right end of chromosome apparently not balanced.

Origin: Gamma irradiation of N2 males.

Recommended use: General balancing, strain construction, strain maintenance, mutant screens.

Reference strain: KR2267, *hIn1[unc-54(h1040)]/unc-75(e950) unc-101 (m1) I.*

Phenotype: Wild type.

Segregants: Wild type, Unc-54 *hIn1* homozygotes, Unc-75 Unc-101.

Growth characteristics: Original isolate homozygous viable with wild-type phenotype; *unc-54* mutation in the reference strain was induced secondarily. Brood size similar to N2 as homozygote and as heterozygote.

Handling: Easy to manipulate. Heterozygous males, and homozygous males of original isolate, mate well. Very rare recombination can occur, which generates deficiencies and duplications.

Marked variants: Morphological: *hIn1[unc-54(h1040)], hIn1[unc-101(sy241)].* Lethal: *hIn1[unc-75(h1041)], hIn1[unc-75(h1042)], hIn1[unc-54(h1040) unc-75[h1041)].*

Derivatives: hDf11, hDf12; hDp131, hDp132.

References: Lee *et al.*, 1994; Zetka and Rose, 1992.

4. *hT1(I;V)*

Summary: Reciprocal translocation, well characterized, very stable. Very effective balancer for left portion of LG I from the left end through *let-80,* and the left portion of LG V from the left end through *dpy-11. hT1(I)* is LG V (left) translocated to LG I (right), disjoins from normal LG I. *hT1(V)* is LG I (left) translocated to LG V (right), disjoins from normal LG V.

Origin: Gamma irradiation of *unc-23 +/+ unc-42 males.*

Recommended use: General balancing, strain maintenance, mutant screens.

Reference strain: KR1037, *unc-13(e51)/hT1 I; dpy-11 (e224)/hT1[unc-42(e270)]V.*

Phenotype: Wild type.

Segregants: Wild type, arrested *hT1* homozygotes, Unc-13 Dpy-11, and large numbers of arrested aneuploid progeny. Recombination occurs occasionally between the *hT1* breakpoint and *unc-42* on *hT1(V),* giving rise to Unc-42 animals. These are of genotype *unc-13(e51)/hT1 I; dpy-11(e224) unc-42(e270)/hT1[unc-42(e270)]V.*

Growth characteristics: Homozygous inviable, cause unknown. Arrests at L3. Brood size in heterozygotes ~75.

Handling: Easy to manipulate. Heterozygous males mate well. Rare exceptional progeny carry one half-translocation as a complex free duplication. Recombination frequency in the unbalanced *unc-101–unc-54* interval on LG I is increased twofold.

Marked variants: hT1[unc-29(e403)].

Derivatives: hDp133(I;V;f).

References: McKim *et al.*, 1988; Howell and Rose, 1990.

5. *hT2(I;III)*

Summary: Reciprocal translocation, well characterized, stable. Effective balancer for left portion of LG I from left end through *unc-101,* and right portion of LG III from right end through *dpy-17*. *hT2(I)* is LG III (right) translocated to LG I (right), disjoins from normal LG I. *hT2(III)* is LG I (left) translocated to LG III (left), disjoins from normal LG III.

Origin: Gamma irradiation of *bli-4(e937)I* males.

Recommended use: General balancing, strain maintenance.

Reference strain: KR1235, *unc-13(e51/hT2 I; dpy-18(e364)/hT2[bli-4(e937)]III*.

Phenotype: Wild type.

Segregants: Wild type, Bli-4 *hT2* homozygotes, Unc-13 Dpy-18, and large numbers of arrested aneuploid progeny.

Growth characteristics: Original isolate homozygous viable with Bli-4 phenotype.

Handling: Easy to manipulate. Heterozygous males, and homozygous males of original isolate, mate well. *dpy-18(h662)* variant is very mildly Dpy as a homozygote. Homozygous Bli-4 phenotype completely suppressed in *dpy-5* and *dpy-18* variants. Rare exceptional progeny carry one half-translocation as a complex free duplication. Mutations have been observed to become unbalanced at low frequency, but the mechanism is not fully understood.

Marked variants: hT2[dpy-5(h659)], hT2[dpy-18(h662)], hT2[unc-54(e190)], hT2[bli-4(e937) unc-29(h1011)], hT2[dpy-18(h662) unc-59(e261)].

Derivative: hDp134(I;III;f).

Reference: McKim *et al.*, 1993.

6. *hT3(I;X)*

Summary: Translocation (rigorous proof of reciprocity lacking), moderately well characterized, very stable. Very effective balancer for left portion of LG I from left end to around *let-363,* and the right portion of LG X from the right end to between *dpy-7* and *unc-3*. *hT3(I)*, which disjoins from normal LG I, is probably LG X (right) translocated to LG I (right). *hT3(X)*, which disjoins from normal LG X, is probably LG I (left) translocated to LG X (left).

Origin: Gamma irradiation mutagenesis of *dpy-5(e61) unc-29(e403)/hT2[dpy-18(h662)] I;+/hT2[bli-4(e937)] III.* Isolated as a lethal mutation balanced by *hT2,* now maintained as a homozygote balanced by *szDp1.*

Recommended use: General balancing, strain maintenance.

Reference strain: KR1879, *hT3[dpy-5(e61) unc-29(e403)](I;X); szDp1(I;X;f).*

Phenotype: Unc-29 (*szDp1* complements *dpy-5* but not *unc-29*).

Segregants: Unc-29, arrested *hT3* homozygotes.

Growth characteristics: Original isolate marked with *dpy-5* and *unc-29*. Homozygous inviable, probably breaks in *let-363(I)*. Heterozygotes exhibit reduced viability, low level of X chromosome nondisjunction (1.2%).

Handling: Easy to manipulate. Rare exceptional progeny carry one half-translocation as a free duplication. Recombination frequency in unbalanced intervals increased on both LG I and LG X.

Marked variants: hT3[dpy-5(e61)].

Derivative: hDp135(I;X;f).

Reference: McKim *et al.,* 1993.

7. *mnC1(II)*

Summary: Dominant crossover suppressor, uncharacterized with regard to structure, very stable. Very effective balancer for right portion of LG II from around *dpy-10* to around *unc-52.*

Origin: X-ray mutagenesis of *unc-4/dpy-10 unc-52.*

Recommended use: General balancing, strain construction, strain maintenance, mutant screens.

Reference strain: SP127, *unc-4(e120)/mnC1[dpy-10(e128) unc-52(e444)].*

Phenotype: Wild type.

Segregants: Wild type, Unc-4, Dpy-10 Unc-52 *mnC1* homozygotes. The homozygotes are short, fat, and paralyzed, whereas the Unc-4 segregants are large and healthy and move forward well, but cannot back up.

Growth characteristics: Homozygotes viable with extremely small broods (average: 7 progeny). Brood size in heterozygotes ~200, with 100% egg hatching.

Handling: Easy to manipulate. Heterozygous male stocks mate well. Very rare recombination gives rise to Dpy non-Unc and Unc non-Dpy progeny. The recombinant chromosomes carried by these progeny are homozygous lethal.

References: Herman, 1978; Sigurdson *et al.,* 1984.

8. *mnDp1(X;V)*

Summary: Translocated duplication, well characterized, does not recombine with normal homologs. Very effective balancer for right portion of LG X from right end through *let-4.*

Origin: ~7500-R X-ray mutagenesis of N2 males.

Recommended use: General balancing, strain construction, strain maintenance, mutant screens.

Reference strain: SP219, *mnDp1(X;V)/+ V; unc-3(e151)X*

Phenotype: Wild type.

Segregants: Wild type, Unc-3, sterile *mnDp1* homozygotes.

Growth characteristics: Brood size of reference strain ~235. Unc-3 progeny constitute 25% of total, and about a third of total are slow-growing, sterile duplication homozygotes.

Handling: Easy to manipulate. Males mate well. *mnDp1* is attached to LG V near the left end, and severely reduces recombination frequency from *unc-60* to *dpy-11*.

References: Herman *et al.,* 1976, 1979; Meneely and Herman, 1981.

9. *mnDp3(X;f)*

Summary: Free duplication, well characterized, does not recombine with normal LG X. Effective balancer for right portion of LG X from around the right end through *unc-9*.

Origin: ~7500-R X-ray mutagenesis of N2 males.

Recommended use: General balancing, strain construction, strain maintenance.

Reference strain: SP123, *unc-3(e151)X; mnDp3(X;f)*.

Phenotype: Wild type.

Segregants: Wild type, Unc-3.

Growth characteristics: Brood size ~275, duplication transmitted to ~65% of progeny.

Handling: Easy to manipulate. Males carrying duplication mate well. Shows some tendency for somatic loss.

Marked variant: mnDp3[sup-10(mn338)].

References: Herman *et al.,* 1976, 1979; Herman, 1984.

10. *mnDp10(X;I)*

Summary: Translocated duplication, well characterized, does not recombine with normal LG X. Effective balancer for right portion of LG X from around the right end through *lin-2*.

Origin: ~7500-R X-ray mutagenesis of N2 males.

Recommended use: General balancing, strain construction, strain maintenance.

Reference strain: SP117, *mnDp10(X;I); unc-3(e151)X*.

Phenotype: Wild type.

Segregants: Wild type, rare Unc-3.

Growth characteristics: Duplication is homozygous viable. Unc-3 animals arise from somatic loss of duplication.

Handling: Easy to manipulate. Males carrying the duplication mate well. *mnDp10* shows some tendency to segregate from the X chromosome in male spermatogenesis.

References: Herman *et al.,* 1979; Meneely and Herman, 1981.

11. *mnDp33(X;IV)*

Summary: Translocated duplication, well characterized, does not recombine with normal X. Effective balancer for small region of left portion of LG X, from *lin-18* to *osm-5* (inclusive).

Origin: ~7500-R X-ray mutagenesis of N2 males.

Recommended use: General balancing, strain construction, strain maintenance.

Reference strain: SP309, *mnDp33(X;IV); unc-20(e112)X.*

Phenotype: Wild type.

Segregants: Wild type, Unc-20, arrested L1 or L2 larvae (duplication homozygotes).

Growth characteristics: Homozygous inviable. ~100% egg hatching, but 25% arrest.

Handling: Easy to manipulate. Males carrying the duplication mate well.

Reference: Herman *et al.,* 1979.

12. *mnDp34-36(II)*

Summary: Independently isolated free duplications with apparently identical genetic extents. Well characterized, do not recombine with normal homologs. Very effective balancers for right portion of LG II from around *unc-52* through *unc-53.*

Origin: ~7500-R X-ray mutagenesis of *mnC1 dpy-10(e128) unc-52(e444)/ unc-4(e120).*

Recommended use: General balancing, strain maintenance.

Reference strains: mnDp34: SP306, *mnC1 dpy-10 unc-52/unc-4 unc-52; mnDp34.* mnDp35: SP307, *mnC1 dpy-10 unc-52/unc-4 unc-52; mnDp35.* mnDp36: SP308, *mnC1 dpy-10 unc-52/unc-4 unc-52; mnDp36.*

Phenotype: Wild type.

Segregants: Wild type, Dpy-10 Unc-52 (*mnC1 dpy-10 unc-52 homozygotes*), Unc-52 (*unc-4 unc-52* homozygotes and *mnC1 dpy-10 unc-52/unc-4 unc-52*), Unc-4 (*unc-4 unc-52; mnDpx*), Dpy-10 (*mnC1 dpy-10 unc-52; mnDpx*).

Growth characteristics: Egg hatching nearly 100%. About 20% of these arrest development as early larvae, and are presumably duplication homozygotes. The duplications are transmitted to about 40% of progeny.

Handling: These duplications tend to segregate from the X chromosome in male spermatogenesis.

Reference: Herman *et al.,* 1979.

13. *nT1(IV;V)*

Summary: Translocation, moderately well characterized, very stable. Very effective balancer for right portion of LG IV from right end through *unc-17,* and for left portion of LG V from left end through *unc-76.*

Origin: Spontaneous.

Recommended use: General balancing, strain maintenance, mutant screens.

Reference strain: MT1000, *unc-5(e53)/nT1 IV; dpy-11(e224)/nT1 V.*

Phenotype: Wild type.

Segregants: Wild type, vulvaless *nT1* homozygotes that make bags of worms, Unc-5 Dpy-11, and large numbers of arrested aneuploid progeny.

Growth characteristics: Brood size in *nT1* heterozygotes ~100.

Handling: Easy to manipulate. Heterozygous males mate well. Vulvaless homozygous hermaphrodites completely unable to mate. Cause of vulvaless phenotype unknown. Translocation may break down spontaneously, but analysis of such events is lacking. Heterozygous strains occasionally begin to segregate large numbers of sick-looking progeny while appearing to remain heterozygous, or they occasionally begin to give larger broods (Schein and Baillie, unpublished results).

Marked variants: nT1[unc(n754dm) let] (previously called DnT1, dominant Unc, recessive Let); *nT1[let(m435)]*.

References: Ferguson and Horvitz, 1985; Clark *et al.*, 1988; Rogalski and Riddle, 1988.

14. *qC1(III)*

Summary: Dominant crossover suppressor, uncharacterized with regard to structure, very stable. Very effective balancer for the left portion of LG III from *tra-1* to at least *dpy-1*.

Origin: 7200-R gamma-irradiation mutagenesis of *unc-32(e189)/dpy-19(e1259)*.

Recommended use: General balancing, strain maintenance.

Reference strain: CB4681, *nDf17/qC1[dpy-19(e1259ts) glp-1(q339)] III*.

Phenotype: Wild type.

Segregants: Wild type, arrested nDf17 homozygotes, sterile *ts* Dpy-19.

Handling: Relatively easy to manipulate. Heterozygous males mate and transfer *qC1*, though perhaps at low frequency. *qC1* fails to complement *glp-1* and *mog-1* mutations.

References: Austin and Kimble, 1989; J. Austin, E. Goodwin, and J. Kimble, pers. comm.; Ha and Baillie, unpublished results.

15. *sC1(III)*

Summary: Dominant crossover suppressor, uncharacterized with regard to structure, very stable. Very effective balancer for an approximately 15-mu portion of LG III from around *unc-45* to near *daf-2*.

Origin: 2000-R gamma-irradiation mutagenesis of N2 males.

Recommended use: General balancing, strain maintenance, mutant screens.

Reference strain: BC4279, *sC1[dpy-1(s2170)] III*.

Phenotype: Dpy-1.

Segregants: Dpy-1 (homozygous strain).

Growth characteristics: Original isolate wild type. Broods approximately wild type in size.

Handling: Easy to manipulate. Heterozygous males, and homozygous males of original isolate, mate well.

Marked variants: sC1[dpy-1(s2171)]; sC1[dpy-1(s2171) let].

Reference: Stewart & Baillie, unpublished results.

16. *sC4(V)*

Summary: Dominant crossover suppressor, uncharacterized with regard to structure, moderately stable. Balances right portion of LG V from *rol-9* to *unc-76.*

Origin: 2000-R gamma-irradiation mutagenesis of *dpy-21/unc-76 rol-9.*

Recommended use: Being characterized and tested: *unc-76–rol-9* genetic distance reduced to 1.8%. Presence of *dpy-21* on *sC4* not confirmed.

Reference strain: BC4586, *sC4 dpy-21/unc-76 rol-9.*

Phenotype: Wild type.

Segregants: Wild type, Unc-76 Rol-9, arrested sC4 homozygotes.

Growth characteristics: Homozygous inviable. Average brood size 117. Cause of homozygous lethal phenotype unknown.

Handling: Easy to manipulate. Heterozygous males mate well.

References: Stewart and Baillie, unpublished results.

17. *sDp2(I;f)*

Summary: Free duplication, well characterized, does not recombine with normal homologs. Very effective balancer for the left portion of LG I from the left end through *unc-15* (just left of *unc-13*).

Origin: 7500-R gamma-irradiation mutagenesis of N2 males.

Recommended use: General balancing, strain maintenance, mutant screens.

Reference strain: KR236, *dpy-5(e61) unc-13(e450)I; sDp2(I;f).*

Phenotype: Unc-13.

Segregants: Unc-13, Dpy-5 Unc-13.

Growth characteristics: Both Unc-13 and Dpy-5 Unc-13 animals are slow growing (generation time at 20°C nearly 5 days). Animals carrying two copies of *sDp2* have never been recovered.

Handling: sDp2-bearing males mate and give some progeny, but are slow growing and do not compete well with non-Dp males in mating.

Derivatives: hDp2–hDp30; hDp59; hDp74–hDp77.

References: Rose *et al.,* 1984; Howell *et al.,* 1987; Howell and Rose, 1990; McKim and Rose, 1990; McKim *et al.,* 1992, 1993.

18. *sDp3(III;f)*

> *Summary:* Free duplication, well characterized, does not recombine with normal homologs. Very effective balancer for left portion of LG III from around *unc-86* through at least *dpy-1* (does not extend to *unc-45*).
>
> *Origin:* 1500-R gamma-irradiation mutagenesis of *dpy-18/eT1 III; unc-46/ eT1 V*.
>
> *Recommended use:* General balancing, strain maintenance, mutant screens.
>
> *Reference strain:* BC986, *eT1(III;V); sDp3(III;f)*.
>
> *Phenotype:* Wild type.
>
> *Segregants:* Wild type, Unc-36 *eT1* homozygotes.
>
> *Handling:* Easy to manipulate. Males mate well. Duplication homozygotes are probably inviable (never recovered).
>
> *Reference:* Rosenbluth *et al.*, 1985.

19. *stDp2(X;II)*

> *Summary:* Translocated duplication, moderately well characterized, not observed to recombine with normal LG X. Very effective balancer for small region in the center of LG X, from around *unc-58* to around *unc-6*.
>
> *Recommended use:* General balancing, strain construction, strain maintenance.
>
> *Reference strain:* RW6002, *+/stDp2 II; unc-18(e81)X*.
>
> *Phenotype:* Wild type.
>
> *Segregants:* Wild type, Unc-18.
>
> *Growth characteristics:* Homozygous inviable
>
> *Handling:* Easy to manipulate. Males carrying one copy of the duplication mate well.
>
> *Reference:* Meneely and Wood, 1984.

20. *szDp1(I;X;f)*

> *Summary:* Complex free duplication, well characterized, does not recombine with normal LG I. Very effective balancer for the left portion of LG I from the left end through *unc-13*. Consists of one half-translocation [*szT1(X)*] from *szT1* maintained in addition to a normal chromosome complement.
>
> *Origin:* Exceptional Unc-3 segregant from *dpy-5/szT1[lon-2] I; unc-3/szT1 X*.
>
> *Reference strain:* KR1577, *dpy-5(e61) unc-13(e450)I; szDp1(I;X;f)*.
>
> *Phenotype:* Wild type.
>
> *Segregants:* Wild-type hermaphrodites, small percentage wild-type males, Dpy-5 Unc-13.

Growth characteristics: Animals carrying two copies of *szDp1* apparently inviable. Duplication strains give rise to spontaneous males through meiotic nondisjunction of the X chromosome.

Handling: szDp1-bearing males either do not mate or are infertile.

Derivatives: hDp31–hDp58; hDp60–hDp73.

References: McKim *et al.,* 1988, 1992, 1993; McKim and Rose, 1990.

21. *szT1(I;X)*

Summary: Reciprocal translocation, well characterized, very stable. Effective balancer for left portion of LG I through *unc-13,* nearly all of LG X from right end to around *dpy-3. szT1(I)* is large segment of LG X (right) translocated to LG I, disjoins from normal LG I. *szT1(X)* is LG I (left) translocated to fragment of LG X (left), disjoins from normal LG X.

Origin: 7000-R gamma-ray mutagenesis of *lon-2(e678)/dpy-8(e1321) unc-3 (e151)* hermaphrodites.

Recommended use: General balancing, strain construction, strain maintenance.

Reference strain: AF1, *+/szT1[lon-2(e678)] I; dpy-8(e1321) unc-3(e151)/szT1 X.*

Phenotype: Wild type.

Segregants: Wild type, Dpy-8 Unc-3, embryonic lethal *szT1* homozygotes, large numbers of embryonic or early larval arrest aneuploid progeny, and about 10% Lon-2 males.

Growth characteristics: Homozygous inviable; breakpoint resulting in lethality must interrupt a gene on LG I, as hemizygous males are viable and fertile. Lon-2 males arise through meiotic nondisjunction of X chromosome. Brood size in heterozygotes ~100.

Handling: Easy to manipulate. Lon-2 *szT1* males mate well. Rare exceptional progeny carry one half-translocation as a complex free duplication. Gives rise spontaneously to rare apparent lethal mutations that may represent fusion of *szT1(X)* and the normal X. Shows threefold enhanced recombination frequency immediately adjacent to right of LG I breakpoint and about twofold enhanced frequency in the *unc-101–unc-54* interval.

Marked variant: szT1[lon-2(e678) unc-29(e403)].

References: Fodor and Deak, 1985; McKim *et al.,* 1988; Howell and Rose, 1990; McKim and Rose, 1990.

22. *γDp1(IV;V;f)*

Summary: Complex free duplication, moderately well characterized, not observed to recombine with either normal homolog. Very effective balancer for right portion of LG IV from around *dpy-4* to around *unc-22,* and left portion of LG V from around *unc-34* through *unc-46.*

Origin: EMS mutagenesis of *unc-22(s7) dpy-26(n199)IV/nT1[unc(n754) let(IV;V)*.

Recommended use: General balancing, strain construction, strain maintenance.

Reference strain: TY156, *unc-30(e191) dpy-4(e1166)IV; yDp1(IV;V;f)*.

Phenotype: Wild type.

Segregants: Wild type, Unc-30 Dpy-4.

Growth characteristics: Brood size ~250. Animals carrying two copies of *yDp1* apparently inviable. The duplication segregates away from X chromosome in male meiosis.

Handling: Easy to manipulate. Males carrying the duplication mate well.

References: DeLong *et al.,* 1987; Plenefisch *et al.,* 1989; Yuan and Horvitz, 1990.

References

Albertson, D. G., and Thomson, J. N. (1982). The kinetochores of *Caenorhabditis elegans. Chromosoma* **86,** 409–428.

Albertson, D. G., and Thomson, J. N. (1993). Segregation of holocentric chromosomes at meiosis in the nematode, *Caenorhabditis elegans. Chromos. Res.* **1,** 15–26.

Austin, J., and Kimble, J. (1989). Transcript analysis of *glp-1* and *lin-12,* homologous genes required for cell interactions during development of *C. elegans. Cell* **58,** 565–571.

Brenner, S. (1974). The genetics of *Caenorhabditis elegans. Genetics* **77,** 71–94.

Bucher, E. A., and Greenwald, I. (1991). A genetic mosaic screen of essential zygotic genes in *Caenorhabditis elegans. Genetics* **128,** 281–292.

Clark, D. V., Rogalski, T. M., Donati, L. M., and Baillie, D. L. (1988). The *unc-22*(IV) region of *Caenorhabditis elegans*: Genetic analysis of lethal mutations. *Genetics* **119,** 345–353.

Clark, D. V., Johnsen, R. C., McKim, K. S., and Baillie, D. L. (1990). Analysis of lethal mutations induced in a mutator strain that activates transposable elements in *Caenorhabditis elegans. Genome* **33,** 109–114.

Coulson, A., Sulston, J., Brenner, S., and Karn, J. (1986). Toward a physical map of the genome of the nematode *Caenorhabditis elegans. Proc. Natl. Acad. Sci. U.S.A.* **83,** 7821–7825.

DeLong, L., Casson, L. P., and Meyer, B. J. (1987). Assessment of X-chromosome dosage compensation in *Caenorhabditis elegans* by phenotypic analysis of *lin-14. Genetics* **117,** 657–670.

Ferguson, E. L., and Horvitz, H. R. (1985). Identification and characterization of 22 genes that affect the vulval cell lineages of the nematode *Caenorhabditis elegans. Genetics* **110,** 17–72.

Fire, A. (1986). Integrative transformation of *Caenorhabditis elegans. EMBO J.* **5,** 2673–2680.

Fodor, A., and Deak, P. (1985). The isolation and genetic analysis of a *Caenorhabditis elegans* translocation (*szT1*) strain bearing an X-chromosome balancer. *J. Genet.* **64,** 143–157.

Greenwald, I. S., and Horvitz, H. R. (1980). *unc-93(e1500):* A behavioral mutant of *Caenorhabditis elegans* that defines a gene with a wild-type null phenotype. *Genetics* **96,** 147–164.

Greenwald, I. S., Sternberg, P. W., and Horvitz, H. R. (1983). The *lin-12* locus specifies cell fates in *C. elegans. Cell* **34,** 435–444.

Herman, R. K., Albertson, D. G., and Brenner, S. (1976). Chromosome rearrangements in *Caenorhabditis elegans. Genetics* **83,** 91–105.

Herman, R. K. (1978). Crossover suppressors and balanced recessive lethals in *Caenorhabditis elegans. Genetics* **88,** 49–65.

Herman, R. K., Madl, J. E., and Kari, C. K. (1979). Duplications in *Caenorhabditis elegans. Genetics* **92,** 419–435.

Herman, R. K., Kari, C. K., and Hartman, P. S. (1982). Dominant X-chromosome nondisjunction mutants of *Caenorhabditis elegans. Genetics* **102,** 379–400.

Herman, R. K. (1984). Analysis of genetic mosaics of the nematode *Caenorhabditis elegans*. *Genetics* **108,** 165–180.

Herman, R. K. (1987). Mosaic analysis of two genes that affect nervous system structure in *Caenorhabditis elegans*. *Genetics* **116,** 377–388.

Herman, R. K., and Kari, C. K. (1989). Recombination between small X chromosome duplications and the X chromosome in *Caenorhabditis elegans*. *Genetics* **121,** 723–737.

Hodgkin, J. (1980). More sex-determination mutants of *Caenorhabditis elegans*. *Genetics* **96,** 649–664.

Hodgkin, J. (1987). A genetic analysis of the sex-determining gene, *tra-1*, in the nematode *Caenorhabditis elegans*. *Genes Dev.* **1,** 731–745.

Hodgkin, J. A., Horvitz, H. R., and Brenner, S. (1979). Nondisjunction mutants of the nematode *Caenorhabditis elegans*. *Genetics* **91,** 67–94.

Horvitz, H. R., Brenner, S., Hodgkin, J., and Herman, R. K. (1979). A uniform genetic nomenclature for the nematode *Caenorhabditis elegans*. *Mol. Gen. Genet.* **175,** 129–133.

Howell, A. M., Gilmour, S. G., Mancebo, R. A., and Rose, A. M. (1987). Genetic analysis of a large autosomal region in *Caenorhabditis elegans* by the use of a free duplication. *Genet. Res.* **49,** 207–213.

Howell, A. M., and Rose, A. M. (1990). Essential genes in the *hDf6* region of chromosome I in *Caenorhabditis elegans*. *Genetics* **126,** 583–592.

Hunter, C. P., and Wood, W. B. (1990). The *tra-1* gene determines sexual phenotype cell-autonomously in *C. elegans*. *Cell* **63,** 1193–1204.

Johnsen, R. C., and Baillie, D. L. (1988). Formaldehyde mutagenesis of the *eT1* balanced region in *Caenorhabditis elegans*: Dose-response curve and the analysis of mutational events. *Mutat. Res.* **201,** 137–147.

Johnsen, R. C., and Baillie, D. L. (1991). Genetic analysis of a major segment [LGV(left)] of the genome of *Caenorhabditis elegans*. *Genetics* **129,** 735–752.

Lee, J., Jongeward, G. D., and Sternberg, P. W. (1994). *unc-101*, a gene required for many aspects of *Caenorhabditis elegans* development and behavior, encodes a clathrin-associated protein. *Genes Dev.* **8,** 60–73.

Marra, M. A., and Baillie, D. L. (1994). Recovery of duplications by drug resistance selection in *Caenorhabditis elegans*. *Genome* **37,** 701–705.

McKim, K. S., Howell, A. M., and Rose, A. M. (1988). The effects of translocations on recombination frequency in *Caenorhabditis elegans*. *Genetics* **120,** 987–1001.

McKim, K. S., and Rose, A. M. (1990). Chromosome I duplications in *Caenorhabditis elegans*. *Genetics* **124,** 115–132.

McKim, K. S., Starr, T., and Rose, A. M. (1992). Genetic and molecular analysis of the *dpy-14* region in *Caenorhabditis elegans*. *Mol. Gen. Genet.* **233,** 241–251.

McKim, K. S., Peters, K., and Rose, A. M. (1993). Two types of sites required for meiotic chromosome pairing in *Caenorhabditis elegans*. *Genetics* **134,** 749–768.

Mello, C. C., Kramer, J. M., Stinchcomb, D., and Ambros, V. (1991). Efficient gene transfer in *Caenorhabditis elegans*: Extrachromosomal maintenance and integration of transforming sequences. *EMBO J.* **10,** 3959–3970.

Meneely, P. M., and Herman, R. K. (1979). Lethals, steriles and deficiencies in a region of the X chromosome of *Caenorhabditis elegans*. *Genetics* **92,** 99–115.

Meneely, P. M., and Herman, R. K. (1981). Suppression and function of X-linked lethal and sterile mutations in *Caenorhabditis elegans*. *Genetics* **97,** 65–84.

Meneely, P. M., and Wood, W. B. (1984). An autosomal gene that affects X chromosome expression and sex determination in *Caenorhabditis elegans*. *Genetics* **106,** 29–44.

Meneely, P. M., and Nordstrom, K. D. (1988). X chromosome duplications affect a region of the chromosome they do not duplicate in *Caenorhabditis elegans*. *Genetics* **119,** 365–375.

Moerman, D. G., and Baillie, D. L. (1979). Genetic organization in *Caenorhabditis elegans*: Fine-structure analysis of the *unc-22* gene. *Genetics* **91,** 95–104.

Moerman, D. G., and Baillie, D. L. (1981). Formaldehyde mutagenesis in the nematode *Caenorhabditis elegans*. *Mutat. Res.* **80,** 273–279.

Moerman, D. G., and Waterston, R. H. (1989). Mobile elements in *Caenorhabditis elegans* and other nematodes. *In* "Mobile DNA" (D. E. Berg and M. M. Howe, eds.), pp. 537–556. American Society for Microbiology, Washington, D. C.

Nelson, G. A., Schubert, W. W., Marshall, T. M., Benton, E. R., and Benton, E. V. (1989). Radiation effects in *Caenorhabditis elegans*. Mutagenesis by high and low LET ionizing radiation. *Mutat. Res.* **212,** 181–192.

Plenefisch, J. D., DeLong, L., and Meyer, B. J. (1989). Genes that implement the hermaphrodite mode of dosage compensation in *Caenorhabditis elegans*. *Genetics* **121,** 57–76.

Riddle, D. L., and Brenner, S. (1978). Indirect suppression in *Caenorhabditis elegans*. *Genetics* **89,** 299–314.

Rogalski, T. M., and Riddle, D. L. (1988). A *Caenorhabditis elegans* RNA polymerase II gene, *ama-1 IV*, and nearby essential genes. *Genetics* **118,** 61–74.

Rogalski, T. M., Bullerjahn, A. M. E., and Riddle, D. L. (1988). Lethal and amanitin-resistance mutations in the *Caenorhabditis elegans ama-1* and *ama-2* genes. *Genetics* **120,** 409–422.

Rose, A. M., and Baillie, D. L. (1980). Genetic organization of the region around *unc-15(I)*, a gene affecting paramyosin in *Caenorhabditis elegans*. *Genetics* **96,** 639–648.

Rose, A. M., Baillie, D. L., and Curran, J. (1984). Meiotic pairing behavior of two free duplications of linkage group I in *Caenorhabditis elegans*. *Mol. Gen. Genet.* **195,** 52–56.

Rosenbluth, R. E., and Baillie, D. L. (1981). The genetic analysis of a reciprocal translocation, *eT1(III;V)*, in *Caenorhabditis elegans*. *Genetics* **99,** 415–428.

Rosenbluth, R. E., Cuddeford, C., and Baillie, D. L. (1983). Mutagenesis in *Caenorhabditis elegans*. I. A rapid eukaryotic mutagen test system using the reciprocal translocation *eT1(III;V)*. *Mutat. Res.* **110,** 39–48.

Rosenbluth, R. E., Cuddeford, C., and Baillie, D. L. (1985). Mutagenesis in *Caenorhabditis elegans*. II. A spectrum of mutational events induced with 1500 R of gamma-radiation. *Genetics* **109,** 493–511.

Rosenbluth, R. E., Rogalski, T. M., Johnsen, R. C., Addison, L. M., and Baillie, D. L. (1988). Genomic organization in *Caenorhabditis elegans*: Deficiency mapping on linkage group V (left). *Genet. Res.* **52,** 105–118.

Rosenbluth, R. E., Johnsen, R. C., and Baillie, D. L. (1990). Pairing for recombination in LG V of *Caenorhabditis elegans*: A model based on recombination in deficiency heterozygotes. *Genetics* **124,** 615–625.

Sigurdson, D. C., Spanier, G. J., and Herman, R. K. (1984). *Caenorhabditis elegans* deficiency mapping. *Genetics* **108,** 331–345

Stewart, H. I., Rosenbluth, R. E., and Baillie, D. L. (1991). Most ultraviolet irradiation induced mutations in the nematode *Caenorhabditis elegans* are chromosomal rearrangements. *Mutat. Res.* **249,** 37–54.

Sulston, J., and Hodgkin, J. (1988). Methods. *In* "The Nematode *Caenorhabditis elegans*" (W. B. Wood, ed.), p. 592. Cold Spring Harbor Laboratory, Cold Spring Harbor, New York.

Yandell, M. D., Edgar, L. S., and Wood, W. B. (1994). Trimethylpsoralen induces small deletion mutations in *Caenorhabditis elegans*. *Proc. Natl. Acad. Sci. U.S.A.* **91,** 1381–1385.

Yuan, J. Y., and Horvitz, H. R. (1990). The *Caenorhabditis elegans* genes *ced-3* and *ced-4* act cell autonomously to cause programmed cell death. *Dev. Biol.* **138,** 33–41.

Zetka, M.-C., and Rose, A. M. (1992). The meiotic behavior of an inversion in *Caenorhabditis elegans*. *Genetics* **131,** 321–332.

PART II

Neurobiology

CHAPTER 8

Genetic Pharmacology: Interactions between Drugs and Gene Products in *Caenorhabditis elegans*

James B. Rand and **Carl D. Johnson**[†]

[*]Program in Molecular and Cell Biology
Oklahoma Medical Research Foundation
Oklahoma City, Oklahoma 73104
[†]NemaPharm, Inc.
Cambridge, Massachusetts 02139

I. Introduction

Compared with other animals, the nematode *Caenorhabditis elegans* has many advantages for mutant isolation and for genetic analysis. Some of these, for example, small size and rapid growth to high density on inexpensive media, simplify the manipulation of large numbers of animals. Others, such as the lack of a muscle-driven circulatory system and the self-fertilizing hermaphroditic mode of reproduction, enable the survival of strains with genetic defects that would be lethal to more complex animals. *C. elegans* is also sensitive to a wide spectrum of bioactive compounds.[1] Although a few compounds with *C. elegans*-specific or nematode-specific actions have been described, the vast majority appear to act on targets that are widely distributed in most or all animals, including humans (or even in most or all eukaryotes). As a result, *C. elegans* has been a popular organism in which to study drug action and there is a substantial body of published work. In this chapter we attempt to extract an underlying feature of this work: the methods that are used in compound-based studies of *C. elegans*. We present general approaches to evaluating the effects of compounds on *C. elegans* growth, development, metabolism, and behavior, we discuss strategies for the isolation and analysis of drug-resistant and hypersensitive mutants, and we describe the use of *C. elegans* for new drug discovery. We also provide, as Table I, a list of some of the compounds already studied in *C. elegans*, along with one or more references in which information about the detection of compound-specific effects can be found. It is hoped the table will expedite the use of compound-specific mutants as genetic markers.

Studies combining bioactive compounds and *C. elegans* can be separated on the basis of experimental strategy. The first strategy employs compounds with known modes of action to characterize particular aspects of *C. elegans* biology in wild-type and mutant animals. Thus, for example, experiments with serotonin-related compounds were used to identify and characterize the components of egg-laying behavior and to analyze mutants with egg-laying defects (Horvitz *et al.*, 1982; Trent *et al.*, 1983; Desai and Horvitz, 1989). The second strategy uses active compounds as screening or selective agents to isolate new drug-resistant or hypersensitive mutants and, thus, to identify genes with altered drug responses. Study of such compound-specific mutants can identify specific drug targets and/ or provide insight into the mechanism of drug action and the sites of drug action. Analysis of mutants resistant to acetylcholinesterase inhibitors and to acetylcholine agonists, for example, has led to the identification of the genes that control acetylcholine synthesis, release, and reception (Rand and Russell, 1984, 1985; Lewis *et al.*, 1980a,b, 1987; Hosono *et al.*, 1989, 1992; Alfonso *et al.*, 1993, 1994). The third strategy involves the use of *C. elegans*, both wild type and selected mutants, to analyze the mechanism of action of uncharacterized or poorly characterized compounds. This has led to the use of *C. elegans* as a primary screen for compounds active against parasitic nematodes (Vanfleteren and Roets, 1972; Simkin and Coles, 1981; Ohba and Ishibashi, 1984; Bennett and Pax, 1986), as well as for specific human pharmaceuticals (Johnson, 1989) and for toxicity testing (van Kessel *et al.*, 1989; Williams and Dusenbery, 1990). In what follows, we discuss methods pertinent to each of the three strategies.

---

[1] In this article the terms *bioactive compound, compound,* and *drug* are used interchangeably to mean a chemical with a recognizable effect on *C. elegans*.

Table I
Representative Drug and Mutant Studies in *Caenorhabditis elegans*[a]

Compound	Site of action	Genes	References
Acetylcholine receptor agonists (e.g., levamisole, nicotine, morantel, pyrantel)	Nicotinic acetylcholine receptor	*unc-29, unc-38, unc-50,* etc.	Brenner, 1974; Lewis *et al.,* 1980a,b, 1987
α-Amanitin	RNA polymerase	*ama-1, ama-2*	Sanford *et al.,* 1983; Rogalski *et al.,* 1988; 1990
Anesthetics (e.g., halothane)	Unknown	*unc-7, unc-9, unc-79, unc-80*	Sedensky and Meneely, 1987; Boswell *et al.,* 1990; Morgan *et al.,* 1990, 1991
Benzimidazoles (e.g., benomyl, nocodazole)	Microtubules	*ben-1*	Chalfie and Thomson, 1982; Driscoll *et al.,* 1989
Caffeine	Phosphodiesterase	*caf-1, caf-2*[b]	Hartman, 1987
Chavicol	Unknown	Unknown	Kawaii *et al.,* 1994
Cholinesterase inhibitors (e.g., aldicarb, lannate, trichlorfon)	Acetylcholinesterase	*cha-1, snt-1, unc-13, unc-17, unc-18,* etc.	Brenner, 1974; Rand and Russell, 1984, 1985; Tomlinson *et al.,* 1985 Hosono *et al.,* 1989, 1992; Nonet *et al.,* 1993; Alfonso *et al.,* 1993, 1994
Fluoride	"Cell signaling"	*flr-1–flr-5*	Katsura, 1993; Katsura *et al.,* 1994
GABA-related (e.g., GABA, muscimol)	GABA receptors, GABA uptake, etc.	*unc-25, unc-30, unc-49,* etc.	Avery and Horvitz, 1990; McIntire *et al.,* 1993a,b
Ivermectin	"Avermectins receptors"	Low level: *che-3, osm-3,* etc. High level: *avr-14, avr-15, etc.*	C. D. Johnson, ACeDB
Nordihydroguairetic acid (NDG)	Lipoxygenase, membrane permeability	*unc-8, ndg-4*	Shreffler *et al.,* 1995
Paraquat (methyl viologen)	Oxidative damage	*mev-1, age-1*	Ishii *et al.,* 1990; Vanfleteren, 1993
Phorbol esters	Protein kinase	*tpa-1*	Miwa *et al.,* 1982; Lew *et al.,* 1982; Tabuse and Miwa, 1983; Tabuse *et al.,* 1989
Serotonin-related drugs (e.g., serotonin, imiprimine)	Serotonin receptors, uptake, etc.	*egl-1, egl-2, cat-4,* etc.	Croll, 1975; Desai and Horvitz, 1989; Avery and Horvitz, 1990; Horvitz *et al.,* 1982; Trent *et al.,* 1983

[a] Some compounds are grouped by their putative function; not all drugs in a given class are listed. The putative targets are, in most cases, based on vertebrate pharmacology, and may not be the only or the primary target of action in *C. elegans.* In addition, there are informal reports of the effects of the following compounds and ions on *C. elegans* (which may be accessed through ACeDB): actinomycin D, avitrol, Bay-K, $CdCl_2$, chloroquine, Cu^{2+}, cycloheximide, cytochalasin D, diltiazem, doxorubicin, emetine, α-endosulfan, fluoroacetic acid, 5-fluorodeoxyuridine, L-glutamic acid diethyl ester, haloperidol, $HgCl_2$, hydrogen peroxide, ionomycin, K252a, ketamine, MK801, mezerein, monoamine oxidase inhibitors, muscarinic agonists, Ni^{2+}, O_2, okadaic acid, ozone, paraherquamide, Pb^{2+}, preocenes, ryanodine, trifluoroperazine, UCF1-C, UCH2000, verapamil, Zn^{2+}.

[b] The genes *caf-1* and *caf-2* have recently been shown to be *osm-3* and *che-3,* respectively (Starich *et al.,* 1995).

II. Use of Drugs as a Method of Phenotypic Analysis

In this section we consider research initiated by analyzing the effects of one or more compounds with known action on wild-type and mutant *C. elegans*. The goal is first to "discover" and then to explore drug effects, to gain information about the control of a particular aspect of nematode behavior or development. Several extensive uses of this line of research have focused on the effects of drugs associated with common neurotransmitters: acetylcholine (Russell *et al.,* 1977; Lewis, 1980a; Nguyen *et al.,* 1995, γ-aminobutyric acid (GABA) (Avery and Horvitz, 1990; McIntire *et al.,* 1993a,b), serotonin (Horvitz *et al.,* 1982; Trent *et al.,* 1983; Desai and Horvitz, 1989; Avery and Horvitz, 1990), dopamine (C. Loer, ACeDB[2]) and, more recently, glutamate (J. Kaplan, ACeDB; C. Bargmann, ACeDB). At one level, this research is similar and complementary to behavioral and electrophysiological studies on other nematodes (del Castillo *et al.,* 1963, 1964; Croll, 1975; Kass *et al.,* 1984; Stretton *et al.,* 1985; Walker *et al.,* 1992; Martin, 1993; Segerberg and Stretton, 1993). The comparison of drug effects between wild type and appropriate mutants, however, adds a new dimension, the exploitation of which has produced significant insights about normal function. Similar studies were used to dissect the functions of a class of touch-receptive neurons (using antimicrotubule drugs: Chalfie and Thomson, 1982) and the initiation of spermiogenesis (Shakes and Ward, 1989).

A compound chosen for this type of study is usually considered "well known"; that is, has been studied in other species, most frequently mammals, and it has a well-defined mode of action and target(s). The effects of most of the compounds, however, had not previously been studied with *C. elegans* or, indeed, with any nematode. The compounds used to analyze neurotransmitter functions have included the transmitters themselves, agonists and antagonists of their receptors, and compounds that block transmitter degradation or uptake. From gene cloning studies, it is clear that the genes that encode the targets of these drugs are homologous to those performing comparable functions in mammals (Driscoll *et al.,* 1989; Rogalski *et al.,* 1990; Arpagaus *et al.,* 1994). The logical corollary that underlies these compound-based studies is that homologous—nematode and mammalian—gene products share similar pharmacological properties. This assumption has received considerable, but not universal, support. In the following section we first present some general approaches and methods for analysis of drug effects and then discuss rationale, assumptions, and common pitfalls.

A. Determining Suitable Parameters for Drug Exposure

Several preliminary issues must be addressed concerning the exposure of the animals to any compound. These include whether the exposure is to be brief or

---

[2] The "ACeDB" designation indicates that these studies have not yet been published formally, but have been reported at international *C. elegans* conferences and/or in the *Worm Breeder's Gazette*; they may be accessed through ACeDB, listed under the investigator's name or the compound.

chronic, whether the exposure will be in liquid medium or on agar plates, and the age of the animals to be treated. If an investigator is examining questions of general toxicity, and the biological "assay" is overall growth or development, then a chronic exposure is most frequently used. Usually, but not necessarily, chronic exposure involves incorporating the compound into the growth agar. If, however, a specific biological aspect is to be studied, for example, paralysis, cessation of pharyngeal pumping, induction of egg laying, or loss of chemotaxis response, then a brief exposure to drug (5–90 minutes) may be more appropriate. Such short exposures have been performed either in liquid or on agar; microtiter plates are particularly useful for such experiments. The age of the animals to be tested is also important, because different developmental stages often have different drug sensitivities and, in some cases, different responses. For protocols involving brief drug exposure, it is important to use synchronous populations and to determine stage-specific effects directly.

Although interactions between drugs and bacteria sometimes occur, in practice the effects of a drug on the bacterial food source are not usually a problem. Liquid cultures are seeded with bacteria under conditions where no further growth occurs. Plate cultures are seeded with bacteria when the drug is present, so if the drug blocked bacterial growth, no lawn would appear. Under such conditions, a concentrated slurry of bacteria can be applied to the agar plate. A greater concern, however, is the effects of bacterial metabolism on the drug, and this is discussed below.

A useful first experiment for assessing the effects of previously unstudied compounds is to place a small amount of pure compound onto an agar plate swarming with wild-type nematodes. Observation of animals at various distances from the site of placement reveals the spectrum of acute effects of the compound. A simple next experiment is to transfer a modest number of eggs or newly hatched larvae (~100) and/or a small number of near-adult or adult worms to concentration series of the drug. Careful observation can reveal the concentration dependence of changes in behavior or growth rate. In a slightly more sophisticated version of the same experiment, aliquots of the culture are removed after various times, and the animals washed free of drug and placed in fresh drug-free cultures. Comparing these cultures with the control can reveal the time dependence and also probe the reversibility of a compound's effects. If multiple stages are used, these experiments also help to determine the age dependence of the compound's effects. Microtiter plates are particularly useful for experiments: they permit many strains and/or drug concentrations to be tested in parallel, while using a mimimum of drug.[3] The results provide a solid basis to guide more focused investigations, including the isolation or analysis of mutants.

---

[3] For 96-well plates, approximately 50 μl of S medium is used per well, containing 0.5 μl of packed *Escherichia coli*. No shaking is necessary, but rigorous methods are necessary to prevent evaporation, such as storing the plates in a sealed box with water-soaked paper towels. *C. elegans* grow well in microtiter plates constructed of polystyrene, but do not grow in polypropylene or vinyl plates.

B. Compound Stability

In all cases, it is necessary to test the stability of the drug under the conditions of anticipated use. Although some drugs are stable to autoclaving, it is generally preferable to add the drug to the medium after autoclaving, as a concentrated stock solution, in for example, dimethyl sulfoxide or 70 to 100% ethanol, or as a filter-sterilized aqueous solution. It is usually more convenient to add the drug to the not-yet-solidified agar before pouring into petri dishes, but it is also possible, for relatively low-molecular-weight compounds, to add a small volume of the drug solution to already poured plates and let the compound diffuse through the plate overnight.

The ideal situation is a compound with extreme chemical stability that is inert to bacterial metabolism. Growth plates containing such drugs may be prepared in bulk, seeded with *E. coli*, and stored at 4°C almost indefinitely, if evaporation is controlled. Unfortunately, because most situations are less than ideal, it is important to test whether "old" (e.g., 1 day to 4 weeks) drug-containing culture medium, solid or liquid, with bacteria or without, has the same efficacy as freshly prepared medium. If it is determined that the drug has a relatively brief (several hours to 2–3 days) period of efficacy, then one is usually limited to protocols using brief, rather than chronic exposure. If the drug has an undesirably short biological half-life, it may be possible that chemically modified derivatives would be more stable.

C. Appropriate Drug Concentration

The concentration of a drug required to produce any effect on living *C. elegans* is often quite high, as much as a thousandfold higher than the drug concentration effective on mammalian cells. If the target of the drug is known, and can be easily assayed (e.g., the inhibition of RNA polymerase II by α-amanitin: Sanford *et al.,* 1983; Rogalski *et al.,* 1990), it is possible to determine whether the effective concentration of the drug in homogenates corresponds to the dose required on intact animals. Large discrepancies in apparent efficacy are generally due to the relative impermeability of *C. elegans*. This may not pose a serious problem: biologically meaningful information and resistant mutants can be obtained even when using an absurdly high (to a pharmacologist) external drug concentration.

Several techniques have been used to improve the solubility or permeability of a drug; these approaches are useful when using drugs of low solubility or high cost. Brief vortexing or sonication at elevated temperature (e.g., 10 minutes at 65°C) are useful for maximizing solubilization under standard conditions. In addition, additives to media that increase solubility may be used. Organic solvents increase the activity of many compounds. *C. elegans* can tolerate modest amounts of common solvents:<2% dimethyl sulfoxide, <4% ethanol, and <2% methanol have little effect on growth or behavior. When solvents are used, it is important to consider and control selective solvent evaporation. With highly volatile solvents, for example, methanol, this is more easily accomplished with liquid media than agar plates. Nonionic detergents have been shown to increase the activity of some compounds: the animals readily tolerate <0.1% Triton X-100. The use of hydroxybutylated cyclodextrins may also help in the solubilization of some drugs. An alternative strategy is to use chemically modified derivatives of a drug; these may alter the solubility, stability, permeability, and/or efficacy of the compound, without changing its target or mode of action. A final strategy, which has yet to be thoroughly explored, is the use of permeable mutants. Mutations that affect cuticle structure (e.g., the collagen-encoding *dpy* and *sqt* genes or the *srf* genes) might affect cuticular permeability and, as a result, the potency of drugs that enter the worm by passing across the cuticle. In fact, some *dpy* mutants appear to be hypersensitive to some drugs (see below), which suggests that a systematic study of this phenomenon could lead to useful new tools for *C. elegans* drug studies.

There are, of course, risks inherent in the study of biological effects using high concentrations of a drug. Some compounds may have nonspecific toxic effects and interactions with alternate targets at high concentrations. After an effect is obtained at high concentration, it is generally advisable to test a wide range of drug concentrations. Dose–response curves using whole animals should be interpreted carefully: the occurrence of diverse effects at different concentrations may indicate that the compound has multiple actions. A prudent approach is to develop a standard protocol using the lowest drug concentration producing a clear, reproducible biological effect. The situation can sometimes be clarified through the analysis of compound-specific mutants.

III. Use of Mutants to Study Mechanisms of Drug Action

We now consider research initiated by isolating mutants with altered sensitivity to compounds already known to have effects on *C. elegans*. Most of these studies involve selections for drug-resistant mutants, but we also include experiments in which preexisting mutants are screened for resistance or hypersensitivity to specific compounds. The resistance selection strategy has been applied with the major classes of antinematode compounds (Brenner, 1974; Lewis *et al.*, 1980, 1987; Rand and Russell 1985; Driscoll *et al.*, 1989; C. D. Johnson, unpublished), as well as with a number of metabolic poisons (Sanford *et al.*, 1983; Rogalski *et al.*, 1990; Tabuse and Miwa, 1983; Hartman, 1987; Williamson *et al.*, 1991). This strategy involves exposing a population of (usually mutagenized) animals to an otherwise lethal concentration of a compound and then choosing the rare individuals able to survive or grow. Mutants hypersensitive to volatile anesthetics have been obtained by screening (Sedensky and Meneely, 1987; Morgan *et al.*, 1991), that is, the direct testing of already available mutant strains with a range of compound concentrations.

The initial intent of many of these efforts was to identify the gene(s) that encodes the compound's target. In principle, mutant selections based on resistance to a toxic compound are relatively straightforward and extremely powerful—an attractive alternative to biochemical purification of targets. The results anticipated from such experiments are unpredictable, however, and are dominated by factors that are often unknown at the start of the experiment, for example, whether the target is encoded by (an) essential gene(s) and whether mutations of nontarget genes can "bypass" the toxic effects of the compound. As a result, resistance selections frequently also detect genes that encode components of physiologically related pathways or that control permeability to the compound.

The likelihood of isolating mutations in the structural gene for a receptor depends on the nature of the drug being used. Resistance to a receptor agonist might merely require loss of the receptor; such loss-of-function mutations are expected to be recessive and relatively common. Resistance to an antagonist, however, might require a specific alteration of the ligand binding domain, which is expected to be dominant and quite rare. Primary analysis—to determine the frequency of mutation and whether the resistance is dominant or recessive—can provide some information about the responsible genes. Nonetheless, in general, secondary analysis using an orthogonal technique, for example, a measurement of enzyme activity, a ligand binding assay or gene cloning is needed to distinguish between different explanations for the altered response.

Drug resistance in parasitic nematodes has been defined operationally as "any growth above the threshold" (Shoop, 1993). For the purposes of *C. elegans* research, we sometimes use a somewhat broader definition, namely, the genetic reversal of any drug-mediated phenotype above the threshold. This definition is useful to investigators studying bioactive compounds that do not block growth. It is also useful for analysis of compound-based effects on specific aspects of *C. elegans* behavior or on a particular target tissue, where genetic reversal of the specific phenotype might not be accompanied by general resistance and/or growth of the animals. In what follows, we often, for clarity, refer only to characteristics of resistance or resistant mutants. Most of these observations are applicable to hypersensitivity and hypersensitive mutants with only minor modification.

A. Selecting for Compound Resistance Mutants

The specific methods for isolation, maintenance, and storage of mutant strains are discussed elsewhere in this book. In addition to the considerations of compound stability and solubility discussed above, the experimental design of a resistance selection requires the choice of a selective concentration. Often, an iterative approach is useful. One should start initially with the lowest concentration of drug that, based on preliminary experiments, gives a good selection. Once a set of resistant strains is identified, and the level of resistance of each has been tested, it may be desirable to repeat the selection at higher drug concentrations.

A second decision involves the phenotype to be selected. As indicated above, some compounds have specific behavioral effects (such as paralysis and inhibition of egg laying) at a relatively low concentration and display acute lethality or complete inhibition of growth at a higher concentration. When trying to isolate resistance mutations, the investigator must choose between measuring resistance by the behavioral phenotype and measuring resistance by survival. There are advantages and potential drawbacks to each approach. Behavioral testing is substantially more laborious, and the number of animals screened is limited by the need to observe individuals. On the other hand, the resulting mutants are more likely to have the desired behavioral specificity. With growth/survival strategies, the number of genomes examined is limited only by the method of culture. Single resistant animals have been isolated by placing 10^3 to 10^5 eggs on compound-containing selection plates. Rarer events, for example, at 1 in 10^8, can be selected in liquid culture.

A potential problem when selecting for survival (rather than growth and reproduction) is the possibility of isolating dauer larvae. This may be viewed as a selection for impermeable animals, and is remedied by using synchronized L3 animals for the selection or by changing to a growth and reproduction selection. A more subtle problem, which must be carefully considered, is that the effect of the compound on growth may result from a nonspecific effect or from an interaction with an alternate target.

A final issue, when mutagenesis is used to increase the frequency of resistance mutations, involves the timing of the application of selection. If progeny of the mutagenized animals are exposed to drug, that is, an F_1 selection, then resistant animals carrying dominant or semidominant mutations will be selected, whereas animals carrying recessive mutations will be lost (unless a second, independent, noncomplementing mutation is also present). If progeny of F_1 animals are exposed to drug (an F_2 selection), then both dominant and recessive resistance mutations will be recovered. If the ratio of recessive to dominant resistance mutations is very large, the interpretation of F_1 selections may require the performance of a no-mutagenesis control selection experiment that measures the background level of spontaneous resistant mutations.

B. Screening for Compound-Resistant or Hypersensitive Mutants

Screening involves the testing of preexisting mutant strains for drug resistance or hypersensitivity. In practice, the investigator can either screen mutants in all known genes; all genes of a given phenotype, for example, all *unc* genes or all chemosensory mutants; or random individual F_2 lines from mutagenized populations. At first glance, screening appears to be not as powerful an approach as selection. The disadvantages of a screen are clear: it is slower and more cumbersome. Nonetheless, there are also several advantages. As populations, rather than individual animals, are being examined, the results are not subject to animal-to-animal variability. In addition, animals from a given strain can be tested at several different drug concentrations; this approach can therefore detect even subtle differences in drug response. Finally, screening is the only method available to identify mutants hypersensitive to a drug, because "suicide-selection" methods, such as penicillin selection in bacteria (Lederberg and Zinder, 1948) and inositol-less death in *Neurospora* (Lester and Gross, 1959), are not yet available in *C. elegans*.

Screening for compound-selective mutants has been successfully applied in a number of cases, most notably in obtaining mutants with selective responses to volatile anesthetics (Sedensky and Meneely, 1987; Morgan *et al.*, 1991). This approach could well be effective for other compounds: many of the genes identified by mutations derived from resistance selections have additional alleles that were isolated based on another phenotype, usually alteration of behavior. As the number of genes identified by mutation in *C. elegans* increases, screening the collection of known mutants for compound-specific effects will become increasingly efficient, and may become the recommended first approach when searching for mutations with altered responses to a novel bioactive compound.

C. Genetic Analysis of Resistant Mutants

1. Dominant or Recessive?

The initial genetic question is whether the resistance is dominant or recessive to sensitivity. That is, what is the phenotype of heterozygotes? It is important to perform the analysis using a range of drug concentrations. Many drug-resistant mutants reported as "dominant" are actually semidominant; that is, heterozygous animals have partial resistance. Semidominant mutations will appear to be either dominant or recessive, depending on the precise drug concentration used. Not only can this effect interfere with the interpretation of gene function; it can lead to spurious complementation results: double heterozygote combinations of nonallelic semidominant mutations may lead to artifactual noncomplementation.

2. Mutation Frequency

The frequency with which drug resistance mutations are recovered is generally informative. This information is obtained by measuring the number of independent resistant strains obtained in experiments using a low density of animals per selection plate (the number of F_1 genomes per plate should be < 1/mutation frequency). The frequency of mutation is then calculated by dividing the number of resistant strains obtained by twice the number of F_1 animals exposed to the selection. From similar experiments it has been estimated that the "average" frequency of gene knockout mutations following standard ethyl methanesulfonate (EMS) mutagenesis is approximately 1 in 10^3 per gene (Herman and Horvitz, 1980). (Spontaneous mutations occur at approximately 300-fold lower frequency.) Recovery of resistant mutants at a frequency appreciably greater than 1 in 10^3 suggests that more than one gene may mutate to confer resistance. It is also estimated that EMS mutagenesis leads to a change of any given nucleotide in the genome with a frequency of approximately 1 in 10^6 (Herman and Horvitz, 1980). Observation of a frequency of resistance considerably less than 1 in 10^6 suggests that multiple independent mutations are required for the resistance phenotype.

Some forms of resistance, which require highly specific changes in single gene products, may be "unavailable" in *C. elegans* or may not be induced by EMS. If no resistant mutants are found after extensive selections following EMS mutagenesis, it may be useful to try other mutagens. Alternately, some insight may be gained by repeating the selections on other nematode species that are easily maintained in the laboratory.

3. Genetic Mapping

In principle, the techniques used for mapping compound-specific mutants are no different than those used to map mutations conferring other phenotypes. In fact, many mutations conferring drug resistance or hypersensitivity also lead to additional phenotypes, such as uncoordinated movement and egg-laying defects. In genetic crosses, these behavioral phenotypes may be more convenient to score than the pharmacological phenotypes; however, the investigator must confirm at some point that the two phenotypes are genetically inseparable and are due to a lesion in a single gene. In other cases, the pharmacological phenotype is the best or the only scorable phenotype, and techniques must be developed to score individual F_1 and/or F_2 progeny unambiguously. One simple approach is to clone individuals and test the resistance characteristics of a sample population of progeny: no resistant animals would be observed only if the cloned animals were homozygous wild type at the resistance locus. In this context, we note that a number of commonly used *C. elegans* marker mutations have been shown to have nonspecific pharmacological effects. For example, *dpy-11* and *sma-1* are hypersensitive to α-amanitin (Rogalski *et al.*, 1988), and *dpy-13* is hypersensitive to aldicarb (J. B. Rand, unpublished); it is therefore prudent to test the resistance/sensitivity of all marker mutants.

D. Phenotypic Analysis of Compound–Specific Mutants

1. Quantitation of Resistance

We believe that it is very important to develop a quantitative assay for resistance/sensitivity to the drug being used. Such quantitation is important for comparing different alleles of a particular gene, for comparing mutations in different genes, or for evaluating the phenotypes of double mutants. In addition, these quantitative methods can be used on wild-type animals to determine the extent to which different behaviors (such as sensory behavior and motor behavior) are affected by a particular drug. A quantitative assessment of resistance requires a quantitative measure of the biological parameter being tested. This permits the determination of the drug concentration that gives a 50% decrease in the measured parameter (EC_{50}), thus providing an overall measure of the sensitivity/resistance of the strain tested.

These determinations are complicated by a behavioral impairment of the mutant strain in the absence of drug. In all cases, therefore, the response of animals to different drug concentrations must be compared with the response of the same strain in the absence of drug.

2. Quantitation by Behavioral Testing

Some behaviors, such as pharyngeal pumping rate, defecation frequency, and egg laying, are easily quantified. Brood size and percentage hatching are also useful quantitative measures. There are also quantitative measures of sensory behaviors such as chemotaxis, based on the accumulation of animals near a local source of attractant (e.g., Bargmann *et al.*, 1993). The relative rate of locomotion and its impairment, that is, "unc-ness," is harder to quantify. There are, however, several ways to quantitate specific aspects of locomotion and/or general body neuromuscular function: a "thrashing" assay, which measures the rate at which waves of body muscle contraction are initiated; a "fractional contraction" assay, which measures the ability of the musculature to contract in response to neurotransmitters; and a "radial diffusion" assay, which measures the overall efficiency of locomotion, regardless of its "style."

The thrashing assay is based on the observation that wild-type *C. elegans* swim more vigorously in liquid than on solid agar. Under these conditions, even uncoordinated animals appear to be capable of the head movements associated with foraging and the initiation of sinusoidal body waves. Age-synchronous animals are transferred to buffer in microtiter wells, and after a short time, the number of head thrashes is counted for 1 to 3 minutes. Even with animals that are immobile on agar, this assay frequently provides quantitative behavioral data (K. G. Miller and J. B. Rand, unpublished). It can also be used to obtain a quantitative measure of drug resistance/sensitivity.

A number of drugs (such as levamisole and acetylcholinesterase inhibitors) cause contraction of the body wall muscles; for such drugs, a "fractional contraction" assay is appropriate (Nonet *et al.*, 1993). Animals, usually young adults, from a synchronous population are exposed to drug in microtiter wells or on agar plates. After a short time (5–30 minutes) the fractional change in the animals' length is measured. Unfortunately, the animals are rarely straight, so a precise visual determination of length is difficult to obtain. This problem can be solved by photographing or videotaping the drug-treated animals, although some difficulty may be encountered when photographing animals in microtiter wells. The length of the animals may then be determined by methods as crude as laying a piece of string on a video monitor, or as complicated as scanning the image into a computer for morphometric analysis.

The "radial diffusion" assay (Epstein *et al.*, 1976) uses agar plates seeded with an annular lawn of bacteria. Animals from synchronous cultures are washed free of bacteria and 50 to 100 are transferred to the center of the plate. The animals are attracted to the bacterial lawn and gradually "diffuse" from the center of the plate to the periphery. Uncoordinated or drug-affected animals move more slowly. To quantitate the assay, at intervals, the fraction of animals remaining near the center of the plate is determined by counting. This value follows first-order kinetics, with a rate constant that is a measure of the overall mobility of the strain. This assay is easily adapted to measure drug effects and resistance. For example, we have shown that the "diffusion rate" of wild-type animals is affected by aldicarb, an acetylcholinesterase inhibitor, in a dose-dependent manner, and that the "diffusion" of aldicarb-resistant mutants is clearly less sensitive to the drug than is that of wild-type animals (J. B. Rand, unpublished). The strength of this procedure is its sensitivity to even slight impairments of coordination. Conversely, it has only limited usefulness with animals that are extremely uncoordinated due to mutation or to drug effects.

3. Quantitation by Measures of Growth and Development

Although overall growth of a cohort of animals can be characterized by simple growth curves (mean length of the animals as a function of age), this method is not usually suitable for assessing the effects of drugs. Most compounds that reduce growth also reduce the synchrony of a population and the fecundity of the adults. Therefore, proper quantitation of growth rate usually requires a functional determination of the generation time.

Growth rate can be measured in several ways. Although unsophisticated, "plate-clearing" determinations are quite useful. A fixed number of animals, generally either eggs or young adults, are transferred to a set of cultures containing different drug concentrations. The cultures are scored daily. The number of days required for the food to be consumed completely provides a crude measure of generation time. In practice, the food is consumed by the progeny of the transferred animals; thus, such assays measure both growth and fecundity.

A more precise and more labor-intensive method involves progeny counting. In this method, small aliquots of buffer ($10\mu l$) containing 200 synchronously hatched 2-hour-old larvae are transferred to drug-containing plates. When such small worms are used, the reproducibility of the aliquots is quite good. Each plate is screened once or twice a day, and the numbers of progeny eggs and larvae on each plate are recorded. The generation time is defined arbitrarily, for example, as the time required to produce a number of progeny equal to the initial inoculum. The growth rate is then defined as the reciprocal of the generation time, and the "relative growth rate" is the ratio of the growth rate in the presence of the drug to the growth rate in the absence of the drug. Although this approach does not distinguish between each of the original animals producing one offspring and only one of the original animals producing many progeny, the results obtained are useful for quantifying drug effects and characterizing resistant mutants.

4. Divergence of Behavioral and Growth Resistance

There are cases in which a mutant is resistant to some of the effects of a particular compound, while being drug sensitive in other ways. For example, *unc-29* mutants are relatively resistant to the paralytic effects of cholinesterase inhibitors (Lewis *et al.*, 1980a), but they are not able to grow and reproduce in the presence of these compounds (Rand and Russell, 1985). Although such situations can lead to confusion, they may also be instructive. It is likely that, for many bioactive compounds, the target is regulated by several different gene products. These may be expressed at different times and/or in different cell types, and any one resistance mutation may affect only a subset of the susceptible gene products and/or cells. It is therefore advisable to develop and use several different paradigms for the assessment of resistance, because discrepancies can provide information about the cellular and temporal expression of the resistance gene.

IV. Use of *Caenorhabditis elegans* for Drug Discovery

Caenorhabditis elegans has long been popular as a primary screen for antinematode drugs—anthelmintics and nematicides (Simkin and Coles, 1981; Ohba and Ishibashi, 1984; Bennett and Pax, 1986). It has also been proposed as a useful screen for general toxicity as well as neurotoxicity (Williams and Dusenbery, 1990; van Kessel *et al.*, 1989). Most of these screens use animals from the wild-type strain only. As it is now known that many human therapeutic targets are encoded by genes with homologs in *C. elegans*, the nematode could also have value for human pharmaceutical discovery. Indeed, one of us has proposed the establishment of a series of *C. elegans*-based screens, using selected mutants that sensitize the assays to compounds with a defined mode of action (Johnson, 1989). To date, however, there are no examples of human drugs or drug classes discovered with such methods.

A. Standard Assay Conditions

The basic considerations relevant to compound screening for drug discovery are the same as those for studies of known drugs: choice of solid or liquid media, compound concentration, solubility and stability, and choice of a desired drug effect. To facilitate the analysis of a large number of compounds in a short time, general strategies amenable to high throughput are required. Most systematic screening is performed in small liquid cultures in either 96-well microtiter plates (50–100 μl per well) or in other multiwell plates. Screens for antinematode drugs are performed at a relatively low concentration, for example, 1 to 10 μg/ml, in media containing solvent, most often 1% dimethyl sulfoxide. The assays are initiated shortly after addition of compound to minimize the impact of compound instability. The selected phenotype is generally either blockage of growth or paralysis. These choices bias the screen toward the selection of relatively potent compounds that might be appropriate for futher commercial development.

Screens for human pharmaceuticals are performed under similar conditions. They need not, however, be constrained by the requirement for activity at low concentration: a compound with weak, but specific, effects on a novel target is a potentially valuable lead compound. Following the discovery of a lead, chemical modification, combined with structure–activity analysis using the human homolog, can frequently be used to generate compounds with the desired potency and specificity.

B. Uses of Compound-Specific Mutants

Compounds that cause behavioral defects or block nematode growth are of little interest as potential human pharmaceuticals. On the other hand, a *C. elegans*-based screen that was biased to detect only compounds that act on a specific target might well find utility as a method for identification of new therapeutic drugs. In some cases, this can be accomplished by judicious use of compound-specific mutants. Mutants selected for resistance to a specific compound, for example, generally display side or cross-resistance (Shoop, 1993) to other compounds with the same or a related mode of action. Thus, a panel of resistant strains can be used to determine if a new compound, with an unknown mode of action, acts similarly to one of the known drugs. Alternately, a mutant that fails to respond to a specific compound might be used to identify other compounds with a similar mode of action. Mutants with defects in egg laying, for example, can be used to determine if compounds act as serotonin agonists or serotonin uptake blockers (Johnson, 1989). Wild-type animals lay eggs in response to both classes of compounds (Horvitz *et al.*, 1982), whereas specific mutants selectively fail to respond either to uptake blockers or to agonists (Trent *et al.*, 1983; Desai and Horvitz, 1989). Finally, by screening for compounds that mimic the effect of particular *C. elegans* mutants, it is possible to select for compounds that act on targets for which no known compounds are yet available. As the level of knowledge of biological properties of *C. elegans* homologs of known and potential new human therapeutic targets expands, we can expect a similar escalation in the use of *C. elegans*-based technologies that facilitate the discovery of new human drugs.

References

Alfonso, A., Grundahl, K., Duerr, J. S., Han, H.-P., and Rand, J. B. (1993). The *Caenorhabditis elegans unc-17* gene: A putative vesicular acetylcholine transporter. *Science* **261**, 617–619.

Alfonso, A., Grundahl, K., McManus, J. R., and Rand, J. B. (1994). Cloning and characterization of the choline acetyltransferase structural gene (*cha-1*) from *C. elegans*. *J. Neurosci.* **14**, 2290–2300.

Arpagaus, M., Fedon, Y., Cousin, X., Chatonnet, A., Bergé, J.-B., Fournier, D., and Toutant, J.-P. (1994). cDNA sequence, gene structure, and *in vitro* expression of *ace-1*, the gene encoding acetylcholinesterase of class A in the nematode *Caenorhabditis elegans*. *J. Biol. Chem.* **269**, 9957–9965.

Avery, L., and Horvitz, H. R. (1990). Effects of starvation and neuroactive drugs on feeding in *Caenorhabditis elegans*. *J. Exp. Zool.* **253**, 263–270.

Bargmann, C. I., Hartwieg, E., and Horvitz, H. R. (1993). Odorant-selective genes and neurons mediate olfaction in *C. elegans*. *Cell* **74**, 515–527.

Bennett, J. L., and Pax, R. A. (1986). Micromotility meter; An instrument designed to evaluate the action of drugs on motility of larval and adult nematodes. *Parasitology* **93**, 341–346.

Boswell, M. V., Morgan, P. G., and Sedensky, M. M. (1990). Interaction of GABA and volatile anesthetics in the nematode Caenorhabditis elegans. *FASEB J.* **4**, 2506–2510.

Brenner, S. (1974). The genetics of *C. elegans*. *Genetics* **77**, 71–94.

Chalfie, M., and Thomson, J. N. (1982). Structural and functional diversity in the neuronal microtubules of *Caenorhabditis elegans*. *J. Cell Biol.* **93**, 15–23.

Croll, N. A. (1975). Indoleaklyamines and nematode behavior. *Can. J. Zool.* **53**, 894–903.

del Castillo, J., de Mello, W. C., and Morales, T. (1963). The physiological role of acetylcholine in the neuromuscular system of *Ascaris lumbricoides*. *Arch. Int. Physiol. Biochim.* **71**, 741–757.

del Castillo, J., de Mello, W. C., and Morales, T. (1964). Inhibitory action of GABA on *Ascaris* muscle. *Experientia* **20**, 141–143.

Desai, C., and Horvitz, H. R. (1989). *Caenorhabditis elegans* mutants defective in the functioning of the motor neurons responsible for egg laying. *Genetics* **121**, 703–721.

Driscoll, M., Dean, E., Reilly, E., Bergholz, E., and Chalfie, M. (1989). Genetic and molecular analysis of a *Caenorhabditis elegans* β-tubulin that conveys benzimidazole sensitivity. *J. Cell Biol.* **109**, 2993–3003.

Epstein, H. F., Isachsen, M. M., and Suddleson, E. A. (1976). Kinetics of movement of normal and mutant nematodes. *J. Comp. Physiol.* **110**, 317–322.

Hartman, P. S. (1987). Caffeine-resistant mutants of *Caenorhabditis elegans*. *Genet. Res.* **49**, 105–110.

Herman, R. K., and Horvitz, H. R. (1980). Genetic analysis of *C. elegans*. *In* "Nematodes as Biological Models" (B. Zuckerman, ed.), Vol. 1, pp. 228–261. Academic Press, New York.

Horvitz, H. R., Chalfie, M., Trent, C., Sulston, J. E., and Evans, P. D. (1982). Serotonin and octopamine in the nematode *C. elegans*. *Science* **216**, 1012–1014.

Hosono, R., Sassa, T., and Kuno, S. (1989). Spontaneous mutations of trichlorfon resistance in the nematode *Caenorhabditis elegans*. *Zool. Sci.* **6**, 667–708.

Hosono, R., Hekimi, S., Kamiya, Y., Sassa, T., Murakami, S., Nishiwaki, K., Miwa, J., Taketo, A., and Kodaira, K.-I. (1992). The *unc-18* gene encodes a novel protein affecting the kinetics of acetylcholine metabolism in the nematode *Caenorhabditis elegans*. *J. Neurochem.* **58**, 1517–1525.

Ishii, N., Takahashi, K., Tomita, S., Keino, T., Honda, S., Yoshino, K., and Suzuki, K. (1990). A methyl viologen-sensitive mutant of the nematode *Caenorhabditis elegans*. *Mutat. Res.* **237**, 165–171.

Johnson, C. D. (1989). The nematode *Caenorhabditis elegans:* A model for the human nervous system. *ICSU Short Rep.* **9**, 32–33.

Kass, I. S., Stretton, A. O. W., and Wang, C. C. (1984). The effects of avermectin and drugs related to acetylcholine and 4-aminobutyric acid on neurotransmission in *Ascaris suum*. *Mol. Biochem. Parasitol.* **13**, 213–225.

Katsura, I. (1993). In search of new mutants in cell-signaling systems of the nematode *Caenorhabditis elegans*. *Genetica* **88**, 137–146.

Katsura, I., Kondo, K., Amano, T., Ishihara, T., and Kawakami, M. (1994). Isolation, characterization and epistasis of fluoride-resistant mutants of *Caenorhabditis elegans*. *Genetics* **136**, 145–154.

Kawaii, S., Yoshizawa, Y., and Mizutani, J. (1994). Effects of chavicol on intracellular calcium in a free-living soil nematode, *Caenorhabditis elegans*. *Biosci. Biotechnol. Biochem.* **58**, 982–985.

Lederberg, J., and Zinder, N. (1948). Concentration of biochemical mutants of bacteria with penicillin, *J. Am. Chem. Soc.* **70**, 4267.

Lester, H. E., and Gross, S. R. (1959). Efficient method for selection of auxotrophs in *Neurospora*. *Science* **139,** 572

Lew, K. K., Chritton, S., and Blumberg, P. M. (1982). Biological responsiveness to the phorbol esters and specific binding of [3H]phorbol 12, 13-dibutyrate in the nematode *Caenorhabditis elegans*, a manipulable genetic system. *Teratogenesis Carcinog. Mutagen.* **2,** 19–30.

Lewis, J. A., Wu, C.-H., Berg, H., and Levine, J. H. (1980a). The genetics of levamisole resistance in the nematode *Caenorhabditis elegans*. *Genetics* **95,** 905–928.

Lewis, J. A., Wu, C. H., Levine, J. H., and Berg, H. (1980b). Levamisole-resistant mutants of the nematode *Caenorhabditis elegans* appear to lack pharmacological acetylcholine receptors. *Neuroscience* **5,** 967–989.

Lewis, J. A., Elmer, J. S., Skimming, J., McLafferty, S., Fleming, J., and McGee, T. (1987). Cholinergic receptor mutants of the nematode *Caenorhabditis elegans*. *J. Neurosci.* **7,** 3059–3071.

Martin, R. J. (1993). Neuromuscular transmission in nematode parasites and antinematodal drug action. *Pharmacol. Ther.* **58,** 13–50.

McIntire, S. L., Jorgensen, E., and Horvitz, H. R. (1993a). Genes required for GABA function in *Caenorhabditis elegans*. *Nautre* **364,** 334–337.

McIntire, S. L., Jorgensen, E., Kaplan, J., and Horvitz, H. R. (1993b). The GABAergic nervous system of *Caenorhabditis elegans*. *Nature* **364,** 337–341.

Miwa, J., Tabuse, Y., Furusawa, M., and Yamasaki, H. (1982). Tumor promoters specifically and reversibly disturb development and behavior of *Caenorhabditis elegans*. *J. Cancer Res. Clin. Oncol.* **104,** 81–87.

Morgan, P. G., Sedensky, M. M., and Meneely, P. M. (1990). Multiple sites of action of volatile anesthetics in *Caenorhabditis elegans*. *Proc. Nat. Acad. Sci.* **87,** 2965–2969.

Morgan, P. G., Sedensky, M. M., and Meneely, P. M. (1991). The genetics of response to volatile anesthetics in *Caenorhabditis elegans*. *Ann. N. Y. Acad. Sci.* **625,** 524–531.

Nguyen, M., Alfonso, A., Johnson, C. D., and Rand, J. B. (1995). Mutants of *C. elegans* resistant to inhibitors of cholinesterase. *Genetics* **140,** 527–535.

Nonet, M. L., Grundahl, K., Meyer, B. J., and Rand, J. B. (1993). Synaptic function is impaired but not eliminated in *C. elegans* mutants lacking synaptotagmin. *Cell* **73,** 1291–1305.

Ohba, K., and Ishibashi, N. (1984). A nematode, *Caenorhabditis elegans*, as test organism for nematicide evaluation. *J. Pest. Sci.* **9,** 91–96.

Rand, J. B., and Russell, R. L. (1984). Choline acetyltransferase-deficient mutants of the nematode *Caenorhabditis elegans*. *Genetics* **106,** 227–248.

Rand, J. B., and Russell, R. L. (1985). Molecular basis of drug-resistance mutations in the nematode *Caenorhabditis elegans*. *Psychopharm. Bull.* **21,** 623–630.

Rogalski, T. M., and Riddle, D. L. (1988). A *Caenorhabditis elegans* RNA polymerase II gene, *ama-1 IV,* and nearby essential genes. *Genetics* **118,** 61–74.

Rogalski, T. M., Bullerjahn, A. M., and Riddle, D. L. (1988). Lethal and amanitin-resistant mutations in the *Caenorhabditis elegans ama-1* and *ama-2* genes. *Genetics* **120,** 409–422.

Rogalski, T. M., Golomb, M., and Riddle, D. L. (1990). Mutant *Caenorhabditis elegans* RNA polymerase II with a 20,000-fold reduced sensitively to α-amanitin. *Genetics* **126,** 889–898.

Russell, R. L., Johnson, C. D., Rand, J. B., Scherer, S., and Zwass, M. S. (1977). Mutants of acetylcholine metabolism in the nematode *C. elegans*. *In* "Molecular Approaches to Eucaryotic Genetic Systems" (G. Wilcox, J. Abelson, and C. F. Fox, eds.), pp. 359–371. Academic Press, New York.

Sanford, T., Golomb, M., and Riddle, D. L. (1983). RNA polymerase II from wild type and α-amanitin-resistant strains of *Caenorhabditis elegans*. *J. Cell Biol.* **258,** 12804–12809.

Sedensky, M. M., and Meneely, P. M. (1987). Genetic analysis of halothane sensitivity in *Caenorhabditis elegans*. *Science* **236,** 952–954.

Segerberg, M. A., and Stretton, A. O. W. (1993). Actions of cholinergic drugs in the nematode *Ascaris suum*. Complex pharmacology of muscle and motorneuron. *J. Gen. Physiol.* **101,** 271–286.

Shakes, D. C., and Ward, S. (1989). Initiation of spermiogenesis in *C. elegans*: A pharmacological and genetic analysis. *Dev. Biol.* **134,** 189–200.

Shoop, W. L. (1993). Ivermectin resistance. *Parasitol. Today* **9**, 154–159.

Shreffler, W., Magardino, T., Shekdar, K., and Wolinsky, E. (1995). The *unc-8* and *sup-40* genes regulate ion channel function in *Caenorhabditis elegans* motorneurons. *Genetics* **139**, 1261–1272.

Simkin, K. G., and Coles, G. C. (1981). The use of *Caenorhabditis elegans* for anthelmintic screening. *J. Chem. Tech. Biotechnol.* **31**, 66–69.

Starich, T. A., Herman, R. K., Kari, C. K., Yeh, W.-H., Schackwitz, W. S., Schuyler, M. V., Collet, J., Thomas, J. H., and Riddle, D. L. (1995). Mutations affecting chemosensory neurons of *Caenorhabditis elegans*. *Genetics* **139**, 171–188.

Stretton, A. O. W., Davis, R. E., Angstadt, J. D., Donmoyer, J.E., and Johnson, C. D. (1985). Neural control of behavior in *Ascaris*. *Trends Neurosci* **8**, 294–300.

Tabuse, Y., and Miwa, J. (1983). A gene involved in action of tumor promoters is identified and mapped in *Caenorhabditis elegans*. *Carcinogenesis* **4**, 783–786.

Tabuse, Y., Nishiwaki, K., and Miwa, J. (1989). Mutations in a protein kinase C homolog confer phorbol ester resistance in *Caenorhabditis elegans*. *Science* **243**, 1713–1716.

Tomlinson, G., Albuquerque, C. A., and Woods, R. A. (1985). The effects of amidantel (BAY d 8815) and its deacylated derivative (BAY d 9216) on *Caenorhabditis elegans*. *Eur. J. Pharmacol.* **113**, 255–262.

Trent, C., Tsung, N., and Horvitz, H. R. (1983). Egg-laying defective mutants of the nematode *C. elegans*. *Genetics* **104**, 619–647.

van Kessel, W. H., Brocades Zaalberg, R. W., and Seinen, W. (1989). Testing environmental pollutants on soil organisms: A simple assay to investigate the toxicity of environmental pollutants on soil organisms, using $CdCl_2$ and nematodes. *Ecotoxicol. Environ. Safety* **18**, 181–190.

Vanfleteren, J. R. (1993). Oxidative stress and ageing in *Caenorhabditis elegans*. *Biochem. J.* **292**, 605–608.

Vanfleteren, J. R., and Roets, D. E. (1972). The influence of some anthelmintic drugs on the population growth of the free-living nematodes *Caenorhabditis briggsae* and *Turbatrix aceti*. *Nematologica* **18**, 325–338.

Walker, R. J., Colquhoun, L., and Holden-Dye, L. (1992). Pharmacological profiles of the GABA and acetylcholine receptors from the nematode, *Ascaris suum*. *Acta Biol. Hung* **43**, 59–68.

Williams, P. L., and Dusenbery, D. B. (1990). A promising indicator of neurobehavioral toxicity using the nematode *Caenorhabditis elegans* and computer tracking. *Toxicol. Ind. Health* **6**, 425–440.

Williamson, V. M., Long, M., and Theodoris, G. (1991). Isolation of *Caenorhabditis elegans* mutants lacking alcohol dehydrogenase activity. *Biochem. Genet.* **29**, 313–323.

CHAPTER 9

Methods of Studying Behavioral Plasticity in *Caenorhabditis elegans*

Timothy N. Gannon and Catharine H. Rankin

Department of Psychology
University of British Columbia
Vancouver, British Columbia, Canada V6T 1Z4

I. Introduction

Behavioral plasticity is the ability of organisms to modify their behavior over time, based on their experience, and is thus critical to the survival of any organism in a changing environment. It allows organisms to adapt to new surroundings and to take better advantage of novel situational variables they may encounter. It is therefore an extremely important ability, and it has attracted much research attention in innumerable organisms and across several disciplines.

Much of the research on plasticity has been characterized by an attempt to integrate information and expertise from a number of these different disciplines within selected invertebrate organisms. Researchers from a variety of fields, including psychology, physiology, biochemistry, genetics, neurobiology, and molecular biology, have been uniting in an effort to investigate "simple systems" in which these approaches are being combined and focused on the general goal of elucidating the cellular, molecular, and genetic basis of behavioral plasticity (for a review, see Carew and Sahley, 1986). These simple system approaches have led to considerable progress in our understanding of the mechanisms underlying adaptive behaviors. The general strategy of such approaches is to try to identify the genes, molecules, channels, ion currents, cells, and neural circuits underlying some form of plasticity and then determine the precise nature of their respective roles in producing the behavior.

The nematode *Caenorhabditis elegans* is a simple system that offers some unique opportunities to explore the cellular, molecular, and genetic mechanisms of behavioral plasticity. It spends its life in the laboratory swimming on the two-dimensional surface of an agar-filled dish (*in situ* it lives in soil), eating *Escherichia coli,* defecating, and laying eggs (if hermaphrodite) or mating (if male). *C. elegans* has several different sense modalities, including mechanosensation (Chalfie and Sulston, 1981; Croll, 1975), chemosensation ("taste") (Dusenbury, 1974; Ward, 1973), chemosensation ("smell") (Bargmann *et al.,* 1993), thermosensation (Hedgecock and Russell, 1975), osmosensation (Culotti and Russell, 1978), and perhaps galvanosensation (Sukul and Croll, 1978) and photosensation (Burr, 1985). *C. elegans* has been shown to respond to chemical compounds, temperature, and electric fields by moving either toward or away from the centers of prepared gradients. In addition, *C. elegans* responds to mechanical stimulation, such as touch and vibration, either by accelerating forward, or by reversing (swimming backward) for some distance and then changing course and resuming forward movement in a new direction.

The *C. elegans* nervous system is extremely simple, relative to other organisms studied. With only 302 neurons, all of which have been completely described in terms of their cell lineage, location, and synaptic connectivity across development, it is one of the simplest multicellular organisms yet to be studied for behavioral plasticity, and it offers the unique opportunity to elucidate the functions of all the neurons involved in a given behavior (Sulston and Horvitz, 1977; Sulston *et al.,* 1983; Chalfie *et al.,* 1985; White *et al.,* 1986). *C. elegans* is also amenable to genetic analyses due to several factors, including its small, almost completely sequenced genome, its hermaphroditic mode of reproduction, and its short reproductive cycle (see other chapters in this volume). Moreover, *C. elegans* is transparent, which allows the use of laser ablation techniques in which identified neurons can be individually killed in a living worm (see Chapter 10 in this volume). Lastly, in addition to all of its behavioral, developmental, neuronal, and genetic simplicity, *C. elegans* has demonstrated the ability to modify its behavior on the basis of experience in a number of experimental paradigms. Thus, in *C. elegans,* several distinct lines of investigation can be integrated to study behavioral plasticity in detail.

As with most organisms, in *C. elegans* this behavioral plasticity can take several forms, ranging from sensory adaptation and response fatigue to simple learning and memory. Response fatigue is one of the simplest forms of behavioral plasticity. After prolonged stimulation, a system can become fatigued, which will result in loss of normal function. Some cells in the system (e.g., muscle cells) simply cannot continue to function at a high level of stimulation and therefore require some time to rest and recuperate to fully recover their normal behavior. Sensory adaptation is a similar form of simple behavioral plasticity. It occurs when a sense organ becomes temporarily and predictably changed in its sensitivity, in response to exposure to particular environmental conditions. Importantly, this change or adaptation is due to changes within the sense organ itself; it is not produced by changes in the remainder of the nervous system (Domjan and Burkhard, 1986). For example, in the human eye the photoreceptor cells (the rods and the cones) require a certain amount of time to fully adapt to dramatic changes in brightness: While these cells are adapting, vision is poor because the cells are *unable* to respond properly and the only thing that will let them recover is time.

In learning, the subject changes its response to a stimulus even though it remains fully capable of responding to the response in its original manner—the sensory receptor cells register the stimulus information, and the system is not fatigued. Traditionally, simple learning has been divided into a number of different subcategories, based on the type of experimental protocol used to elicit the behavioral change. Although these distinctions have the positive effect of making learning more accessible by defining various protocols of study, they also have the unfortunate consequence of suggesting that the cellular correlates of these phenomena are distinct. This need not be the case: These classifications are based solely on experimental protocol; there is no reason why they must be mechanistically distinct.

One such protocol distinction made by learning theorists is between nonassociative and associative forms of learning. Nonassociative learning is a consequence of the application of only a single type of stimulus, and it is further subdivided into habituation and sensitization. Habituation is defined as a decrement in response due to the repeated application of a stimulus (Thompson and Spencer, 1966; Groves and Thompson, 1970). This decrement in response is distinguished from sensory adaptation or motor fatigue on the basis that the subject habituates to a stimulus despite the fact that it remains fully capable of sensing the stimulus and of making the muscle movements required for the response. This quality is usually demonstrated by dishabituation, in which the subject's responsiveness is rapidly recovered by the application of a single novel or noxious stimulus (Thompson and Spencer, 1966; Groves and Thompson, 1970). In contrast, sensory adaptation and response fatigue can recover only through the passage of time. Sensitization is characterized by an elevation of responsiveness over baseline nondecremented levels by the application of a novel or noxious stimulus (Thompson and Spencer, 1966; Groves and Thompson, 1970).

Associative learning, on the other hand, is based on the pairing of two events and is divided into classical and operant conditioning. Classical conditioning (i.e., Pavlovian conditioning) enables organisms to take advantage of the orderly sequence of events in the environment and to learn which stimuli tend to go with or predict other events. In classic conditioning, a conditioned stimulus (CS, e.g., a bell), which initially elicits no response, is paired with an unconditioned stimulus (US, e.g., some food), which initially (with no prior training) does elicit a predictable response called the unconditioned response (UR, e.g., salivation). The most important characteristic of the CS–US relationship is the predictive power of the CS to signal the occurrence of the US (Rescorla and Holland, 1976). After a number of CS–US presentations (training), the CS (the bell) acquires the ability to elicit the same response as the US (the food), and this newly acquired response is called the conditioned response (CR, e.g., salivation). Thus, stimuli and responses whose properties do not depend on prior training are called *unconditioned,* and stimuli and responses whose properties do depend on training are called *conditioned* (Domjan and Burkhard, 1986). In operant (or instrumental) conditioning, the reinforcer is response contingent, which means that presentations of reinforcing stimuli (e.g., food, shock) depend on the prior occurrence of some designated responses (e.g., bar press). Thus the animal learns an association between the response it emits and the consequences or reinforcement of that response (Carew and Sahley, 1986; Domjan and Burkhard, 1986; Mackintosh, 1974). For example, if a certain behavior (e.g., bar press) is regularly rewarded by some pleasurable stimulus (e.g., food), then this association will be learned and the behavior that is reinforced (bar press) will be repeated.

A second distinction learning theorists have made is based on the duration of the behavioral change, which is reflected by the duration of an organism's memory for the learning. Memory can be divided into short-term memory, which lasts minutes to hours, and long-term memory, which lasts 24 hours and longer. The assumption behind this distinction is that short-term changes are the result of alterations in the existing "machinery" of the cell, whereas long-term changes are the result of modifications in gene expression.

Caenorhabditis elegans has been shown to exhibit many of the above forms of behavioral plasticity ranging from sensory adaptation to learning, including habituation, sensitization, and classical conditioning. *C. elegans* also exhibits both short-term and long-term memory. The first aim of this chapter is to provide a survey of the research done on behavioral plasticity in *C. elegans.* This overview is organized around the experimental protocols used, beginning with the simplest forms of plasticity, and it includes a description of the different methods and apparatus used, along with a brief summary of some of the results and conclusions. It is important to realize that studying behavioral plasticity is really just an extension of studying behavior in general and, therefore, one must become familiar with the standard behavioral assays used to define and describe the behavior within each paradigm. In an important sense the behavior, or in this case the behavioral change, *is* the method, and thus it demands description. The second aim of this chapter is to focus explicitly on the tap withdrawal learning protocol in sufficient detail such that a researcher could then set up the equipment, implement the procedures, and begin addressing some of the major issues in the area.

II. Behavioral Plasticity Paradigms for *Caenorhabditis elegans*

A. Taste Adaptation: Track Analysis

The first form of behavioral plasticity studied in *C. elegans* is the simple sensory adaptation of its taste sense. Sustained exposure of *C. elegans* to a chemical attractant leads to a reversible loss of the response to that attractant and to other related molecules (Ward, 1973; Bargmann *et al.,* 1990). The first research where this form of response plasticity was discovered (Ward, 1973) used a "track analysis" assay to identify and define the behavior.

The basic technique of track analysis is to try to determine how a worm finds its way to the center of a gradient. In this technique, an organism is placed onto an agar plate of constant depth and uniform water content. Then, as the worm moves about, it leaves an easily discriminable track which can be photographed and enlarged for later analysis. These tracks preserve significantly more than just the positional history of the organism. The sinusoidal waves produced on the agar also provide a considerable amount of information about the nature of the whole-body waveforms that propel the worms along (Croll, 1975).

This track analysis assay requires first the establishment of defined and reproducible gradients of attractants (Ward, 1973). Radial gradients were established in 8-cm petri plates by spreading 3 to 4 ml of melted 1.5% agarose (BDH, electrophoresis grade) in buffer [0.01 M N-2-hydroxyethylpiperazine-N'-2-ethanesulfonic acid (Hepes), pH 7.2, 0.25% Tween 20]. The agarose stabilizes the liquid against convection and also provides a medium through which the worms can swim rapidly. After the agarose cooled, 5 μl of attractant was twice applied to the center of the plate, at time intervals adjusted to give a gradient that does not flatten at the center. Gradients of identical shape were established for molecules with different diffusion coefficients by adjusting the time allowed for diffusion inversely to the diffusion coefficient. The worms, one per plate, were transferred directly to the assay plates from the growth plates with sharpened applicator sticks. After the desired tracking time, the worms were killed in their tracks by inversion of the plates over a few drops of chloroform. The tracks were recorded permanently by placing the plate on a sheet of Kodak Kodalith Ortho Type 3 film in a dark room and exposing it to parallel light from an enlarger, thus making a contact negative of the plate. The tracks were subsequently analyzed from prints or direct projection of the negatives (Ward, 1973).

Ward (1973) found that for many ions the tracks were directed up the gradient toward high concentrations and, therefore, the behavioral response is positive chemotaxis. Several hundred chemicals were screened at concentrations up to 10 mM and strong attraction was found to several inorganic salts, cAMP, cGMP, and basic pH, and weaker attraction was found to several amino acids. It was also found that the worms' behavior followed a cyclical pattern: First, a worm would swim toward the center of the plate, where the concentration was the highest; the worm would remain in the center for a certain time, depending on the concentration of attractant (the lower the concentration of attractant, the less time the worm would spend in the center); then the worm would swim away from the center, toward the periphery of the plate, only to return to the center some time later and so repeat the cycle. It is believed that this cyclical behavior is due to sensory adaptation. The worms' sensation of the attractant adapts after a specified amount of time, and this sensory adaptation eliminates the chemotactic response (i.e., the worms no longer remain in the center of the gradient). After some time out of the high-concentration area, the adaptation weakens and the chemotaxis behavior resumes (i.e., the worms return to the center of the gradient).

B. Taste Adaptation: Tethered Worm Protocol

Another method of showing sensory adaptation in *C. elegans* is to use a different assay for the worm's taste response. This assay involves tethering the worm in a flowing stream of solution so that chemical stimulation can be controlled at the same time behavior is recorded (Dusenbury, 1980). In this technique the worm was held in place by the tail with a suction pipet. Behavior was instantly recorded with a polygraph through the use of two pairs of 1-cm^2 light sensors (solar cells) connected to a multichannel recorder. An enlarged image (100× magnification) of the worm was projected onto a field containing the solar cells. One pair of cells was positioned at the tail end of the worm image (near the tip of the pipet) and detected large-amplitude movements; the other pair was positioned near the head of the worm image and detected movements of smaller amplitude. The detectors were then connected in such a way that there was a downward deflection of the polygraph pen if the shadow of the worm fell across one detector, and an upward deflection of the pen if the shadow fell on the corresponding detector on the opposite side. Several types of behavior, including forward and backward waveforms, could then be detected as the solutions were manipulated by the experimenter. It was found that pauses, curls, coils, and reversal bouts all tended to occur more often when a favored (more attractive, e.g., 50 nM NaCl) solution was replaced with a more neutral (less attractive, e.g., no NaCl) solution. The two primary advantages of this technique are that it allows the experimenter to control the timing of the stimulus presentation to the worm and that the worm's behavioral events are recorded in a relatively high time resolution.

Taking advantage of this technique's superior time resolution, Dusenbury (1980) showed that at least this one form of chemoadaptation occurs fairly rapidly: The dramatic increase in reversal frequency decays back to normal about 1 minute following a larger NaCl concentration decrease, and even more rapidly on a smaller change. This technique also demonstrates that there is an inverse relationship between the strength of the stimulus, in this case the concentration change of the solutions, and the rate of adaptation. Interestingly, this technique also demonstrates that this reversal behavior tends to adapt several times more slowly when it is initiated by an increase in concentration of a chemical, as opposed to a decrease in concentration.

C. Olfactory Adaptation: Track Analysis

In addition to responding to dissolved compounds, *C. elegans* can chemotax to volatile odorants, including organic alcohols, ketones, esters, ethers, and aromatic molecules (Bargmann *et al.,* 1990). This olfactory assay to similar to the taste assay described above; however, whereas the water-soluble molecules take some hours to diffuse across the agar, the volatile attractants, such as isoamyl alcohol, can be presented simply by suspending them over the agar immediately before the assay (Bargmann *et al.,* 1993). This suspension was accomplished by placing a drop of the odorant onto the lid of the plate, not in any direct physical contact with the agar. The worms then immediately oriented their movement so that they accumulated directly underneath the drop of attractant. But the worms will not remain at the attractant source indefinitely, because the worms eventually adapt to the odorant and the odorant eventually evaporates. To deal with this problem, all animals within about 0.5 cm of the attractant source were anesthetized with sodium azide (1 *M*, 1 μl), which was placed at the attractant center. As a control, a much weaker attractant, surrounded by an equal radius of anesthetic, was placed at the opposite end of the plate. In the above experiment, a "chemotaxis index" was calculated such that the difference between the total number of animals at the attractant and the total number of animals at the counterattractant was divided by the total number of animals in the assay. This index could therefore vary from 1.0 (perfect attraction) to −1.0 (perfect repulsion). It was found that after 60 minutes in such assays, with sodium azide, the chemotaxis index reached a plateau and did not increase significantly thereafter (Bargmann *et al.,* 1993).

This olfactory sense has exhibited plasticity (Colbert and Bargmann, pers. comm.). Prolonged exposure to volatile odorants leads to a loss of the odorant response, in the form of sensory adaptation. After their analysis of the chemosensory cells through the use of laser ablation and behavioral mutants, Bargmann *et al.* (1993) argued that the worms' response to volatile odorants is probably distinct from that to water-soluble molecules.

D. Experience-Dependent Thermotaxis

The two assays used to study thermosensation (Hedgecock and Russell, 1975) are also both used to study how this behavior adapts under certain conditions. The first assay of thermotaxis described by Hedgecock and Russell (1975) measured the accumulation pattern of the worms on a linear thermal gradient. First, a stable and reproducible linear temperature gradient was established by connecting two thermostatically regulated water baths, 5 and 35°C by a long, thin aluminum plank (61 × 10 × 1.3 cm) tightly bolted at each end to an aluminum cube (10 × 10 × 10 cm) in a bath. Various 9-cm petri plates were then placed on this aluminum gradient at regular intervals (centered at 12.9, 17.6, 22.8, and 27.1°C); each plate was thus positioned at a progressively warmer or cooler temperature, and each plate thus exhibited within itself, a warmer and a cooler side. In the analysis, each plate was scored for worms migrating to the warmer half of the plate, worms migrating to the cooler half of the plate, and worms choosing neither.

The second assay described by Hedgecock and Russell (1975) used track analysis to record the worms' behavior within a radial gradient. The individual worms (grown at 20°C) were placed on 9-cm plastic plates which were inverted at room temperature. Then glacial acetic acid (melting point 16.6°C) was placed at the center of the bottom of each plate, creating a stable radial temperature gradient within which the worms could move. It was found from both techniques that when grown at temperatures from 16 to 25°C and placed on a thermal gradient, *C. elegans* migrates to its growth temperature and then moves isothermally.

This response is not quite so simple, however, as it has been shown to be plastic and experience dependent. Thermotaxis changes under a range of conditions involving starvation and overcrowding (Hedgecock and Russell, 1975). If a worm is raised under starvation conditions then this migration is reversed: The worm will disperse from its cultivation temperature. Also, if a worm is nutritionally deprived at its "preferred" temperature long enough, its preference will change and it will develop the dispersion response. This transition from attraction behavior to dispersion behavior occurs approximately 4 to 6 hours after the onset of starvation.

In addition, temperature shift experiments have been done that demonstrate that the preferred temperature can be reset, without starvation, in a period of hours; this is called *reacclimation* (Hedgecock and Russell, 1975). Worms shifted from 16 to 25°C as newly laid eggs behave, when tested as adults, like normally raised 25°C worms. The same is true in the reverse condition: Adults from downshifted eggs (from warm to cold) behave like cold-raised worms. When shifted as young adults, the worms' thermal preferences change rapidly over the first 2 to 4 hours and then more slowly thereafter, with similar time courses for both upshifted and downshifted worms.

Genetic analyses of thermotaxis have led to the hypothesis that migration to a preferred temperature may be guided by two opposing drives: one for upward and one for downward thermal migration (Hedgecock and Russell, 1975). Mutants have been isolated with phenotypes consistent with this idea; some are cryophilic (prefer colder temperatures) and some are thermophilic (prefer warmer temperatures), respectively. Interestingly, the thermal response of the thermophilic mutants is still strongly affected by the growth temperature, whereas the response of the cryophilic mutants is not. This distinction suggests that only the "upward" drive is plastic, and mediates the above adaptive behaviors.

A worm must be well fed to engage in positive thermotaxis, which is defined as the migration of the animals to their cultivation temperature (Mori, pers. comm.). Thus, in the above single-animal assays, a brief starvation (2 hours) will induce a strong dispersion from the starvation temperature, whereas a longer starvation (4 hours) will lead to a decrease in this response. Animals were fed at 25°C until adulthood (i.e., the animals were fully acclimated to 25°C), then starved at 25°C for either 2 or 4 hours, and then their thermotaxis was assayed individually on 9-cm plates. Another two groups of animals were acclimated to 15°C and then starved at 15°C for 2 and 4 hours, respectively. In all cases, the fraction of animals that avoided the starvation temperature was higher with 2-hour starvation than with 4-hour starvation (Mori, pers. comm.).

E. Taste-Conditioning Paradigm

Taste conditioning exhibits many of the qualities of associative learning, specifically classical conditioning (Kumar *et al.,* 1989). This protocol involves the use of chemoattractant ions (Na$^+$ and Cl$^-$) as the conditioned stimuli and *E. coli* (food) as the unconditioned stimuli. The animals are conditioned by exposing them to a constant concentration of one ion paired with the food source and the other ion presented in the absence of the food.

The concentrations of Na$^+$ and Cl$^-$ ions were first adjusted in pilot experiments to 2.0 *M* NaCH$_3$COO and 2.5 *M* NH$_4$Cl such that there was no significant difference in the preference of native animals for either gradient center. Prior to testing, the animals were washed three times with distilled H$_2$O in a conical centrifuge tube to ensure that the worms were free of contamination from either the ions or the food. The testing consisted of placing approximately 200 of the conditioned animals between the gradients of each ion (counterbalanced for order) and allowing them 1.5 hours to migrate to the gradient center of their choice. The test plates were then placed into a refrigerator for at least 30 minutes. This refrigeration cooled the animals so that they were no longer active and thus facilitated the counting process. Only those worms within 20 mm of the gradient center were considered to have preferred a particular ion. Immediately after one CS–US pairing, the worms demonstrated a preference for the ion paired with the food. This protocol has been used to show that *C. elegans* can learn both excitatory relationships, such as when a CS predicts food and the animal learns to approach it, and inhibitory relationships, such as when a CS predicts an unpleasant substance (i.e., garlic) and the animal learns to avoid it. Several other factors and variables in this protocol have been and continue to be studied, such as the effect of food deprivation (deprivation improves test performance), the rate of memory loss, effects of using different ions, effect of punishment versus reward, and comparisons between the aforementioned inhibitory and excitatory relationships (van der Kooy, pers. comm.).

F. Mechanosensation: Tap Withdrawal Protocol

Although there has been little mention of learning in *C. elegans* literature, it was not until the development of the tap withdrawal protocol that learning and memory were directly and systematically studied in the worm (Rankin *et al.*, 1990). Possibly the first documented description of learning in *C. elegans* was of a simple protocol developed by Croll (1975). He watched the behavior of worms as they bumped into glass bends that were scattered onto the surface of the agar. As time went on, and as the worms experienced more successive collisions, they became progressively less responsive, probably due to some form of adaptation or habituation. A more direct description of habitutation came from the "light-touch" protocol (Chalfie and Sulston, 1981). In this technique, the heads and tails of individual worms were directly stimulated with a stroke from a light hair. The response of the worms to this light touch also tended to wane as time went on, in a manner conducive to habituation. But it was only in the tap withdrawal protocol where the observed learning was further characterized and methodically studied in detail.

The tap withdrawal protocol measures the responses of a worm to a series of successive taps, or trains of taps, given to the side of an agar-filled dish (described below). The taps/trains cause the worm's environment to momentarily vibrate, and this provokes the adult worm to swim backwards for some distance. Unlike the instances of habituation just described, this technique produces a quantifiable measure of the magnitude of this reversal response due to the consistent nature of the stimuli produced by the mechanical tapping device. It is the habituation of this reversal response to the vibration that is central to the tap withdrawal protocol.

The following sections describe and discuss the various experiments and techniques applied within the tap withdrawal protocol. The first section describes in detail the apparatus and method general to these experiments. The succeeding sections present several important variations on this protocol, complete with explanations of their significance.

1. Apparatus and Method

The experimental apparatus (Fig. 1) consists of a stimulus generator, an electromagnetic relay that drives a wire tapper, a resting plate connected to a plastic resting arm, a micromanipulator, a dissecting microscope with under lighting, a video camera, a videocassette recorder (VCR), a color monitor, and a time–date generator (Rankin *et al.*, 1990). A worm is placed in the center of a 4-cm petri plate filled with 10 ml of NGM agar, and this dish is placed onto the resting plate (which is an inverted petri plate lid). The resting plate is connected by a plastic resting arm to the micromanipulator (Marzhauser Model MM33), which enables the experimenter to make smooth, precise movements and adjustments to the plate's position under the microscope (Wild M3Z, Wild Leitz Canada) using fine and coarse dials. This fine control of movement is necessary because

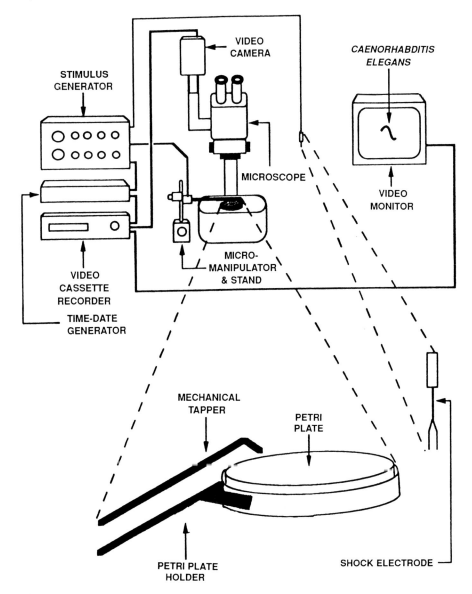

Fig. 1 Apparatus for studying the tap withdrawal response. Adapted, with permission, from Mah (1991).

the field of observation is much smaller than the plate, and therefore the plate continually must be moved to keep the worm under observation. The relay that drives the tapper is connected to a Grass S88 stimulus generator, which allows for easy regulation of stimulus delivery and timing. The wire tapper is connected to the relay and is positioned halfway up the side wall of the dish to deliver vibratory stimuli (of approximately 1 to 2 N per tap), which are transmitted through the dish and the agar to stimulate the worm. For single taps, the generator is set to deliver a 25-millisecond pulse to the relay. A train of taps consists of six 25-millisecond pulses delivered at 8.5 Hz for 600 milliseconds.

The worms standardly used in these experiments are *C. elegans* var. Bristol (strain N2) maintained on NGM agar at room temperature ($20 \pm 2°C$) with *E. coli* (strain OP50) as food (techniques described by Brennar, 1974). Synchronous age groups (or colonies) are established by allowing several adults to lay eggs on *E. coli*-seeded plates for about 1 to 3 hours. At the beginning of every month, a new colony of worms of the original strain is thawed, to control for any genetic variability over time. The agar plates on which the worms are grown are freshly poured every 1 to 2 weeks. If the plates are too old they become dehydrated, and the agar begins to pull away from the sides of the dish, which is a problem because it allows the worms the opportunity to move into the space between the dish and the agar, where they can no longer be monitored or scored. It is also important to check that the plate is healthy before any worms from it can be used. If there is any contamination (e.g., some bacterial growth) on the plate, the worms should not be used. Sometimes an unusually large number of eggs were laid when the colony was made and this results in an overcrowded colony. The worms on these plates are often somewhat starved and, thus, should not be used. These plates can be recognized by an unusually large number of worms, little food, and large clusters of larval worms, often several worms deep, scattered on the plate.

An individual worm is selected off one of the 4-day-old colony plates with a sharp pick and placed onto a test plate, which usually contains no food. The advantage of using a plate without food is that the worm behaves differently on and off food, and thus a plate without food ensures a homogeneous environment (plates with food are usually quite heterogeneous, with large regions of the surface without food). On the other hand, laser-ablated animals are usually trained on plates with food, because these animals are directly placed on individual plates with food immediately after surgery.

As the worm moves along the agar surface, one must manually track the worm such that its behavior will be recorded by a video camera connected to the microscope. The video camera (Panasonic Digital 5100) is connected, through the VCR (Panasonic AG1960), to a 10-in. color monitor (NEC Model No. PM-1271A) in such a way that the recorded image appears "live" on the screen. The time–date generator (Panasonic WJ-810) is used to superimpose a digitial stopwatch and time–date display on the video record, which is important for marking the presentation of each stimulus. The image of the worm is then kept in the center of the screen through adjustments of the micromanipulator. It has been found that $160\times$ ($16\times$ objective lens with $10\times$ ocular lens) magnification is the ideal, as it maximizes visual discrimination while maintaining the worm image at a manageable size for video tracking.

The stimuli are then presented to the worm in a manner appropriate to that particular experiment and the worm's behavior is recorded. The timing of the stimuli can be controlled manually (although it is recommended that for longer stimulus intervals, i.e., 60 seconds, an experimenter have a "reminder" timer that signals the arrival of the next stimulus) or it can be automated with the Grass S88 generator. The advantage of automation is the assurance of a reliable and consistent stimulus. The advantage of manual control is that the presentation of each stimulus can be slightly modified to accommodate the behavior of the worm. For example, if a worm is spontaneously reversing when the stimulus is presented, then that data point must be discarded, and a manually given stimulus can be slightly delayed to avoid such an occurrence. For longer interstimulus intervals (ISIs), like 60 seconds, manual stimulus presentation is preferred for that reason, but for shorter ISIs, like 10 seconds, both the difficulties in coordinating the stimulus delivery and the tracking device at the same time and the increased relevance of a "few-second" delay make the automated approach more appropriate.

Once the experiment is run and video-recorded, the behavior is ready to be scored. Using stop-frame video analysis, each worm's behavior is individually scored by tracing its body from the video image onto a transparent acetate sheet, going frame by frame through the tape. The adult worm usually (90–95% of the time) responds to the tap with a reversal response, with the size and number of the responses decreasing as stimuli are repeated through the habituation run. In a typical reversal response, a stopped or forward-moving worm moves backward for a distance (usually less than one or two worm lengths) and then either remains still or reinitiates forward movement in a new direction. To score the response, a person notes the pre- and posttap positions of the worm, and then traces the total distance the worm reversed (i.e., track length) onto the acetate sheet. It is important to note that the worm maintains the same waveform as it reverses (i.e., the head will pass along the same path as the tail); this is an extremely important positional reference when recording the length of a reversal.

In some cases, a worm responds with a forward acceleration rather than a reversal. In a typical acceleration response, a stopped or forward-moving worm either initiates forward movement or increases its speed, respectively. Generally, in standard experiments with adult worms, these acceleration responses are simply scored as missing data points (an adult worm accelerates to tap only about 5% of the time). In other circumstances or protocols, such as with larval or laser-ablated animals, the acceleration response occurs more often and is therefore scored. In these cases, if a worm accelerates after the tap, the acceleration is scored by measuring the distance the worm moves (i.e., track length) during the 1-second interval before the tap and subtracting it from the distance the worm moves during the 1-second interval after the tap. It is important to note that the reversal response and the acceleration response are two qualitatively different outcomes which cannot easily be compared.

These "scored" tracings are then digitized using a digitizing tablet (Summa Graphics Bit Pad Plus) that is interfaced with a Macintosh SE microcomputer and Mac Measure software. The values from this program, representing the reversal/acceleration magnitude, can then be directly transported into a statistical package for data analysis. The frequency of reversals and accelerations is also an important measure of the behavior of the worm, and it is scored simply by counting the number of instances of either response.

2. Learning Paradigms Using the Tap Withdrawal Protocol

a. Habituation

To study habituation, an experimenter places an individual adult (4-day-old) worm onto a plate that usually contains no food, using a platinum wire pick, and allows the worm time (usually 2 minutes) to adjust to its new surroundings. A specific number of taps or trains are then delivered to the worm at a consistent ISI. Regardless of the parameters chosen (within reason), the worm will express a decrement in responding to the stimulus—it will habituate. The habituation curves for reversal responses all show the standard habituation pattern of an initial, sharply descending slope followed by a more gradual, almost flat slope that is known as the asymptote (Rankin and Broster, 1992) (Fig. 2). The habituation curves for acceleration responses have a similar general shape, but are flatter. The levels of these parameters (number of stimuli, taps/trains, and ISI) affect the shape and time course of the habituation curve and are thus purposely selected for each individual experiment, to maximize the expression of the effect being studied. The reversal response is graded such that the distance reversed is larger to stronger stimuli; thus trains, which are a more intense stimuli than taps, result in larger reversal responses. This larger response size provides more room to see the effects of variables on the rate and degree of habituation. Results of studies on the effect of ISI, like those in Fig. 2, show that habituation is more pronounced and faster with a shorter ISI (10 seconds) than with a longer ISI (60 seconds). Finally, the more stimuli that are delivered, the more complete the habituation; however, whether continuing stimulation after asymptote is reached has any effect is currently unknown (Rankin and Broster, 1992).

b. Dishabituation

To test for dishabituation, the worm must first be habituated and then be given a dishabituating stimulus. In this protocol, the dishabituating stimulus is a brief train of electric shocks, generated by the Grass S88 stimulator. The shocks are delivered using a hand-held spanning electrode with wires placed into the agar on either side of the worm, about three to four worm widths apart. The two forks of the electrode thus span perpendicularly over the animal, piercing the agar about one worm width away on each side of the cuticle, at about the middle of the worm's length. Importantly, neither fork of the electrode actually contacts the cuticle; the shock is transmitted solely through the agar. The train

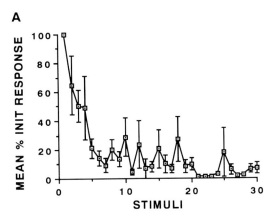

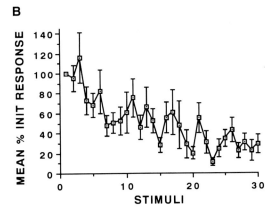

Fig. 2 (A) Habituation curve for 10 second ISI. Habituation of response amplitude is expressed as a mean percentage of the initial response for 30 stimuli delivered at a 10-second ISI; $n = 20$. (B) Habituation curve for 60-second ISI. Habituation of response amplitude is expressed as a mean percentage of the initial response for 30 stimuli delivered at a 60-second ISI; $n = 20$. Adapted, with permission, from Rankin and Broster (1992).

of shocks usually consists of 10-millisecond shocks of 60 V at 10 PPS (pulses per second) for 600 milliseconds. Following this dishabituating stimulus an additional set of stimuli, such as another 10 taps, are given to assess the effect of the shock on the habituation. Normally, there is significant dishabituation as evidenced by the increase in response amplitude following the shock.

c. Spontaneous Recovery from Habituation

Spontaneous recovery from habituation is analyzed by monitoring the worm's response to some additional test stimuli presented at different intervals after the last training stimulus. These recovery stimuli are generally given at much longer intervals to gauge the worm's spontaneous recovery from habituation. In our experiments, a typical set of recovery stimuli would be at 30 seconds, 5 minutes, 10 minutes, 20 minutes, and 30 minutes following the last training stimulus (Rankin and Broster, 1992; Broster and Rankin, 1994).

Using this recovery paradigm, *C. elegans* was shown to recover spontaneously from habituation (Rankin and Broster, 1992). The amount and nature of the recovery were dependent on the times of the test stimuli and the ISI of the habituation training (Rankin and Broster, 1992). Spontaneous recovery from habituation is greater and much more rapid with shorter ISIs (10 seconds) than with longer ISIs (60 seconds). The rate of recovery of animals that had reached asymptotic response levels differed from that of animals still in the descending portion of the habituation curve. The worms still in the descending portion of the curve recovered significantly more rapidly than the "asymptotic" worms.

d. Sensitization

Sensitization has also been demonstrated in *C. elegans*, although it has not been studied in detail comparable to habituation. To study sensitization, worms in the experimental group were given a pair of baseline single taps 2 minutes apart. Then, after 2 more minutes they were given a stronger stimulus of a train of taps. Finally, again after a 2-minute delay, they were given another pair of test taps 2 minutes apart (Rankin *et al.*, 1990). A control group was set up that received five single taps, each 2 minutes apart. It was found that the experimental group exhibited a significantly larger response than the control group following the stronger stimulus on the fourth and fifth stimuli, and thus the train of taps produced short-term sensitization.

e. Long-Term Memory Testing

Long-term retention of habituation has been demonstrated in which worms retain habituation training for at least 24 hours (Rankin *et al.*, 1990). In this protocol, all worms receive a standard baseline block of 20 stimuli at a 10-second ISI on day 1. The experimental group then received four additional training blocks of 20 stimuli at a 10-second ISI, with each group separated by 1 hour. On day 2 all worms were given a single test block of 20 stimuli at a 10-second ISI. Although the mean reversal amplitudes of the control and experimental worm groups on day 1 were the same, the experimental group had significantly lower responses (i.e., showed greater retention of habituation) than the control group on day 2. Thus, *C. elegans* is capable of 24-hour retention of habituation.

f. Ontogenetic Analysis of Learning

Depending on its particular stage of development and complement of cells, *C. elegans* has an increasing propensity to reverse in response to tap as it ages. Whereas adult worms reverse more than 90% of the time, larval animals reverse about 50% of the time and accelerate about 50% of the time (Chiba and Rankin, 1990). As a result, developmental studies of learning in the tap withdrawal reflex are more difficult than studies using only adult worms because the accelerations and reversals are two qualitatively different outcomes that cannot be easily compared. To study learning in the tap withdrawal reflex during and including larval development, the laser can be used to ablate the neurons responsible for the acceleration response in larval animals (Wicks and Rankin, 1995). Once those neurons (the tail-touch neurons: PLMR and PLML) are killed, the worm always reverses to tap, and thus developmental analyses of learning are possible (Gannon and Rankin, in preparation). The nature of the habituation as the worm ages can also be studied by running worms at various ages beyond 4 days. In a study investigating the nature of habituation in worms at days 4, 7, and 12, it was found that both spontaneous and reflexive movements were smaller in older worms than in younger worms (Beck and Rankin, 1993).

g. Other Experimental Designs

Much further research has been done to characterize more clearly the nature of habituation in C. elegans. By studying the behavioral effects of laser-ablating selected sensory neurons and interneurons, much has been learned about the nature of the neural circuit underlying the behavior (Wicks and Rankin, 1995). With the identification of the neural circuit underlying the response comes the opportunity to study the role of individual neurons in various forms of learning. It is our hope that these laser studies will lead to an understanding of the role of each cell in habituation of the tap withdrawal reflex.

Work is also underway to develop mutant screens for these behaviors so that detailed genetic analyses can begin. Already, there has been much research devoted to the cross-testing of mutants identified in many of the other behavioral plasticity paradigms, in a search for common mechanisms underlying the various forms of behavioral adaptation. In addition, C. elegans is conducive to several other means of analysis including pharmacology, and the advent of new technologies has made some electrophysiological methods feasible (see Chapter 11 in this volume).

III. Conclusion

In this chapter we discussed in some detail the methods of studying behavioral plasticity in C. elegans. Both the methods and the behaviors that they study are numerous and varied, but they are not without their commonalities. In each case, an adaptive behavior has been singled out and studied by modifying some existing behavioral plasticity protocol to suit C. elegans. The plasticity is there; the challenge is to develop methods to study it.

Given C. elegans' relatively simple behavioral repertoire, these methods are not easy to devise. It requires some creativity to adapt the protocols and definitions that are so entrenched in the mammalian literature and that have such rich behaviors to draw from, to an organism as simple as C. elegans. In fact, until recently it was assumed that *C. elegans* was *too* simple, that it *must* be all hard-wired.

Yet, it is this simplicity that is also *C. elegans'* greatest strength. It is this simplicity that distinguishes *C. elegans* from the other organisms previously studied and graces it with such unique advantages. *C. elegans* can learn, and it appears to follow many of the same rules as the "higher" organisms do, from the general shape and time course of habituation to the predictions of classical conditioning. Its simplicity, with only 302 neurons, allows us to ask questions we could not ask in more complex organisms. Its simplicity allows us to be more concrete and offers the potential for understanding the role of every neuron involved in a given behavior. It grants us the potential to understand how neural circuits integrate information to produce behavior and how this behavior can be modified by experience. In addition, its small, well-studied genome gives us a tremendous advantage in identifying compounds involved in behavioral plasticity. Its simplicity also makes it especially attractive as a system where several different perspectives and disciplines can be integrated at a fine level of analysis. This interdisciplinary aspect of *C. elegans* is only now beginning to be used. As more becomes known, and as technologies continue to improve, this integration of approaches and further exploitation of *C. elegans'* simplicity will become more complete.

C. elegans is not *too* simple, but it is simple enough.

References

Bargmann, C. I., Hartwieg, E., and Horvitz, H. R. (1993). Odorant selective genes and neurons mediate olfaction in *C. elegans. Cell* **74,** 515–527.

Bargmann, C. I., Thomas, J. H., and Horvitz, H. R. (1990). Chemosensory cell function in the behavior and development of *C. elegans. Cold Spring Harb. Symp. Quant. Biol.* **Vol. LV,** 529–538.

Beck, C. D. O., and Rankin, C. H. (1993). Effects of aging on habituation in the nematode *Caenorhabditis elegans. Behav. Proc.* **28,** 145–164.

Brenner, S. (1974). The genetics of *C. elegans. Genetics* **77,** 71–94.

Broster, B. S., and Rankin, C. H. (1994). The effects of changing interstimulus interval during habituation in *Caenorhabditis elegans. Behav. Neurosci.* **108,** 1019–1029.

Burr, A. H. (1985). The photomovement of Caenorhabditis elegans, a nematode which lacks ocelli. Proof that the response is to light not radiant heating. *Photochem. Photobiol.* **41**(5), 577–582.

Carew, T. J., and Sahley, C. L. (1986). Invertebrate learning and memory: From behavior to molecules. *Ann. Rev. Neurosci.* **9,** 435–487.

Chalfie, M., and Sulston, J. E. (1981). Developmental genetics of the mechanosensory neurons of *C. elegans. Dev. Biol.* **82,** 358–370.

Chalfie, M., Sulston, J. E., White, J. G., Southgate, E., Thomson, J. N., and Brenner, S. (1985). The neural circuit for touch sensitivity in *C. elegans. J. Neuroscience,* **5**(4), 956–963.

Chiba, C. M., and Rankin, C. H. (1990). A developmental analysis of spontaneous and reflexive reversals in the nematode *C. elegans. J. Neurobiol.* **21**(4), 543–554.

Croll, N. A. (1975). Components and patterns in the behavior of the nematode *C. elegans. J. Zool. Lond.* **176,** 159–176.

Culotti, J. G., and Russell, R. L. (1978). Osmotic avoidance defective mutants of the nematode *C. elegans. Genetics* **90,** 243–256.

Domjan, M., and Burkhard, B. (1986). "The Principles of Learning and Memory" Belmont, Wadsworth.

Dusenbury, D. B. (1974). Analysis of chemotaxis in the nematode *C. elegans* by countercurrent separation. *J. Exp. Zool.* **188,** 41–48.

Dusenbury, D. B. (1980). Responses of the nematode *C. elegans* to controlled chemical stimulation. *J. Comp. Physiol.* **136,** 327–331.

Groves, P. M., and Thompson, R. F. (1970). Habituation: A dual process theory. *Psychol. Rev.* **77,** 419–450.

Hedgecock, E. M., and Russell, R. L. (1975). Normal and mutant thermotaxis in the nematode *C. elegans. Proc. Natl. Acad. Sci. U.S.A.* **72**(10), 4061–4065.

Kumar, N., Williams, M., Culotti, J., and van der Kooy, D. (1989). Evidence for associative learning in the nematode *C. elegans. Soc. Neurosci. Abstr.* **18,** 532.

Mackintosh, N. J. (1974). "The Psychology of Animal Learning" Academic Press, London.

Mah, K. B. (1991). "An Analysis of the Tap Withdrawal Response in Male *Caenorhabditis elegans*" Unpublished M. A. Thesis, Department of Psychology, University of British Columbia, Canada.

Rankin, C. H., and Broster, B. S. (1992). Factors affecting habituation and recovery from habituation in the nematode *C. elegans. Behav. Neurosci.* **106**(2), 239–249.

Rankin, C. H., Beck, C. D. O., and Chiba, C. M. (1990). *C. elegans:* A new model system for the study of learning and memory. *Behav. Brain Res.* **37,** 89–92.

Rescorla, R. A., and Holland, P. C. (1976). Some behavioral approaches to the study of learning. *In* "Neural Mechanisms of Learning and Memory" (M. R. Rosenweig and E. L. Bennett, eds.), pp. 165–192. Cambridge, MIT Press.

Sukul, N. C., and Croll, N. A. (1978). Influence of potential difference and current on the electrotaxis of *C. elegans. J. Nematol.* **10**(4), 314–317.

Sulston, J. E., and Horvitz, H. R. (1977). Post-embryonic cell lineages of the nematode, *Caenorhabditis elegans. Dev. Biol.* **56,** 110–156.

Sulston, J. E., Schierenberg, E., White, J. G., and Thomson, J. N. (1983). The embryonic cell lineage of the nematode *Caenorhabditis elegans. Dev. Biol.* **100,** 64–119.

Thompson, R. F., and Spencer, W. A. (1966). Habituation: A model phenomenon for the study of neuronal substrates of behavior. *Psychol. Rev.* **173,** 16–43.

Ward, S. (1973). Chemotaxis by the nematode *C. elegans:* Identification of attractants and analysis of the response by use of mutants. *Proc. Natl. Acad. Sci. U.S.A.* **70**(3), 817–821.

White, J. E., Southgate, E., Thomson, J. N., and Brennar, S. (1986). The structure of the nervous system of the nematode *Caenorhabditis elegans. Philos. Trans. R. Soc. Lond.* **314,** 1–340.

Wicks, S. R., and Rankin, C. H. (1995). Integration of mechanosensory stimuli in *Caenorhabditis elegans. J. Neurosci.* **15,** 2434–2444.

CHAPTER 10

Laser Killing of Cells in
Caenorhabditis elegans

Cornelia I. Bargmann[*] and Leon Avery[†]

[*]Programs in Developmental Biology, Neuroscience, and Genetics
Department of Anatomy
University of California
San Francisco, California 94143
[†]Department of Biochemistry
University of Texas Southwestern Medical Center
Dallas, Texas 75235

I. Overview

One way to study cell function is to eliminate the cell and observe subsequent developmental or behavioral abnormalities in the animal. In *Caenorhabditis elegans,* this is usually accomplished by killing individual cells or groups of cells with a laser microbeam. Laser killing has been used to determine the functions of many mature cell types, including neurons involved in locomotion, feeding, mechanosensation, and chemosensation (Chalfie *et al.*, 1985; Avery and Horvitz, 1989; Bargmann and Horvitz, 1991a; Bargmann *et al.*, 1993). These studies have been practical because only a few cell types appear to be absolutely required for viability (J. Sulston, pers. comm.; Avery and Horvitz, 1987; Bargmann and Horvitz, 1991b).

Laser ablation can also be used to ask how cells interact during development. Signaling and inductive interactions between cells can be examined by removing one cell and observing the development of the remaining cells. Killing the distal tip cells of the somatic gonad causes premature differentiation of the germ line, showing that the somatic gonad is required for maintenance of the germ line in an undifferentiated state (Kimble and White, 1981). Another form of cell interaction that can be observed is regulation to replace a killed cell (Sulston and White, 1980). If the precursor to the gonadal cell is killed, a second cell becomes the anchor cell, but the uterine cells usually generated by the second cell are absent (Kimble, 1981). Postembryonic cell interactions in the developing gonad, the hermaphrodite vulva, and the male tail have been particularly well characterized using laser killing (Sulston and White, 1980; Kimble, 1981; Kimble and White, 1981; Chamberlin and Sternberg, 1993). Other cells have been found to regulate specific aspects of each other's development, such as cell migrations and axon outgrowth (Walthall and Chalfie, 1988; Thomas *et al.*, 1990; Li and Chalfie, 1991; Garriga *et al.*, 1993).

The developmental potential of cells in the early embryo has also been explored by killing cells with a laser (e.g., Sulston *et al.*, 1983; Priess and Thomson, 1987; Schnabel, 1994). These experiments are particularly useful because classic embryological manipulations like transplantations and microdissections have only been possible for the first few blastomeres of the *C. elegans* embryo.

Laser killing can assist in the interpretation of mutant phenotypes in several ways. If a cell interaction or cell function has been defined by killing a cell, genes that affect that cell may be identified by isolating mutants with phenotypes similar to cell killing (Ferguson and Horvitz, 1985; Austin and Kimble, 1987; Bargmann *et al.*, 1993). In addition, killing cells in mutant animals can provide insights into the defects associated with a mutation (Waring and Kenyon, 1990; Bargmann and Horvitz, 1991b; Mello *et al.*, 1992).

Laser ablation can also be used to probe cell function in nematode species that are not accessible to genetic analysis. Laser killing of vulval cell precursors has been used to elucidate cell interactions in *Mesorhabditis* and *Teratorhabditis* nematodes (Sommer and Sternberg, 1994).

Individual cells can be killed in *C. elegans* by damaging them with a laser microbeam focused through the objective of a microscope. The first apparatus used for this purpose was developed by John White (Sulston and White, 1980). Subsequent technical refinements have made this technique easier and more reproducible (J. G. White, pers. comm.; Avery and Horvitz, 1987). The laser beam is focused in three dimensions on a single spot in the field of view of a microscope. A cell of interest is aligned with the laser beam. Damage to the cell and adjacent structures can be visualized through the microscope during and after the operation. These methods can be applied to any cell, but this discussion is biased toward neurons because of the expertise of the authors.

II. Identifying Cells in *Caenorhabditis elegans*

Identifying cells unambiguously is probably the most difficult part of the laser operation. Rigorous identification of a cell type can be accomplished by following cell lineages through embryonic or postembryonic divisions (Sulston and Horvitz, 1977; Kimble and Hirsh, 1979; Sulston *et al.*, 1980, 1983). This approach is practical if a cell can be killed soon after its birth; it is the only method that works well for many blast cells in the embryo. Following cell divisions can be very time consuming, but, fortunately, most cells in *C. elegans* are found in reproducible positions. Therefore, for many cell types a combination of morphological cues and position can be used to identify the cells in wild-type animals without following cell lineages.

The nuclei of different cell types have characteristic appearances by Nomarski microscopy (Fig. 1). Hypodermal nuclei and gut nuclei have a "fried egg" appearance; they are round and smooth in texture with a large, prominent nucleolus. Neuronal nuclei are smaller and round, lack prominent nucleoli, and have a punctate nucleoplasm ("pepperoni" appearance). Muscle nuclei are oblong, are intermediate in size between neuronal and hypodermal nuclei, and have a punctate nucleoplasm and a small nucleolus.

The optimal time for finding a cell varies depending on the particular cell type. Most cells are most easily seen using Nomarski microscopy in very young larvae. As the animals age, optical interferences makes visualization of cells in deep focal planes more difficult. Many neurons can be identified at the beginning of the first larval stage (L1) (Fig. 2). In the pharynx, nuclei may be easier to see in the L2 stage. Cells in the pharynx can be identified by using the diagrams in Fig. 3. The pharynx and nerve ring do not change much during postembryonic development.

Once postembryonic divisions begin (about 5 hours after hatching), it may be necessary to stage the animals carefully or follow cell lineages to identify cells unambiguously in the body and tail. Embryonic and postembryonic blast cells are described in detail in Sulston *et al.* (1983) and Sulston and Horvitz (1977). A few stages can be learned as starting points for following lineages, including the 28-cell stage in the embryo (Fig. 4), the Bα/β/γ/δ stage in the male tail, and the 12-cell stage at the hermaphrodite vulva (Sulston and Horvitz, 1977).

Some cells cannot be identified reliably by position because of natural variability in their location. The most difficult areas are (1) the posterior lateral ganglia in the head (AIN, RIC, AIZ, ADEso, AVD) (2) the anterior socket and sheath cells in the head (AMSo, ILsh, ILso, OLQso) (3) postembryonic neurons in the tail, and (4) postembryonic neurons in the ventral nerve cord.

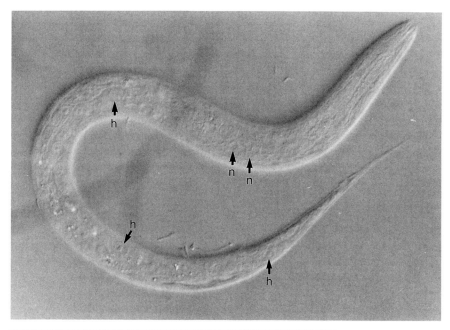

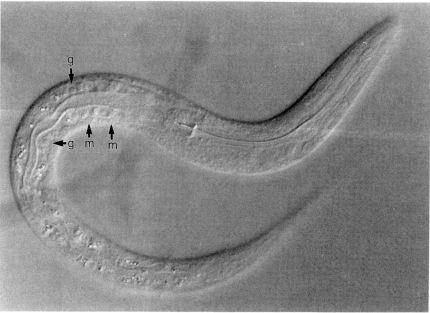

Fig. 1 Appearance of different cell types. L1 animal viewed by Nomarski optics under a 100×
Neuflour objective (Zeiss). h, hypodermal nucleus; n, neuronal nucleus; g, gut nucleus; m, muscle nucleus.

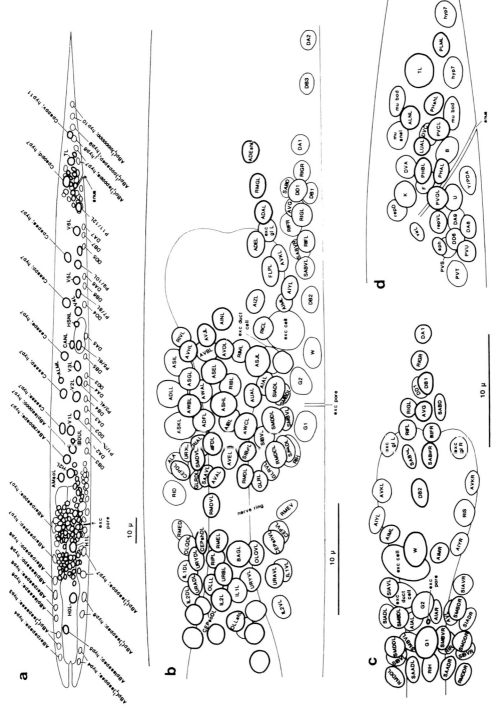

Fig. 2 Positions of nuclei in L1 larvae. (a) Positions of nuclei in L1 larvae (left lateral view). (b) Neuronal nuclei in the head (left lateral view). (c) Neuronal nuclei in the tail (ventral view). (d) Neuronal nuclei in the head (left lateral view). Anterior is to the left. In a, b, and d, only the left lateral nuclei and the medial nuclei are shown. Most right lateral nuclei occupy positions similar to those of their homologs on the left side; the exceptions are found most on the ventral side (see c). The thickness of the nuclear outline is inversely related to the depth of the nucleus within the worm (e.g., in b, lateral nuclei have thick outlines and medial nuclei have thin outlines). Reprinted, with permission, from Sulston et al. (1983).

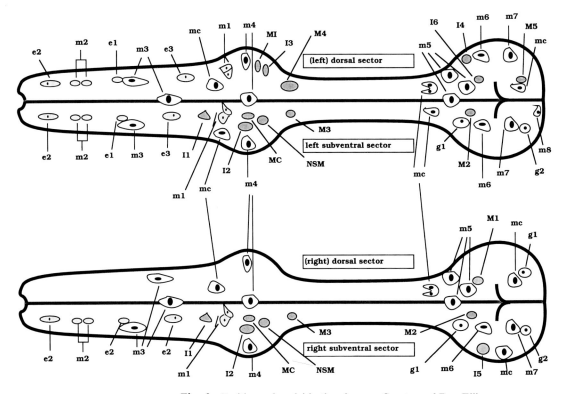

Fig. 3 Positions of nuclei in the pharynx. Courtesy of Ron Ellis.

It is easiest to learn the position of particular cells in animals in which a few cell types are labeled. For example, a few cells in the nerve ring and a few cells in the tail are stained with the fluorescent dye fluorescein isothiocyanate (FITC) (Hedgecock *et al.*, 1985). Simultaneous observation of Nomarski images and fluorescent images of these cells can be used to learn their positions. Once these cells are familiar, it can be relatively simple to identify adjacent cells. Similarly, fixed animals can be doubly stained with an antibody and 4',6-diamidino-2-phenylindole (DAPI, which strains all nuclei). Comparison of the fluorescent images can be used to learn the position of a cell that can be subsequently be sought in live animals. Some useful staining techniques and antibodies are listed

Fig. 4 Embryonic nuclei. (a) Twenty-eight-cell embryo 100 minutes, left dorsal aspect. (b) Embryo, 260 minutes, dorsal aspect, superficial nuclei. (c) Embryo, 270 minutes, ventral aspect, superficial nuclei. Anterior is at top. The thickness of the nuclear outline is inversely related to the depth of the nucleus within the worm. Reprinted, with permission, from Sulston *et al.* (1983). For detailed descriptions of embryonic and postembryonic cell divisions, see Sulston and Horvitz (1977), Kimble and Hirsh (1979), and Sulston *et al.* (1983).

a

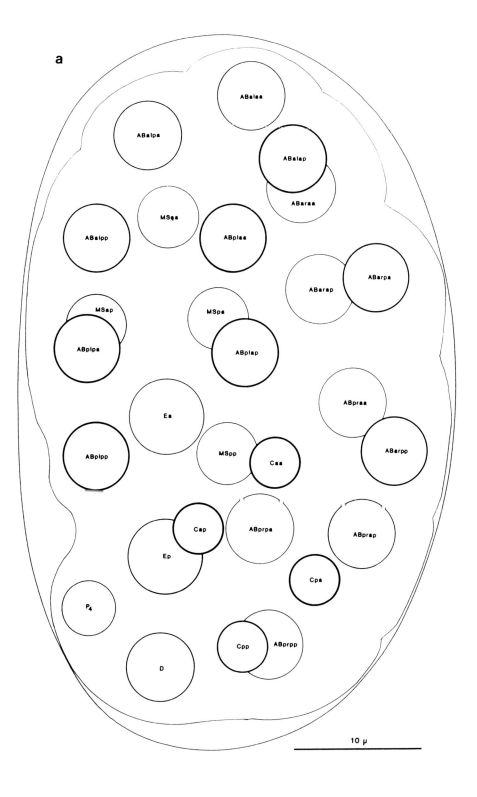

10 μ

b

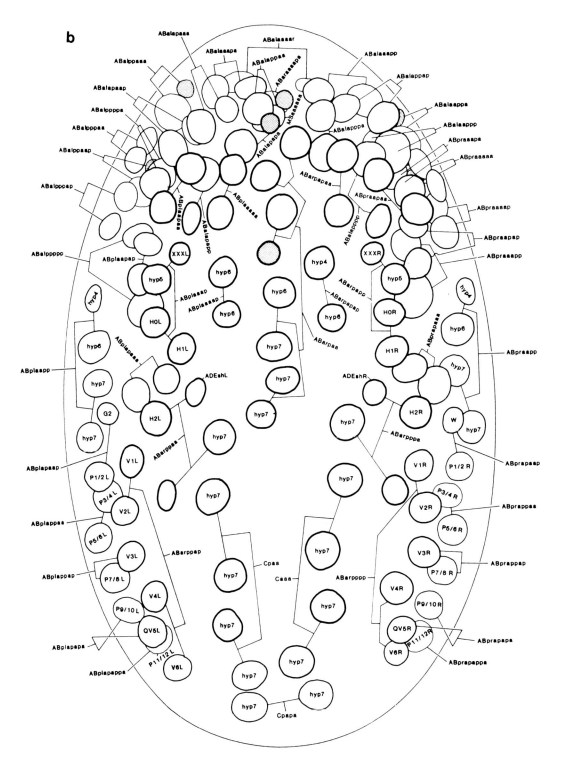

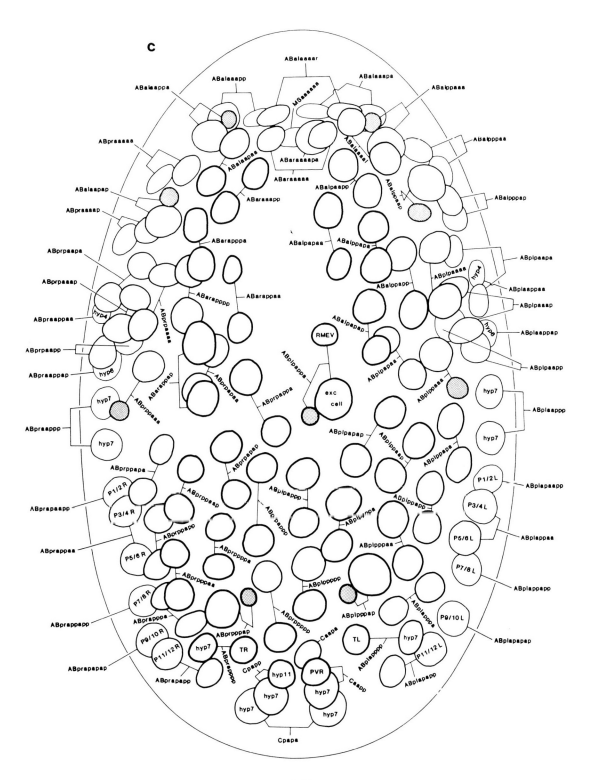

c

233

in Chapter 16 of this volume. In the future, cell identifications should be assisted by the availability of promoter fusions with the green fluorescent protein (gfp) of the jellyfish *Aequorea victoria* (Chalfie *et al.,* 1994). Cells expressing gfp can be examined simultaneously by Nomarski microscopy and fluorescence in live animals.

Visualizing cells that contain any of these markers by fluorescence microscopy can damage or kill these cells and adjacent cells, so fluorescence microscopy should be avoided during the laser operation procedure. Fluorescent markers, however, may be used at the end of an experiment to confirm the deaths of operated cells or the survival of nearby cells.

III. Practical Aspects of Laser Ablation

A. Theory

When a laser microbeam is fired at a *C. elegans* nucleus, at least three things happen: deposition of energy in the nucleus, followed by transport, followed by energy-induced damage. In this drama deposition is the hero; it places the energy with remarkable precision just where you aim the beam. Transport is the villain; it moves the energy from where it was deposited to other places, such as cells or structures you are trying not to hurt. Damage is the dark mystery. Almost nothing is known about how laser energy destroys a *C. elegans* nucleus. Energy deposited in the irradiated nucleoplasm eventually takes the form of increased temperature and pressure, either of which can denature proteins, break DNA, and so on. We can plausibly assume that damage is a steeply increasing nonlinear function of energy, as the rate of a chemical reaction will increase exponentially with temperature. Thus if the energy is doubled, damage is much more than doubled. In fact, for this discussion we assume it is the peak pressure or temperature experienced at a given point that determines how much damage happens there.

1. Energy Deposition

There are two leading candidate mechanisms for the deposition of energy. The first and most obvious is direct absorption of the laser light. Light enters the specimen from above in a broad symmetrical cone. For example, using an objective with a numerical aperture of 1.30, light is focused onto the specimen from angles up to 80° from the axis. It exits below in a similar cone. One might expect that absorption would drop off in the same way. In fact, one can do much better if there is nonlinear absorption. For example, if the wavelength is 440 nm, and if the specimen absorbs poorly at 440 nm but well at 220 nm, there will be two-photon absorption at sufficiently high light intensities. Two-photon absorption goes as the square of the light intensity, so energy deposition by this mechanism drops as the inverse fourth power of distance from the focus. Simple calculations suggest that the light intensity in typical *C. elegans* laser ablation experiments is indeed high enough for multiphoton absorption.

The second candidate mechanism for energy deposition is mechanical. Refractive index gradients within the nucleoplasm deflect the light. Because light has momentum, particles that deflect the light also recoil. The effect in this case is to compress higher-refractive-index materials into the focus of the beam. Optical tweezers use a benign version of this same effect to manipulate microscopic objects (Ashkin *et al.*, 1987). The boundary of the compressed region will be the edge of the spot to which the laser light is focused.

The net effect of either multiphoton absorption or refractive compression is increased pressure and temperature. Absorption directly causes a temperature increase, and the temperature increase, by expanding the heated material, causes a pressure increase. Compression directly causes a pressure increase, and the work done in compressing the material is partly turned into heat. In either case, the initial size of the high-pressure and -temperature region is about the same as the size of the spot to which the laser beam is focused. The laser light can be focused to a spot whose diameter is about the same as the wavelength of the laser light, typically about 400 nm. This is very small, even compared with the smallest of *C. elegans* nuclei (2000 nm). Energy can thus be deposited very precisely.

2. Transport

Unfortunately, although energy can be deposited very precisely, it can also move. Energy that moves away from the site of deposition can cause damage distant from that site. This is obviously undesirable if one is trying to kill a single cell. Thus operations should be done in such a way as to minimize transport.

a. Pressure

Mechanical energy is transported away from the beam focus by sound waves or, if the pressure is high enough, supersonic shock waves. If the beam is symmetrical, these waves will be roughly spherical, and the peak energy experienced at a point will be inversely proportional to the square of its distance from the focus. If the laser beam is not uniform, pressure jets may form; these will not dissipate as quickly with distance.

b. Heat

Heat is transported by diffusion. It is useful to start by considering two extremes: heat deposited continuously at a point over a long time, and heat deposited at a point during a very brief pulse. For the long-term case, heat diffusing away from the point source will reach a steady state, where the temperature increase is inversely proportional to distance from the source. Thus, if the temperature is 200°C above ambient 200 nm from the source, it will be 100°C above ambient 400 nm from the source. In contrast, if heat is deposited in a very brief pulse, steady state will not be achieved. The heat will gradually diffuse away, and temperature at a distance from the source will increase, reach a peak, and then decrease. The peak temperature increase for this case is proportional to the inverse cube of distance from the source. Thus, if a peak temperature of 200°C above ambient is achieved 200 nm from the source, a peak increase of 25°C will be achieved 400 nm away.

On the basis of these considerations, it is better to deposit heat in brief pulses, with sufficient time for dissipation between pulses. A pulse can be considered brief if it is much shorter than the time required for heat to diffuse a distance of the radius of the spot in which it is deposited, about 200 nm, as described above. The time to diffuse an average (root mean squared) distance r is $t = r^2/(6D)$, where $D = 10^{-3}$ cm²/s is the diffusion coefficient of heat in water. Thus, a pulse is brief if it lasts much less than 70 nanoseconds and long if it lasts much longer.

The first system for laser killing of C. elegans cells, introduced by John White (White and Horvitz, 1979; Sulston and White, 1980), used a dye laser excited by the light from an electric discharge through a gas. The typical pulse length was 500 nanoseconds. In 1984 White began using a dye laser excited by a nitrogen laser, with a pulse length of 0.2 nanosecond. He discovered that a lower-energy pulse could be used than with the discharge-excited laser and that damage was more localized. This result is understandable from the above discussion. During the 500-nanosecond pulse, heat was diffusing away as it was deposited. To get the same peak temperature, it was necessary to put in more energy. This energy heated up and damaged a larger region.

The most widely used laser systems employ nitrogen laser-excited dye lasers with 3-nanosecond pulse lengths. Three nanoseconds is much less than 70 nanoseconds, so these pulses are expected to work as well as the 0.2-nanosecond pulses of White's first nitrogen laser. Our experience confirms this expectation.

These calculations also show that heat dissipates rapidly between pulses. Typical lasers used for killing C. elegans cells cannot fire faster than once in 50 milliseconds. Even at this maximum rate the heat from one pulse will dissipate before the next is fired.

3. Summary

For maximum precision in laser killing, energy transport must be minimized. We make three recommendations, which make theoretical sense and are borne out in practice:

1. Make the laser irradiation uniform and symmetrical to minimize pressure jets.

2. Use brief light pulses to minimize heating distant from the beam focus.

3. Use many low-energy pulses rather than a few high-energy ones to minimize damage distant from the focus, as damage is probably a steeply increasing function of pressure and temperature.

B. The Laser Apparatus

A laser ablation system consists of a laser, a microscope, and some optics to direct the beam of the laser into the microscope objective. The microscope and the laser can be bought off the shelf. It is also possible to buy coupling optics, but they are expensive and not much easier to set up or use than homemade optics.

Detailed instructions for setting up a laser ablation apparatus (including a parts list) are currently available on the Internet from eatworms.swmed.edu by anonymous FTP, gopher, or World-Wide-Web client programs such as NCSA Mosaic.

1. Components

a. Microscope

The microscope is the most important (and most expensive) part of the laser ablation system. It must be of the type used for cell lineage analysis: a compound microscope with Nomarski differential interference contrast optics and an objective of sufficient quality that individual nuclei can be easily identified. To focus the laser beam, this objective should have a numerical aperture of at least 1.25. You should also get a low-power objective to use in finding the worms. The low-power objective does not need differential interference contrast optics.

The microscope must have an optical port through which the laser beam can enter. One solution is to purchase the optics for epifluorescence illumination and bring the laser light in through the port to which the excitation light source would usually be attached. A beam splitter is needed to reflect the laser light down into the specimen while allowing light transmitted up through the specimen to reach the eyepiece so that you can see what you are doing. A barrier filter is also necessary to prevent reflected laser light from reaching the eyepiece. With the wavelengths typically used, the beam splitter and barrier filter from a fluorescein filter set work well. The excitation filter of the set, which is between the light source and the beam splitter, should be removed. An ocular micrometer reticle should be installed in one of the eyepieces. It will be used in locating the focus of the laser during killing (see Section III,C).

b. Laser

The laser should be a dye laser pumped by a nitrogen laser. The pulse energy necessary to kill cells is roughly 5 mJ. Higher pulse energies are useful, as one can improve the uniformity of illumination of the specimen by using only the center of the beam. In addition, there may be energy losses in the microscope.

For example, in some microscopes the laser beam passes through the analyzer on its way to the specimen, decreasing the energy by a factor of 2.

Lasers have the potential to cause eye damage and should be treated with respect. The main safety problems come in setting up and aligning the laser. Ultraviolet safety glasses should be worn if the laser is opened so that the UV beam is exposed. You cannot wear glasses to block the visible beam, as you need to see it to align it, but you should avoid looking up the beam and avoid specular reflections off mirrors, microscope slides, and so on. (Diffuse reflections, e.g., from a piece of paper, are not dangerous.)

c. Optics

The coupling optics do two things. First, they shape the beam so that it enters the specimen from the full available range of angles and comes to a focus at a point in the image plane. Second, they allow beam location and angle to be adjusted by moving lenses and mirrors, rather than microscope and laser. Lenses and mirrors can be mounted in optical positioning equipment that allows fine, stable, continuous adjustment. As six separate adjustments are necessary to make the laser system operate properly, stable adjustment is important. The design of the coupling optics is the single most important factor in determining how convenient the laser system will be to use. The coupling optics are far less expensive than the laser and microscope, so even a lavish system does not increase the overall cost much.

Figure 5 shows the lenses used to shape and focus the beam. The most important lens is the microscope objective. Years ago virtually all microscope objectives were designed to produce an image of the specimen 160 mm behind the objective. Figure 5a shows a laser ablation system based on this type of microscope. Lens y focuses the beam to a point within the image, so that it will focus to a corresponding point within the specimen. Lens y can be moved along the beam axis to adjust the focus of the laser so that it corresponds to the visible image. If lens y is moved toward the laser, the focus will move upward in the specimen. Today, many microscopes use infinity-corrected objectives: All the rays of light from a single point in the specimen exit the objective parallel (Fig. 5b). The laser light cannot be focused to a point in the image, because no image is formed. In this case one uses an additional lens (z in Fig. 5b) to form an image.

To determine whether your microscope forms an image, use the low-power objective to focus the condenser so that you see a sharp image of its image-plane diaphragm. Close the image-plane diaphragm and open the diffraction-plane diaphragm as far as possible. Turn the microscope light up all the way, and take the polarizer, analyzer, and any filters out of the light path. Finally, put in place the beam splitter that will be used to reflect laser light into the objective. If you now turn the room lights off and hold a white card outside the port through which laser light is destined to enter, you will see a beam of light coming out of the microscope. If the beam gets narrower as you move the card away from the microscope, your microscope forms an image. You can locate the image

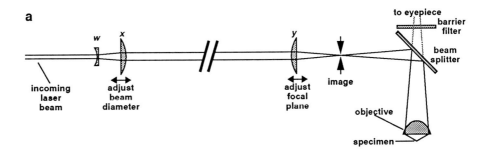

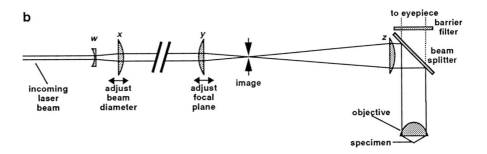

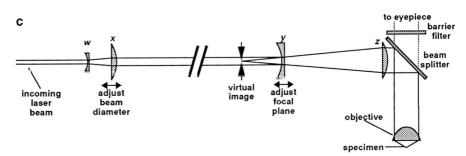

Fig. 5 Optics for laser ablation. (a) Optics for use with a microscope objective that forms an image 160 mm away. Lenses *w* and *x* form a Galilean telescope. Beam diameter can be changed by moving lens *x*. Lens *y* focuses the beam to a point in the image of the specimen, so that it will also focus to a point within the specimen itself. The distance between *x* and *y* is larger in proportion to other distances than shown. This is indicated by a break in the beam. The beam splitter reflects blue laser light into the specimen while passing longer-wavelength light to the eyepiece so that the worm can be seen. The barrier filter prevents stray laser reflections from reaching the eyepiece. (b) Optics for use with a microscope objective that forms an image at infinity. This arrangement is identical except for the addition of a new lens *z*. With this type of objective, all the rays from a point in the specimen come out parallel, so that there is no image plane. Lens *z* form an image in which the laser beam can be focused. Lens *z* may be an additional lens you insert, or it may be part of the microscope. It may be more complex than a single lens. (c) A variation, useful if there is not enough space for the arrangement shown in b. Lens *y* is now concave instead of convex, and causes the laser light to diverge to the right of the lens as if it were emanating from a point (the virtual image) to the left.

approximately by finding the place where the beam narrows to a point (actually, a tiny image of the diaphragm). If the beam diameter stays the same or increases as you move the card away from the microscope, you need an extra lens as in Fig. 5b.

It is important that laser light enter the specimen from the widest possible range of angles, which means that beam diameter must be at least large enough to illuminate the entire objective. (To determine whether the beam diameter is large enough, unscrew the high-power objective from its mount, then compare the size of the spot of laser light on a card held under the hole with the opening in the back of the objective.) Lenses w and x form a simple Galilean telescope that allows the beam diameter to be adjusted. If lens x is moved slightly toward the laser, the beam will diverge slightly as it leaves the telescope, so that its diameter will be larger at lens y and the objective. If the beam is larger than the objective, only the center will enter. Thus, as lens x is moved toward the laser, less of the light enters the objective, so that the illumination becomes weaker, a useful way of adjusting the intensity. It also improves the uniformity of the illumination, as the center of the beam is the most uniform. Intensity can also be adjusted by interposing neutral density filters in the beam or, for very small changes in intensity, microscope slides.

Of course, unlimited variations on these arrangements are possible. For example, the light path in Fig. 5b can be shortened by using a concave lens instead of a convex lens (Fig. 5c). In our example, we place a mirror between y and z to bend the light path so that the laser can be more conveniently placed on a desktop.

2. An Example

Figure 6 shows the arrangement of the laser, microscope, and coupling optics in a laser ablation system similar to that in use in one of our laboratories. The laser combination is a VSL-337 nitrogen laser with a DLM-110 dye laser, both from Laser Science Incorporated. These lasers are small, self-contained, and relatively inexpensive (about $6000 at the time of writing). The dye solution is 5 mM coumarin 120 (7-amino-4-methylcoumarin) in ethanol. With this dye, the laser produces 3-nanosecond pulses of 440-nm light with an energy of about 30 mJ. The coupling optics are a telescope (Laser Science Incorporated) for adjusting beam diameter (lenses w and x of Fig. 5), a 50-mm focal length planoconvex lens (Newport Optical) to focus the beam to a point in an image of the specimen (lens y of Fig. 5), and a mirror (Oriel Corporation) to direct the beam into the microscope. The microscope is a Zeiss Axioskop with epifluorescence optics. The Axioskop uses infinity-corrected optics, so our system is most similar to that of Fig. 5b. In this case lens z of Fig. 5b corresponds to two lenses within the microscope that form the epifluorescence condenser.

Laser light enters through the port on which an arc lamp would normally be mounted for excitation of fluorescence. On the Axioskop this port is at the back

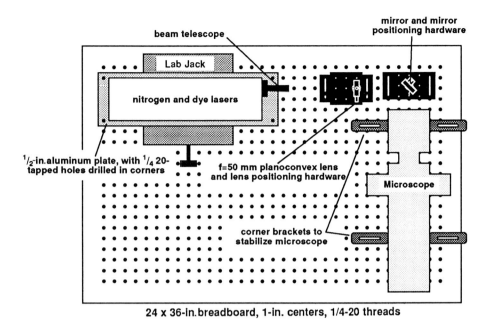

Fig. 6 Mechanical arrangement of the laser, microscope, and coupling optics.

of the microscope, 30 cm above the table top, so the laser and coupling optics are elevated on steel rods (Fig. 7), mounted in rod holders that allow crude adjustment of the height. The mirror is placed in a mount that allows fine adjustment of its angle. The lens mount allows fine adjustment of its position in the plane perpendicular to the beam. (Rods, rod holders, and mounts are from newport and Oriel.) These adjustments are used for aligning the angle at which the beam enters the microscope and the location in the specimen at which it comes to a focus. The lens mount is fastened to a translation stage (Newport Optical) that allows fine movement along the beam axis, which moves the focus up and down in the specimen. All these components are stably mounted on an optical breadboard (Technical Manufacturing Corp.).

C. Cell Killing

1. Prepare Slide

Agar for slide consists of 5% agar in M9 (for 1 liter of M9: 3 g KH_2PO_4, 6 g Na_2HPO_4, 5 g NaCl, 1 ml 1 M $MgSO_4$). This stock is autoclaved and stored in small (5-ml) aliquots, sealed with Parafilm to prevent dehydration. Individual aliquots of agar are melted in a microwave or over a flame. Melted agar can be kept at 65°C for up to 2 days.

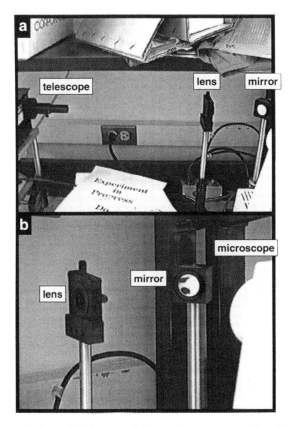

Fig. 7 Photographs of the optical elements. (a) The telescope, mounted on the laser, corresponds to lenses w and x in Fig. 5. The lens corresponds to lens y of Fig. 5. Lens z of Fig. 5b is inside the microscope. The mirror (not shown in Fig. 5) is between lenses y and z. The lens, mirror, and laser are mounted on steel posts. The lens and mirror mounts allow their positions to be adjusted. (b) Closeup showing the lens, mirror, and back of the microscope.

Sodium azide 3–10 mM (anaesthetic) is added to the melted agar. Azide arrests development, so it should be omitted if cell lineages will be followed. Azide is also usually omitted if embryonic cells will be killed.

Slide preparation is shown in Fig. 8. A drop of melted agar is placed on a slide and flattened into a pad. Two slides with a single thickness of tape are used as guides for flattening the agar into a pad, so the final thickness of agar is the same as that of the tape. Prepare the slide immediately before use.

2. Place Worms on Slide at Dissecting Microscope

Work quickly. Place 1 μl of M9 on the agar. Quickly pick up about 5 to 15 L1 worms with a platinum wire and elute them into the drop of M9 with gentle

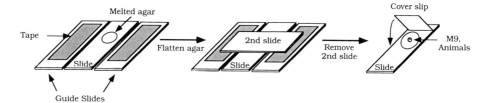

Fig. 8 Slide preparation. Melted agar is placed on the surface of the slide. A second slide is used to flatten the agar into a thin pad. The thickness of the agar pad is set using two guide slides to which a piece of tape has been attached. After liquid and worms have been placed on the slide, a coverglass is placed on the slide.

shaking. Count the worms in the liquid, then place a coverslip on the slide. Make a drawing of the worms on the slide. This drawing will be a guide for finding the worms under the compound microscope at the laser.

It is possible to mount all of the worms in a small region, in which case a drawing is unnecessary. After releasing the worms into the drop of M9, use an eyelash to draw the worms and a small amount of liquid apart from the original drop of M9. When the coverslip is placed on the slide, the worms will remain together in one area.

Prepare a set of control animals from the same plate. These animals should be placed in azide and rescued at the same time as the operated animals.

To facilitate cell identifications, slides should be prepared so that most animals are oriented exactly on their left or right sides, as shown in Figs. 1 to 3. Animals will take this orientation if they are swimming actively when the coverslip is placed on the agar. For best results, (1) prepare slides very quickly (2) treat animals gently, and (3) limit the amount of liquid on the slide to 1 to 2 μl.

If slide preparation is slow, many worms will be mounted so that their dorsal or ventral side is uppermost. If this orientation is desirable, use the higher recommended azide concentrations and place the coverslip on the slide *after* the worms have been anesthetized by the azide (this takes only a few minutes). Shift the coverslip very slightly after it is in place. Many of the worms should lodge in a ventral-up or dorsal-up position.

If cells are being killed in the embryo, mount embryos of the appropriate stage. If early embryos (<50 cells) are desired, they should be released from gravid hermaphrodites. Elute about 10 hermaphrodites into 10 μl of M9 on a microscope slide (without agar). As the animals swim in the liquid, cut them in half with a sharp razor blade by pressing them onto the glass slide. Eggs will be released into the liquid. Using a capillary pipet, move the eggs onto an agar pad without azide. To prevent air bubbles from forming, extra M9 can be placed on the slide before the coverslip is added. Cell lineages can be followed or cells killed as desired.

3. Use the Laser

To find the position of the laser spot, fire the laser using the manual control or the foot pedal and focus on the coverslip. When the laser is focused in the plane of the coverslip, it will make a small hole in the glass (Fig. 9a). Move the micrometer in the eyepiece until it is aligned with the laser spot. Now the sample can be moved so that the same part of the micrometer is over the cell of interest, and firing the laser will hit that cell.

Set the laser power by adding or removing neutral density filters between the laser and the scope. To kill neurons, add filters until the laser can just make a small hole in the coverslip. To kill larger cells such as hypodermal cells, reduce the neutral density filters so that the beam is about twice as intense. To kill large founder cells in the embryo, the beam should be about eight times as intense as needed to break holes in the coverslip. At these power levels, it should take between 20 and 200 laser bursts to kill a cell. If cell damage is observed more rapidly, neutral density filters should be used to reduce the beam intensity.

Find animals using the diagram prepared above (not necessary if the worms are all in one place). Animals may move during the recovery process, so it is best to kill the same cell or group of cells in all of the animals on a single slide. When killing cells, it is best to start by killing cells on the far side of the animal. Any nonspecific damage induced by firing the laser through the animal should be visible in the closer planes of focus. Animals in 3 mM azide can be kept on the slide for approximately 1 hour, after which nonspecific cell damage and toxicity are observed. At 10 mM azide, animals should be kept on the slide no longer than 15 minutes.

Make sure to consider eye safety throughout this procedure. Avoid looking at the laser beam or direct reflections of the laser beam. Exposure to the beam can be reduced by keeping the external mirrors and lens in a protective housing. With a properly installed barrier filter in the filter set, no reflections of the beam should reach the eyepiece.

4. Monitor Damage

After laser killing any one of the following kinds of damage may be considered sufficient to kill the cell (Fig. 9b):

Nucleus disappears

Nucleus takes on a buttonlike appearance characteristic of programmed cell death (Sulston and Horvitz, 1977).

Nucleus changes in refractive index and cell boundary becomes clearly visible.

Scar from laser transects nucleus.

Damage may take up to 30 minutes to develop but is usually visible within 1 minute of the operation. Discard the animal if a basement membrane is punctured (recognized as the sudden appearance of a fluid-filled pocket that expands near

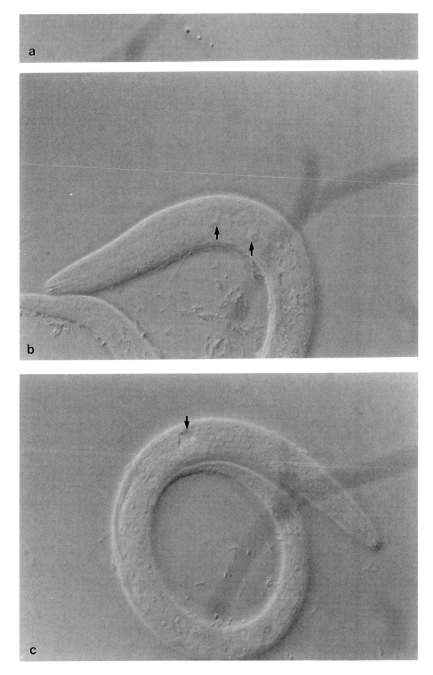

Fig. 9 Laser damage. (a) Damage to the glass coverslip, used to locate the laser spot. (b) Damaged nuclei following laser operations (arrows). (c) A ruptured basement membrane (note the fluid-filled cavity).

the site of ablation, Fig. 9c). Discard all animals in which the cuticle is punctured (visible as oozing or bubbling of material from the animal near the site of the operation).

Kill all undesired animals on the slide by puncturing the cuticle with the laser. To break the cuticle, fire the laser at the underside of the coverslip over the worm (this causes a small explosion). Puncturing the cuticle is easiest in the posterior part of the animal. If all extra animals are killed, the rescue step is easier because only desired animals are viable.

5. Rescue Animals

Draw 1 to 2 μl of M9 into a drawn-out capillary pipet. Slide the coverslip off the slide very gently, by gliding and not by pressing down on the coverslip. If this is done smoothly, the worms will remain in place and can be located using the diagrams prepared at the beginning. The worms are very vulnerable and dehydrated at this point.

Using suction, release a bit of liquid from the capillary pipet, draw the worm into the pipet, and release the worm onto a seeded NGM plate. The worm should start moving again within an hour or two and will be an adult in 3 days. Confirm the specificity of the operation as described below.

IV. Experimental Design and Controls

Interpreting the result of laser killing depends on the answers to two questions: Has the operated cell lost all function? Have additional cell types been damaged? Because the nucleus is the structure most easily visualized by Nomarksi optics, laser damage is usually assessed by the appearance of the nucleus; however, cells may maintain some function even in the absence of a nucleus. For example, when the nuclei of the touch cells are killed in the third larval stage, touch cell processes and function are maintained in the adult (Chalfie *et al.*, 1985).

Killing cells early in development maximizes the chances that they will lose function. In general, killing a cell nucleus in the first larval stage appears to eliminate cell function by the adult stage. For several types of neuronal cells, functional data and electron microscopy confirm that neuronal processes lose function within 24 to 48 hours if the nucleus is damaged by the laser in the first larval stage (Avery and Horvitz, 1987, 1989; Bargmann and Horvitz, 1991a).

Alternatively, the precursor of the cell of interest can be killed during development so that the cell is never generated. This approach often leads to the elimination of several cell types. It is especially important to examine adjacent cells for any changes in cell fate when precursor cells are killed. Most cell interactions are confined to a short period (minutes to hours), so the timing of cell killing is particularly important when cell interactions take place.

In addition to technical issues, two classes of intellectual problems limit the interpretation of cell killing results:

1. *Redundant functions.* In several cases, a particular defect is observed only when several cell types are all killed together (Avery and Horvitz, 1989; Bargmann and Horvitz, 1991b; McIntire *et al.,* 1993). Therefore, killing one cell may reveal only a subset of the functions of that cell.

2. *Multiple effects of one cell.* If a cell participates in several distinct biological processes, some effects may be hard to observe. For example, if a cell is essential for viability, it may not be possible to determine whether it functions in a particular behavior. Also, the death of one cell may have indirect effects on the development, survival, or functions of other cell types.

A. Assessing Damage to the Operated Cell

Verification is essential for every laser operation. The amount and timing of damage required to eliminate a given cell are determined empirically, using the following guidelines:

1. Closely observe the cell of interest and adjacent cells for 5 to 10 minutes after the laser observation.

2. Confirm cell death 1 hour to 1 day after the operation (remount the animal on a slide, search for the killed cell, and examine cells in the vicinity).

3. Confirm cell identity and cell death by some method other than observing the nucleus, if possible. For example, if an antibody is known to recognize the cell of interest or nearby cells, animals can be stained with the antisera after laser killing of the cell. Other functions of the cell may also be assessed. These experiments often require that the animal be killed and may be practical only after the end of the experiment.

4. If possible, compare the results of killing a cell and killing precursors to that cell.

B. Unintended Damage

The simplest way to establish that cells adjacent to the killed cell are intact is to observe their appearance and function directly. After killing a cell, antibodies or assays specific for adjacent cells should be used to determine whether those cells are normal. If an effect of killing a cell is seen, it is also useful to kill all of the surrounding cells and not the cell of interest. This control can ensure that the intended cell is responsible for a particular effect.

Difficulties in interpretation arise if the death of a cell leads to retarded development or small size, as accidental damage to the pharynx or cuticle will retard development. To verify that a specific cell death retards development, the protocols can be modified to minimize nonspecific effects of the operation.

Reducing the amount of time the animals spend on azide to less than 15 minutes leads to faster and more efficient recovery from anesthesia. Short times under azide should be used for any protocol in which development is slowed. Reducing the power from the laser beam by using neutral density filters decreases unintended damage from the laser, so minimal laser energy should be used in all experiments.

V. Future Directions

Laser killing can be a precise and versatile tool for eliminating specific cells in an animal. Its usefulness is limited, however, because of the difficulty of identifying each cell, particularly during development, and because of the small numbers of animals that can be generated. Several emerging techniques may be useful for killing defined cells in larger numbers of animals.

A. Degenerin Expression

Dominant alleles of *mec-4* and *deg-1* lead to the deaths of subsets of neurons (Chalfie and Wolinsky, 1990; Driscoll and Chalfie, 1991). These two genes encode related transmembrane proteins ("degenerins") that are similar to the amiloride-sensitive epithelial sodium channel; the dominant alleles may produce hyperactive or unregulated channel proteins. Expression of a dominant allele of *mec-4* under the control of different promoters leads to the death of cells in which it is expressed (M. Driscoll, pers. comm.; A. V. Maricq and C. I. Bargmann, unpublished). If a promoter exists for a cell type of interest, a *mec-4* fusion gene can be used to produce a line of transgenic worms that lack those cells. A similar technique is being developed using the cell death genes *ced-3* and *ced-4*. (S. Shaham, pers. comm.).

B. Photoablation

The heat and free radicals generated by illumination of fluorescent molecules are able to damage nearby cellular components. Cells that are filled with fluorescent dyes may be susceptible to damage after illumination with wavelengths that excite the fluorescent molecules. This technique is easier than laser ablation, so larger numbers of animal can be generated. Unlike expression of *mec-4*, the time of death can be controlled by the time of illumination. Amphid sensory neurons filled with the fluorescent dye FITC are killed following a long (60-second) illumination at high power (1000×) with a mercury lamp (C. I. Bargmann, and J. H. Thomas, unpublished observations). Short or low-power illuminations do not cause as much damage. At least some of the FITC-filled neurons lose function after this treatment, as evidenced by behavioral defects; however, the behavioral defects are more severe than those observed if the same cells are killed with a laser, suggesting that the procedure damages additional cells. More defined damage can be produced by limiting fluorescent illumination to a small area using a diaphragm in the fluorescent light path. Refinement is needed to make this protocol useful. It is possible that it can also be used for cells that express the jellyfish green fluorescent protein (Chalfie *et al.*, 1994).

Acknowledgments

We thank John Sulston and Ron Ellis for allowing us to include Figs. 2 and 4 and Fig. 3, respectively, and David Raizen, Piali Sengupta, and Scott Clark for their comments on this manuscript. This work was supported by USPHS grants DC-01393 (to C.I.B.) and HL-46154 (to L.A.). C.I.B. is a Lucille P. Markey Scholar and a Searle Scholar.

References

Ashkin, A., Dziedzic, J., and Yamane, T. (1987). Optical trapping and manipulation of single cells using infrared laser beams. *Nature* **330**, 769–772.

Austin, J., and Kimble, J. (1987). *glp-1* is required in the germ line for regulation of the decision between mitosis and meiosis in C. elegans. *Cell* **51**, 589–599.

Avery, L., and Horvitz, H. R. (1987). A cell that dies during wild-type C. elegans development can function as a neuron in a ced-3 mutant. *Cell* **51**, 1071–1078.

Avery, L., and Horvitz, H. R. (1989). Pharyngeal pumping continues after laser killing of the pharyngeal nervous system of *C. elegans. Neuron* **3**, 473–485.

Bargmann, C. I., and Horvitz, H. R. (1991a). Chemosensory neurons with overlapping functions direct chemotaxis to multiple chemicals in *C. elegans. Neuron* **7**, 729–742.

Bargmann, C. I., and Horvitz, H. R. (1991b). Control of larval development by chemosensory neurons in *Caenorhabditis elegans. Science* **251**, 1243–1246.

Bargmann, C. I., Hartwieg, E., and Horvitz, H. R. (1993). Odorant-selective genes and neurons mediate olfaction in *C. elegans. Cell* **74**, 515–527.

Chalfie, M., and Wolinsky, E. (1990). The identification and suppression of inherited neurodegeneration in *Caenorhabditis elegans. Nature* **345**, 410–416.

Chalfie, M., Sulston, J. E., White, J. G., Southgate, E., Thomson, J. N., and Brenner, S. (1985). The neural circuit for touch sensitivity in Caenorhabditis elegans. *J. Neurosci.* **5**, 956–964.

Chalfie, M., Tu, Y., Euskirchen, G., Ward, W., and Prasher, D. (1994). Green fluorescent protein as a marker for gene expression. *Science* **263**, 802–805.

Chamberlin, H., and Sternberg, P. (1993). Multiple cell interactions are required for fate specification during male spicule development in Caenorhabditis elegans. *Development* **118**, 297–324.

Driscoll, M., and Chalfie, M. (1991). The *mec-4* gene is a member of a family of *Caenorhabditis elegans* genes that can mutate to induce neuronal degeneration. *Nature* **349**, 588–593.

Ferguson, E. L., and Horvitz, H. R. (1985). Identification and characterization of 22 genes that affect the vulval cell lineages of the nematode Caenorhabditis elegans. *Genetics* **110**, 17–72.

Garriga, G., Desai, C., and Horvitz, H. (1993). Cell interactions control the direction of outgrowth, branching and fasciculation of the HSN axons of Caenorhabditis elegans. *Development* **117**, 1071–1087.

Hedgecock, E. M., Culotti, J. G., Thomson, J. N., and Perkins, L. A. (1985). Axonal guidance mutants of Caenorhabditis elegans identified by filling sensory neurons with fluorescein dyes. *Dev. Biol.* **111**, 158–170.

Kimble, J. (1981). Alterations in cell lineage following laser ablation of cells in the somatic gonad of Caenorhabditis elegans. *Dev. Biol.* **87**, 286–300.

Kimble, J., and Hirsh, D. (1979). The postembryonic cell lineages of the hermaphrodite and male gonads in Caenorhabditis elegans. *Dev. Biol.* **70**, 396–417.

Kimble, J. E., and White, J. G. (1981). On the control of germ cell development in Caenorhabditis elegans. *Dev. Biol.* **81,** 208–219.

Li, C., and Chalfie, M. (1991). Organogenesis in C. elegans: Positioning of neurons and muscles in the egg-laying system. *Neuron* **4,** 681–695.

McIntire, S., Jorgensen, E., Kaplan, J., and Horvitz, H. (1993). The GABAergic nervous system of Caenorhabditis elegans. *Nature* **364,** 337–341.

Mello, C., Draper, B., Krause, M., Weintraub, H., and Priess, J. (1992). The pie-1 and mex-1 genes and maternal control of blastomere identity in early C. elegans embryos. *Cell* **70,** 163–176.

Priess, J. R., and Thomson, J. N. (1987). Cellular interactions in early C. elegans embryos. *Cell* **48,** 241–250.

Schnabel, R. (1994). Autonomy and nonautonomy in cell fate specification of muscle in the Caenorhabditis elegans embryo: A reciprocal induction. *Science* **263,** 1449–1452.

Sommer, R. J., and Sternberg, P. W. (1994). Changes of induction and competence during the evolution of vulva development in nematodes. *Science* **265,** 114–118.

Sulston, J. E., and Horvitz, H. R. (1977). Post-embryonic cell lineages of the nematode, Caenorhabditis elegans. *Dev. Biol.* **56,** 110–156.

Sulston, J. E., and White, J. G. (1980). Regulation and cell autonomy during postembryonic development of Caenorhabditis elegans. *Dev. Biol.* **78,** 577–597.

Sulston, J. E., Albertson, D. G., and Thomson, J. N. (1980). The Caenorhabditis elegans male: Postembryonic development of nongonadal structures. *Dev. Biol.* **78,** 542–576.

Sulston, J. E., Schierenberg, E., White, J. G., and Thomson, J. N. (1983). The embryonic cell lineage of the nematode Caenorhabditis elegans. *Dev. Biol.* **100,** 64–119.

Thomas, J., Stern, M., and Horvitz, H. (1990). Cell interactions coordinate the development of the C. elegans egg-laying system. *Cell* **62,** 1041–1052.

Walthall, W. W., and Chalfie, M. (1988). Cell-cell interactions in the guidance of late-developing neurons in Caenorhabditis elegans. *Science* **239,** 643–645.

Waring, D., and Kenyon, C. (1990). Selective silencing of cell communication influences anteroposterior pattern formation in C. elegans. *Cell* **60,** 123–131.

White, J., and Horvitz, H. (1979). Laser microbeam techniques in biological research. *Electro-Optical Systems Design AUG.*

CHAPTER 11

Electrophysiological Methods

Leon Avery,[*] David Raizen,[*] and Shawn Lockery[†]

[*] Department of Biochemistry
University of Texas Southwestern Medical Center
Dallas, Texas 75235
[†] Institute for Neuroscience
University of Oregon
Eugene, Oregon 97403

I. Introduction

This chapter has two aims. First, we describe one method, the electropharyngeogram (EPG), in sufficient detail that a *Caenorhabditis elegans* researcher unfamiliar with electrophysiological methods could set up the apparatus and get useful results. Second, we describe more generally for researchers familiar with electrophysiological methods how they may be applied to *C. elegans*. We do not describe methods for electrophysiological investigation of *C. elegans* sperm (see Chapter 12).

II. The Electropharyngeogram

Most *C. elegans* electrophysiology so far has been done on the pharynx. There are three main reasons for this.

First, the pharynx is clearly visible by Nomarski differential interference contrast microscopy. Although single muscle cells cannot be seen, it is easy to distinguish the three major groups that make up most of the volume of the pharynx: the corpus—six binucleate muscle cells, the isthmus—three binucleate muscle cells, and the terminal bulb—seven mononucleate muscle cells (Albertson and Thomson, 1976). This means that muscle motions are easily correlated with electrical events.

Second, the pharynx can be exposed simply by cutting the head away from the rest of the worm (see Section II,B). Dissected pharynxes are useful for drug and ion substitution studies, as the solution has direct access to the muscle basal membrane. They are also potentially useful for recording from individual identified muscle cells, although this potential has been little exploited.

Third, pharyngeal muscle cells are excitable polarized myoepithelial cells. Together with the hypodermis, intestine, and parts of the genitalia, they form the continuous epithelium that topologically separates the pseudocoelom from the outside world (White, 1988). Their electrical activity generates transepithelial currents that can be recorded even in an intact worm (Raizen and Avery, 1994). These recordings, made from the outside of the intact animal, are analogous to electrocardiograms or electroencephalograms recorded from humans. We call them electropharyngeograms (EPGs).

A. Theory

As in other fast muscles, contraction in pharyngeal muscle is controlled by changes in membrane electrical potential. But pharyngeal muscle cells are polarized, with apical and basal faces (White, 1988). The apical membrane faces the pharyngeal lumen. The basal membrane, which faces the pseudocoelom, seems to generate the active voltage changes that control muscle contraction (Byerly and Masuda, 1979; Raizen and Avery, 1994). It is also the membrane onto which pharyngeal neurons synapse (Albertson and Thomson, 1976). The apical membrane, in contrast, seems to passively follow basal membrane changes.

Consider what happens at the beginning of a muscle action potential. At first the basal membrane potential is negative: The cytoplasm is at a lower voltage than the pseudocoelom. Suddenly a pulse of current flows through the basal membrane into the cell, raising the voltage of the cytoplasm above that of the pseudocoelom. (By analogy with other muscles, this current pulse probably flows through voltage-activated sodium or calcium channels.) Now, the total voltage difference between the cytoplasm and pseudocoelom must be the same along any path that connects them, including the long path that goes from the cytoplasm across the apical membrane, out the mouth, through the surrounding fluid, and finally across the cuticle and hypodermis back into the pseudocoelom (Fig. 1). As all the solutions in this path conduct electricity well, most of the voltage difference will appear across membranes (represented by capacitors in Fig. 1): the apical membrane of pharyngeal muscle or the apical and basal membranes of the hypodermis (represented by a single capacitor for simplicity). Biological membranes are capacitors: Any voltage difference between the two faces of a membrane is accompanied by a proportional difference in charge. Thus, when pharyngeal muscle is excited, a pulse of current must flow out of the mouth to charge the apical membranes and hypodermis.

From this analysis one can deduce several useful facts about the EPG. First, the total charge that comes out of the mouth during a current pulse (which can be measured by measuring the area of the current peak) will be proportional to the change in voltage across the basal membrane. Second, the current at any point in time will be proportional to the rate of change of basal membrane potential. Thus, fast voltage changes will cause brief, big current pulses, but slow voltage changes will cause small, long-lasting, generally undectable currents. Third, the total charge that comes out of the mouth during a current pulse will be proportional to the capacitance of that part of the apical membrane whose voltage changes. As capacitance is proportional to membrane area, bigger worms give bigger signals.

B. How to Record an Electropharyngeogram

Use a 5-ml syringe filled with silicone vacuum grease to make a 1- to 2-cm-diameter circle on a 35 × 50-mm glass coverslip (Carolina Biological Supply). Put 200 to 400 μl of saline in the circle. We generally use either *Ascaris* saline

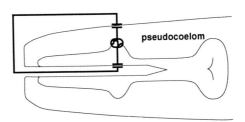

Fig. 1 Equivalent circuit of the pharynx.

or Dent's saline (Table I and Section III,B), but the saline composition is not important when recording from intact worms. Add several worms. Healthy adult worms produce the biggest currents. Drugs may be added to the saline; the most useful is 10 m*M* serotonin, which induces rapid pumping and somewhat sedates the worm.

Suction pipets are pulled from borosilicate glass capillaries (1.0-mm o.d., 0.5-mm i.d.) Use capillaries without an internal filament, because the filament may prevent a good seal with the worm. The tip should have an opening 20 to 40 μm in diameter, depending on the size of the worm. When it is filled with saline (Table I), the pipet should have a resistance between 200 kΩ and 1 MΩ. Mount the pipet in a holder with a tubing port through which suction can be applied (World Precision Instruments), attached to a 5-ml syringe. Wrap a 5- to 10-cm length of a grounded silver/silver chloride electrode helically around the pipet from the base to within 3 mm of the tip (Fig. 2a). (To make a silver/silver chloride electrode, dip the tip of a silver wire in chloride bleach for 5 minutes, then rinse it with distilled water). Lower the pipet tip into the bath until the tip

Table I
Solutions for Electrophysiological Recording

	Extracellular salines		
	Ascaris saline	Dent's saline	Tet's saline
Sodium chloride (m*M*)	4.0	140.0	137.0
Sodium acetate (m*M*)	125.0		
Potassium chloride (m*M*)	24.5	6.0	5.0
Calcium chloride (m*M*)	5.9	3.0	1.0
Magnesium chloride (m*M*)	4.9	1.0	5.0
Hepes[a] (m*M*)	5.0	5.0	5.0
Glucose (m*M*)			10.0
pH	7.4	7.4	7.2
Osmolarity (mOsm)	323	285	302
	Internal solution		
Potassium gluconate (m*M*)	136.5		
Potassium chloride (m*M*)	17.5		
Sodium chloride (m*M*)	9.0		
Magnesium chloride (m*M*)	1.0		
Hepes (m*M*)	10.0		
EGTA (m*M*)	0.2		
pH	7.2		
Osmolarity (mOsm)	311		

[a] Hepes, 4-(2-hydroxyethyl)-1-piperazineethanesulfonic acid; EGTA, ethylene glycol bis(β-aminoethyl ether)-*N,N'*-tetraacetic acid.

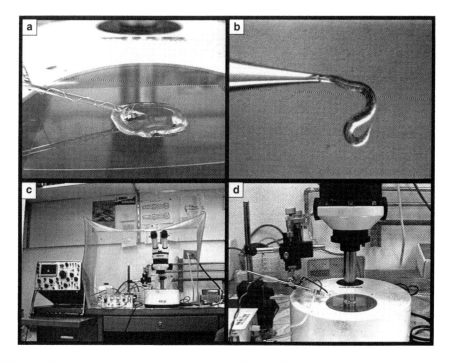

Fig. 2 Electropharyngeogram electrodes and minirig. (a) Electrode and bath during recording. The bath is about 15 mm in diameter. (b) A worm with its head trapped in the pipet for recording. The worm is slightly more than 1 mm long. (c) Complete rig with dissecting microscope, micromanipulator, microelectrode amplifier, Faraday cage, and oscilloscope. (d) Closeup of the microscope and micromanipulator.

is submerged and the ground electrode contacts the liquid, then apply suction to fill the pipet with solution until it contacts the pipet electrode.

You are now ready to capture a worm. Move the mouth of the pipet close to the nose of a worm and apply gentle suction, gradually increasing until the worm is sucked up to the pipet. If the worm is held by the side or the tail, blow it away from the pipet with slight positive pressure and try again. A few attempts are usually necessary to capture the nose (Fig. 2b). Once the nose is captured, raise the pipet slightly above the coverslip to decrease the chance that the worm will escape by pushing against the glass. You should now see electrical signals on the amplifier output with every pump.

It is also possible to record EPGs from dissected pharynxes. Place a few worms in a vacuum grease-confined drop of Dent's or similar saline (Table I) on a coverslip as above. (Dissected pharynxes, unlike intact worms, are sensitive to the ionic composition of the saline. See Section III,B). Cut the head away from the rest of the worm by slicing transversely through the body with a No. 15 surgical knife blade (Fig. 3). The worms move energetically throughout this

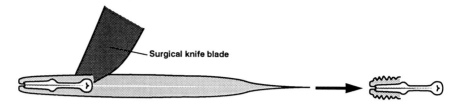

Fig. 3 Pharynx dissection. The worm is cut transversely through the body just behind the pharynx with a surgical knife. (The knife blade is actually much larger relative to the worm than pictured.) The tail section, consisting of everything posterior to the pharynx, is discarded. The smaller head section contains the pharynx. The muscles underlying the head cuticle contract, exposing most of the pharynx.

process (and who can blame them?), but with a little practice about half of these dissections are successful in cutting the terminal bulb away from the intestine. The isolated head segment contains the entire pharynx and nerve ring. It is initially covered by a hood of cuticle and body wall muscle extending to the back of the terminal bulb. On dissection, the body wall muscles contract, conveniently crumpling the hood and exposing the nerve ring and posterior pharynx. You can improve the exposure of the pharynx by including 1 μM levamisole in the bath. Levamisole is an acetylcholine agonist that excites body wall muscles (Lewis *et al.*, 1987; Fleming *et al.*, 1993), thus increasing their contraction. At this concentration it has no detectable effect on the pharynx (Avery and Horvitz, 1990; our unpublished observations). Serotonin at a concentration of 1 μM will stimulate vigorous pumping.

C. Interpretation

Figure 4 shows a portion of a typical normal EPG that corresponds to a single pharyngeal pump, that is, a contraction followed by a relaxation (Raizen and Avery, 1994). The record has been filtered as described in Section II,F to remove low-frequency noise. This record has three phases: the E or excitation phase, when the basal membranes of pharyngeal muscle cells depolarize; the P or plateau phase, during which the membrane potential remains depolarized and contraction proceeds; and the R or repolarization phase, when the membrane potential returns to negative values, initiating muscle relaxation. In addition, we call the time between two pumps the I or interpump phase. E phase consists of two closely spaced positive spikes, often overlapping, the first usually smaller than the second. R phase consists of two negative spikes, a large one followed by a small one. P phase is defined as the period between the last E-phase spike and the first R-phase spike. During rapid pumping (induced by serotonin, for instance) there are few or no spikes during P phase. During slow pumping, in contrast, there is typically a series of negative P phase spikes as shown in Fig. 4. I phase contains occasional positive spikes. These are rare in wild-type but much more frequent in some mutant backgrounds.

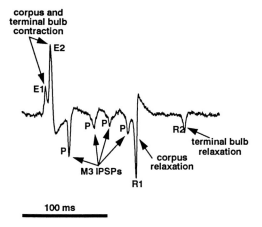

Fig. 4 Typical normal electropharyngeogram.

The origins of most of these features have been determined (Raizen and Avery, 1994). The first R-phase spike is caused by the repolarization of corpus muscles, and the second by repolarization of terminal bulb muscles. Negative P-phase spikes and positive I-phase spikes reflect changes in muscle membrane potential caused by synaptic input from pharyngeal motor neurons: the P-phase spikes from M3 motor neurons (Raizen and Avery, 1994), and the I-phase spikes probably from MC neurons (Raizen and Avery, unpublished). The E-phase spikes are less well understood. They immediately precede contraction and clearly result from excitation of pharyngeal muscles, but we do not know why there are two or to what extent they depend on the nervous system. E and R spikes are therefore useful for studying muscle excitability. P-phase spikes are currently the most useful for studying synaptic function.

D. Video Correlation

It is often necessary to correlate electrical events with movement, for example, to ask whether a particular electrical transient may cause a movement. This can be done by making a simultaneous video recording of the movements of the animal and an oscilloscope display of the electrical events (Raizen and Avery, 1994). A video camera is focused on the screen of an oscilloscope connected to the output of the recording amplifier. The small size of oscilloscope screens requires this camera to be equipped with a macro lens; we found the cheapest option to be a camcorder (e.g., the Sony Handyman CCD-FX310). A second video camera attached to the microscope records the worm's movements. You should choose a microscope camera with a sync input that allows it to be synchronized to the oscilloscope camera. The two cameras are connected to the inputs of a video mixer, which produces a single video image that combines the two pictures. The combined image can be made in several different ways; we usually split the screen into upper and lower halves, one displaying the worm and the other the oscilloscope. The output of the mixer is recorded by a videocassette recorder. Slow-motion or stop-frame analysis of the tape later allows analysis with a time resolution of $\frac{1}{60}$ second (Avery, 1993).

E. Electronics

The currents that flow in and out of the mouth can be measured in either of two ways. First, they can be measured directly with a low-impedance current-following amplifier. An ideal current follower (also known as a current-to-voltage converter) acts like a short-circuit in that it passes current between its two inputs without a voltage drop (Fig. 5). Its output is a voltage proportional to the current flowing from one input to the other. In practice one uses a voltage-clamp amplifier—a current follower with the ability to produce a voltage difference between its inputs on command. When the command voltage is set to zero, a voltage-clamp amplifier becomes a current follower. The ability to set a nonzero voltage can be used to correct for junction potentials caused by slight differences in ion concentrations. In addition, voltage-clamp amplifiers intended for electro-

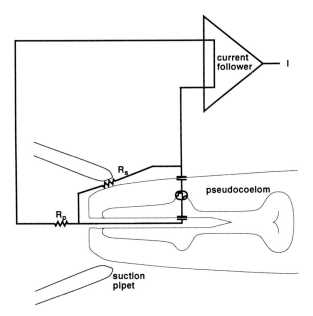

Fig. 5 Equivalent circuit of the electropharyngeogram recording arrangement. This figure shows the recording configuration in voltage-clamp mode, where currents are recorded with a low-impedance current-following amplifier diagrammed internally as a short-circuit. In current-clamp recording the current follower is replaced with a high-impedance voltage amplifier, which acts roughly as an open circuit.

physiology typically have other built-in features useful for recording EPGs, such as variable output gain, a low-pass filter, and series resistance correction. In this voltage-clamp mode, where the voltage difference between the pharyngeal lumen and the bath is held constant and the current that passes between them measured, one typically records peak currents of 300 to 500 pA flowing into the mouth during corpus relaxation (the first R-phase spike) in gravid adult hermaphrodites.

In the second recording mode the currents generated by pharyngeal electrical activity are measured indirectly with a high-impedance AC-coupled voltage amplifier. In this configuration, the current that flows out of the mouth is unable to flow through the amplifier (because of its high input impedance), and instead must flow across the seal (R_s in Fig. 5) between the pipet and the worm's cuticle, producing a voltage drop. For example, if the seal resistance is 10 MΩ and the peak current 400 pA, the voltage amplifier will record a peak voltage of 4 mV. This current-clamp recording mode has one advantage over voltage-clamp: the simplicity and low cost of the amplifier. It has one main disadvantage: Because the seal resistance is variable, absolute spike amplitudes are not meaningful. (In addition, because the noise characteristics of the simplest voltage amplifiers are not as good as those of the feedback circuitry used in voltage-clamp amplifiers, they are not as good for measuring small signals.) Nevertheless, it is usually the timing and relative sizes of spikes that are most informative. Current-clamp recording is therefore nearly as informative as voltage-clamp. It is undoubtedly the simplest way to get started.

F. Noise

Figure 6a shows a typical EPG recorded in voltage-clamp mode from a normal worm. Figures 6b and c show a crude separation of the signal in Fig. 6a into slow and fast components. The current transients or spikes (Fig. 6b) result from fast changes in muscle membrane potential as described in Section II,A. The slow changes (Fig. 6c) may result from a variety of uninteresting sources: changes in the resistances and capacitances of the circuit caused by movement of the body or pharyngeal muscles, junction potentials caused by the mixing of solutions of slightly different composition, drift in the internal components of the amplifier, and so on. These slow changes are complex and poorly understood.

The practical effect of low-frequency noise is that only the spikes can be interpreted. It is convenient when analyzing EPGs to filter the signal to remove frequency components below about 5 Hz (high-pass filtering); this attenuates the slow noise and leaves the spikes easily visible, although slightly distorted. Unfortunately, even the slowest signals have some high-frequency component. Signals should be high-pass filtered only after making a permanent record, and the unfiltered signal should be examined to make sure that apparent transients are not merely a residue of unusually large slow changes.

High-frequency noise is better understood. It is caused by the imperfect seal between the worm and the pipet. This seal is represented by a resistor R_s in Fig.

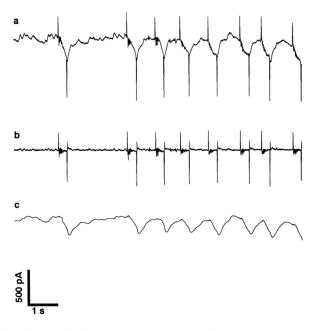

Fig. 6 Dissection of the electropharyngeogram into low- and high-frequency components. (a) A typical electropharyngeogram. (b) High-frequency component of a, obtained by high-pass filtering with a time constant of 10 milliseconds. This component is caused mostly by electrical events in pharyngeal muscle. (c) Low-frequency component of a, obtained by low-pass filtering with a time constant of 100 milliseconds. This component comes from many sources, such as drift in the electronic components and probably motions of the worm and the pharynx.

5, which shows an equivalent circuit of worm's head from which an EPG is being recorded in voltage-clamp configuration. Any resistor produces thermal noise (Johnson noise). The current noise is inversely proportional to the square root of the resistance. Therefore a tight seal, meaning higher resistance, produces less noise. The seal resistance is variable from worm to worm and from minute to minute. Increased suction improves the seal, but too much suction compresses the worm and makes it act strange. (For example, pumping may be inhibited). Seals of 10 MΩ can usually be achieved on intact worms without bad effects. A 10 MΩ seal will produce peak-to-peak noise of 5 to 10 pA (assuming the signal is filtered to exclude frequencies above 1000 Hz as described below). Even small spikes are clearly visible above this noise when recording from a large worm. If, however, the seal is poor, or the worm is small (e.g., because of mutation or chronic drug treatment), or you need to see small currents, high-frequency noise can be a serious problem.

High-frequency noise can be reduced by a low-pass filter, which blocks fast signal changes. Of course, such a filter also distorts the spikes if its cutoff frequency is too low. We have found 1000 Hz to be a good cutoff frequency. If you store your recordings in a computer, the computer should be told to sample at at least twice the filter cutoff frequency. For example, a signal filtered at 1000 Hz should be sampled at least 2000 times a second.

G. A Practical Exercise: The Minirig

Our current electrophysiology setup, or rig, includes an inverted microscope with Nomarski differential interference contrast optics, two hydraulic joystick micromanipulators, two AC voltage amplifiers, a patch-clamp amplifier, and analog storage oscilloscope, a computer with data acquisition hardware and software, and the video equipment described above (see Section II,D). To a geneticist interested in doing a little electrophysiology, buying and setting up such a heap of equipment may be a forbidding prospect. In fact, most of this is unnecessary to record simple EPGs.

To demonstrate what can be done with the simplest setup, we put together the EPG rig shown in Fig. 2c. Figure 2d is a closeup of the microscope, amplifier, and manipulator. To screen out environmental noise, these components are inside a small Faraday cage made by folding $\frac{1}{8}$-in. mesh hardware cloth. The cage is connected to the ground lead of the amplifier. The bottom of the cage is a sheet of aluminum foil. The front can be closed by leaning a rectangle of hardware cloth against it. The microscope light power cord (not visible in the figure) must be grounded; otherwise it will act as an antenna, picking up noise from outside and bringing it into the cage. (You should first make certain that the lamp power supply is designed in such a way as not to create a short-circuit when one of its output leads is grounded.) Furthermore, the AC current passed through the lamp is itself a source of noise; it must be turned off while recording. Alternatively, you can buy a DC power supply for about $200. With the DC power supply the animals can be watched while the recording is made. In this case your body will shield the front if you touch a finger to the cage as you lean over the microscope.

This minirig can be put together for a little over $3000 at current prices (Table II). As pictured, it is not complete, because there is no way to record results. For pilot experiments a Polaroid oscilloscope camera can be used to photograph signals saved on the oscilloscope. For real work, however, some sort of electronic storage is essential. Although there are many possible ways of making permanent recordings, a computer is the most practical. With data acquisition hardware and software a suitable computer costs between $3000 and $4000. The total cost of a practical minirig is therefore about $7000.

III. Patch-Clamping

A. The Slit-Worm Preparation

For patch-clamp recordings from neurons, whole worms are immobilized by gluing them to an agarose-coated coverslip. The coverslip is prepared by pressing

Table II
Minirig Components

Component	Manufacturer	Price
SM1 stereomicroscope[a]	Oriental Scientific Import[a]	$1080
P15 AC microelectrode amplifier	Grass Instrument	570
M3301L manual manipulator, with steel base plate, magnetic base, and microelectrode holder	World Precision Instruments	934
453 dual-beam oscilloscope (used, obtained from local electronics surplus store)	Tektronix	500
Total		$3084

[a] The stereomicroscope shown in Fig. 2 is a Wild M5A; however, we have also used the Oriental Scientific SM1, and it will work for this purpose.

a single drop of hot 1% agarose between two coverslips (24 × 50 mm Corning No. 1). The top coverslip is carefully drawn away, leaving a moist agarose film on the bottom coverslip. At this point one must work quickly to finish before the agarose film dries. Ten to twenty worms are transferred to the coverslip using a fine paint brush ($\frac{10}{0}$ Grumbacher, 178). Worms are glued by applying a tiny amount of adhesive (Vetbond, 3M Animal Care Products) at several points on one side of each animal using a fine glass pipet. Pipets are made in advance by breaking the tip of a glass microelectrode pulled on a conventional electrode puller from 1.0-mm-o.d., 0.5-mm-i.d. capillary tubing. After it is broken, the diameter of the tip is about half the diameter of the worm. The back end of the pipet is held in a mouth tube and loaded by immersing the tip of the pipet in a fresh puddle of glue and sucking gently.

Gluing is done under a dissecting microscope (50×) by following individual worms with the pipet and then, at just the right moment, blowing out a drop of glue. With practice, the drop lands on the agarose, barely touching the side of the worm's head and neck. Moisture in the agarose film polymerizes the glue almost instantly. A second drop placed more posteriorly secures the midbody and tail. It is generally best to glue as many worms as possible before the agarose dries, as the final posture of the worm, and the success of the subsequent dissection, is hard to predict. As soon as enough worms are immobilized, the coverslip is doused with M9 buffer (Hodgkin and Sulston, 1988) to prevent further drying. The coverslip is washed several times in buffer to remove unglued worms and debris, then placed in a recording chamber containing physiological saline (see below). A convenient recording chamber can be made by gluing a large coverslip (35 × 50 mm Fisher No. 2) to the bottom of a plexiglass plate into the center of which a rectangular opening just smaller than the coverslip has been cut (Fig. 7). For stability, the coverslip is recessed into the bottom of the plate so that only the plate touches the microscope stage.

Neurons are exposed using a fine tungsten needle to make a small tear in the cuticle at the level of the nerve ring. The position of the needle is adjusted with a

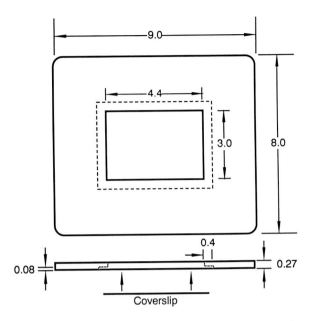

Fig. 7 Schematic drawing of a simple recording chamber. A rectangular hole is cut in a plexiglass plate. A coverslip is glued (epoxy cement) over the hole on the underside of the plate. Dimensions are in centimeters.

micromanipulator so that it is perpendicular to the long axis of the worm and approximately parallel to the bottom of the recording chamber. Internal pressure is partially relieved by making a small opening in the midbody, well away from the head. The needle is then moved to the level of the nerve ring and the point is inserted until it is just through the cuticle. For the needle to penetrate, the worm must be firmly glued on the opposite side of the body; otherwise there is nothing to push against. The cuticle is torn by gently moving the needle several micrometers anteriorly or posteriorly until a small bleb, perhaps 5 μm across, appears. The needle is then withdrawn while the bleb grows into a neuron-filled bouquet two to three times its original size. This may take a minute or two. If the hole is too big, or the internal pressure is too high, the entire nerve ring and pharynx come out, and one must start over on a new worm. After exposure, the neurons are not free-floating, but remain attached mechanically to the rest of the nervous system by connective material and by their processes in the neuropil of the nerve ring. Exposing the neurons in this way disrupts the positional cues by which *C. elegans* neurons are normally identified. In the future, however, it should be possible to identify neurons in the bouquet by using transgenic animals in which particular types of neurons express green fluorescent protein (Chalfie *et al.,* 1994).

The tungsten needle is made by an electrolytic sharpening process. First, a short length of tungsten wire (127 μm in diameter) is threaded down the length of a 23-gauge syringe needle until about 1 cm of wire protrudes from the end of the needle.

Crimping the needle keeps the wire from slipping. The needle is held in a vertical manipulator just above the solution. One lead of a variable AC power supply (0–10 V, 10 A) is connected to the needle and the other lead is connected to a saturated sodium nitrite solution by a graphite electrode. The wire is then dipped repeatedly into the solution to a depth of 1 or 2 mm. This eventually produces a gradual taper because more material is removed from the tip than from further back along the wire. Sharpening is complete when the tip diameter is less than 0.5 μm. A single needle is good for 5 to perhaps 25 worms. Shallower tapers yield sharper tips but are quickly bent by the tough cuticle; steeper tapers yield duller but longer-lasting tips.

B. Physiological Saline Solutions for *Caenorhabditis elegans*

Two strategies are generally used to device a saline solution for electrophysiological recording. The first is to determine the chemical composition of the extracellular fluid and to make a solution with the appropriate concentrations of the major inorganic ions. This approach is unlikely to work in *C. elegans* because it would be hard to obtain a large enough sample of uncontaminated extracellular fluid from such a small organism. The second strategy is trial and error, starting with salines from other species. One then varies the concentration of individual ions in dissected preparations, using an easily observable physiological response to determine the effect. We began with the physiological saline based on a chemical analysis of the extracellular fluid of *Ascaris suum* (Hobson *et al.*, 1952), another nematode, but this solution produced abnormal pharyngeal pumping and EPGs without postsynaptic potentials, suggesting failure of the nervous system. Two solutions that gave essentially normal pumping, Dent's saline and Tet's saline, are listed in Table I. Abnormal pumping in *Ascaris* saline could be due to its relatively high potassium concentration, which is well above that of the other two. One possibility is that high external potassium affects pumping by making the reversal potential for potassium more positive, thereby depolarizing pharyngeal neurons and muscles. The levels of potassium that produce normal pumping in *C. elegans* are consistent with the levels found in chemical analyses of the extracellular fluid in earthworms and other annelids that probably inhabit a similar fluid environment (Drewes and Pax, 1973; Nicholls and Kuffler, 1964).

The composition of the solution in the patch pipet depends on the type of recording to be made and the type of channels to be studied. For example, in a cell-attached recording, the pipet is often filled with the solution that bathes the preparation, whereas in a whole-cell recording (in which the membrane patch under the pipet is ruptured to obtain access to the inside of the cell), the pipet may contain a solution meant to mimic the composition of the cytoplasm. A detailed discussion of formulating pipet solutions is beyond the scope of this chapter (but see Kay, 1992). It is, however, worth noting, that many patch-clamp specialists report anecdotally that the relative osmolarity of the pipet solution and the extracellular solution can be important. A pipet solution 5 to 10 mOsm hypertonic with respect to the extracellular solution is believed to promote seal formation and to facilitate rupture of the membrane when establishing the whole-cell recording configuration. On the other hand, a pipet solution 10 to 15% hypotonic with respect to the extracellular solution is believed to make the seal between the cell and the pipet more reliable and more stable (Kay, 1992; Hamill *et al.*, 1981).

C. The Patch-Clamp Setup

An inverted compound microscope is recommended for dissection and electrophysiological recordings of *C. elegans* neurons because of the extra working distance it provides above the preparation. With a long-working-distance condenser, working distances of 2 cm are typical. High magnification (at least 400× to 640×) is required to observe the progress of the dissection and to position the patch pipet, as the cell body of a typical *C. elegans* neuron is only 2 µm in diameter. The objectives, too, must have a long working distance because neurons must be viewed through two coverslips, the agarose film, and possibly several layers of other neurons. We use a 40× (0.75 NA) water immersion objective with a working distance of 1.9 mm (Ziess 44 00 91). Because the objective is an immersion lens, a drop of water is placed between the objective and the bottom of the recording chamber with a syringe. Dry lenses with adequate working distances do not provide enough resolution because they have comparatively low numerical apertures. Magnification is increased by 16× eyepieces. A range of lower-power objectives, beginning at 4×, is helpful for selecting the best worm to dissect and for centering and rotating the worm in the field of view. The preparation is viewed using differential interference contrast optics.

The mechanical and electronic requirements for patch-clamping *C. elegans* neurons are the same as for patch-clamping other cells, and have been described in detail already (Sakmann and Neher, 1983; Rudy and Iverson, 1992). At this writing, an electrophysiology setup for patch-clamping *C. elegans* neurons costs about $75,000. The most expensive item is an inverted compound microscope with epifluorescence and differential interference contrast optics (about $30,000). It is important to have the best optics possible, as the ability to see the cells and the membrane patch inside the pipet (see below) is a limiting factor in making the recording. It is also wise to invest in a good micromanipulator for holding the patch-clamp pipet (about $5000), as less expensive manipulators are prone to drift.

D. Patch-Clamp Pipets

Because *C. elegans* neuron cell bodies are typically only 2 µm in diameter, we use pipets pulled from thick-walled borosilicate glass tubing (1.2-mm o.d., 0.69-mm i.d.), as thick-walled glass forms smaller openings more readily than thin-walled glass (Brown and Flaming, 1986). Any of a number of widely available pullers will suffice (e.g., Sutter Instruments, David Kopf Instruments, Narashige USA). With an intracellular solution in the pipet (Tet's solution, Table I), the pipet resistance is 5 to 7 MΩ, but this is only a rough guide to the size of the opening because pipet resistance is influenced by other aspects of pipet shape (Sakmann and Neher, 1983, pp. 37–52). The opening of the pipet is approximately 0.7 μm as measured from scanning electron micrographs. In some preparations (e.g., *C. elegans* sperm; see Chapter 12 in this volume), smoothing the pipet tip by fire-polishing promotes seal formation, but in *C. elegans,* polishing does not seem to matter.

E. Patch-Clamp Recordings

A typical experiment proceeds as follows. The tip of the pipet is filled by immersing it in the pipet solution and applying negative pressure to the back of the pipet for 10 to 15 seconds. The pipet is then backfilled with more pipet solution from a syringe. The pipet solution should be carefully filtered beforehand (pore size 0.22 μm). The pipet is then mounted in the manipulator, and positive pressure is applied to the back of the pipet to keep the tip clean as the pipet is lowered into the bath and brought up to the cell. At this point, the pipet holding potential is set to 0 mV and the current is set to zero by balancing the junction potential. We usually select a neuron on the margin of the bouquet because alignment of the cell and pipet is crucial and these cells are easiest to see. The pipet is then advanced against the cell as far as possible without the cell slipping off the tip. The positive pressure is then released, and if necessary, negative pressure is applied using a mouthpiece. Sometimes the seal forms instantly; other times it takes up to a minute. Seal resistance in either case may continue to increase for several minutes. In a recent series of experiments, the success rate for seal formation was 91% and the average seal resistance was 9.6 GΩ. Inside-out excised patches can be made in the usual way (Hamill *et al.,* 1981), by first establishing a gigaohm seal, then retracting the pipet to tear the patch away from the cell. It is not yet known whether whole-cell recordings can be made reliably from *C. elegans* neurons, though they can be made from *C. elegans* sperm (see Chapter 12 in this volume).

A systematic study of the types of channels *C. elegans* neurons have is just beginning. Nevertheless, three general remarks are possible: (1) The great majority of cell-attached patches on ring neurons exhibit single-channel currents. With an intracellular solution in the pipet, channel activity is observed at a holding potential of 0 mV. This shows that some channels are active when the patch membrane is at the resting potential; these channels may contribute to the cell's resting potential. It also provides evidence for a nonzero resting potential, because if the resting potential were 0 mV, little or no ionic current would flow, as the concentrations of ions on either side of the patch membrane are approximately equal. The indication of a resting potential suggests the dissection procedure and the choice of saline preserve fundamental aspects of neuronal function. (2) Many of the channels are voltage dependent, as the probability of being open changes with the holding potential. For example, the open probability of the channels in Fig. 8 increases as the holding potential is made more positive with respect to the bath. In the cell-attached configuration, positive holding potentials hyperpolarize the patch. Thus, these channels appear to be activated by hyperpolarization, a characteristic feature of an inwardly rectifying potassium current (Katz, 1949). (3) The current carried by a single channel is sometimes large enough to change the membrane potential of the neuron significantly. At a holding potential of +80 mV, prolonged closures sometimes occur, revealing an exponential (rather than stepwise) decline in the current (Fig. 8, arrowhead). This reflects the discharging of the whole-cell membrane capacitance, which can occur only if the cell's voltage changes. In a cell-attached patch, only the voltage of the pipet is clamped. The voltage of the cell is in fact free to change when a channel in the patch (or elsewhere in the cell) opens. In large cells, the input resistance is generally so low that the effect of a single channel is negligible, but in small cells the input resistance can be so large that a single channel can strongly affect the membrane potential. Thus, the observation that single-channel currents can change the membrane potential of *C. elegans* neurons suggests that their input resistance is comparatively high, a fact that should be possible to confirm using whole-cell patch-clamp recording.

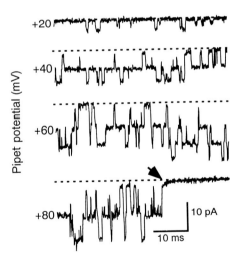

Fig. 8 Single-channel currents recorded from a neuron in the cell-attached patch configuration. Downward deflections represent inward current. The numbers at the left are pipet potential with respect to the bath (in mV) and the dotted lines indicate zero current. The pipet contained the intracellular solution in Table I. Open probability increased when the patch was hyperpolarized by making the pipet potential more positive. At 80 mV, prolonged closures sometimes occurred revealing an exponential (rather than stepwise) relaxation of the current (arrowhead). This suggests that current flowing through a single ion channel is sufficient to alter the membrane potential of the neuron.

IV. Further Reading

The main purpose of this chapter has been to describe how standard electrophysiological and patch-clamp techniques can be used to record from neurons and muscles in *C. elegans*. Additional technical information is available from many sources. A brief bibliography is given below.

A. General Electrophysiological Techniques

1. Purves, R. D. (1981). "Microelectrode Methods for Intracellular Recording and Ionophoresis." Academic Press, New York.

2. Brown, K. T., and Flaming, D. G. (1986). "Advanced Micropipette Techniques for Cell Physiology." Wiley, New York.

3. "The Axon Guide for Electrophysiology & Biophysics Laboratory Techniques." Axon Instruments, Foster City, CA.

B. Patch-Clamp Techniques

1. Sakmann, B., and Neher, E. (1983). "Single-Channel Recording." Plenum, New York.

2. Rudy, B., and Iverson, L. E. (1992). "Methods in Enzymology," Vol. 207: "Ion Channels." Academic Press, San Diego.

3. Chad, J., and Wheal, H. (1991). "Cellular Neurobiology: A Practical Approach." Oxford, New York.

References

Albertson, D. G., and Thomson, J. N. (1976). The pharynx of *Caenorhabditis elegans*. *Phil. Trans. R. Soc. Lond.* **B275,** 299–325.

Avery, L., and Horvitz, H. R. (1990). Effects of starvation and neuroactive drugs on feeding in *Caenorhabditis elegans. J. Exp. Zool.* **253,** 263–270.

Avery, L. (1993). The genetics of feeding in *Caenorhabditis elegans. Genetics* **133,** 897–917.

Brown, K. T., and Flaming, D. G. (1986). Advanced Micropipette Techniques for Cell Physiology. Wiley, New York.

Byerly, L., and Masuda, M. O. (1979). Voltage-clamp analysis of the potassium current that produces a negative-going action potential in *Ascaris* muscle. *J. Physiol.* **288,** 263–284.

Chalfie, M., Tu, Y., Euskirchen, G., Ward, W. W., and Prasher, D. C. (1994). Green fluorescent protein as a marker for gene expression. *Science* **263,** 802–805.

Drewes, C. D., and Pax, R. A. (1973). Neuromuscular physiology of the longitudinal muscle of the earthworm, Lumbricus terrestris I. Effects of different physiological salines. *J. Exp. Biol.* **60,** 445–452.

Fleming, J. T., Tornoe, C., Riina, H. A., Coadwell, J., Lewis, J. A., and Satelle, D. B., (1993). Acetylcholine receptor molecules of the nematode *Caenorhabditis elegans. EXS* **63,** 65–80.

Hamill, O. P., Marty, A., Neher, E., Sakmann, B., and Sigworth, F. J. (1981). Improved patch-clamp techniques for high resolution current recording from cells and cell-free membrane patches. *Pflugers Arch.* **391,** 85–100.

Hobson, A. D., Stephenson, W., and Eden, A. (1952). Studies on the physiology of *Ascaris lumbricoides* II. The inorganic composition of the body fluid in relation to that of the environment. *J. Exp. Biol.* **29**, 22–29.

Hodgkin, A. L., and Rushton, W. A. H. (1946). The electrical constants of a crustacean nerve fibre. *Proc. Soc. Lond.* [*Biol*] **133**, 444–479.

Hodgkin, J. A., and Sulston, J. E. (1988). Methods. *In* "The Nematode *Caenorhabditis elegans*" (W. B. Wood, ed.), pp. 587–606. Cold Spring Harbor Laboratory, Cold Spring Harbor, New York.

Katz, B. (1949). Les constantes electriques de la membrane du muscle. *Arch. Sci. Physiol.* **2**, 285–299.

Kay, A. R. (1992). An intracellular medium formulary. *J. Neurosci. Methods* **44**, 91–100.

Lewis, J. A., Elmer, J. S., Skimmings, J., McLafferty, S., Fleming, J. T., and McGee, T. (1987). Cholinergic receptor mutants of the nematode *Caenorhabditis elegans*. *J. Neurosci.* **7**, 3059–3071.

Nicholls, J. G., and Kuffler, S. W. (1964). Extracellular space as a pathway for exchange between blood and neurons in the central nervous system of the leech: Ionic composition of glial cells and neurons. *J. Neurophysiol.* **27**, 645–671.

Raizen, D. M., and Avery, L. (1994). Electrical activity and behavior in the pharynx of *Caenorhabditis elegans*. *Neuron* **12**, 483–495.

Rudy, B., and Iverson, L. E. (1992). Ion Channels. *In* "Methods in Enzymology," **207**, Academic Press, San Diego.

Sakmann, B., and Neher, E. (1983). "Single Channel Recording." Plenum, New York.

White, J. G. (1988). The anatomy. *In* "The Nematode *Caenorhabditis elegans*" (W. B. Wood, ed.), pp. 81–122. Cold Spring Harbor Laboratory, Cold Spring Harbor, New York.

PART III

Cell Biology
and Molecular Biology

CHAPTER 12

Cell Biology of Nematode Sperm

Steven W. L'Hernault[*] and Thomas M. Roberts[†]

[*]Department of Biology
Emory University
Atlanta, Georgia 30322
[†]Department of Biological Science
Florida State University
Tallahassee, Florida 32306

I. General Introduction

In this chapter, we review methods that have been developed for working with the amoeboid sperm of nematodes. Although the sperm from a number

of species have been examined, we confine our discussion to the free-living
Caenorhabditis elegans and the pig parasite *Ascaris suum.* Each of these experimental systems offers the investigator certain strengths and weaknesses, and the
type of contemplated experiment determines which is most suitable. *Ascaris*
sperm are more easily obtainable in large quantity and are, therefore, more
suited for biochemical studies. Furthermore, the *Ascaris* sperm is much larger
than its *C. elegans* counterpart, allowing easier light microscopic analyses (Fig.
1). The superb genetics and ease in obtaining DNA clones containing desired
gene sequences make *C. elegans* the system of choice for genetic and molecular
biological studies. Much evidence indicates that the sperm of these two systems
share important similarities, and data obtained in one are frequently applicable
to the other. Consequently, although the rest of this volume concerns principally
C. elegans, we feel this chapter requires discussion of both *C. elegans* and *Ascaris*
sperm because much of our understanding of amoeboid sperm cell biology has,
in fact, been obtained from *Ascaris.*

II. *Caenorhabditis elegans*

A. Introduction to Reproductive Biology and Spermatogenesis

The unusual method of reproduction used by *C. elegans* permits ready recovery
of mutations that affect spermatogenesis. *C. elegans* exists principally as a self-
fertile hermaphrodite in which internal fertilization is extraordinarily efficient;
in young animals, virtually every sperm fertilizes an oocyte, and the resulting
shelled eggs are laid on the agar growth plate (Ward and Carrel, 1979). Mutant
hermaphrodites containing defective sperm lay oocytes and are self-sterile; mating these mutants to wild-type males permits recovery of the mutation from

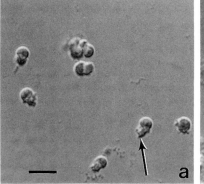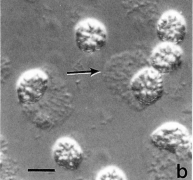

Fig. 1 *Caenorhabditis elegans* (a) and *Ascaris* (b) spermatozoa. The arrow points at the pseudopod
of a representative cell. Bar = 10 μm. Nomarski differential interference contrast optics.

resulting outcross progeny. This simple screen has identified more than 58 genes that appear to affect spermatogenesis (Hirsh and Vanderslice, 1976; Ward and Miwa, 1978; Argon and Ward, 1980; Ward *et al.*, 1981, 1982, 1983; Nelson *et al.*, 1982; L'Hernault *et al.*, 1987, 1988, 1993; Shakes and Ward, 1988, 1989a,b; L'Hernault and Arduengo, 1992; Varkey *et al.*, 1993). Standard methods, described elsewhere in this volume, can then be employed to obtain DNA clones containing mutationally defined *spe* gene sequences (e.g., L'Hernault and Arduengo, 1992; L'Hernault *et al.*, 1993). Much of spermatogenesis and how it is affected in various mutants can be studied both *in vivo* and *in vitro*, which permits direct microscopic inspection of this process as it is occurring. Unlike nearly all other *C. elegans* cells, homogeneous sperm can be obtained in sufficient quantities to permit biochemical analyses (Klass and Hirsh, 1981; Nelson *et al.*, 1982). Recently, we have proven that it is possible to patch-clamp *C. elegans* sperm cells at many stages during their differentiation (Machaca *et al.*, 1993). Consequently, *C. elegans* spermatogenesis can be studied by a combination of genetic, molecular biological, cytological, ultrastructural, patch-clamp electrophysiological, and biochemical techniques.

Wild-type *C. elegans* spermatogenesis has been studied in detail by others (Wolf *et al.*, 1978; Ward *et al.*, 1981, 1982). The $4N$ primary spermatocyte buds off the rachis (a central syncytial cytoplasmic core) after entering pachytene and undergoes the first meiotic division. Subsequent development of the primary spermatocyte can occur *in vitro* in the absence of any exogenously supplied hormones or any type of accessory cell such as the Sertoli cell that is required for mammalian spermatogenesis (reviewed in, for instance, Skinner *et al.*, 1991). Secondary spermatocytes either completely separate or stay linked by a cytoplasmic bridge as they undergo the second meiotic division to yield a total of four haploid spermatids. Asymmetrical cytoplasmic partitioning places all ribosomes and virtually all of the actin, tubulin, and myosin of the spermatocyte into the residual body during formation of haploid spermatids. Resulting sessile apolar spermatids are activated to form motile bipolar spermatozoa in a 5- to 10-minute differentiation process. These spermatozoa crawl by extension of a single motile pseudopod (Fig. 1). Unlike other amoeboid cells, nematode spermatozoa lack actin and contain instead a cytoskeleton composed of major sperm protein (MSP) filaments. The relative simplicity of nematode spermatozoan motility might reveal important clues about the general principles of amoeboid cell motility (reviewed by Heath, 1992).

B. Large-Scale Culture of Worms and Isolation of Males

1. General Comments

Growth plates support large quantities of worms; however, the synchrony required to purify males from a mixed male/hermaphrodite population is difficult to achieve under these conditions. Thus, liquid culture techniques have been developed, using procedures modified from published methods (Klass and Hirsh, 1981; Nelson *et al.,* 1982; S. Ward, unpublished).

Liquid culture of *C. elegans* is usually performed in medium that does not contain antibiotics or other agents to inhibit growth of contaminating organisms. Consequently, extreme care is required to avoid contamination with bacteria, yeasts, or molds, which adversely affects synchrony of worms growth, yield of worms, and separation of males from hermaphrodites. Rigorous sterile technique within a laminar-flow hood is required. Precautions to employ include the following:

1. Wear gloves. Spray them with 95% ethanol to wet the entire surface and allow them to dry within the laminar-flow hood before handling cultures. Repeat this sterilization step frequently, especially when performing worm filtration steps. Be sure to keep ethanol-soaked gloves away from a lit Bunsen burner!

2. Autoclave and dry all glassware. Seal growth flasks with a silicone sponge closure. Cover the entire neck and top of growth flasks with aluminum foil prior to autoclaving. Liquid cultures occasionally require checking during the growth phase. Always use a fresh, sterilized silicone sponge closure when resealing the flask; it is nearly impossible to put a used sponge back onto a flask without compromising sterility.

3. Manipulations involving worm cultures and their fractionation must be performed within a laminar-flow hood surface sterilized by wiping down with 70% ethanol prior to use.

4. Use either sterile, individually wrapped disposable pipets or reusable ones that have been cotton plugged prior to autoclaving.

5. Flame sterilize the neck of all open bottles and flasks before and after transfer of contents. One exception to this rule is made for the cholesterol stock solution (see Section III,C,1), which is made up in ethanol and, consequently, is not flamed because of fire/explosion hazard.

2. Equipment

Forced-air incubator set at the appropriate temperature (20°C is standard). The internal dimensions of the incubator must accommodate the orbital shaker.

Orbital shaker with speed control and clamps for flasks (7744 series, Bellco Glass, Vineland, NJ, or equivalent).

Vacuum line attached to a side-arm flask trap and suitable for solution aspiration (tubes should be held within the sterile laminar-flow hood during aspirations).

Adjustable-speed tabletop centrifuge with a swinging-bucket rotor capable of holding 50-ml conical tubes.

Pair of large forceps suitable for manipulating worm filters (described below). The tips of these forceps are dipped in ethanol and flame sterilized before each use; they are referred to as "sterile forceps" below.

a. Sterilized Glassware

1- and 2-liter baffled flasks (2542 series, Bellco)

250- and 50-ml screw-cap centrifuge bottles

Silicone sponge closures for plugging flasks (2004 series, Bellco)

5-, 10-, and 25-ml serological pipets

Pasteur pipets

b. Worm Filters

Stretch a square of Nitex nylon bolting cloth (TETKO, Elmsford, NY) over a 13-cm plastic embroidery hoop and tighten with a stainless-steel screw (usually, the screw sold with the hoop must be replaced). Carefully trim the Nitex cloth so that little protrudes from the embroidery hoop. At least one 20-μm- and one 35-μm-mesh-diameter filter are required for each 250-ml culture; two of each size for each culture are recommended. Label the hoops by engraving the mesh diameter into the frame with a hot needle. Each hoop filter is supported within a 15-cm glass petri dish by a triangle created from three equal lengths of 4-mm-diameter glass rod that have been fire polished on their ends (Fig. 2). Before use, sterilize the hoop/petri dish/glass rod assemblies, referred to below as "worm filters," by soaking for 5 minutes in 70% ethanol, shaking out the ethanol, and drying under an ultraviolet germicidal lamp in a hood. After the ethanol has evaporated, put on sterile gloves and place the petri dish lid on the bottom containing the hoop. Exposure to ultraviolet light will eventually cause the bolting cloth to become brittle and fall apart and, thus, should be minimized. After use, immerse the filters in Alconox detergent solution, scrub with a (all plastic) bottle brush, and rinse thoroughly in deionized water.

3. Solutions

WG medium: See Section IV,B,1. This is usually aliquoted into sterile 250-ml bottles.

M-9 salts (see Chapter 1)

Density gradient medium: Use either Renograffin-60 (Squibb Diagnostics; available from your local pharmacy) diluted 1 part to 1.5 part M-9 or 30% Ficoll in M-9. Renograffin is cheaper, and it is also easier to use because it has a lower viscosity than Ficoll.

Food bacteria: *Escherichia coli* strain NA22 or P90C in WG medium at 2–3 × 10^{11} cells/ml (A_{550} ~200). These bacteria can be prepared by any suitable means, including growth in a fermenter. The bacterial food must be free of contamination.

0.625 M NaOH

Bleach: Clorox is most consistent. Use plain laundry bleach, lacking scents, additional fabric brighteners, or other additives. Hypochlorite (the active ingredi-

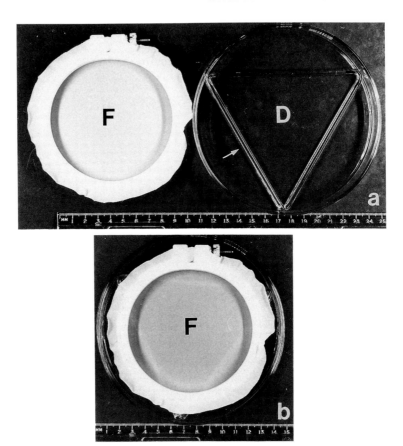

Fig. 2 Filter unit for purification of *C. elegans* males from hermaphrodite/male mixed cultures. (a) Nitex cloth is tightly stretched over a plastic embroidery hoop to form the filter unit (F). A triangle prepared from 4-mm glass rod (arrow) supports the filter unit within a 15-cm glass petri dish (D). (b) The filter unit is placed within the petri dish and buffer is added so that the Nitex cloth is wetted. The glass rod triangle forms a void between the bottom of the petri dish and the underside of the filter, and worms that can crawl through the mesh collect in this space. The ruler at the bottom of the figure shows the scale.

ent in bleach) is unstable, and old bleach will not dissolve worm carcasses as effectively as fresh bleach.

4. Detailed Protocol

In *C. elegans,* males arise occasionally by spontaneous nondisjunction of the X chromosome, and it is possible to create stocks that are ~50% males by setting up matings of males to hermaphrodites on growth plates. Mating efficiency, however, is very low in liquid medium, so that it is not practical to use wild-type worms for large-scale production of males. In liquid medium, males are most easily prepared from *him-5(e1490) V* cultures. This mutant produces ~45% males without a requirement for mating (Hodgkin *et al.,* 1979), and its sperm are cytologically indistinguishable from wild-type sperm (Ward *et al.,* 1981). Sperm from *spe* and *fer* mutants are usually obtained from *him-5* double-mutant strains.

1. Allow a clean 6-cm plate stock of worms to grow to saturation. Using a flame-sterilized spatula, transfer a 0.5-cm² chunk of this plate to ten to twelve 10-cm growth plates that have 12 spots (lawns) of P90C bacteria. Grow until the bacterial lawns have cleared and worms have begun to starve.

2. Examine the plates under a dissecting microscope for the presence of contamination and discard any contaminated plates. Working in a laminar-flow hood and wearing sterile gloves, carefully rinse the surfaces of the plates with WG using a Pasteur pipet. Pool the plate rinses in a 1-liter baffled flask and bring the total volume to 200 ml of WG. Add 50 ml of bacteria.

3. Place the flask on an orbital shaker in a 20°C incubator and grow for 2–3 days. Growth of this culture will not be synchronous, but this does not matter as long as many gravid hermaphrodites are obtained. (If too many worms were inoculated, many dauers and few gravid hermaphrodites will be present. Usually, such a culture can be salvaged by following steps 4–6 (below), resuspending ~20% of the packed worm volume in 200 ml of WG, adding 50 ml bacteria, and starting again at step 4).

4. Pellet the adults by settling at 1 g in 250-ml conical centrifuge bottles for 10 minutes. Alternatively, for small volumes, worms can be pelleted by centrifugation in a swinging-bucket rotor at 55*g* for 2 minutes.

5. Aspirate and discard the supernatant and transfer the worm-containing pellet to a 50-ml conical centrifuge tube. Resuspend the worms in M-9. Pellet by centrifugation at 55*g* for 2 minutes in a swinging-bucket rotor.

6. Aspirate and discard the supernatant. Adjust worm volume so that no more than 15 ml of packed worms is in each 50-ml centrifuge tube. Add M-9 to bring volume to 20 ml and add 13 ml Renograffin-60. Put a screw cap on the tube and mix well by gentle inversion.

7. Centrifuge at 475*g* for 10 minutes. Carefully remove tubes from the centrifuge. Under these conditions, worms will float at the top of the tube and bacteria and worm debris will pellet.

8. Recover the worms by careful aspiration with a Pasteur pipet and place in a 50-ml conical centrifuge tube. Fill the tube with M-9, invert to mix, and centrifuge at 55*g* for 2 minutes. (The worms should pellet, but if too much Renograffin-containing solution was carried over, the worms will not pellet well. If this happens, dilute further with M-9 and repeat the centrifugation step.) Aspirate and discard the supernatant.

9. Add 10 ml of bleach/NaOH mixture (make fresh by mixing 10 ml bleach with 35 ml 0.625 *M* NaOH; Emmons *et al.,* 1979) per milliliter of packed worms,

not to exceed a total of 35 ml per 50-ml conical tube. Vortex at top speed for 4 minutes. The solution will change color and become yellow/brown as the worms dissolve toward the end of this 4-minute vortex procedure, releasing the unaffected eggs. Pellet the eggs by centrifugation at 55g for 1 minute. Aspirate and discard the supernatant. The pellet should be white; if it is brown or has a brown layer at the top, resuspend in 10 ml of bleach/NaOH mixture, vortex at top speed for no more than 1 minute, and centrifuge (as above). Do not do more than two bleach/NaOH treatments as the eggs will be adversely affected. If two treatments do not work, it is likely that there are many dauers or bacterial spores in the culture. Dauers are killed by bleach/NaOH treatment but they are not easily dissolved. Bacterial spores, especially of certain wild *Bacillus* species, are not necessarily killed by this treatment. If you have *Bacillus* contamination, it is best to start again from plates (step 1).

10. Resuspend the eggs in M-9 and pellet for 1 minute at 55g. Aspirate and discard the supernatant. Repeat this step one time so the eggs have been rinsed a total of two times.

11. The yield from this procedure is usually around 1 ml of eggs per 5 ml of packed, gravid hermaphrodites. Each milliliter contains ~4 × 10^6 eggs, assuming no significant contamination. Resuspend each milliliter of eggs in a small volume of WG, place in a 1-liter baffled flask using a Pasteur pipet, bring the volume up to 80 ml WG/ml of eggs (do not exceed 1.5 ml of eggs per 1-liter flask), and place on an orbital shaker for 16 to 24 hours. All the stages of embryogenesis are present within an egg sample and they hatch at different times; however, because this step is performed without the addition of food, newly hatched larvae arrest at the L$_1$ stage and do not grow. This step is essential to synchronize the culture, and larvae can be held without food for several days. A small aliquot of eggs should be spotted onto sterile NGM worm growth plate to check for contamination. The following day, this plate should contain only larvae and no contamination.

12. Remove an aliquot from the baffled flask and check the hatch rate by visual inspection under a dissecting microscope. Pellet the larvae by centrifugation at 55g for 1 minute. Aspirate and discard the supernatant. Resuspend the larvae in M-9, pellet once more, and aspirate the supernatant. This rinse step reduces the level of dauer pheromone, which was secreted by starving larvae and can cause the culture to enter the dauer stage on feeding (Golden and Riddle, 1982).

13. A standard worm growth culture consists of 0.5 ml L$_1$ larvae (2 × 10^6 viable larvae), 200 ml WG, and 50 ml of food bacteria in a 2-liter baffled flask. Place this culture on an orbital shaker for 80 to 96 hours at 20°C.

14. Perform steps 4–8 to separate the worms from bacteria and debris.

15. Remove the cover from a 35-μm worm filter and fill the petri dish with M-9 buffer until it just wets the Nitex cloth. Remove worms from the centrifuge tube with a Pasteur pipet and drip them onto the 35-μm worm filter; do not exceed 10 ml of packed worms per filter. Put the petri dish lid on the worm filter

and allow it to sit undisturbed for 30 minutes. Adult hermaphrodites are wider than larvae or males and they are retained by the 35-μm worm filter.

16. Pick up the 35-μm worm filter with sterile forceps and place it on the inside of the sterile petri dish lid. Remove the filtrate and process as described in step 17. Place the 35-μm worm filter back in the petri dish and add M-9 until the Nitex cloth is just wet. Repeat step 16 to determine if any additional males are obtainable. If there are additional males, process them as described in step 17. Be careful because sometimes a few hermaphrodites will get through the 35μm filter if you give them enough time! Pick up the 35μm worm filter with sterile forceps and transfer to the inside of the sterile petri dish lid. Hold the filter at an angle, and squirt sterile M-9 with a Pasteur pipet to dislodge the hermaphrodites from the filter. These hermaphrodites can be used to prepare eggs according to step 9 and start a new liquid culture(s).

17. Using a dissecting microscope, check an aliquot of the 35-μm filtrate for larvae and, if present, transfer filtrate onto a dry 20-μm worm filter and adjust the volume with M-9 so that the bottom of the Nitex cloth is barely wetted. Put the petri dish lid on the worm filter and allow it to sit undisturbed for 30 minutes. Check the retained males for absence of larvae by examining an aliquot under a dissecting microscope. Pick up the 20-μm worm filter with sterile forceps and transfer to the inside of the sterile petri dish lid. Hold the filter at an angle, and squirt sterile M-9 with a Pasteur pipet to dislodge the worms from the filter. Pellet the males by centrifugation at 55g for 2 minutes. There are $\sim$3 $\times$ 10^5 males per packed milliliter.

18. Aspirate and discard the supernatant. Resuspend the male worms in WG and transfer to a 1-liter flask. Bring the total volume of WG to 100 ml and add 10 ml bacteria per milliliter of packed males. Shake culture for 24 hours.

19. Repeats steps 4 to 8 and, if hermaphrodites and/or larvae are present, steps 15 to 17. Typically, the worm population will be greater than 95% male at this point and is suitable for the preparation of sperm.

C. Sperm Isolation

1. General Comments

Greater than 50% of the cells in a mature *C. elegans* male are sperm. Most of its sperm are held as arrested spermatids, but spermatocytes of all stages are also present. The procedure described below relies on the fact that sperm are one of the few *C. elegans* cells that are not physically connected to adjacent cells to form a tissue (Wolfe *et al.*, 1978; Ward *et al.*, 1981). Consequently, when *C. elegans* males are squashed under hydraulic force, they burst open and release their sperm into the surrounding medium under conditions where other tissues remain relatively intact. This permits straightforward purification of near-homogeneous sperm, the vast majority of which are in the spermatid stage. The steps listed below are not performed as sterile techniques. It is, however, advisable to wear gloves because squash medium contains phenylmethylsulfonyl fluoride (PMSF), which is poisonous and should not be allowed to contact one's skin.

2. Equipment

Adjustable-speed tabletop centrifuge with a swinging-bucket rotor capable of holding 50-ml conical tubes.

Laboratory press (i.e., Model C, Fred S. Carver, Menomonee Falls, WI).

Two $\frac{1}{2}$-in. Plexiglas squash plates. The top plate is 6.5×8.5 in. and the bottom plate is 7.25×9.5 in. Around the three sides of the face of the bottom plate, a channel $\frac{3}{8}$ in. wide and $\frac{3}{8}$ in. deep is milled into the Plexiglas, $\frac{1}{8}$ in. from the edge. On the fourth side (which is 7.25 in. wide), a channel $\frac{1}{2}$ in. wide and $\frac{3}{8}$ in. deep is milled into the Plexiglas, $\frac{1}{4}$ in. from the edge. The top plate fits onto the bottom plate within the perimeter of the channels.

Three layers of 10-μm Nitex bolting cloth (TEKTO) stretched across one 11-cm embroidery hoop, referred to below as a sperm filter (see Fig. 2).

50-ml disposable conical centrifuge tubes with screw caps.

3. Solutions

See Section IV,B for formulas. Per milliliter of males to be squashed, the following volumes of solutions are required:

50 ml of squash medium (MSM containing 1 mg/ml bovine serum albumin and 1 mM PMSF)

35 ml of monovalent free sperm medium (MSM) MSM with polyvinylpyrrolidone (PVP)

5 ml of SM with PVP

10 ml of 10% Percoll density gradient medium (Pharmacia Biotech, Piscataway, NJ) in MSM with PVP

4. Detailed Protocol

1. Resuspend a 1-ml pellet of packed males in 10 ml of squash medium in a 50-ml conical glass centrifuge tube. Allow to settle at $1g$ for 10 minutes and remove supernatant down to 2-ml mark on the calibrated tube. Only 1 ml of males can be squashed at a time. Additional males can be maintained in M-9 in a glass centrifuge tube until they are squashed; the tube should be gently inverted every few minutes for aeration.

2. Place many small drops of worms on the bottom Plexiglas squash plate with a Pasteur pipet and allow to settle for 1 minute. Place the top Plexiglas squash plate onto the bottom plate and place the two-plate "sandwich" into the laboratory press.

3. Jack the press up rapidly until the gauge reads 13,000 psi and leave for 30 seconds. Slowly allow the pressure to drop by turning the release valve. It might be necessary to continue pumping the jack during pressure release for it to occur slowly, over the course of about 1 minute. Examine the squash plate "sandwich" under a dissecting microscope to ensure that nearly all males have been effectively squashed and released their sperm. If most males appear intact, repeat this step.

4. Remove the top plate and rinse surface with squash medium onto bottom plate. Thoroughly rinse bottom plate and pool into a petri dish. Pour the squashed worms through the 10-μm sperm filter and rinse with 25 ml squash medium.

5. Put 10 ml of 10% Percoll in a 50-ml conical centrifuge tube. Gently layer the filtrate containing sperm on top of the Percoll cushion. Mix the interface gently with a Pasteur pipet to remove the sharp boundary. Pellet the sperm by centrifugation at 475g for 10 minutes. The centrifuge should be slowly brought up to speed over 1 minute.

6. Aspirate and discard the supernatant. Resuspend the pelleted sperm in 25 ml MSM with PVP. Count the sperm in an aliquot with a hemocytometer. Note the percentage that have a pseudopod, indicating that they have activated.

7. Pellet the sperm by centrifugation at 475g for 10 minutes. Resuspend in SM with PVP at 1×10^8 sperm/ml.

8. Sperm that are to be used for biochemical experiments (i.e., samples for gel electrophoresis) should be stored as frozen pellets. This usually involves placing an aliquot containing 3×10^7 sperm in a 1.5-ml conical microcentrifuge tube and briefly subjecting it to centrifugation to pellet cells. Discard the supernatant and freeze the tube containing the pellet in either a dry ice/ethanol bath or liquid N_2. Resuspend this packed volume of cells (approximately 480 μg of protein) in 100 μl of Laemmli sample buffer. We run 3 μl (=15 μg) per gel lane on a Bio-Rad Protean II minigel (Bio-Rad Laboratories, Hercules, CA), and this works well either for an analytical gel or if the gel is to be Western blotted. For maximum resolution of all proteins, use a 10 to 20% gradient gel. A typical protein pattern (on a standard sized gel) can be seen in Fig. 5 of Ward *et al.* (1986).

9. Sperm that are to be used for electron microscopy should be resuspended in SM without PVP during step 7 because PVP interferes with cell fixation.

D. Alternative Method for Large-Scale Sperm Isolation

This method allows preparation of spermatids that can be stored as viable cells at −100°C and thawed when needed. Neither author has had experience with this method, and we are indebted to Dr. B. Phelps and Dr. S. Ward for providing this unpublished protocol.

1. Prepare males as described above in Section II,B,4.

2. Resuspend males in 5 ml of PSM with protease inhibitors. Pellet by centrifugation at 600g for 2 minutes. Aspirate and discard supernatant.

3. Transfer worms to a glass petri dish with a Pasteur pipet and chop for about 10 minutes with a clean, new razor blade (rinse in ethanol and wipe dry).

4. Pour 10 ml of PSM with protease inhibitors onto the worms and gently mix. Pour chopped worms over a 10-μm mesh Nitex sperm filter (see Fig. 2). Rinse the petri dish with a fresh 2-ml aliquot of modified SM with protease inhibitors, and pour over 10-μm mesh sperm filter.

5. Transfer filtrate to a 15-ml conical centrifuge tube. Rinse petri dish with 2 ml of PSM with protease inhibitors. Underlay with 1 ml of 50% Percoll (in PSM).

6. Pellet the cells by centrifugation at 600g for 1 minute. Aspirate and discard the supernatant. Resuspend the pelleted sperm in 1 ml of PSM for each aliquot that is to be frozen.

7. Vortex and transfer a 1-ml aliquot to each 1.5-ml conical microcentrifuge tube. Pellet the spermatids at 750g for 3 minutes in a microcentrifuge.

8. Aspirate and discard the supernatant. Add 1 ml of freezing medium (see Section IV,B,4) and place tubes at 4°C for 15 to 20 minutes.

9. Place in freezer at -100°C.

10. For use, the tube containing spermatids is quickly thawed in a 20°C water bath. Spermatids are pelleted by centrifugation at 750g for 3 minutes in a microcentrifuge. The cells are resuspended in nutrient PSM buffer, which is changed every 16 to 18 hours, if necessary.

E. Small–Scale Isolation of Sperm

1. General Comments

For many types of cell biological and electrophysiological experiments, it is not necessary to isolate large quantities of *C. elegans* sperm. Hand dissection of males is usually performed in these circumstances, and each male can release up to several thousand sperm (Fig. 3). It is also possible to obtain 200 to 300 sperm from a hermaphrodite.

2. Solution

Working SM solution containing either PVP or bovine serum albumin (BSA) is used.

3. Detailed Protocol

1. Pick L$_4$ male worms to a NGM growth plate (see Chapter 1 for preparation of NGM growth plates) that has been spotted with bacteria, and allow to grow 2 to 3 additional days at 20°C in the absence of hermaphrodites (adjust growth time depending on temperature). Under these conditions, large quantities of spermatids accumulate within the seminal vesicle.

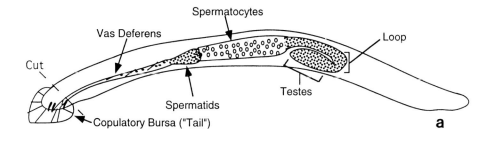

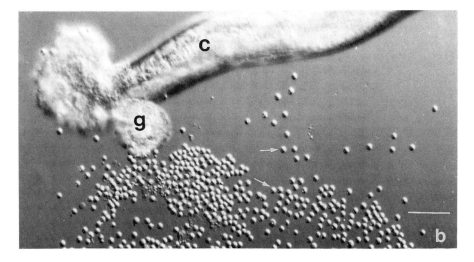

Fig. 3 *Caenorhabditis elegans* male and its dissection to obtain sperm. (a) Simplified diagram of a *C. elegans* male showing only reproductive organs; the male is approximately 1 mm in length and 50 μm in diameter (after Klass *et al.*, 1976). (b) Nomarski differential interference contrast photomicrograph of a portion of a dissected *C. elegans* male. The male tail was cut as shown in (a), and many spermatids (arrows point to two examples), as well as part of the gonad (g), have been extruded from the carcass (c). Bar = 50 μm.

2. Pick males (from step 1) or late L4–young stage adult hermaphrodites to a bacteria-free NGM growth plate and allow to crawl around for about 5 minutes so worms are freed of external bacteria.

3. Worm dissections are performed while viewing under a dissecting microscope (see Fig. 3). For cytological analyses of males, place one to three worms in a 7-μl drop of SM with PVP or BSA on a specially cleaned glass microscope slide (see Section V) containing SM (choice of BSA or PVP supplement in SM depends on subsequent steps, see below). Two narrow ~2.5-cm beads, applied from a 5-ml Vaseline-packed syringe through a 20-gauge hypodermic needle "grease gun" (*warning:* a metal file should be used to completely blunt the needle to avoid the possibility of accidental Vaseline injection into the investigator,

which can require surgery to correct!), are applied ~1.5 cm apart to the glass slide. Sperm can be released by cutting just in front of the tail, which will open up the seminal vesicle and release sperm (see Fig. 3). Alternatively, cutting just posterior to the pharynx will frequently release an intact seminal vesicle, which can then be cut open. For cytological analyses of hermaphrodites, dissect out the spermatheca and cut it open. Dissections of either males or hermaphrodites are performed with two 20-gauge hypodermic syringe needles. The needles can either be held directly or mounted on the ends of 1-ml syringes. It is not necessary to remove the carcass for most types of cytological analyses.

4. Spermatozoa are obtained from the spermatheca of a hermaphrodite because conversion from spermatids normally occurs during sexual maturation. Males, however, accumulate large quantities of spermatids within their seminal vesicle, and these must be activated to become spermatoza. This can be achieved naturally by permitting males to mate with hermaphrodites for a period (3–7 hours, for instance; Ward and Carrel, 1978), because during ejaculation, spermatids are activated to become spermatozoa and many are retained by the male. More commonly, one of several *in vitro* activators are employed. A number of compounds capable of activating spermatids have been described (Nelson and Ward, 1980; Ward *et al.,* 1983; Shakes and Ward, 1988, 1989b), but there are two that are more commonly employed: monensin and Pronase. Either of these activators can routinely cause 80 to 95% of spermatids to activate into spermatozoa (Ward *et al.,* 1983). Usually, the activator is placed in SM prior to performing the dissection in step 3. If Pronase is employed, SM should be supplemented with PVP, whereas either BSA or PVP can be used with monensin. Efficacy of monensin as a sperm activator is dependent on pH of the surrounding medium. At pH 7.8, 40 nM monensin will efficiently activate spermatids, whereas at pH 7.0, 200 nM monensin is required. Pronase activation does not show sensitivity to pH of the surrounding medium (Ward *et al.,* 1983).

5. A 22-mm^2 coverslip is gently lowered on the preparation after completion of the dissection. Viewing of live cells is best performed by Nomarski differential interference contrast. Although the cells can be seen by conventional phase contrast microscopy, very little detail is visible in these 6-μm cells. Activation (conversion of spermatids to spermatozoa) usually begins within 5 minutes of exposure of spermatids to inducing compound.

6. Sometimes, it is necessary to change the medium in which the sperm were released. This can be performed by placing a small drop of the desired solution at one open (i.e., not sealed with Vaseline) edge of the coverslip and touching a small square of filter paper to the opposite open edge to replace the solution bathing the sperm.

F. Preparation for Electron Microscopy

1. Solutions

1 ml primary fixative (see Section IV,B,5 for formula)
100 mM sodium cacodylate buffer, pH 7.3.

Several milliliters of 1% low-gelling-temperature agarose (FMC BioProducts, Rockland, ME) equilibrated to 37°C.

2. Detailed Protocol

1. Perform dissection as described above in Section II,E,3, except use a depression slide instead of a conventional microscope slide. The best dissections will result in a slight tear of the seminal vesicle, releasing the spermatids, which will form a "cloud" of spermatids in congealed seminal fluid that remains close to the carcass. You can make this tear with the needle, if necessary. This makes the subsequent finding of spermatids following embedding for electron microscopy much easier.

2. Add 100 μl primary fixative. Fix for 1 hour at room temperature in a moist chamber (sealed petri dish with damp paper towels inside). Transfer the moist chamber containing the carcasses to 4°C and fix overnight if this is convenient.

3. Using a drawn-out Pasteur pipet, remove as much of the fixative as possible and discard. Rinse the dissected worms in three changes of 100 mM cacodylate buffer, pH 7.3. Withdraw as much of the last buffer change as possible and enrobe the testes in 1% low-gelling-temperature agarose (in water, equilibrated in a water bath to 37°C prior to use). The agarose "noodle" makes subsequent handling much easier and it can be marked by injecting a small volume of India ink. Fixed sperm can be stored at 4°C at this stage for several days without adverse effects.

4. Any one of a number of standard electron microscopy protocols (e.g., Ward *et al.*, 1981) can be followed for subsequent osmication, dehydration, and embedding.

G. Future Directions

It is possible to apply patch-clamp technology to study *C. elegans* spermatogenesis. Electrophysiology is performed according to standard biophysical techniques (see Sherman-Gold, 1993), except that the patch pipet must have a very small internal diameter because these sperm are tiny. So far, these techniques have been used to study voltage-gated ion channel distribution and function during spermatogenesis.

1. Sperm are obtained by hand dissection (described above) in SM or any of a variety of modified SMs. The dissection is performed in a 30 × 10-mm petri dish containing 2 ml of buffer. The cells are viewed either by phase contrast or bright field, because Newton interference colors caused by strain birefringence in the plastic dish make Nomarski differential interference contrast annoying to use.

2. Electrodes are pulled from borosilicate glass (Corning 7052) using a programmable puller (Sacha-Flaming, P-87, Sutter Instruments, San Rafael, CA).

The pipets are fire polished and have a resistance in the range 20 to 40 MΩ. Standard techniques are employed, and the patch-clamp is established with gentle suction from a hand-operated syringe. It is possible to successfully record from spermatocytes, residual bodies, spermatids, and spermatozoa.

3. Data are collected with a patch-clamp amplifier (Model EPC-7, List Instruments, Darmstadt-13, Germany), bandlimited at 0 to 1000 Hz, and stored on a consumer-grade VHS videocassette recorder. Data are analyzed using an oscilloscope (Model 430, Nicolet Instruments, Madison, WI) and an IBM-AT-grade (or higher) computer.

III. *Ascaris suum*

A. Introduction to Sperm

Ascaris offers three principal advantages over *C. elegans* for the study of sperm cell biology. A robust *Ascaris* male contains ~5×10^7 spermatids in its seminal vesicle, compared with 3×10^3 in a virgin *C. elegans* male. The volume of each spermatid from *Ascaris* is about 10-fold greater than its counterpart from *C. elegans* (see Fig. 1). Activation in *Ascaris* produces motile spermatozoa with a highly ordered cytoskeleton composed of MSP filaments grouped into long, branched fiber complexes that can be viewed in real time in live cells by light microscopy. The interested reader should consult Roberts *et al.* (1989) for more details on the motility of this cell. The ease of obtaining large volumes of cells and the organization of the MSP-based motile apparatus have allowed the biochemical properties of MSP and its role in motility to be studied in ways that would be very difficult with *C. elegans.* The features that distinguish these two species, however, also necessitate different techniques for isolating and handling their sperm.

B. Collection and Handling of Males

1. Procedures

Ascaris suum is a parasite of the small intestine of hogs and, thus, must be collected at a pork slaughterhouse. Infection rates are usually low (e.g., 3–5% of the hogs at a slaughterhouse in Moultrie, GA, are infected) so large commercial operations that process several hundred hogs per day are more reliable sources of material, but often less convenient, than smaller facilities.

Most commercial slaughterhouses allow investigators to search for nematodes before discarding the small intestine. Because *Ascaris* adults are large (10–20 cm long) their presence can usually be detected by inspection of the intact intestine. Worms are removed by cutting open the gut and squeezing out its contents. The size ranges of adult male and female worms overlap, but the sexes can be distinguished by stroking the animal's cuticle. Males respond by curling their tail, a behavior normally used to clasp the female during copulation. *Ascaris* eggs are infective to humans, so females should be discarded at the slaughterhouse.

Transport males to the laboratory in warm (39°C) phosphate-buffered saline supplemented with 10 mM NaHCO$_3$. Maintenance of temperature and bicarbonate concentration during transport is critical to sperm viability; thus, we recommend an insulated, 3- to 4-liter container for transport. Maintain males in the laboratory in an incubator at 39°C in transport buffer supplemented with 1% glucose and 1% yeast extract. Change the buffer twice daily to minimize bacterial growth.

2. Precautions

a. Infection

Even with conscientious attempts to sex worms at the slaughterhouse an occasional female will return to the laboratory and stray eggs will make their way onto collection gear (and personnel). Eggs require a 14-day embryonation period before they are infective. To avoid infection clean all vessels, glassware, dissecting tools, and work areas with acetone. This dissolves the lipid coat on the egg surface that protects the egg from desiccation and, thus, destroys the embryo.

b. Allergic Reaction

Ascaris contains a potent allergen that elicits an immediate hypersensitivity reaction in some investigators. Workers prone to severe allergies should avoid handling worms and depart rooms where dissections are being conducted. Otherwise, wear latex gloves and perhaps also a surgical mask when working with live worms

C. Isolation and Handling of Sperm

1. General Comments

The large size of *Ascaris* males allows sperm to be isolated by dissection of individual animals. The meter-long testis resides in the posterior half of the animal. Most of the gonad consists of threadlike tissue packed into the pseudocoelomic cavity. Spermatids are stored in the prominent seminal vesicle (2–3 mm in diameter × 2–4 cm in length) at the proximal end of the gonad near the tail of the male. The procedure outlined here is designed for isolation of spermatids, although earlier stages of spermatogenesis can also be obtained from more distal regions of the testis.

2. Detailed Protocols

Note that temperature maintenance is critical to sperm viability. Warm all buffers and labware to 39°C before starting dissection. Work quickly and keep isolated cells in an incubator or water bath as much as possible.

1. Use dissecting scissors to make a cross-sectional cut in the anterior half of a male, then slit open the body wall longitundinally. Practice is often necessary to avoid puncturing the seminal vesicle when making the longitudinal incision. For the novice, it is best to consult any number of parasitology dissection manuals, such as Cable (1958), or medical parasitology texts, such as Neva and Brown (1994), for *Ascaris* anatomy. Further details on the anatomy of *Ascaris* testes can be found in Nelson and Ward (1981).

2. Use forceps to pull out the proximal portion of the testis (the entire organ need not be removed from the worm). A gentle tug will separate the vas deferens (the narrow region proximal to the seminal vesicle) from the cloaca. Free the seminal vesicle by cutting the gonad about 1 cm distal to the point where the narrow testis joins the seminal vesicle.

3. Hold the seminal vesicle over a collection tube (e.g., a 1.5-ml microcentifuge tube) containing HKB buffer (see Section IV,C,1) at 39°C, snip open the opposite end of the tissue, and allow the contents to drip into the tube. The sperm from 1 to 10 males, depending on intended use (see below), can be collected in one 1.5-ml tube.

4. Wash the cells two times by centrifugation for 2 to 3 seconds at 10,000g and resuspension in warm HKB. The cells can be used immediately or frozen in liquid nitrogen and stored at −70°C.

D. Sperm Activation

1. General Comments

Ascaris spermatids undergo activation *in vitro* when treated with an extract of the vas deferens. The pattern and timing of activation of spermatids from *Ascaris* and *C. elegans* are very similar; however, monensin, a potent activator of *C. elegans* spermatids, has no effect on *Ascaris,* and vas deferens activator from *Ascaris* does not affect cells from *C. elegans*. Only Pronase (see above) activates spermatids from both species.

2. Detailed Protocol

1. Dissect the vas deferens from several males. This glandular tissue, about 5 to 7 mm long, can usually be saved from gonads used for sperm isolation. After removing the spermatids from the seminal vesicle, snip off the vas deferens and place it in a small tube on ice. The tissue can be used immediately or stored at −70°C.

2. Prepare an extract by homogenizing five vas deferens per milliliter of HKB buffer in a tight-fitting tissue grinder. Centrifuge the extract for 3 minutes in a microcentrifuge. Store aliquots (50–100 μl) of the supernatant at −70°C. This material will remain active for at least 6 months.

3. Isolate sperm from the desired number of males as described above. For most cytological experiments one male provides sufficient material and washing can be omitted. Add 10 to 20 μl of vas deferens extract, mix the contents of the tube thoroughly by inversion, and incubate at 39°C for 5 to 10 minutes.

4. Check a sample of cells by light microscopy. Proper activation results in extension of actively ruffling pseudopods by more than 90% of the cells. *Ascaris* sperm crawl efficiently on a variety of substrates including glass microscope slides cleaned by soaking in 95% ethanol and dried just before use, coverslips used without cleaning, and recently glow-discharged, carbon-coated electron microscopy grids. Cells remain motile for at least 1 hour on these substrates provided that fresh HKB buffer is added at 15- to 20-minute intervals.

3. Troubleshooting

There are four principal causes of poor sperm activation:

1. Improper temperature maintenance: As emphasized above, spermatids from worms not maintained at ~39°C after collection fail to activate.

2. Worm age: Activation of cells from males kept more than 24 hours after collection is inconsistent.

3. Lability of activator: Aliquots of vas deferens extract should be thawed and kept on ice before use and discarded within 3 hours of thawing.

4. Bicarbonate concentration of buffer: *Ascaris* sperm are bicarbonate dependent. The pH of the HKB buffer used for sperm isolation and activation should be checked periodically. Best results are obtained with buffer adjusted to pH 7.1 by bubbling with gaseous CO_2. Cylinders that contain 80% N_2/balance CO_2 from commercial suppliers are suitable.

E. Fixation for Electron Microscopy and Immunolabeling

1. General Fixation for Electron Microscopy

The MSP cytoskeleton in *Ascaris* sperm is extraordinarily labile so special care must be taken when preparing cells for electron microscopy (EM) or for various labeling procedures. The following technique provides excellent morphological preservation and provides sperm that can be sectioned in known orientation (parallel to the plane of the substrate). The fixed cells are also suitable for immunogold tagging, immunofluoresence, or other labeling procedures.

1. Use a "grease gun" (see Section II,E,3) to apply two parallel strips of Vaseline or silicon grease to a microscope slide. Place 4×4-mm pieces of coverslips between the two strips and warm the slide to 39°C.

2. Pipet activated cells onto the coverslips. Allow 2 minutes for the cells to settle and attach to the substrate, then cover with an 18×18-mm coverslip.

3. Fix cells by perfusion of 2.5% glutaraldehyde, 0.2% tannic acid, 0.05% saponin (Maupin and Pollard, 1983) in HKB buffer through the chamber. Omit tannic acid if the cells are to be used for immunolabeling experiments. Cytological preservation is best with glutaraldehyde fixation, but occasionally an antibody will not label aldehyde-fixed tissue, so it is less useful for immunofluorescence.

4. After fixation for 30 minutes, wash by perfusion with several drops of HKB. For labeling experiments, cells should be treated with 0.5% Triton X-100 for 15 minutes, washed, and incubated in a solution to block unreacted aldehyde groups (e.g., 5 mM glycine or lysine; three treatments with freshly prepared 10 mM sodium borohydride). Proceed with appropriate labeling protocol.

5. For EM, transfer coverslips containing fixed sperm to aluminum weighing dishes, cell side up. Tack down coverslips by pressing down on a dab of silicon grease. Osmication, en bloc staining with uranyl acetate, dehydration, and embedding in resin of choice can be carried out in the weighing dish.

6. After polymerization of the resin, peel away the weighing dish and cut out blocks of resin with the coverslip on one face with a jeweler's saw. Remove the coverslip by immersing the block in liquid nitrogen. Use forceps to remove the fragments of broken glass. The cells are embedded at the exposed surface of the resin.

7. Examine the surface of the block under a dissecting microscope. Mark a region of suitable cell density by etching a small square in the block surface with a needle.

8. Use Superglue to mount the block on an aluminum stub (diameter suited to fit into microtome chuck); trim away excess resin with a jeweler's saw using the etch marks as guides. Final trim for sectioning with a razor blade.

2. Simultaneous Demembranation/Fixation

Preparations particularly well suited for examination and labeling of the sperm cytoskeleton can be obtained by substitution of HKB buffer containing 1% glutaraldehyde plus 0.5% Triton X-100 as the fixative in the protocol above. Such treatment lyses the pseudopodial plasma membrane, extracts soluble proteins from the pseudopod, and fixes the MSP filaments. Thus, the cytoskeleton can be examined by EM to analyze the organization of its constituent filaments and is exposed for labeling with antibodies or other reagents (for example, see Roberts and King, 1991).

F. Cellular Fractionation and MSP Isolation

1. General Comments

Dissection of 200 *Ascaris* males yields 5 to 10 ml packed volume of sperm, which is a sufficient amount of material for cellular fractionation. The procedure outlined below is designed for isolation of MSP, but can also be used as a starting point for isolation of other cellular components and scaled up or down as needed.

Ascaris sperm contain two isoforms of MSP, designated α and β, that contain 126 amino acids and differ at only four residues. β-MSP is fivefold more abundant than α-MSP, slightly smaller (14,160 Da vs 14,302 Da), and less basic (pI 8.3 vs pI 8.9) (King *et al.*, 1992). The charge difference is sufficient to separate the two isoforms by cation-exchange chromatography.

2. Detailed Protocol

1. Resuspend cells pelleted in 1.5-ml microcentrifuge tubes in 0.5 ml HKN buffer (see Section IV,C,2) containing 0.1 mM PMSF.

2. Lyse cells by five freeze–thaw cycles, pool lysate, and homogenize by 10 strokes in a tight-fitting tissue grinder.

3. Centrifuge at 10,000g for 5 minutes at 4°C. The particulate material pellets in two distant layers. The whiter bottom layer contains refringent granules (an organelle of unknown function found in the cell body of *Ascaris* sperm) and nuclei. The fluocculent upper layer of the pellet is enriched in membrane-bound organelles (mitochondria, membranous organelles, and vesicles of plasma membrane).

4. Save the supernatant. Add 0.5 ml of HKN buffer and resuspend the upper layer of the pellet using gentle suction from a Pasteur pipet.

5. Transfer the resuspended membrane-enriched fraction to a fresh tube and repeat steps 3 and 4 twice. If desired, store the membrane-enriched pellet at −70°C for later use.

6. Centrifuge the pooled supernatant at 100,000g. This yields a small amber pellet that contains membrane-bound vesicles and small protein particles of unknown function. MSP constitutes about 40% of the protein in the supernatant (S100).

7. Load S100 onto a Sephadex G-75 superfine column (2.5 × 200 cm) equilibrated with HKN buffer and run at a flow rate of ~0.25 ml/min. Collect 5-ml fractions and monitor A_{280}. Elution of MSP-enriched fractions can be detected as an abrupt rise in A_{280} at about 17 hours. MSP yield is ~85% with ~90% purity under these conditions. The column should be cleaned and repacked after five or six runs.

8. Pool the MSP-enriched fractions and concentrate to 25 to 30 mg/ml total protein. Prodimem membranes (10,000 molecular weight cutoff) and Amicon pressure dialysis cells work equally well.

9. Purify and separate α- and β-MSP by cation-exchange chromatography. The following are two suitable methods:

   a. Sepharose S fast-flow cation-exchange column equilibrated with 10 mM Na_2HPO_4/NaH_2PO_4, pH 6: Load 30 to 40 mg total protein and wash with equilibration buffer. Elute with a pH and salt step gradient increasing NaCl from 0 to 25 mM in 5 mM increments and then increasing pH from 6 to 6.5. β-MSP elutes in 15 mM NaCl, pH 6; α-MSP at 25 mM NaCl, pH 6.5

b. High-performance cation-exchange liquid chromatography on a Waters 1×7.5-cm SP-5PW column equilibrated with 5 mM NaH_2PO_4, pH 6. Load 5 to 6 mg total protein. Wash with equilibration buffer for 5 minutes at a flow rate of 1 ml/min. Elute in a 1%/min linear gradient of 0 to 100 mM Na_2HPO_4/NaH_2PO_4, pH 7. β-MSP elutes at ~18 minutes followed by α-MSP at ~25 minutes.

10. Concentrate purified proteins by vacuum dialysis against 10 mM Na_2HPO_4/NaH_2PO_4, pH 6.7, aliquot as desired, and store at $-70°C$. The extinction coefficient (0.1%, 280 nm, 1 cm) for MSP is 0.9 (King et al., 1992). We have found that the protein can be concentrated to 100 mg/ml (~7 mM) without loss of solubility and stored for at least 1 year without significant loss of in vitro polymerization activity.

G. Assembly of MSP Filaments in Vitro

1. General Comments

Until recently, investigation of the structure and assembly properties of MSP filaments was hampered by inefficient in vitro polymerization techniques. For example, in 10 mM phosphate buffer pH 6.7, MSP at 3 mM (42 mg/ml) is required to obtain filament formation detectable by EM. A serendipitous discovery, however, revealed that water miscible alcohols such as ethanol, methanol, n-propanol, isopropanol, and 2-methyl-2,4-pentanediol at 20 to 40% induce assembly in vitro of purified MSP monomer into filaments that are indistinguishable from native filaments observed in lysed and stabilized sperm (King et al., 1992). α- and β-MSP form filaments independently. Neither nucleoside triphosphates nor specific inorganic ions are required for assembly, and the process occurs over a broad range of pH (5.7–9.5) and temperature (2–39°C). The critical concentration for assembly in 10 mM KH_2PO_4, pH 6.7, is 0.1 mM MSP. Alcohol-induced polymerization is fully reversible; filaments disasseable when alcohol is removed and reassemble when alcohol is added back.

2. Reagents and Solutions

Stock MSP at 5 to 20 mg/ml in 10 mM KH_2PO_4, pH 6.7

Reagent-grade absolute ethanol

Glutaraldehyde diluted from stock solution obtained in sealed glass ampoules from commercial sources (e.g., Electron Microscopy Sciences, Ft. Washington, PA) to 2% in 25% cthanol

3.7% uranyl acetate in 27% ethanol (store protected from light and prepare fresh every 30 days)

3. Detailed Protocol

1. Prepare a stock solution of MSP at 5 to 20 mg/ml in 10 mM KH$_2$PO$_4$, pH 6.7; purified protein works best but MSP obtained by Sephadex G-75 chromatography is also suitable. Subsequent steps should be carried out at 22 to 24°C.

2. Add 1 vol of reagent-grade absolute ethanol to 3 vol of the MSP stock. A total volume of 50 to 100 μl is suitable for most applications.

3. Mix rapidly by drawing up and expelling the MSP–ethanol solution with a wide-bore tip affixed to a Pipetman or equivalent. Filament assembly is indicated by a rapid (within 2–3 seconds) increase in viscosity of the solution. Subsequent procedures depend on the desired application. For example, fixed filaments can be obtained by centrifugation of the assembly cocktail at 10,000g for 2 minutes. Resuspend the pellet by quick addition of 25% ethanol containing 2% glutaraldehyde. The following steps, modified from the procedures of Valentine *et al.* (1968), should be used for preparation of negatively stained filaments by EM.

4. Transfer the assembly cocktail to a small vessel such as the cap of a microcentrifuge tube. Hold a piece of carbon-coated, freshly cleaved mica at one end with forceps and float the carbon film at the opposite end onto the surface of the filament solution.

5. Withdraw the mica and wash the filaments adhering to the carbon film by floating for 2 to 3 seconds on a drop of 27% ethanol in 10 mM KH$_2$PO$_4$.

6. Withdraw the mica and, working quickly, float the carbon onto a solution of 3.7% uranyl acetate in 27% ethanol.

7. Gently free the carbon film, leaving it floating on the surface of the staining solution. Discard the mica.

8. Pick up the carbon film from underneath on a rhodium-coated, 400-mesh copper EM grid. Wick off excess stain with the torn edge of a piece of filter paper, air-dry, and examine by EM. Specimens prepared in this way are also suitable for shadowing by conventional methods.

MSP filaments are 10-nm in diameter and composed of two subfilaments wrapped around each other in a right-handed helical sense. Negatively stained filaments can be recognized by their characteristic diameter and by the appearance of a series of dots (stain-filled cavities in the filament lattice) spaced at 9-nm intervals along the long axis of the filament. Most preparations also contain macrofibers, groups of three or more complete filaments wound around one another in a left-handed helical fashion. See King *et al.* (1992, 1994) for a complete description of filament structure.

IV. Solutions

A. Stock Solutions

1. Primary Stock Solutions

The following stock solutions can be used to prepare many of the *C. elegans* and *Ascaris* working solutions discussed in this chapter:

1 M 4-(2-hydroxyethyl)-1-piperazineethanesulfonic acid) (Hepes), do not adjust pH

1 M MgSO$_4$

2.5 M KCl

5 M NaCl

1 M CaCl$_2$

1 M choline chloride

0.5 M glucose

1 M KH$_2$PO$_4$, pH 6.0

1 M K citrate, which is 95 mM Citric acid and 0.9 M K$_3$ citrate, pH ~6.1

1 M NaHCO$_3$

13 mM cholesterol in ethanol

100 mM PMSF in ethanol, store at $-20°C$.

All stock solutions except PMSF and cholesterol should be sterilized by autoclaving.

2. 100× Trace Metal Stock Solution

2.5 mM FeSO$_4$

2.5 m M ethylenediaminetetraacetate, disodium salt

1 mM MnCl$_2$

1 mM ZnSO$_4$

1 mM CuSO$_4$

Aliquot and autoclave this stock solution. Wrap bottles of stock solution with aluminum foil to protect from light.

3. Sperm Activators

a. Monensin

Monensin is made up at 1 mM stock in dimethyl sulfoxide and stored as small aliquots at $-20°C$. The working concentration depends on the pH of the surrounding medium, but is in the range 40 to 1000 nM.

b. Pronase

A 10× Pronase stock solution is made up at 20 mg/ml in 1 mM HCl and stored at $-80°C$. The working concentration is 200 μg/ml.

B. *Caenorhabditis elegans* Working Solutions

1. Worm Growth (WG) Medium

Start with a flask containing ~900 ml of sterile, distilled water. Add each sterile stock solution in the order shown below, swirling between additions. The cholesterol does not dissolve properly so the solution should be swirled again before final aliquoting into 250-ml sterile bottles.

Final concentration	Amount of stock solution
10 mM NaCl	2 ml
10 mM KH$_2$PO$_4$	10 ml
10 mM K Citrate	10 ml
1X trace metals	10 ml
3 mM CaCl$_2$	3 ml
3 mM MgSO$_4$	3 ml
13 μM cholesterol	1 ml
Distilled water	961 ml

2. Sperm Medium (SM) Salts

Final concentration	Amount of stock solution
50 mM Hepes	50 ml
1 mM MgSO$_4$	1 ml
25 mM KCl	25 ml
45 mM NaCl	45 ml
5 mM CaCl$_2$	5 ml
Distilled water	849 ml

Adjust the pH to either 7.0 or 7.8, depending on the experiment, prior to bringing volume up to 1 liter. To prepare complete medium, supplement with either 10 mg/ml PVP (average molecular weight, 40,000) or 1 mg/ml BSA (Fraction V). The solution osmolarity should be about 220 to 230 mOsm.

3. Monovalent Free Sperm Medium (MSM)

Final concentration	Amount of stock solution
50 mM Hepes	50 ml
1 mM MgSO$_4$	1 ml
70 mM choline chloride	70 ml
5 mM CaCl$_2$	5 ml
Distilled water	874 ml

This solution is adjusted to pH 6.5 prior to bringing volume up to 1 liter, and 10 mg/ml PVP (average molecular weight, 40,000) is added for some applications.

4. Phelp's Sperm Medium (PSM)

Final concentration	Amount of stock solution
45 mM choline chloride	45 ml
25 mM KCl	25 ml
1 mM MgSO$_4$	1 ml
5 mM glucose	10 ml
Distilled water	919 ml

Adjust the pH to 7.0 prior to bringing volume up to 1 liter, and add 10 mg/ml BSA for most applications. Nutrient PSM contains 1 mg/ml yeast extract, and it is filter sterilized before use. PSM with inhibitors contains 1 mM PMSF, 2 μg/ml antipain, and 1 μg each of leupeptin, chymostatin, and pepstatin A (all available from Calbiochem–Novabiochem, San Diego, CA). Unlike the other solutions, freezing medium is PSM that lacks BSA and contains 5% glycerol and 1% dimethyl sulfoxide (both should be tissue culture-grade reagents). (B. Phelps and S. Ward, pers. comm.).

5. Primary Fixative for Electron Microscopy

Prepare a 10× SM stock and adjust pH to 7.0 (sometimes pH 7.8 is used for sperm activation studies) with NaOH. Aldehydes are purchased in sealed glass ampoules that should only be used for preparing stock solutions for 1 day after they have been opened). For 5 ml of primary fixative for electron microscopy:

100 μl 10× SM, pH 7.0 (without either PVP or BSA)
312 μl 16% paraformaldehyde (Electron Microscopy Sciences, or equivalent)
625 μl 8% glutaraldehyde (Polysciences, Warrington, PA, or equivalent)
3.963 ml deionized water

C. *Ascaris suum* Working Solutions

1. HKB Buffer

Final concentration	Amount of stock solution
50 mM Hepes	50 ml
65 mM KCl	38.5 ml
10 mM NaHCO$_3$	10 ml
Distilled water	901.5 ml

Adjust the pH to 7.6 prior to bringing volume up to 1 liter. This buffer is required for use with live sperm because of the cell's bicarbonate dependence. Before, use, adjust pH to 7.1 by bubbling gaseous CO$_2$ into the solution.

2. HKN Buffer

Final concentration	Amount of stock solution
50 mM Hepes	50 ml
65 mM KCl	38.5 ml
10 mM NaCl	2 ml

Adjust the pH to 6.7 prior to bringing volume up to 1 liter. This buffer is used for cellular fractionation and protein purification. Replacement of the bicarbonate in HKB makes the solution less pH-labile.

V. Materials

Glass slides are prepared for cytology by the following procedure:

1. Place slides in a Copeland jar containing Alconox laboratory detergent that is dissolved in hot water. Place in a bath ultrasonicator and clean for at least 10 minutes.
2. Rinse thoroughly and soak in 1 N HCl for 1 hour.
3. Rinse in deionized water and air-dry.

Slides prepared in this manner will frequently, but not always, allow analysis of crawling *C. elegans* spermatozoa. Recently, it was discovered that if slides are soaked in 10 N NaOH overnight at room temperature prior to step 1, crawling of spermatozoa is more reliably obtained (D. Royal and D. Soll, pers. comm.).

Acknowledgments

Research was supported by National Institutes of Health Grant GM-40697 and National Science Foundation Grant IBN-9305058 to S.W.L. and National Institutes of Health Grant GM-29994 to T.M.R. The authors thank S. Ward, B. Phelps, D. Royal, and D. Soll for communicating unpublished data.

References

Argon, Y., and Ward, S. (1980). *Caenorhabditis elegans* fertilization-defective mutants with abnormal sperm. *Genetics* **96,** 413–433.

Cable, R. M. (1958). "An Illustrated Laboratory Manual of Parasitology" 4th ed. Burgess Publishing, Minneapolis.

Emmons, S. W., Klass, M. R., and Hirsh, D. (1979). Analysis of the constancy of DNA sequences during development and evolution of the nematode *Caenorhabditis elegans*. *Proc. Natl. Acad. Sci. U.S.A.* **76,** 1333–1337.

Golden, J. W., and Riddle, D. L. (1982). A pheromone influences larval development in the nematode *Caenorhabditis elegans*. *Science* **218,** 578–580.

Heath, J. P. (1992). A worm's eye view of motility. *Curr. Biol.* **2,** 301–303.

Hirsh, D., and Vanderslice, R. (1976). Temperature-sensitive developmental mutants of *Caenorhabditis elegans*. *Dev. Biol.* **49,** 220–235.

Hirsh, D., Oppenheim, D., and Klass, M. (1976). Development of the reproductive system of *Caenorhabditis elegans*. *Dev. Biol.* **49,** 200–219.

Hodgkin, J., Horvitz, H. R., and Brenner, S. (1979). Nondisjunction mutants of the nematode *Caenorhabditis elegans*. *Genetics* **91,** 67–94.

King, K. L., Stewart, M., Roberts, T. M., and Seavy, M. (1992). Structure and macromolecular assembly of two isoforms of the major sperm protein (MSP) from the amoeboid sperm of the nematode, *Ascaris suum. J. Cell Sci.* **101,** 847–857.

King, K. L., Steward, M., and Roberts, T. M. (1994). Supramolecular assemblies of *Ascaris suum* major sperm protein (MSP) associated with amoeboid cell motility. *J. Cell Sci.* **107,** 2941–2949.

Klass, M. R., Wolf, N., and Hirsh, D. (1976). Development of the male reproductive system and sexual transformation in the nematode *Caenorhabditis elegans*. *Dev. Biol.* **52,** 1–18.

Klass, M. R., and Hirsh, D. (1981). Sperm isolation and biochemical analysis of the major sperm protein from *Caenorhabditis elegans*. *Dev. Biol.* **84,** 299–312.

L'Hernault, S. W., Shakes, D., Hogan, E., and Ward, S. (1987). Genetic analysis of spermatogenesis in the nematode *Caenorhabditis elegans. Genetics* **116**, s32. [Abstract]

L'Hernault, S. W., Shakes, D. C., and Ward, S. (1988). Developmental genetics of chromosome I spermatogenesis-defective mutants in the nematode *Caenorhabditis elegans. Genetics* **120**, 435–452.

L'Hernault, S. W., and Arduengo, P. M. (1992). Mutation of a putative sperm membrane protein in *Caenorhabditis elegans* prevents sperm differentiation but not its associated meiotic divisions. *J. Cell Biol.* **119**, 55–68.

L'Hernault, S. W., Benian, G. M., and Emmons, R. B. (1993). Genetic and molecular characterization of the *Caenorhabditis elegans* spermatogenesis defective gene *spe-17. Genetics* **134**, 769–780.

Machaca, K., DeFelice, A. L., and L'Hernault, S. W. (1993). Segregation of ion channels during *C. elegans* sperm differentiation. *Mol. Biol. Cell* **4**, 29a (abstract).

Maupin, P., and Pollard, T. D. (1983). Improved preservation and staining of HeLa cell actin filaments, clathrin-coated membranes and other cytoplasmic structures by tannic acid-glutaraldehyde-saponin fixation. *J. Cell Biol.* **96**, 51–62.

Nelson, G. A., and Ward, S. (1980). Vesicle fusion, pseudopod extension and amoeboid motility are induced in nematode spermatids by the ionophore monensin. *Cell* **19**, 457–464.

Nelson, G. A., and Ward, S. (1981). Amoeboid motility and actin in *Ascaris lumbricoides* sperm. *Exp. Cell Res.* **131**, 149–160.

Nelson, G. A., Roberts, T., and Ward, S. (1982). *Caenorhabditis elegans* spermatozoan locomotion: Amoeboid movement with almost no actin. *J. Cell Biol.* **92**, 121–131.

Neva, F. A., and Brown, H. W. (1994). "Basic Clinical Parasitology" 6th ed. Appleton and Lange, Norwalk, Connecticut.

Roberts, T. M., Sepsenwol, S., and Ris, H. (1989). Sperm motility in nematodes: Crawling movement without actin. *In* "The Cell Biology of Fertilization" (H. Schatten and G. Schatten, eds.), pp. 41–60. Academic Press, San Diego.

Roberts, T. M., and King, K. L. (1991). Centripetal flow and directed reassembly of the major sperm protein (MSP) cytoskeleton in the amoeboid sperm of the nematode, *Ascaris suum. Cell Motil. Cytoskel.* **20**, 228–241.

Shakes, D. C. (1988). A genetic and pharmacological analysis of spermatogenesis in the nematode *Caenorhabditis elegans.* Ph.D. Thesis. Johns Hopkins University.

Shakes, D. C., and Ward, S. (1989a). Mutations that disrupt the morphogenesis and localization of a sperm-specific organelle in *Caenorhabditis elegans. Dev. Biol.* **134**, 307–316.

Shakes, D. C., and Ward, S. (1989b). Initiation of spermiogenesis in *C. elegans. Dev. Biol.* **134**, 189–200.

Sherman-Gold, R. (ed.) (1993). "The Axon Guide for Electrophysiology & Biophysics Laboratory Techniques" Axon Instruments, Foster City, California.

Skinner, M. K., Norton, J. N., Mullaney, B. P., Rosselli, M., Whaley, P. D., and Anthony, C. T. (1991). Cell-cell interactions and the regulation of testis function. *Ann. N. Y. Acad. Sci.* **637**, 354–363.

Valentine, R. C., Shapiro, B. M., and Stadtman, E. R. (1968). Regulation of glutamine synthetase XII. Electron microscopy of the enzyme from *E. coli. Biochemistry* **7**, 2143–2152.

Varkey, J. P., Jansma, P. L., Minniti, A. N., and Ward, S. (1993). The *Caenorhabditis elegans spe-6* gene is required for major sperm protein assembly and shows second site non-complementation with an unlinked deficiency. *Genetics* **133**, 79–86.

Ward, S., and Miwa, J. (1978). Characterization of a temperature sensitive fertilization-defective mutant of the nematode *Caenorhabditis elegans. Genetics* **88**, 235–303.

Ward, S., and Carrel, J. S. (1979). Fertilization and sperm competition in the nematode *Caenorhabditis elegans. Dev. Biol.* **73**, 304–321.

Ward, S., Argon, Y., and Nelson, G. A. (1981). Sperm morphogenesis in wild-type and fertilization-defective mutants of *Caenorhabditis elegans. J. Cell Biol.* **91**, 26–44.

Ward, S., Roberts, T. M., Nelson, G. A., and Argon, Y. (1982). The development of motility of *Caenorhabditis elegans* spermatozoa. *J. Nematol.* **14**, 259–266.

Ward, S., Hogan, E., and Nelson, G. A. (1983). The initiation of spermatogenesis in the nematode *Caenorhabditis elegans. Dev. Biol.* **98**, 70–79.

Ward, S., Roberts, T. M., Strome, S., Pavalko, F. M., and Hogan, E. (1986). Monoclonal antibodies that recognize a polypeptide antigenic determinant shared by multiple *Caenorhabditis elegans* sperm-specific proteins. *J. Cell Biol.* **102,** 1778–1786.

Wolf, N., Hirsh, D., and McIntosh, J. R. (1978). Spermatogenesis in males of the free living nematode *Caenorhabditis elegans*. *J. Ultrastruct. Res.* **63,** 155–169.

CHAPTER 13

Blastomere Culture and Analysis

Lois G. Edgar

Department of Molecular, Cellular, and Developmental Biology
University of Colorado
Boulder, Colorado 80309

I. Introduction: Uses and Limitations of the System

In studying embryos of many species, methods of fragmenting and culturing embryonic tissues or cells have been useful for addressing questions of blastomere autonomy in early and later embryogenesis, for exposure to drugs or other agents that perturb specific processes, and for direct labeling of DNA or RNA. For *Caenorhabditis elegans* workers, the small size of the embryo and the impermeability of the chitinous eggshell and inner vitelline membrane have made such experiments difficult. A method of permeabilization and blastomere isolation, a culture system that will support further cellular development and differentiation, and assay methods for assessing the degree of development and its relative normality after experimental manipulation are minimal requirements for a satisfactory *C. elegans* embryonic culture system. Methods of isolating early blastomeres have included crushing of the eggshell and extrusion (Laufer *et al.*, 1980; Schierenberg, 1987), laser ablation of neighboring blastomeres within an intact eggshell (Sulston *et al.*, 1983; Priess and Thomson, 1987), laser puncturing of the eggshell producing extrusion (Schierenberg, 1987), and digestion of the eggshell followed by shearing or manual stripping of the vitelline membrane (Cowan and McIntosh, 1985; or Edgar and McGhee, 1988, respectively). This last method is described in detail below. Permeabilization of complete embryos can be achieved by the same methods; in addition, one-cell embryos within the shell can be permeabilized to certain drugs such as cytochalasin D by gentle pressure on an overlying coverslip (Hill and Strome, 1990), although older embryos are resistant.

Normal development of *C. elegans* embryos follows an invariant cell lineage, with characteristic asymmetrical divisions, division times, and cleavage planes. The first four cleavages generate a set of founder cells for specific tissues (Fig. 1). Cell proliferation continues to about 500 cells (approximately 5 hours postfertilization at 25°C), followed by a period of rapid morphogenesis and elongation without much further cell division from 5 to 7 hours after fertilization (Fig. 2). Hatching occurs at 12 hours.

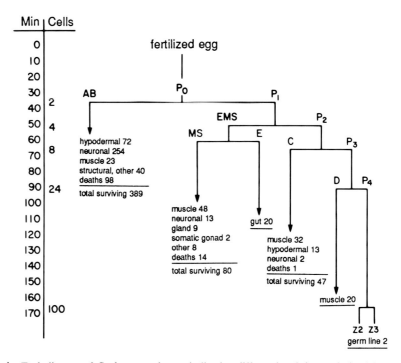

Fig. 1 Early lineage of *C. elegans* embryos, indicating differentiated tissues derived from each of the eight founder cells. (Reprinted with permission from Wood, 1988.)

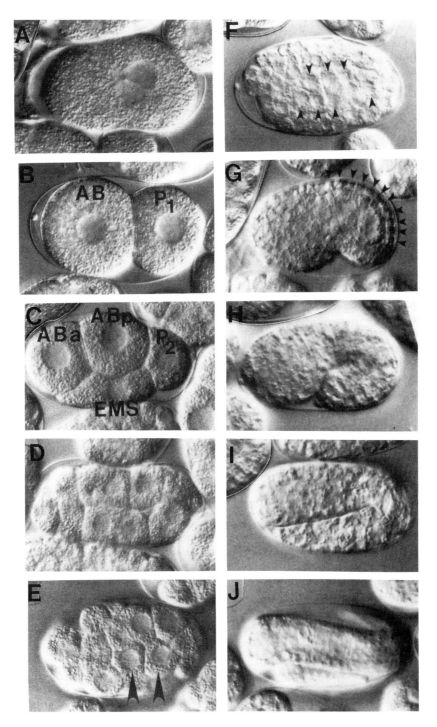

Fig. 2 Embryonic development of *C. elegans* within the eggshell. (A) One-cell stage; (B) two-cell stage; (C) four-cell stage; (D) 16-cell stage; (E) onset of gastrulation at 28 cells (arrowheads indicate the two E cells); (F) midproliferation stage (arrowheads indicate E cells in gut primordium); (G) late comma stage (arrowheads indicate hypodermal cells at dorsal midline); (H) 1.5-fold stage, with elongation beginning; (I) 2-fold stage; (J) pretzel or 3-fold stage. Anterior left, dorsal top in all photos. Photos by Francine Storfer-Glazer.

The media and simple culture chambers described in this chapter will support cell division of intact embryos without a vitelline membrane from the one- or two-cell stage to approximately the normal cell number of 550 cells as assayed by nuclear counts, although at a division rate about 50% slower than normal. Even without the enclosure of the vitelline membrane, early blastomeres divide along the characteristic axes, with the normal relative timing of divisions, and with the appropriate asymmetrical cleavages for their lineage-specific patterns. The nuclear movements in the early P and EMS blastomeres, in which the P1 and P2 nuclei move toward the AB and EMS contact boundaries, also appear normal.

At the 16- to 18-cell stage, an embryo devitellinized at two cells appears as an elongate "neck" of P1 derivatives ending in a small ball of 4 C cells, reflecting the longitudinal division axes in the P lineage. The 16 AB descendants, attached at the MS end, form a larger ball as a result of their spiral cleavage pattern (Figure 3). In favorable embryos, cell movements apparently originating in the E cells are observed at the 28-cell stage when gastrulation would normally occur, bringing the C cells into contact with MS blastomeres. At this stage, the embryo rounds up, in a process similar in appearance to compaction in the mouse blastula. Definable morphogenesis does not occur, however, probably because the lack of vitelline membrane enclosure precludes the usual cell contacts (Schierenberg and Junkersdorf, 1993). Furthermore, if the removal of the vitelline membrane is performed before 8 to 12 cells, correct specification of early blastomeres can be impaired by loss of specific normal cell contacts (Schnabel, 1991, 1994). Although the cuticle does not form around the embryo, cuticular blebs can occasionally be seen. Twitching is sometimes observed, indicating muscle differentiation. Histochemical or antibody staining and observation of gut granules reveal patches of contiguous cells expressing differentiation markers for muscle, hypodermis, germ cells, and gut, representing the proper number of cells appropriate for differential tissues (Fig. 4). By the criteria of increasing antibody staining and cell integrity, the embryos will live about 48 hours before cells begin to lyse.

In culture, variations in embryo viability can be due to the medium quality, the physiological state of the mothers, and unavoidable variability in the permeabilization procedure. A fraction of devitellinized embryos inevitably die early due to rough handling; however, in a good preparation, more than 90% of intact devitellinized embryos will continue division and differentiation, and the yield from a single preparation can be 100 to 200 embryos. In less optimal preparations, cell division will often stop one to two divisions early, at approximately 300 cells, but differentiation generally still proceeds. Separation of blastomeres or drug treatments reduce survival. Embryos devitellinized during early cleavages may show aberrant cleavage patterns due to compression in the permeabilization pipet. Cells that have just divided may rejoin and subsequently undergo a tetrapolar cleavage, which erases P-lineage differentiation. Despite such caveats, this method allows one to produce a large number of permeabilized staged embryos at the dissecting microscope relatively quickly, making possible statistically sig-

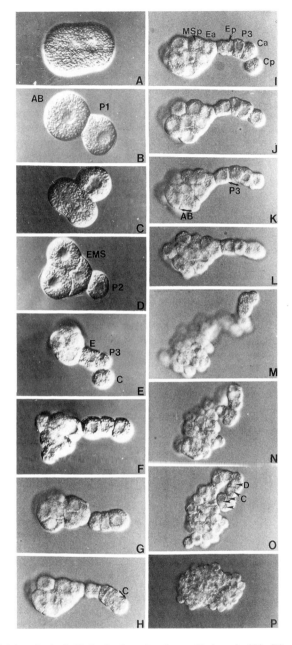

Fig. 3 Early divisions in devitellinized cultured embryos. Embryo in (G)–(P) was cultured in the presence of 200 μg/ml α-amanitin; embryos cultured with or without α-amanitin behave indistinguishably up to about 100 cells. Founder cells and their progeny are labeled in some of the panels; double-ended arrows indicate cleavage axes. (A) First cleavage, $t = 0$ (approximately 40 minutes after fertilization); (B) 2-cell stage, 10 minutes; (C) second cleavage, AB cell dividing, 20 minutes; (D) 4-cell stage, 25 minutes; (E) 8-cell stage, 57 minutes; (F) 12-cell stage, with eight AB cells, four P lineage cells, 73 minutes; (G) 12-cell stage, 81 minutes; (H) C division, 93 minutes; (I) 15-cell stage, 97 minutes; (J–L) 16- to 24-cell stages with P3 and the eight ABs dividing, 105, 110, and 120 minutes, respectively; (M) 187 minutes; (N) 200 minutes; (O), 230 minutes, note gastrulation-like movements beginning (in M) at 46 cells (32 AB, 4C; D, P4, 4E, 4 MS cells), in which P-lineage cells move to contact MS and Eaa; (P) same embryo after 16 hours showing α-amanitin arrest at approximately 100 cells. See Fig. 4D for an embryo cultured overnight without drug treatment.

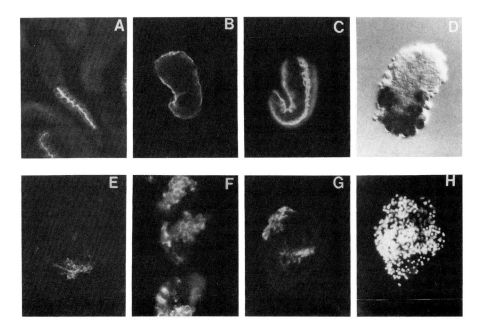

Fig. 4 Antibody staining for differentiated tissue markers in normally developing embryos (A, B, C) and embryos devitellinized at 2–4 cells and cultured overnight (E, F, and G). (A, E) Monoclonal antibody J126 (S. Strome), specific to gut; (B, F) monoclonal antibody J130 (S. Strome) to an early hypodermal protein; (C, G) monoclonal antibody 5.6.1.1 (David Miller) to myosin heavy chain A; (D) cultured embryo viewed with Nomarski, stained for β-galactosidase expression from Ce MyoD–lacZ fusion construct specific for body muscle precursors (from M. Krause); (H) cultured embryo DAPI stained for nuclei.

nificant numbers of embryos in experiments in which variations are inevitable. See Edgar and McGhee (1988), Goldstein (1992, 1993), and Edgar *et al.* (1994) for experimental uses of embryonic culture.

II. Embryo Devitellinization and Blastomere Isolation

In the procedure described here, embryos are stripped of the eggshell and vitelline membranes by chitinasing the eggshell and mechanically stripping off the vitelline membrane. Batches of up to about 200 embryos can be prepared at the dissecting microscope, although if staged embryos are selected, the yield becomes lower; for example, a good preparation yields 20 to 40 two-cell embryos. Blastomeres may be isolated manually following this denuding. The procedure takes from 15 to 40 minutes, depending on the number of worms cut.

A. Materials

Gravid well-fed hermaphrodites: Worms (raised at 16°C) in their second day of laying give the maximum yield of early embryos. Such cultures are best maintained by transferring agar chunks daily from starved L1 plates and retransferring no more than 200 worms to a fresh plate at L3 or L4.

Equipment: Dissecting microscope, lightly siliconized depression slide (two- or three-well types with a shallow depression are convenient); No. 15 scalpel and handle or two 22-gauge syringe needles; mouth pipet apparatus and drawn-out capillaries of proper size; damp box; pipetters; culture slides or chambers (see next section); eyelash mounted on toothpick.

Solutions: Egg salts and egg salts with tetramisole (Sigma T1512, optional); freshly made 1 : 9 solution of NaOCl (Fisher SS 290-1) in egg salts; embryonic growth medium (EGM); silicon oil (Sigma M6884 or Dow Corning) or Voltalef 3S oil, chitinase–chymotrypsin solution. See Section VII for formulations.

B. Procedure

1. Transfer 40 to 80 gravid worms to a 50 to 100-μl drop of egg salts in one well of the depression slide. Add 50 μl of egg salts with tetramisole (approximately 100 μl/ml), then cut worms roughly in half with the scalpel or two syringe needles used like scissors, working at the dissecting microscope. Many eggs will be released by cutting, and additional eggs can be recovered by breaking uncut uteri with the pipet tip or a glass needle.

2. Collect embryos of desired stages in a mouth pipet with small-diameter capillary and transfer them to a 100μl drop of NaOCl solution in the other depression well. Incubate for 2.5 to 3 minutes.

3. Meanwhile, set up a 30-μl drop of EGM, a 30-μl drop of egg salts, and a 15-μl drop of chitinase–chymotrypsin covered with 3 μl silicon oil on the same depression slide. Transfer the embryos quickly through the EGM and egg salt rinses and into the chitinase–chymotrypsin drop. Eggshell digestion will normally take 4 to 8 minutes and is evident when the embryos round up slightly; three-cell embryos will have a cloverleaf shape. Staging can be done during this digestion.

4. Move embryos through a 30-μl rinse drop of EGM and into a 30-μl drop of EGM under silicon oil. Remove the vitelline membrane by drawing individual embryos in and out of a narrow-bore pipet, slightly smaller than the embryo diameter, which shears the tough membrane and strips it off.

5. If isolated blastomeres are needed, separate cells of two-, three-, or four-cell embryos with an eyelash or a fine glass needle.

6. Transfer to fresh EGM in culture chambers (see Section III).

C. Notes

1. Tetramisole (Sigma T1512, a 10 mg/ml stock solution in H_2O diluted to approximately 100 μl/ml in egg salts) addition is optional; this drug paralyzes the worms and makes cutting easier. Cut immediately: if too contracted, the worms will not release many eggs. Use a fresh scalpel blade each day, as they corrode quickly.

For maximum yield, more eggs can be released by treating cut worms for approximately 1 minute with an equal volume of NaOCl solution added directly to the cutting drop. As soon as eggs are released, add the same volume of EGM as NaOCl used to prevent further egg damage. This treatment will kill pronuclear stages and damage one-cell embryos. The 3-minute NaOCl treatment is still necessary before treating with chitinase for a uniform digestion.

For eggs earlier than two-cell stage, in which the shell is still somewhat permeable, add an equal volume of EGM as soon as the worms are cut. After this, many can survive the 3-minute NaOCl and chitinase treatment, and some will still be at the one-cell stage after chitinase treatment and removal of the vitelline membrane if you work fast.

2. The most satisfactory transfer pipets are made from SMI Micropipettor 5- to 30-μl capillaries (Fisher 21-380-9C), by double-pulling over a very small flame. This is done by first heating and pulling gently to make a thin center section, next cooling briefly, and then reheating more gently while keeping the capillary under tension for the final pull. The ideal pull produces a pipet with a distinct shank and a narrow gradually tapering section of about $\frac{3}{4}$ to 1 in.. A small gas burner can be made by mounting a large syringe needle in a cork, with a screw clamp on the tubing to adjust gas flow. Before use, break the capillary to the desired tip, about 100 to 150 μm (three or four times egg diameter) by pinching between your thumbnail and fingertip. Keep the pipet diameter small to minimize liquid transfer. If eggs stick to the inside of the pipet, many can be recovered by flushing with the NaOCl solution or the EGM as you go along. Expect to change pipets frequently, and have a good supply pulled before a working session.

3. If the chitinase digestion does not work within 8 minutes, it will probably not work at all. The most common problems are the hypochlorite and the physiological state of the worms (first-day laying seems to give tougher eggs). Hypochlorite should be an unexpired batch, and it usually becomes poor a month or so before the expiration date. Keep the stock refrigerated in a dark vented bottle, filled to near the top. Mix a 3-ml tube just before starting, and keep it on ice; it will work for about 3 hours and should then be replaced.

After enzyme treatment and especially after permeabilization, the embryos are quite sticky and will clump; this can be minimized by pipetting only a few at a time. Small clumps can be broken up by expelling from the pipet with a little force a few times.

4. Permeabilization pipets are pulled by hand in the same manner as the transfer pipets, using Kwik-fil injection capillaries (1B100F-4 from World Preci-

sion Instruments, Sarasota, FL). The inner thread seems to help cut the vitelline membrane. The ideal pull gives a long gradual taper in the thin section so that it can be cut to the diameter desired. Pipets are cut with a fresh scalpel blade on Parafilm under the dissecting scope. An adaptor for the mouth pipet can be made with small-bore Tygon tubing threaded onto a syringe needle attached to a mouth tube. Fill the pipet tip with EGM back to the wider bore and test on the first batch of chitinased embryos; recut the pipet tip if it is too small. The ideal size will vary according to the age of the embryo you are trying to get: the very early stages are more fragile and need a slightly larger bore; embryos larger than eight cells compress with less damage and will often come out of the larger pipets with the vitelline membrane intact. Such nonpermeabilized embryos continue to develop to the hatching stage.

Use a syringe on the mouth pipet for filling and cleaning permeabilization pipets; the actual permeabilization is done by mouth air pressure. Pipets can sit in air for several hours without drying out, as the bore is so small, but as they dry they will eventually clog. Store pipets (a good one is worth guarding and will last several weeks) by flushing the tip several times with distilled water and suspending the pipet tip in a tube of sterile distilled water or 0.1 M HCl, using a tape "flag" on the pipet so that it does not sink in completely.

If the pipet is right, it takes only a few minutes to permeabilize a batch of embryos by individually sucking them into the pipet and gently expelling them. They will emerge more or less compressed depending on the inner diameter of the pipet, but round up again with a few minutes. If there is a lot of lysis with permeabilization, either the digestion was incomplete or the pipet bore was too small. As the cell membranes are quite labile for 4 to 5 minutes after cleavage, embryos devitellinized during and just after cleavage may lyse or blastomeres may fuse, later undergoing an abnormal tetrapolar cleavage. If critical, check during an experiment and eliminate such embryos.

The following criteria indicate both a good preparation and a good batch of culture medium: (a) embryos show very little lysis, initially or after overnight culture; (b) embryos continue to divide on schedule; (c) intact embryos after overnight incubation have more than 300 cells, and ideally more than 500; (d) gut granules are visible under polarized light in more than 90% of these embryos (if gut granules are missing, this can usually be attributed to an early tetrapolar cleavage as noted above).

5. A fine eyelash (a traditional electron microscopy tool) mounted on a toothpick with glue is the most satisfactory tool for rapid manual blastomere separation; a glass needle also works, but breaks easily. Eyelashes can be cleaned with alcohol and a tissue. Blastomeres will lyse if separated just after a division; 5 to 10 minutes after cleavage is the best time for successful manipulations, unless you need earlier separations. AB/P1 separations are easiest; three- and four-cell embryos can be separated if the permeabilization pipet is the right bore to squeeze them into a single row of cells temporarily. Alternatively, to get P2 and

EMS blastomeres, P1 can be separated after the first division and EMS/P2 after the second. P-lineage blastomeres can be recognized by relative size and their linear arrangement. With low yield, MS, E, P3, and C can be separated from the four descendants of an initial isolated P1 blastomere.

III. Culture Methods

For overnight culture, or observation over several hours, several types of culture chambers have proved useful. The simplest is Teflon-coated immunology slides with multiple wells (Cel-Line HTC Super-cured, available in many configurations from Cel-Line Associates, Newfield, NJ) with 30 to 100 μl of EGM pipetted onto a well and covered with 3 μl of silicon oil. Embryos can be observed by dissecting scope or at 10× or 16× on the compound microscope without a coverslip and subsequently recovered or manipulated further. Alternatively, a coverslip can be added to an oil-covered drop of 10 to 20 μl EGM, so that the drop does not spread beyond the boundaries of the well; however, such embryos are almost impossible to retrieve.

A second way of making a coverslipped chamber is to use a gelatin-subbed slide with spacer strips to raise the coverslip: $\frac{1}{2}$-in. 3M Drafting Transfer Tape, available from art supply stores, makes a good spacer. Embryos are pipetted into 5 to 10 μl EGM on the subbed slide and covered with 3 μl silicon oil. The coverslip is applied gently, then pressure-sealed to the tape before the oil reaches the tape. The open ends are sealed with oil or thin plastic wrap. Again, it is hard to retrieve these embryos. This mount works well at 40× but is too thick for 100×.

For viewing at 100× using an inverted microscope, a very satisfactory culture chamber consists of an aluminum or plastic slide 25 mm × 75 mm × 5 mm, drilled with a 16-mm-diameter central hole. This hole is covered on the bottom with a 20-mm^2 coverslip (acid-washed and baked) sealed with vacuum grease. Thirty microliters of EGM is pipetted on, embryos are added, and the slide is quickly sealed to prevent evaporation, using a 16-mm^2 coverslip with several 2-μl drops of silicon oil pipetted around it to seal. If slides are moved carefully, embryos or fragments will stay fairly well put and can be identified by their position, although they should be well separated initially.

All types of preparations should be kept in a damp chamber when not being observed. Damp paper towels in a plastic box, with risers such as plastic pipets to keep the slides from getting wet, work well. Incubate at 16°C rather than 20°C for optimum viability.

IV. Drug Treatments

After removal of the vitelline membrane, embryos can be easily treated with various drugs by adding the drug to the medium. Cytochalasin D, aphidicolin, nocodazole, α-amanitin, and blockers of nucleic acid or protein synthesis have been used in various protocols (Edgar and McGhee 1988; Edgar et al., 1994; Edgar, unpublished results). Dosage should be titrated by the physiological effects in the medium used. Particularly in the case of α-amanitin, high doses are needed to produce saturation effects in rich medium, as much of the drug seems to be absorbed to components of the medium. When removing embryos from drug exposure, pipet them through several rinses.

Embryos can also be permeabilized to drugs without chitinase treatment and removal of the vitelline membrane. For this method, treat embryos for 1 minute in 1 : 9 NaOCl solution on the depression slide. At 1 minute add an equal volume of EGM to block the hypochlorite. Using a gelatin-subbed slide with two 3M tape spacer strips, put the embryos into a 3- to 5-μl drop of EGM between the tape strips, add a coverslip, and seal it to the tape by pressure with a dissecting needle. Press down gently on the coverslip with the needle while adding 30 μl EGM at the top edge. This should stick the embryos to the slide. To permeabilize the embryos, press harder on the coverslip until the embryos flatten slightly and rebound when released, repeating two or three times. Nonpermeabilized embryos will develop to hatching; permeabilized embryos usually make monsters. Permeabilization can be monitored by adding 0.0002% Nile blue A (make stock in 10% EtOH) to the medium; this vital dye is taken up only by permeabilized embryos and collects in the gut cells. Once the embryos are fixed to the slide and permeabilized, fresh medium with or without drugs can be flushed through the open ends of the chamber by adding liquid at one side and pulling through with a tissue at the other. When changing the medium, use several 30-μl flushes. Fixation and staining can be done in the same manner.

One advantage to this preparation is the embryos remain stuck (with luck) to the gelatin, so that individual embryos can be followed through a procedure. The caveats are that permeabilization may be uneven from embryo to embryo; remnants of the shell and vitelline membrane may prevent rapid and equal access of the drug to all cells; and in some embryos the vitelline membrane appears to reseal, as occasionally a hatching L1 with a blue gut is observed if Nile blue is present.

V. Radioactive Labeling

Both UMP and UTP labeled with ^{3}H or ^{32}P are readily taken up by embryos after removal of the vitelline membrane (Edgar et al., 1994); one supposition as to how the triphosphate gets in is that cell membranes may be slightly leaky.

Radioactive labeling requires extreme care, as working with small numbers of embryos must be done under the dissecting scope and it is virtually impossible to avoid all mouth pipetting. Likewise, wearing gloves makes the manipulation very difficult and probably increases the chance of contamination. It can be done most safely by using the Cel-Line slides and moving embryos in small batches

from drop to drop. A plastic shield should be fitted around the dissecting microscope for labeling with ^{32}P. The mouth pipet should be fitted with a cotton plug
or a very long tube, and care should be taken never to overfill the glass tip.

═══════ VI. Fixation and Cytochemistry

A. Fixation Methods

The method of choice for fixation of devitellinized embryos is paraformaldehyde with glutaraldehyde. This method gives the best morphology for further
Nomarski observations, and allows one to keep track of a small number of the
embryos. If ethanol fixation is required, as for certain antibodies, it should follow
a brief (1-minute) paraformaldehyde fixation to attach the embryos to a slide.
Embryos can be either slide-mounted at the time of fixation or, as is often
desirable after culture in which individual embryos have been followed, fixed in
place in the culture chamber.

1. Fixation in Place

Very gently pipet 1 to 2 vol of fix solution (see Section VII; 3% paraformaldehyde is preferable with this method because of dilution) around the edges of
the EGM drop containing the embryos, so as not to disturb them. Alternatively,
pipet embryos into 50-μl drops of 2.25% fix on a Teflon slide, separating them
as desired for identification. Covering with oil is not necessary for the short
fixation. Fix at room temperature or on an aluminum block on ice for 3 to 5
minutes. For antibodies, room temperature for 5 minutes generally works well.
After fixation, carefully remove approximately half the liquid and replace with
phosphate buffer; do this at least three times. This should be done with the
mouth pipet if you do not want to shift the embryos; if all embryos in a drop are
equivalent, you can use a Pipetman. Keep in a damp box until further processing.

2. Fixation with Attachment to a Slide

These preparations are easier to handle then loose embryos, although sometimes antibody staining is more successful if the embryos are not flattened.

On a gelatin-subbed slide, identify the area to be used by scribing a circle on
the back with a diamond-point pencil, and pipet 3 to 5 μl fix solution (2.25%
paraformaldehyde) on the subbed side. Pipet the embryos into the fix, let them
settle, remove liquid if the volume is large, then cover the drop with a small
coverslip about 5 mm^2 (cut with a diamond point from a larger coverslip). As
the liquid spreads to the point where the embryos flatten slightly, press lightly
on the coverslip with a dissecting needle if the embryos are not contacting the
slide (sometimes crystals or lumps need to be flattened). If there is too much

liquid, pull off some with a tissue; if too little, work fast! Quickly add $30\mu l$ additional fix to float up the coverslip. Fix for 5 minutes at room temperature (fixation time can be modified for specific methods). After floating the coverslip, it can be pressed down again lightly with a needle to stick floating embryos to the slide, to transfer those stuck to the coverslip back to the gelatin, or to flatten for procedures such as nuclear counts. After fixing, transfer the slide to a Coplin jar containing phosphate buffer or phosphate-buffered saline (PBS) (depending on the procedure), making sure the coverslip slides off on immersion. Slides can be collected and held at this point, as long as a day or two in the refrigerator.

3. Ethanol or Methanol Fixation

Use the procedure above, and after attaching the embryos to the slide with a small coverslip and pressure, fix the slide in a Coplin jar of ethanol or methanol at 4°C for 10 minutes. Further treat by air-drying or by rehydration through an alcohol–buffer series: 2 minutes each 95%, 90%, 75%, 50%, 30%, PBS or phosphate buffer.

B. Immunostaining

Devitellinized and cultured embryos that are healthy, or even drug treated, can be successfully stained for many markers of differentiated tissue types using fairly standard methods. The methods below were originally adapted from Strome (Strome and Wood, 1983). Various dilutions of primary and secondary antibodies, incubation times, and incubation temperatures should be tested to optimize staining with the particular antibodies being used.

Embryos on slides are treated in a standard manner by wiping around the previously marked specimen area and incubating in 30- to 50-μl drops in a damp box; washes can be done in Coplin jars. Embryos in drops can be handled by removing and adding liquid or by transferring into fresh drops using the mouth pipet.

1. In a Coplin jar, permeabilize fixed embryos to antibodies by treating 5 minutes in 0.5% Triton X-100 in PBS.

2. Rinse in PBS.

3. On the slide, block with normal goat serum (or serum corresponding to the secondary antibody) diluted with an equal volume of 0.1% Triton–PBS (TPBS) for 1 hour at room temperature or 30 minutes at 37°C.

4. Replace with primary antibody diluted appropriately in TPBS and incubated as appropriate for the particular primary antibody.

5. Wash 3×15 minutes in PBS or TPBS in a Coplin jar at room temperature.

6. Repeat blocking step if background has been high.

7. Incubate on the slide with secondary antibody diluted in TPBS, normally 45 minutes to 2 hours at room temperature. Secondary antibodies from Jackson Laboratories (West Grove, PA) work well.

8. Wash at least 3 × 10 minutes in PBS.

9. Proceed with development of secondary antibody if using peroxidase or phosphatase systems.

10. Stain nuclei with 0.5 to 1 μg/ml 4',6-diamidino-2-phenylindole dihydrochloride (DAPI) in PBS for 5 mintues, if desired.

11. At this point, loose embryos can be observed under an inverted microscope or coverslipped, or mounted to slides with a 1-minute paraformaldehyde fix as described above. If refixed, rinse in PBS before sealing.

12. Mount in Gelutol or other glycerol mounting medium.

C. Cytochemical Staining

1. β-Galactosidase

Embryos are handled on slide mounts or in drops, exactly as for antibody staining, with paraformaldehyde fixation giving the best morphology. Following fixation and a rinse in PBS of 5 minutes or longer, incubate with β-galactosidase stain solution (see Section VII) at room temperature in a damp box. The time of staining will vary with different markers. Follow with DAPI staining as above, and mount.

2. Gut Esterase:

Fix only 3 minutes, on ice; wash 5 minutes in 125 mM phosphate buffer (4°C), and stain in a drop of pararosaniline stain solution (see Section VII) on ice for no more than 2 hours. Rinse, DAPI stain 5 minutes, and mount.

3. Combinations

Most of these staining methods can be combined successfully, although their order is important. Gut esterase is very labile, and if stained for, this should be the first procedure. If esterase staining is used in combination with β-galactosidase blue staining (the American flag effect), the esterase staining should be stopped by a PBS rinse before it gets very red, so as not to obscure the β-galactosidase precipitate. β-galactosidase stain is then added and incubated for the appropriate length of time. Unfortunately, esterase and antibody staining cannot be combined, as the esterase staining solution seems to destroy antigenicity.

Antibody staining should follow the β-galactosidase staining if a visible light system is used. A peroxidase-conjugated secondary antibody works well. Alternatively, if a polyclonal primary antibody is used as a marker, β-galactosidase can be stained using a mouse monoclonal anti-β-galactosidase (Promega Z3781), diluted 1:300 and incubated 3 to 4 hours at room temperature, 37°C for 1 hour, or 4°C overnight, followed by a fluorescent secondary antibody. Two primary antibodies can be incubated together if conditions are the same; otherwise do the longer incubation first. The two secondaries can be incubated together.

VII. Solutions and Culture Media

The following formulations have proved satisfactory with the procedures detailed in preceding sections. EGM (embryonic growth medium) has been developed and modified over several years; a simplified version suitable for short-term culture is included as well as the current optimal version.

Egg Salts.   118 mM NaCl; 48 mM KCl; glass-distilled H_2O. Autoclave. This salt mixture is preferable to M9 for cutting worms or for NaOCl dilutions, as it is more physiologically isotonic than M9 for embryos.

Egg Salts with Tetramisole.   100 μg/ml tetramisole, from 5 mg/ml stock solution.

Egg Buffer.   118 mM NaCl; 48 mM KCl; 2 mM CaCl$_2$; 2 mM MgCl$_2$; 0.025 mM 4-(2-hydroxyethyl)-1-piperazineethanesulfonic acid (Hepes, pH 7.4); glass-distilled H_2O. Filter-sterilize or autoclave before adding sterile Hepes. Permeabilized embryos will be relatively happy for an hour in this buffer.

Chitinase–Chymotrypsin Solution.   Chitinase, 5 units (the best currently available is *Serratia marcescens* chitinase, 30% protein grade, Sigma C7809; Sigma C1525, 60% protein grade from *Streptomyces griseus,* also works quite well); α-chymotrypsin (Sigma type II, C4129), 10 mg; egg salts, 1 ml; penicillin–streptomycin (Sigma P3539), 10 μl. Mix on ice, let sit several hours or overnight, centrifuge if cloudy, and filter-sterilize. Store refrigerated. This works better after a day or so, and can be frozen in 100-μl aliquots for convenience.

Embryonic Growth Medium (EGM), 10 ml.

Polyvinylpyrrolidone (*PVP*)	50 mg
L-Tyrosine	0.5 mg
Stock salts	840 μl
0.25 M Hepes, pH 7.4	1000 μl
Inulin (5 mg/ml in H_2O)	1000 μl
Amino acid stock	1250 μl
Tissue culture-grade H_2O	1320 μl
Fetal bovine serum (FBS)	4000 μl
LPSR-1 (Sigma L9263)	1000 μl
(*Optional:* Reduce FBS to 3 ml if LPSR-1 is used.)	
Penicillin–streptomycin (Sigma P3539)	100 μl
Galactose stock	100 μl
Base mix	100 μl
L-Glutamine (14 mg/ml in H_2O, mix fresh)	100 μl
BME vitamins (Sigma B6891)	50 μl
0.5 M Na$_2$HPO$_4$	40 μl

Pyruvic acid (14 mg/ml in H$_2$O, mix fresh)	20 μl
1 M MgSO$_4$	20 μl
1 M CaCl$_2$ (optional)	20 μl
Lactate syrup (Sigma L4263)	10 μl
Trace minerals (optional)	10 μl
Chicken egg yolk dilution or cholesterol 3-sulfate stock	50 μl

Use tissue culture-grade chemicals (e.g., Sigma). Weigh PVP and tyrosine into a tube and add other components in the order listed with egg yolk last. Let sit on ice 1 to 3 hours, centrifuge at 5000 rpm for 5 to 10 minutes, and filter-sterilize. Store refrigerated; medium is good for a month or longer.

Because this recipe is a tissue culture medium "made from scratch," it is complicated; however, stock solutions can be made up once in several years and frozen or refrigerated as designated below. A batch of medium takes less than an hour to put together, and will last more than a month refrigerated.

Stock Solutions for EGM.

1. Stock Salts (100 ml): 70 ml 1 M NaCl, 30 ml 1 M KCl. Use tissue culture-grade H$_2$O and autoclave. Refrigerate.

2. Base mix (100 ml): tissue culture-grade H$_2$O, 100 ml; adenine, 100 mg; ATP, 10 mg; guanine, 3 mg; hypoxanthine, 3 mg; thymine, 3 mg; xanthine, 3 mg; uridine, 3 mg; ribose, 5 mg; deoxyribose, 5 mg. Autoclave and refrigerate. Good indefinitely.

3. Amino acids (100 ml): tissue culture-grade H$_2$O, 100 ml; DL-α-alanine, 90 mg; L-arginine, 100 mg; L-asparagine, 50 mg; L-cysteine (free base), 24 mg; glycine, 40 mg; L-histidine (free base), 50 mg; DL-isoleucine, 50 mg; L-leucine, 25 mg; L-lysine, 15 mg; DL-methionine, 30 mg; DL-phenylalanine, 50 mg; L-serine, 40 mg; DL-threonine, 120 mg; L-tryptophan, 4 mg; DL-valine, 40 mg. Filter sterilize, aliquot at 1250 μl in Eppendorf tubes for convenience, and store at $-20°$C.

4. Trace mineral stock (1000$\times$): tissue culture-grade H$_2$O 100 ml; ZnSO$_4$.7H$_2$O (5 $\times$ 10^{-3}M) 144 mg; FeSO$_4$.7H$_2$O (1 $\times$ 10^{-3}M) 28 mg; MnSO$_4$.H$_2$O (5 $\times$ 10^{-3}M) 85 mg; Na$_2$SeO$_3$ (1 $\times$ 10^{-4}M) 1.7 mg. Filter-sterilize and store refrigerated. Replace when precipitate is seen.

5. PVP: polyvinylpyrrolidone MW 40,000 (Sigma P0930). If PVP is not tissue culture-grade, dialyze several grams against distilled H$_2$O for 1 to 2 days and lyophilize. Store at room temperature or $-20°$C. The Sigma P0930 can be dissolved at 50 mg/ml in tissue culture-grade H$_2$O and used to replace 1 ml of the H$_2$O in the recipe; filter, sterilize, and store this stock solution at 4°C.

6. Inulin: 5 mg/ml (Sigma I3754) in tissue culture-grade H$_2$O. Inulin (not insulin), like the PVP, adds osmolality. Autoclave to dissolve. Refrigerate or keep at room temperature. This solution tends to precipitate at 4°C, or to grow things at room temperature.

7. Galactose: 100 mg/ml in tissue culture-grade H$_2$O. Autoclave, aliquot to 1 ml, and freeze; refrigerate after thawing.

8. Fetal bovine serum (FBS): Heat treat at 56°C for 30 minutes. The quality of serum is critical, and if not good, embryos tend to bleb at early cleavages and lyse. You may need to try several batches; however, you need so little that a tissue culture laboratory may be willing to let you try their serum. Freeze in 3- or 4-ml aliquots at −20°C.

9. LPSR-1: Low-protein serum replacement with extra growth factors. Its use is optional but may improve the medium somewhat, depending on your batch of serum.

10. Water: Quality of H_2O is very important, so either buy certified tissue culture-grade H_2O or get some from a tissue culture laboratory.

11. Egg yolk: Separate yolk of an egg, roll on paper towel to remove all white, and mix an aliquot $1:1$ with sterile H_2O, as otherwise it is too thick to pipet. Although this sounds arcane, it is a source of cholesterol and carrier lipoproteins, and apparently important for hypodermal cell development, as hypodermal cells detach in low-cholesterol media. Cholesterol 3-sulfate (Sigma C9523) seems to work nearly as well; make a stock at 25 mg/ml in 30% ethanol. This will not dissolve completely but can used as a slurry. Store at 4°C.

12. Additonal Notes: For convenience, freeze serum, amino acids, and LPSR-1 in aliquots for one batch of medium. Small aliquots of vitamins, galactose, and base mix can be refrigerated several months once thawed. A few components, as noted, must be mixed fresh.

This is a trial-and-error medium based on earlier *C. elegans* media (Laufer *et al.*, 1980), mouse embryonic culture medium, and Leibovitz's L-15 medium, an insect tissue culture medium. The osmolality without PVP, inulin, and serum is 291 m*M*, the same as for the standard tissue culture medium M199, but embryos seem to do much better with these additives, so that one suspects that normal osmolality within the vitelline membrane is very high. The L-15 medium works reasonably, although not as well as EGM, in a mixture of 600 μl L-15 (Gibco 320-1415 liquid, 430-1300 dry), 100 μl inulin mix, 100 μl 0.25 *M* Hepes (pH 7.4), 200 μl FBS per milliliter. Add 10 μl base mix and 5 μl egg yolk or cholesterol for better results.

A quick trial of medium can be made by cracking eggs under a coverslip in medium and observing early cleavages in partial embryos or isolated blastomeres. There should be continuing division without much delay, and very little membrane blebbing at division. Blebbing and early lysis are probably serum problems, but may be due to high divalent cations. Ca^{2+} and Mg^{2+} can be reduced or omitted to control blebbing at division. If blastomeres are observed to shrink or swell, overall osmolarity may be adjusted by 5 to 20 m*M* with stock salts. Refrigerated medium sometimes looks contaminated because cholesterol precipitates out over several days; if the embryos are not dying, the medium can be refiltered and used.

Minimal EGM. This simplified version is suitable for short-term culture of permeabilized embryos, for example, in preparation for fixation or for a few hours. It does not support development as satisfactorily for overnight culture as EGM. For 10 ml: PVP, 50 mg; inulin (5 mg/ml), 1 ml; stock salts, 840 μl; 0.25 M Hepes (pH 7.4), 1 ml; FBS, 4 ml; penicillin–streptomycin, 100 μl; galactose (100 mg/ml), 100 μl; lactate syrup, 10 μl; glutamine, (14 mg/ml), 100 μl; pyruvic acid (14 mg/ml), 20 μl; H_2O, 2830 μl.

2.25% Paraformaldehyde Fix (20 ml). Add 2 drops 1 M NaOH to 10 ml H_2O, heat to boiling, and let cool to about 70°C. Meanwhile, weigh 450 mg paraformaldehyde, add to the cooled H_2O, and swirl to dissolve. Add 10 ml 250 mM phosphate buffer, pH 7.2 to 7.4. Filter through Whatman paper and add 80 μl 25% glutaraldehyde (or equivalent) to 0.1% final glutaraldehyde concentration. This will keep about a week in the refrigerator.

Gelatin-Subbed Slides. Hydrate 2% gelatin (Sigma G1890 seems best) in H_2O for a few minutes, then melt at 65°C. Put 15 μl on one end of a slide with a Pipetman, and draw a second slide lengthwise as if making a blood smear, to give an even coating. Air-dry, preferably several weeks for best sticking. This formulation will not kill embryos.

β-Galactosidase Stain (1 ml). 250 mM phosphate buffer (pH 7.2–7.4), 500 μl; H_2O, 378 μl; 1 M $MgCl_2$, 10 μl; 1% sodium dodecyl sulfate, 4 μl (for subsequent antibody staining, substitute Triton X-100 at final concentration of 0.1%); Fe stock (100 mM potassium ferrocyanate, 100 mM potassium ferricyanate, in H_2O; freeze aliquots, store current stock at 4°C), 50 μl; 2% X-gal in dimethyl sulfoxide (store at −20°C), 12 μl. Mix fresh on day of use.

Esterase Stain (1 ml). 4% $NaNO_2$ (stock good 1 week at 4°C), 50 μl; pararosaniline [stock: stir 400 mg pararosaniline HCl (Sigma P1528) with 8 ml H_2O overnight, add 2 ml concentrated HCl, and stir several hours; centrifuge and filter; best after aging at several weeks at 4°C], 50 μl; 2.8% Na_2HPO_4, 1 ml; 0.2 M NaOH, 20 μl; α-naphthyl acetate (20 mg/ml in acetone), 2 μl. Mix $NaNO_2$ and pararosaniline to diazotize; then add other components in order given. Keep on ice; stain is good for about 1 hour.

References

Cowan, A. E., and McIntosh, J. R. (1985). Mapping the distribution of differentiation potential for intestine, muscle, and hypodermis during early development in *Caenorhabditis elegans. Cell* **41**, 923–932.

Edgar, L. G., and McGhee, J. (1988). DNA synthesis and the control of embryonic gene expression in *C. elegans. Cell* **53**, 589–599.

Edgar, L. G., Wolf, N., and Wood, W. B. (1994). Early transcription in *Caenorhabditis elegans* embryos. *Development* **120**, 443–451.

Goldstein, B. (1992). Induction of gut in *Caenorhabditis elegans* embryos. *Nature* **357**, 255–257.

Goldstein, B. (1993). Establishment of gut fate in the E lineage of *C. elegans:* The roles of lineage-dependent mechanisms and cell interactions. *Development* **118**, 1267–1277.

Hill, D., and Strome, S. (1990). Brief cytochalasin-induced disruption of microfilaments during a critical interval in 1-cell *C. elegans* embryos alters the partition of developmental instructions to the 2-cell embryo. *Development* **108**, 159–172.

Laufer, J., Bazzicalupo, P., and Wood, W. B. (1980). Segregation of developmental potential in early embryos of *Caenorhabditis elegans*. *Cell* **19,** 569–577.

Priess, J. R., and Thomson, J. N. (1987). Cellular interactions in early *C. elegans* embryos. *Cell* **48,** 241–250.

Schierenberg, E. (1987). Reversal of cellular polarity and early cell-cell interaction in the embryo of *Caenorhabditis elegans*. *Dev. Biol.* **122,** 452–463.

Schierenberg, E., and Junkersdorf, B. (1992). The role of eggshell and underlying vitelline membrane for normal pattern formation in the early *C. elegans* embryo. *Dev. Biol.* **202,** 10–16.

Schnabel, R. (1991). Cellular interactions involved in the determination of the early *C. elegans* embryo. *Mech. Dev.* **34,** 85–100.

Schnabel, R. (1994). Autonomy and nonautonomy in cell fate specification of muscle in the *Caenorhabditis elegans* embryo: A reciprocal induction. *Science* **263:** 1449–1452.

Strome, S., and Wood, W. B. (1983). Generation of asymmetry and segregation of germline granules in early *C. elegans* embryos. *Cell* **35,** 15–25.

Sulston, J. E., Schierenberg, E., White, J. G., and Thomson, J. N. (1983). The embryonic cell lineage of the nematode *Caenorhabditis elegans*. *Dev. Biol.* **100,** 64–119.

Wood, W. B. (1988). In *"The Nematode Caenorhabditis elegans"* Cold Spring Harbor Laboratory Press, Cold Spring Harbor, New York.

CHAPTER 14

Whole-Mount *in Situ* Hybridization for the Detection of RNA in *Caenorhabditis elegans* Embryos

Geraldine Seydoux and Andrew Fire

Department of Embryology
Carnegie Institution of Washington
Baltimore, Maryland 21210

I. Introduction

In situ hybridization to RNA is an effective tool for the analysis of gene expression during development. This technique is particularly important for

Caenorhabditis elegans, as isolation of RNA from specific tissues or developmental stages is generally not possible in this organism (see Chapter 20 in this volume). In addition, the availability of the complete cell lineage (Sulston and Horvitz, 1977; Kimble and Hirsh, 1979; Sulston *et al.,* 1983) and the reproducibility of cell positions from one animal to the next allow RNA expression patterns to be analyzed at the level of individual cells.

A number of *in situ* hybridization protocols have been developed for the detection of RNA in squashed, dissected, or sectioned tissues of *C. elegans* (Hecht *et al.,* 1981; Klass *et al.,* 1982; Edwards and Wood, 1983; Costa *et al.,* 1988; Schedin *et al.,* 1991; MacMorris and Blumenthal, 1993; Patel and Mancillas, pers. comm.). More recently, protocols using whole-mount preparations of *C. elegans* have also been described (e.g., Mitani *et al.,* 1993; Evans *et al.,* 1994; Chapter 15 in this volume). By preserving the three-dimensional structure of the specimen, whole-mount preparations facilitate the identification of specific cells and the analysis of complex expression patterns. In this chapter, we describe a protocol for detection of RNA in whole-mount *C. elegans* embryos. This procedure is based on protocols for *Drosophila* (Tautz and Pfeifle, 1989; as modified by Patel and Goodman, pers. comm.), which make use of highly sensitive digoxigenin-labeled probes.

Other methods for studying patterns of gene expression in *C. elegans* include the use of reporter fusions (see Chapter 19 in this volume) and immunocytochemistry (see Chapter 16 in this volume). Each method reveals distinct aspects of gene expression. Reporter fusions reflect the ability of *cis*-acting sequences to direct expression of a reporter; it should be noted, however, that not all expression patterns are faithfully reproduced in reporter constructs (G. S. and A. F., unpublished observations). Immunocytochemistry and *in situ* hybridization provide independent means for determining expression patterns. While immunocytochemistry reveals the pattern of protein accumulation, *in situ* hybridization reveals that of RNA. Discrepancies between protein and RNA distributions provide a starting point for studies of post-transcriptional control (e.g., Wightman *et al.,* 1993; Evans *et al.,* 1994).

The different methods for determining expression patterns have different technical requirements. Reporter fusions require the isolation of transcriptional control regions. Immunocytochemistry requires the production of proteins for immunization, followed by the generation of specific antibodies. In contrast, *in situ* hybridization requires simply that the coding region of a gene of interest be isolated.

II. Materials

A. Reagents

Antidigoxigenin Fab fragment, rhodamine labeled (Boehringer-Mannheim, Catalog No. 1207-750)

Antidigoxigenin Fab fragments, alkaline phosphatase labeled (Boehringer-Mannheim, Catalog No. 1093-274).

Bovine serum albumin (BSA, fraction V, Sigma, A7906).

Commercial bleach (5.25% sodium hypochlorite solution, Clorox).

4′,6-diamidino-2-phenylindole dihydrochloride (DAPI, Sigma, D9542).

DNA from salmon testes (Sigma, D1626).

Formaldehyde (37%, Fisher, F79-500).

Formamide (Boehringer-Mannheim, 100-731).

Glycerol (Boehringer-Mannheim, 100-649).

Glycine (Sigma, G4392).

Glycogen (Boeringher-Mannheim, 901-393).

Heparin (Sigma, H3393).

4-(2-hydroxyethyl)-1-piperazineethanesulfonic acid (Hepes, Boehringer-Mannheim, 242-608).

Levamisole (Sigma, L9756).

NaN_3 (Sigma, S-2002).

4-Nitroblue tetrazolium chloride (NBT, Boehringer-Mannheim, 1383-213).

p-Phenylenediamine (Sigma, P6001).

Poly-L-lysine (Sigma, P1525).

Polyoxyethylene–sorbitan monolaurate (Tween 20, Sigma, P1379).

Proteinase K (Boehringer-Mannheim, 161-519).

Taq DNA polymerase (Promega, M1861).

Tris (Boehringer-Mannheim, 604-205, 812-854).

Triton X-100 (Sigma, X-100).

5-Bromo-4-chloro-3-indolyl-phosphate (X-phosphate, Boehringer-Mannheim, 1383-221).

B. Stock Solutions

Diethyl pyrocarbonate (DEPC) treatment of solutions is not needed. Solutions are stored at −20°C unless otherwise indicated.

10× dNTP mix: Digoxigenin-11-dUTP (DIG-dUTP) premixed with other nucleotides (1 mmole/liter dATP, 1 mmole/liter dCTP, 1 mmole/liter dGTP, 0.65 mmole/liter dTTP, 0.35 mmole/liter DIG-dUTP) (Boehringer, 1277-065).

10× PBS: 80 g NaCl, 2 g KCl, 6.1 g anhydrous Na_2HPO_4, 2 g KH_2PO_4, H_2O to 1 liter. Autoclave and store at room temperature.

10× Taq buffer: 500 mM KCl, 100 mM Tris–HCl (pH 9.0 at 25°C), 1% Triton X-100.

20× SSC: 3M NaCl, 0.3 M Na$_3$citrate·2H$_2$O. Store at room temperature.

Mounting medium: 70% glycerol, 1 mg/ml p-phenylenediamine (pH 9).

Polylysine solution: 0.3% polylysine in water.

C. Working Solutions

These solutions are prepared on the day of use.

Formaldehyde fixative solution: 1× phosphate-buffered saline (PBS), 0.08 M Hepes (pH 6.9), 1.6 mM MgSO$_4$, 0.8 mM ethylene glycol bis(β-aminoethyl ether)-N,N,N',N'-tetraacetic acid (EGTA), 3.7% formaldehyde.

Hybridization buffer for cDNA-derived probes: 100 μg/ml autoclaved salmon sperm DNA, 50 μg/ml heparin, 0.1% Tween 20, 50% formamide, 5× SSC.

Hybridization buffer for oligonucleotide probes: 100 μg/ml autoclaved salmon sperm DNA, 50 μg/ml heparin, 0.1% Tween 20, and appropriate concentrations of formamide and SSC as described in Section III,D.

Hypochlorite solution: 1 N NaOH, 1 : 10 dilution of commercial bleach.

PBT: 1× PBS, 0.1% BSA, 0.1% Triton X-110.

PTw: 1× PBS, 0.1% Tween 20.

Staining solution: 100 mM NaCl, 5mM MgCl$_2$, 100 mM Tris, pH 9.5; 0.1% Tween 20; 1 mM levamisole. Levamisole is a potential inhibitor of endogenous phosphatases.

TTBS: 150 mM NaCl, 50 mM Tris–HCl, pH 7.8, 0.1% BSA, 0.1% Tween 20.

D. Slides and Other Materials

Carter's rubber cement (Dennison Stationary Products).

Coverslips for freeze-cracking (No. 1$\frac{1}{2}$; 24 × 50 mm; Thomas Scientific, Catalog No. 6663K94).

Incubation dishes: Unless otherwise noted, all washes and incubations are done in Wheaton staining dishes (Thomas, Catalog No. 8541-H15), which can hold 18 slides in 150 ml.

Parafilm squares cut to 20 × 20 mm.

Slides (75 × 25 mm, Cel-Line Associates, Catalog No. 10-2066 brown autoclavable coating). These slides have three square wells (14 × 14 mm) surrounded by a thin hydrophobic coating similar in thickness to a $C.$ $elegans$ embryo. This coating supports the coverslip during freeze-cracking and facilitates incubation with small volumes of staining solutions. Only the two outside wells are used. Wells are subbed with polylysine on the day of use: 50 μl of polylysine solution is allowed to settle on slides for 10 to 20 minutes; excess solution is wiped off and slides are baked at 60°C for 10 minutes.

III. Procedure

A. Overview

A mixed population of *C. elegans* embryos are attached to microscope slides, permeabilized by freezing, and fixed with methanol and formaldehyde. Embryos are then incubated overnight with a digoxigenin-labeled, single-stranded DNA probe, followed by extensive washes to remove excess probe. Fluorescent or enzyme-linked antidigoxigenin antibodies are used to visualize the hybridized probe. The entire procedure requires approximately 1.5 days from harvest of embryos to probe visualization.

B. Collection of Embryos

1. Worms are grown on a lawn of *Escherichia coli* strain OP50 on NGM agar plates (100 × 15 mm). For the wild-type strain N2, each plate is started with 20 adult hermaphrodites, which are allowed to grow until all their progeny have started to lay eggs. Ten such plates yield enough embryos for approximately 30 individual wells. Chunks of agar on plates should be avoided, as these can interfere with the freeze-cracking step.

2. Gravid hermaphrodites and their laid eggs are washed off the plates in water, and collected into a 15-ml conical tube. After centrifugation (1700 rpm for a sufficient time to pellet embryos and adults, approximately 1 minute), most of the water above the pellet is removed.

3. The worm pellet is resuspended in 10 ml of hypochlorite solution and incubated at room temperature for 3 minutes with some agitation. Worms are recovered by centrifugation and incubated in fresh hypochlorite solution for another 3 minutes (Incubation times may vary depending on the type of bleach used.) Embryos are protected by their eggshell from hypochlorite digestion, whereas larvae and adults are dissolved by this treatment.

4. When carcasses of larvae and adults are no longer visible in the dissecting microscope, embryos are washed twice in 15 ml of PBS, before resuspension in a small volume of PBS (0.5 ml or less).

C. Permeabilization and Fixation of Embryos

1. Embryos are transferred to the polylysine-coated slides using a micropipet (15 μl of embryos in PBS are sufficient to cover a 14 × 14 mm square well).

2. Freeze-cracking of embryos is performed as described in Chapter 16 in this volume. Briefly, embryos are overlaid with a glass coverslip and frozen by placing the slides on an aluminum block that has been precooled on dry ice. The coverslips are then quickly snapped off, and the slides are immediately immersed in 100% methanol at −20°C for 5 minutes.

3. Slides are transferred to 100% methanol at room temperature for 5 minutes and then rehydrated at room temperature as follows:

One 1-minute wash in 90% MeOH in H$_2$O
One 1-minute wash in 70% MeOH in PBS
One 1-minute wash in 50% MeOH in PBS
Two 5-minute washes in PTw

4. At this point, a proteinase K digestion step can be incorporated. Such a step may be necessary to increase the accessibility of low-abundance messages expressed after the lima bean stage (Pete Okkema, pers. comm.). For earlier stages, however, proteinase K treatment is not recommended. Each batch of proteinase K needs to be titrated to determine proper incubation conditions. (Typically, a 15-minute incubation in a 1μg/ml solution in PTw at room temperature is sufficient if needed.) Proteinase K digestion is stopped by incubating for 2 minutes in 2 mg/ml glycine in PTw, followed by two 5-minute washes in PTw. (If protease digestion is not necessary, proceed directly from step 3 to step 5.)

5. Embryos are fixed by incubation at room temperature for 20 minutes in formaldehyde fixative solution.

6. To remove formaldehyde, embryos are washed extensively at room temperature as follows:

Two 5-minute washes in PTw
One 5-minute wash in 2 mg/ml glycine in PTw
Three 5-minute washes in PTw

D. Probe Synthesis

We have used two types of single-stranded DNA probes: probes derived from cloned cDNAs and synthetic oligonucleotides. The cDNA-derived probes are used to detect mRNAs derived from specific genes. These probes are synthesized by multiple cycles of primer extension in the presence of digoxigenin–dUTP, using a cloned cDNA as a template ("asymmetric PCR," Patel and Goodman, 1992). The oligonucleotide probes are suitable for detecting abundant RNAs containing a defined sequence such as poly (A)+ RNAs [using an oligo (dT) probe] and SL1-bearing RNAs (using an anti-SL1 probe). These probes are end-labeled with terminal transferase and digoxigenin–ddUTP.

1. Preparation of Single-Stranded Probes from Cloned cDNA

This procedure is from Patel and Goodman (1992).

1. Plasmid DNA (2–5 μg) containing the cDNA insert is linearized using an appropriate restriction enzyme. For antisense probes, a unique restriction site

5' to the insert is used. This digested DNA will be amplified using an antisense primer at the 3' end of the insert. For sense (control) probes, a unique restriction site 3' to the insert is used. The digested DNA will be amplified using a sense primer at the 5' end of the insert. (Inserts of up to 2 kb are labeled efficiently.)

2. Digested DNA is extracted once with phenol/chloroform and once with chloroform, precipitated with 3 vol of 100% EtOH, and resuspended in TE at a final concentration of 100 to 200 μg/ml.

3. The following reagents are mixed in a 0.5-ml Eppendorf tube:

Water	7.0 μl
10× Taq buffer	2.5 μl
25 mM MgCl$_2$	1.5 μl
10× dNTP mix	5.0 μl
Primer[1] (30 ng/μl)	5.0 μl
Digested DNA (100–200 μg/ml)	2.0 μl
Mineral oil	40 μl

4. Mixed reagents are boiled for 5 minutes before adding 2.0 μl of a 1:8 dilution in water of 5 units/μl Taq polymerase stock (1.25 units total).

5. The labeling reaction is incubated for 35 thermal cycles as follows: 95°C for 45 seconds, 55°C for 30 seconds (lower temperature for primers less than 20 nucleotides), 72°C for 1 minute.

6. H$_2$O (75 μl) is added to the reaction below the oil, and 90 to 95 μl of the diluted reaction is transferred to a new tube.

7. Ten microliters of 1 M NaCl, 10 μg of glycogen, and 3 vol of 100% EtOH are added to the diluted reaction. After 30 minutes at −70°C, the reaction is centrifuged at 15,000 rpm for 10 minutes. The pellet is washed in 70% ethanol, dried, and resuspended in 300 μl of hybridization buffer.

8. The probe is boiled for 1 to 2 hours. This step reduces the length of the probe for efficient penetration of embryos.

9. Probe production is assayed using the following protocol. One microliter of probe in hybridization buffer is mixed with 5μl of 5× SSC, boiled for 5 minutes, and cooled on ice. One microliter of this mixture is spotted on a nitrocellulose strip. Several dilutions of a prelabeled control DNA (1 ng to 1 pg/μl; Boehringer-Mannheim) are also spotted for comparison. The strip is baked for 30 minutes in a vacuum oven at 80°C, washed once in 2× SSC and twice in PBT, and blocked for 30 minutes in PBT. The strip is then incubated for 30 to 60 minutes with alkaline phosphatase–anti-DIG antibody diluted 1:2000 in PBT. After three 10-minute washes in PBT and two 5-minute washes in staining solution, the strip is developed in staining solution containing 4.5 μl NBT/ml and 3.5 μl X-phosphate/ml. Spots should be visible within minutes. Spot intensities of

---

[1] For cDNAs cloned in Bluscript, we use the following primers (21-mers):

"T3" = 5'-ACT AAA GGG AAC AAA AGC TGG-3'
"T7" = 5'-ACT CAC TAT AGG GCG AAT TGG-3'.

the probe and control dilutions are compared to determine the concentration of the probe.

10. Probes can be stored at $-20°C$ in hybridization buffer for several weeks.

2. Synthesis of Oligonucleotide Probes

Synthetic oligonucleotides are end-labeled using terminal transferase and digoxigenin–ddUTP (Boehringer-Mannheim sells a 3′ end-labeling kit, Catalog No. 1362372; we have used these reagents on gel-purified oligonucleotides). Labeled oligonucleotide probes are resuspended to 0.5 μg/ml in hybridization buffer. The percentage of formamide and concentration of SSC in the hybridization buffer are adjusted for each oligonucleotide to give a melting temperature (T_m) of 52°C, using the following formula (Davis *et al.*, 1986):

$$T_m = 16.6 \log[M] + 0.41[P_{gc}] + 81.5 - B/L - 0.65[P_f]$$

where M is the molar concentration of Na (maximum of 0.5) P_{gc} is the percentage of G and C bases in the oligonucleotide, B is 675 for synthetic oligonucleotides up to 100 bases in length, L is the length of the probe in bases, and P_f is the precentage concentration of formamide. A T_m of 52°C allows for efficient hybridization at 37°C.

E. Prehybridization

1. Fixed embryos are incubated for 10 minutes in a 1 : 1 mixture of hybridization buffer and PTw, followed by a 10-minute incubation in undiluted hybridization buffer. (These incubations are done at room temperature.) During this time, a separate aliquot of hybridization buffer is heated in a boiling water bath for 10 minutes and cooled on ice.

2. Embryos are pretreated in this freshly heated hybridization buffer for 1 to 2 hours at the temperature to be used for probe hybridization (48°C for cDNA-derived probes and 37°C for oligonucleotide probes).

F. Hybridization

1. cDNA-derived probes can be used undiluted (original 300 μl, approximately 5 μg/ml) or up to ninefold diluted depending on the abundance of the transcript. In general, the probe is diluted threefold for moderately abundant messages (e.g., *skn-1* mRNA) and up to ninefold for very abundant messages (e.g., *unc-54* mRNA, *lacZ* mRNA derived from a multiple-copy array). Oligonucleotide probes are used at a concentration of 0.5 μg/ml.

2. The probe is boiled for 10 minutes, then cooled on ice.

3. Slides are removed from the prehybridization buffer, and excess buffer is wiped off while keeping the embryos wet.

4. Thirty microliters of diluted probe is added to each well. Each well is then covered with a square Parafilm coverslip (20 × 20 mm), which is sealed onto the slide with rubber cement.

5. Slides are incubated in a sealed humidity chamber overnight at 48°C (for cDNA-derived probes) or 37°C (for oligonucleotide probes).

G. Posthybridization Washes

After hybridization, Parafilm coverslips are removed with forceps while keeping the slides submerged in hybridization solution. Embryos are then washed with gentle agitation (e.g., 40–60 rpm in shaker with 17-cm radius) as follows:

1. Washes for cDNA-derived Probes

Two 15-minute washes in hybridization solution at 48°C

Two 15-minute washes in 3 parts hybridization solution/2 parts PTw at 48°C

Two 15-minute washes in 1 part hybridization solution/4 parts PTw at 48°C

Two 15-minute washes in PTw at 48°C

Two 20-minute washes in PBT at room temperature

2. Washes for Oligonucleotide Probes

One 10-minute wash in hybridization solution at 37°C

Two 10-minute washes in TTBS at room temperature

H. Probe Detection

Two types of labels are available for detection: marker enzymes such as alkaline phosphatase (AP) and fluorescent tags such as rhodamine or fluorescein. AP-mediated detection is highly sensitive, but results in a signal with limited subcellular resolution. In contrast, fluorescence detection is generally less sensitive but allows more defined subcellular resolution. For these reasons, we prefer to use AP-mediated detection to identify cells expressing specific mRNAs, and fluorescence detection to determine the subcellular localization of relatively abundant RNAs.

1. AP-Mediated Detection

1. Thirty microliters of the diluted AP–anti-DIG antibody conjugate (1 : 2500 in PBT, 0.3 unit/ml) is applied to each well. Each well is then covered with a

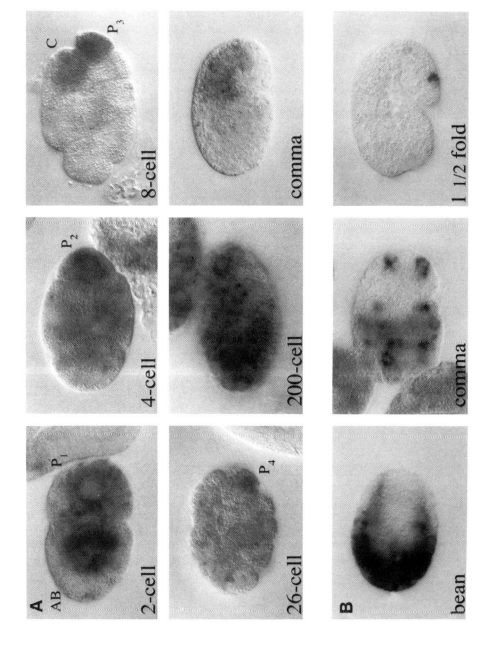

square Parafilm coverslip and incubated in a humidity chamber for 2 hours at room temperature.

2. Embryos are washed four times for 10 minutes in PBT. (If an oligonucleotide probe was used, embryos are washed twice for 10 minutes in TTBS instead.)

3. Embryos are incubated twice for 5 minutes in freshly made staining solution.

4. Thirty microliters of staining solution with 4.5 μl NBT/ml, 3.5 μl X-phosphate/ml, and 1 μg DAPI/ml is applied to each well. Slides are kept in the dark during the color reaction. The signal should appear after 20 minutes to 1 hour depending on the probe. The color reaction is monitored under the microscope to avoid background and is stopped by washing embryos twice in PBS.

5. Embryos are mounted in 5 to 10 μl of a 70% glycerol solution and covered with a glass coverslip.

2. Fluorescence Detection

1. Thirty microliters of rhodamine–anti-DIG antibody conjugate (0.2 mg/ml with 1 μg DAPI/ml) is applied to each well. Each well is then covered with a square Parafilm coverslip and incubated in a humidity chamber for 2 hours at room temperature.

2. Embryos are then washed four times for 10 minutes in PBT. (If an oligonucleotide probe was used, embryos are washed twice for 10 minutes in TTBS instead). For increased sensitivity, a secondary antibody can also be used.

3. Embryos are mounted in 5 to 10 μl of mounting medium and covered with a glass coverslip.

IV. Double Labeling

To facilitate the identification of cells in whole-mount embryos, it is often useful to label specific cells using antibodies or other markers. Here, we describe

---

Fig. 1 Hybridization of cDNA-derived probes to whole-mount embryos. Hybridized probes were visualized using an antidigoxigenin antibody coupled to alkaline phosphatase, which uses NBT and X-phosphate as substrates to give a dark color. (A) Embryos hybridized with a probe derived from *CeIF,* a gene encoding a product related to the eukaryotic translation factor eIF4-A. Maternal *CeIF* RNA (2-cell stage to 26-cell stage) is rapidly lost from somatic cells but maintained in the P lineage. This distribution is typical of many maternal RNAs (Seydoux and Fire, 1994). Embryonically transcribed *CeIF* RNA (26-cell stage to comma) is intially ubiquitous, but becomes restricted to gut cells by the comma stage. Anterior is to the left, dorsal is up. The *CeIF* cDNA was provided by D. Roussell and K. Bennett (Roussell and Bennett, 1992). (B) Embryos hybridized with a probe derived from cm14g5, a cDNA encoding a product related to histone H1. The expression pattern of this gene changes rapidly after the onset of morphogenesis. Identity of staining cells has not been determined. Anterior is to the left. Bean stage embryo: dorsal view. All other embryos: lateral view. cm14g5 was provided by P. Wohldman and R. Waterson (Waterson *et al.,* 1992).

the use of an anti-P-granule antibody to label the P cells (P1–P4) and their germ cell descendants (Z2 and Z3) (Strome and Wood, 1982) in embryos that have been subjected to the *in situ* hybridization protocol described above. In theory, any antibody could be used in a similar manner, provided that its epitope is not destroyed by the hybridization procedure.

1. After completing the detection step but before mounting the embryos in glycerol, the embryos are subjected to three 10-minute washes in TTBS.

2. Embryos are incubated for 2 hours at room temperature with an FSE-labeled anti-P-granule antibody (diluted 1:400 in TTBS; we use FSE-conjugated OIC1D4 from Janet Paulsen and Susan Strome).

3. Embryos are washed twice for 5 minutes in TTBS, before mounting in 5 μl of mounting medium. P-granule staining should be seen in most embryos. Strong alkaline phosphatase staining can quench the fluorescence of the anti-P-granule antibody conjugate.

V. Interpretation

A. Generality of the Technique

We have used this protocol to analyze the expression pattern of 21 genes expressed during embryogenesis (Seydoux and Fire, 1994). We find that the protocol allows the visualization of RNA in well-preserved embryos from the one-cell stage to the pretzel stage (Fig. 1). In general, RNAs are detected in the cytoplasm of cells, with the exception of embryonically transcribed RNAs, which can sometimes be detected in nuclei when they are first transcribed in early blastomeres. Low-abundance RNAs expressed after the lima bean stage can be difficult to detect; proteinase K digestion of embryos prior to hybridization can be helpful in such cases (P. Okkema, pers. comm.). Although the protocol was developed to detect RNAs in embryos, preliminary results suggest that it will also be applicable for detecting RNAs in larvae and adults (G. S. and A. F., unpublished data).

B. *lacZ* Fusion RNAs

Because of their great abundance, RNAs derived from chromosomally integrated *lacZ* fusions are an excellent target for *in situ* hybridization. When first transcribed, these RNAs accumulate in two nuclear foci, which may correspond to the sites of transcription on the two homologous chromosomes that carry the array (Seydoux and Fire, 1994). The appearance of these "double dots" can help determine the earliest onset of transcription for a gene of interest. Double dots can occasionally also be seen for endogenous RNAs, but are in general more difficult to detect. In contrast to endogenous RNAs that quickly accumulate in

Table I

Problem	Cause	Solution
Nonspecific staining: patchy or uniform staining on the surface of embryos and/or staining of all nuclei	Embryo clumping	Limit hypochlorite treatment to minimum time needed for removal of adult and larval carcasses. Before transferring the embryo suspension to the slide, use a micropipet to blow air in the suspension to break any clumps.
	Poor freeze-cracking step	Embryos should be in small volume of PBS (15 μl for a 14 × 14-mm well). Avoid having small pieces of agar on the slide. Use more than one well for each experiment (four wells usually guarantee at least one good freeze-crack).
Nonspecific staining: faint staining all over embryos	Excessive probe concentration	Reduce concentration of probe. (Concentrations in the range 0.5–2.5 ng/μl are recommended for most RNAs.)
Nonspecific staining: faint staining in extruded portions of embryos	This appears to be an intrinsic property of the Boehringer antidigoxigenin AP-conjugated antibody	Only intact embryos should be examined.
No signal	Oversquashed embryos	Do not press too hard on the coverslip when freezing the embryos.
	Proteinase K over- or underdigestion	Vary concentration and/or duration of proteinase K digestion *Note:* Proteinase K digestion can boost the signal obtained from RNAs in lima bean stage and older embryos. Proteinase K digestion is not recommended for pregastrulation embryos.
	Low probe concentration	Increase probe concentration.
No embryos left on slide	Poor freeze-cracking step	Reduce volume of PBS used in freeze-cracking step.
	Not enough polylysine	Slides are best when subbed with polylysine solution the day of the *in situ* hybridization.

the cytoplasm after their initial appearance in the nucleus, *lacz* fusion RNAs remain predominantly nuclear and appear quite labile until the 26-cell stage (Seydoux and Fire, 1994). After that stage, *lacZ* fusion RNAs accumulate in the cytoplasm and become more stable, often perduring longer than endogenous RNAs. This behavior of *lacZ* fusion RNAs may be due to the long, intronless coding region of the *lacZ* gene.

C. Background versus Authentic Staining

A common problem associated with the protocol presented here is the high incidence of nonspecific sticking of the probe to embryos. Often, up to 50% of all wells in an experiment exhibit some form of nonspecific staining. This problem may be due to variability in the permeabilization of embryos introduced during the freeze-cracking step. Fortunately, this nonspecific staining is easily distinguished from authentic staining. Nonspecific staining usually appears within 10 minutes in the color reaction as dark purple patches on the surface of embryos or in nuclei. The best way to distinguish authentic staining from nonspecific staining is to compare staining patterns obtained from both antisense and sense probes. Any staining common to both probes is likely to be due to nonspecific background. In our experience, successful hybridization with sense probes yields embryos with no staining at all.

VI. Troubleshooting

In Table I, we list suggestions to limit the occurrence of nonspecific staining and other common problems.

Acknowledgments

We are grateful to Nipam Patel, who encouraged us to develop *in situ* hybridization for *C. elegans* embryos and generously shared his protocols and expertise. We thank Tom Evans, David Greenstein, Vincent Guacci, Mike Krause, Shohei Mitani, Pete Okkema, Neela Patel, and Jorge Mancillas for advice; Susan Strome for her anti-P-granule antibodies; David Bird, Dave Hsu, Edward Kipreos, Verena Plunger, Jim Priess, Ann Sluder, Deborah Roussell, Karen Bennett, Patty Wohldmann, and Bob Waterston for DNA clones; and Bill Kelly and Peter Okkema for critical reading of the manuscript. G.S. is a Helen Hay Whitney Foundation Postdoctoral Fellow. A.F. is a Rita Allen Foundation Scholar. Work in this laboratory was supported by the National Institutes of Health (Grant R01 GM-37706) and by the Carnegie Institution of Washington.

References

Costa, M., Weir, M., Coulson, A., Sulston, J., and Kenyon, C. (1988). Posterior pattern formation in *C. elegans* involves position-specific expression of a gene containing a homeobox. *Cell* **55,** 747–756.

Davis, L. G., Dibner, M. D., and Battey, J. F. (1986). In "Basic Methods in Molecular Biology" Elsevier, New York.

Edwards, M. K., and Wood, W. B. (1983). Location of specific messenger RNAs in *C. elegans* by cytological hybridization. *Dev. Biol.* **97**, 375–390.

Evans, T. C., Crittenden, S. L., Kodoyianni, L., and Kimble, J. (1994). Translational control of maternal *glp-1* mRNA establishes an asymmetry in the *C. elegans* embryos. *Cell* **77**, 183–194.

Hecht, R. M., Gossett, L. A., and Jeffery, W. R. (1981). Ontogeny of maternal and newly transcribed mRNA analyzed by in situ hybridization during development of *C. elegans*. *Dev. Biol.* **83**, 374–379.

Kimble, J., and Hirsh, D. (1979). Post-embryonic cell lineages of the hermaphrodite and male gonads in C. elegans. *Dev. Biol.* **70**, 396–417.

Klass, M., Dow, B., and Herndon, M. (1982). Cell-specific transcriptional regulation of the major sperm protein in *C. elegans*. *Dev. Biol.* **93**, 152–164.

MacMorris, M., and Blumenthal, T. (1993). In situ analysis of *C. elegans* vitellogenin fusion gene expression in integrated transgenic strains-effects of promoter mutations on RNA localization. *Gene Expression* **3**, 27–36.

Mitani, S., Du, H., Hall, D. H., Driscoll, M., and Chalfie, M. (1993). Combinatorial control of touch receptor neuron expression in *Caenorhabditis elegans. Development* **119**, 773–783.

Patel, N. H., and Goodman, C. S. (1992). Preparation of digoxigenin-labeled single-stranded DNA probes. *In* "Non-radioactive Labeling and Detection of Biomolecules" (C. Kessler, ed.). Springer-Verlag, Berlin.

Roussell, D. L., and Bennett, K. L. (1992). *Caenorhabditis* cDNA encodes an eIF-4A-like protein. *Nucleic Acids Res.* **20**, 3783.

Schedin, P., Hunter, C., and Wood, W. B. (1991). Autonomy and non-autonomy of sex determination in triploid intersex mosaics of *C. elegans. Development* **112**, 833–879.

Seydoux, G., and Fire, A. (1994). Soma-germline asymmetry in the distributions of embryonic RNAs in *C. elegans. Development*, 2823–2834.

Strome, S., and Wood, W. (1982). Immunofluorescence visualization of germ-like specific cytoplasmic granules in embryos, larvae and adults of *Caenorhabditis elegans. PNAS* **79**, 1558–1562.

Sulston, J. E., and Horvitz, H. R. (1977). Postembryonic cell lineages of the nematode *Caenorhabditis elegans. Dev. Biol.* **56**, 110–156.

Sulston, J. E., Shierenberg, E., White, J. G., and Thomas, J. N. (1983). The embryonic cell lineage of the nematode *Caenorhabditis elegans. Dev. Biol.* **100**, 64–119.

Tautz, D., and Pfeifle, C. (1989). A nonradioactive *in situ* hybridization method for the localization of specific RNAs in *Drosophila* embryos reveals translational control of the segmentation gene *hunchback. Chromosoma* **98**, 81–85.

Waterson, R., Martin, C., Craxton, M., Huynh, C., Coulson, A., Hillier, L., Durbin, R., Green, P., Shownkeen, R., Halooran, N., Metzstein, M., Hawkins, T., Wilson, R., Berks, M., Du, Z., Thomas, J., Thierry-Mieg, J., and Sulton, J. (1992). A survey of expressed genes in *Caenorhabditis elegans. Nature Genet.* **1**, 114–123.

Wightman, B., Ha, I., and Ruvkun, G. B. (1993). Postranscriptional regulation of the heterochronic gene *lin-14* by *lin-4* mediates temporal pattern formation in *C. elegans. Cell* **75**, 855–862.

CHAPTER 15

Fluorescence *in Situ* Hybridization for the Detection of DNA and RNA

Donna G. Albertson, Rita M. Fishpool, and Philip S. Birchall

MRC Laboratory of Molecular Biology
Cambridge CB2 2QH, England

I. Introduction

Both the location and distribution of nucleic acid sequences in genomes and in cells can be visualized by hybridization of labeled probe DNAs to cytological preparations of chromosomes or tissues. With the introduction of nonisotopically labeled nucleotides that could be incorporated into cloned DNAs by enzymatic methods *in vitro,* it became possible to detect the site of hybridization quickly using antibodies that recognized the modifying group on the nucleotides incorporated into the probe DNA. More recently, nucleotides labeled with a fluorescent molecule have been incorporated into probes by *in vitro* enzymatic reactions and the site of hybridization can then be visualized directly. As fluorescence *in situ* hybridization provides a rapid and high-resolution method for mapping genes, it is being used increasingly for mapping cloned DNAs to chromosomes and for the ordering of clones in large-scale genome projects. On the other hand, physically mapped clones can also be used to label chromosomes for analysis of such biological processes as chromosome segregation, pairing in meiosis, and interphase nuclear order. Nonisotopic methods of hybridization are also ideally suited to visualization of mRNA distributions in tissues, because the signal can be detected in thick specimens, in contrast to isotopic methods that require thin specimens for detection by autoradiography.

There are two elements to consider in any *in situ* hybridization method: tissue preparation and probe labeling. The specimens must be fixed so that the target nucleic acids are held in place and the morphology must be maintained, even when subjected to harsh treatments, such as denaturation of the DNA. Probe molecules, however, must still be able to penetrate well. Probe labeling is also of critical importance, because, unlike other methods of hybridization to matrix-bound nucleic acids, when hybridizing to cytological material the number of target molecules may be as few as two to four on chromosomes, and they may be distributed throughout a large volume in the cytoplasm of cells. Depending on the application, there appear to be different optimal fixation protocols, methods of labeling probes, and amounts of modified nucleotide to incorporate. Often these parameters can be determined only empirically. Therefore, when starting out, it is best to select a large repetitive target, such as the ribosomal genes, present in about 100 copies on the chromosome and transcribed in all cells. Almost always, once a signal has been obtained, it is possible to make it bigger and better by practice and by minor adjustment to the protocol to suit a particular application. This is not so easily done, if no signal is seen.

II. Nucleotides and Stains Used for Fluorescence *in Situ* Hybridization

The earliest work on fluorescence *in situ* hybridization with *Caenorhabditis elegans* was done using biotin–dUTP (Albertson, 1984a, 1985) and later digoxigenin (DIG)–dUTP, detecting the site of hybridization by immunofluorescence. Current work uses fluorescently labeled nucleotides almost exclusively for labeling probes, and these are visualized directly. Table I lists the modified nucleotides that have been used for *in situ* hybridization with *C. elegans*. The list is not exhaustive, and there are a number of other modified nucleotides in common use for fluorescence *in situ* hybridization that would probably be suitable. Note that both biotin- and DIG-labeled probes can be visualized by antibodies labeled with any of the fluorochromes listed in Table I, and when used for immunofluorescence, their spectral properties will be similar, but may differ slightly. In addition, the site of hybridization of biotin- and DIG-labeled probes can be visualized by bright-field microscopy. The use of these methods for studying the tissue distribution of mRNA is described in Chapter 14 in this volume.

When probes are hybridized to DNA, the chromosomes or nuclei can be counterstained with one of the fluorescent stains listed in Table II. By comparing the spectral properties of the fluorescently labeled nucleotides and the DNA counterstains, combinations can be chosen for detection of several probes simultaneously. Up to seven probes have been detected when probes were labeled with two different fluorochromes and the hybridization signals recorded by fluorescence ratio imaging (Ried *et al.*, 1992).

III. Sources of Target Material for Hybridization

A. Metaphase Chromosomes

In *C. elegans* hermaphrodites, the diploid number of chromosomes is 12, there being five pairs of autosomes and a pair of sex chromosomes. In males, the diploid number is 11, as males arise by nondisjunction of the X chromosomes and carry only a single copy of this chromosome. Mitotic chromosomes are found most readily in cells undergoing the early embryonic cleavage divisions, and metaphase spreads can be visualized by squashing embryos on glass microscope slides (Albertson *et al.*, 1979). The chromosomes are nearly uniform in size, and in the earliest divisions, chromosomes, approximately 5 μm in length, can be seen. As development proceeds, however, the chromosomes appear more condensed and uniform in size. *C. elegans* chromosomes are holocentric; that is, at metaphase the kinetochore forms along the length of the chromosome, rather than at a single locus. Therefore, the chromosomes lack any visible primary constriction that demarcates the centromere of monocentric chromosomes (Albertson and Thomson, 1982). Additionally,

Table I
Fluorescent Nucleotides Used for *in Situ* Hybridization

| Nucleotide[a] | Manufacturer | Spectral properties[b] | | Microscopy | | |
| | | Absorbance maximum (nm) | Emission maximum (nm) | Conventional fluorescence illumination, mercury lamp | | Confocal laser scanning illumination, Kr/Ar laser |
				Excitation	Emission	Excitation (nm)
Fluorescein–dUTP Fluorescein–12-dUTP	Boehringer-Mannheim	495	520	Blue	Green	488
Rhodamine–dUTP Rhodamine–4-dUTP	Amersham, "FluoroRed"	545	575	Green/yellow	Orange	568
Cy3–dCTP Cy3.29–amido-13-dCTP	Biological Detection Systems	552	565	Green/yellow	Orange	568
Cy5–dCTP Cy5.29–amido-13-dCTP	Biological Detection Systems	650	667	Green/yellow	Infrared[c]	647

[a] Chemical formula available in some cases from manufacturer's data sheets.
[b] Data from manufacturer's specification sheets.
[c] Requires electronic imaging device, such as photomultiplier or cooled CCD camera.

Table II
Fluorochromes Used for Staining Nucleic Acids

| | Spectral properties[a] | | Microscopy | | Confocal laser scanning illumination, Kr/Ar laser |
| | | | Conventional fluorescence illumination, mercury lamp | | |
Stain	Absorbance maximum (nm)	Emission maximum[b] (nm)	Excitation	Emission	Excitation (nm)
DAPI	359	461	Near UV	Blue	Not suitable
Hoechst 33258	346	460	Near UV/violet	Blue/green	Not suitable
Propidium iodide	536	617	Green/yellow	Red	488 or 568

[a] Haugland (1994).
[b] Emission maxima when bound to DNA.

as banding patterns are generally absent, there are few features to distinguish one linkage group from another. This has necessitated the development of cytological methods for distinguishing both linkage groups and also the left–right orientation of the chromosome (Albertson, 1984a, 1985).

B. Meiotic Chromosomes

Another source of chromosomes for *in situ* hybridization may be found in adult hermaphrodites. The two reflexed arms of the gonad contain many nuclei progressing through meiotic prophase, the least mature near the distal tip cell. Proximally, the nuclei arrest in diakinesis with highly condensed bivalents, prior to fertilization. In the distal arm, synapsed chromosomes are arrayed around a large central nucleolus, and although visible as distinct chromosomes, they are rarely obtained well spread and distinguishable. Hybridization of probes to meiotic chromosomes, however, can be accomplished with sufficient resolution to distinguish whether two probes are linked on a chromosome or a single probe hybridizes at one or multiple sites, due to alterations in chromosome pairing, resulting from a chromosome rearrangement or mutation (Albertson, 1993).

C. Whole Embryos or Animals

The small size and transparency of embryonic, larval, and adult stages of *C. elegans* make hybridization to whole animals or embryos feasible. By combination of fluorescence *in situ* hybridization with confocal imaging, the distribution of nucleic acid sequences in nuclei and tissues of the organism can be determined at high resolution. Methods for hybridization to embryos, larvae, and adults immobilized on glass microscope slides or in suspension have been developed (Albertson and Thomson, 1993; Birchall, 1993).

IV. Applications

A. Mapping Genes on Metaphase Chromosomes

As the metaphase chromosomes are generally featureless, the identification of both the chromosomes and the left–right orientation along the chromosome is accomplished by hybridization of previously mapped probes together with the probe being mapped (Albertson, 1985). In addition, genetically characterized chromosome rearrangements that result in morphological changes to the karyotype that are easily visualized cytologically can be used to distinguish one linkage group from another. By combining a number of chromosome rearrangements, a mapping strain (CB3740, available from the *Caenorhabditis* Genetics Center) was constructed that allows a number of linkage groups to be distinguished using hybridization of a ribosomal gene probe to distinctively label the right ends of linkage groups I (*eDf24*) and II (*eDp20*). Linkage groups IV and X together are distinguished as the double-length translocation chromosome, *mnT12(IV;X),* as shown in Figs. 1 and 2, see color plate for Fig. 2. To map a DNA clone, it is first hybridized to *eDf24;eDp20;mnT12* chromosomes together with the ribosomal gene probe. If the unmapped clone hybridizes to either linkage group I or II, then the position along the chromosome can be assigned as the percentage distance from the genetic left end of the chromosome. Hybridization to the long *mnT12* chromosome indicates that the cloned DNA maps to either linkage group IV or X, whereas hybridization to one of the two unmarked chromosomes indicates that the cloned DNA is located on linkage group III or V. In these

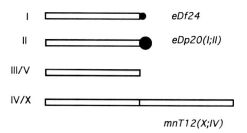

Fig. 1 Karyotype of *eDf24;eDp20(I;II);mnT12(X;IV).* An idiogram of the metaphase karyotype of *eDf24;eDp20(I;II);mnT12(X;IV)* is drawn. The ribosomal deficiency, *eDf24,* results in a loss of most of the ribosomal gene cluster on linkage group I; therefore hybridization of the ribosomal DNA probe gives a small signal on this chromosome. Hybridization of the ribosomal DNA probe to *eDp20(I;II)* gives a large signal. The distinctive hybridization signals of the ribosomal probe on these rearrangement chromosomes identified the right ends of linkage groups I and II, while X and IV together are recognized as the double-length chromosome. The small circle indicates the position of the ribosomal deficiency, *eDf24,* and the large circle indicates the ribosomal duplication *eDp20(I;II).*

latter cases, a second hybridization experiment is necessary to distinguish between these alternatives using a marker for one of the possible chromosomes. Finally, it is necessary that the cloned DNA be mapped with a marker on the same chromosome so that the left–right orientation of the position can be determined. The location of the center of the hybridization site on ten or more chromosomes is plotted and the position determined as a range of percentage distances along the chromosome from the left end (Albertson, 1985).

B. Mapping Chromosome Rearrangement Breakpoints to the Physical Map

As most chromosome rearrangements are homozygous lethal, they are maintained as heterozygotes. Analysis of rearrangement breakpoints, by hybridization of physically mapped probes thought to be near the genetically defined rearrangement breakpoints to the rearranged metaphase chromosomes, would be difficult, because the embryonic metaphases will have different karyotypes (heterozygous for the rearrangement, or homozygous for either the rearrangement or the balancer chromosome). The meiotic prophase nuclei of the heterozygous, rearrangement-bearing hermaphrodites, however, are a source of nuclei of defined genetic composition (rearrangement/balancer), and the pattern of hybridization of probes to these nuclei can be predicted from the genotype of the animal. Because the chromosomes are normally synapsed in pachytene nuclei, only one hybridization signal is normally expected from a probe. In animals carrying a rearranged chromosome, the pattern of hybridization can be altered (Albertson, 1993). To map a free duplication, for example, probes mapping in or near the duplicated regions are hybridized to meiotic prophase nuclei. If a probe is included in the duplication, then two hybridization signals will be seen; probes not included in the duplication result in only one hybridization signal (Figs. 3a and b). In a similar fashion, it is possible to map deficiencies or translocation breakpoints when the rearranged chromosomes no longer pair with a normal homologous region, because the site or sites of hybridization of the probe on the meiotic prophase nuclei will be spatially distinct (Figs. 3a and c, see color plate for parts b and c).

C. Distribution of Nucleic Acid Sequences in Whole Organisms

In the previous applications, fluorescence *in situ* hybridization was used to generate maps and no attempt was made to preserve the three-dimensional morphology of the organism, as chromosomes are most easily visualized in flattened specimens. The physically mapped probes may also be used to study questions of chromosome biology (Albertson and Thomson, 1993) or the tissue distribution of messenger RNA (Fig. 4), and in these applications it is desirable to maintain the three–dimensional architecture of the nucleus or cell.

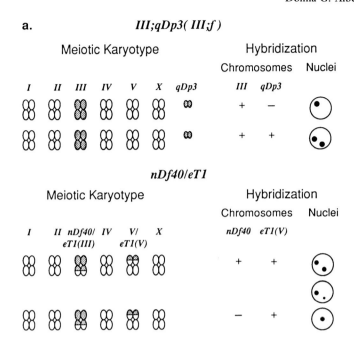

Fig. 3 Mapping chromosome rearrangements on meiotic chromosomes. (a) Idiograms of the meiotic karyotypes of oocytes in hermaphrodites heterozygous for two chromosomal rearrangements, *qDp3* (Austin and Kimble, 1987) and *nDf40* (Hengartner *et al.*, 1992), and the predicted patterns of hybridization expected on meiotic prophase nuclei. Chromosomes carrying linkage group III are shaded. The rearrangement, *qDp3*, is a duplication of part of linkage group III and is present in addition to the normal linkage group III bivalent. It is cytologically visible as a smaller chromsome. Two hybridization signals will be seen with YAC probes included in *qDp3;* otherwise only one signal is seen. The deficiency, *nDf40*, is balanced by *eT1(III;V)*. The rearrangement, *eT1*, is a reciprocal translocation involving linkage groups III and V. In +/*eT1* animals, the half-translocation, *eT1(V)*, which includes the right half of linkage group III, pairs with and disjoins from linkage group V. Therefore, hybridization of YAC probes for the right half of linkage group III will result in two hybridization signals. In *nDf40/eT1* animals the deficiency chromosome pairs with and disjoins from *eT1(III)*. Because the deficiency, *nDf40*, maps to the right half of linkage group III, hybridization of YAC probes from the right half of linkage group III that are included in the deficiency will result in only a single hybridization signal, rather than two. If a YAC is partially included in the deficiency, one hybridization signal may appear smaller than the other one. (b, see color plate) Hybridization of a YAC to linkage group III and *qDp3* chromosomes at diakinesis. The *qDp3* chromosome is easily identified by its small size compared with the 6 bivalents. Different shades of red false color in the hybridization signals are due to the intensity differences in the blue false color in the chromosome. Bar = 5 μm. (c, see color plate) Hybridization of YACs to meiotic prophase nuclei from *nDf40/eT1* hermaphrodites. The right half of linkage group (LG) III is carried on *eT1(V)* in this strain, and so pairs and disjoins from the wild-type copy of LG V, while the left half of LG III on *eT1(III)* pairs and disjoins from *nDf40*. Therefore, YACs mapping to the right half of LG III will hybridize to two sites on meiotic prophase nuclei (top). The inclusion of a YAC in the deficiency is indicated by the presence of only one hybridization signal from the YAC (middle), while a YAC partially included in the deficiency (bottom) may show one normal-sized hybridization signal and one visibly smaller signal. Bar = 5 μm.

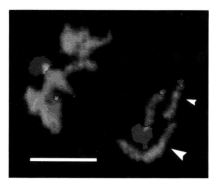

Fig. 2 Mapping the cosmid K10B4 on metaphase chromosomes. Embryo squashes were prepared as described in Section VI,A and were hybridized with the ribosomal probe, pCe7, and the cosmid, K10B4, labeled by nick translation with biotin–dUTP. The site of hybridization was detected with rabbit anti-biotin and Texas red-labeled goat anti-rabbit antibodies. Chromosomes were stained with Hoechst 33258. The slides were viewed with a conventional fluorescence microscope and the individual Hoechst 33258 and Texas red images were recorded with a microchannel plate-intensified CCD camera, stored digitally, then merged and displayed in false color using a Bio-Rad MRC600 workstation (Albertson *et al.,* 1991). Blue, Hoechst 33258; red, Texas red. The cosmid was assigned to linkage group II because it was located on the same chromosome as the large hybridization signal, characteristic of the hybridization of pCe7 to the ribosomal genes on the right end of *eDp20*. The *mnT12(X;IV)* chromosome can be identified by its length (large arrowhead) and the *eDf24* chromosome by the hybridization signal from pCe7 (small arrowhead). The three chromosomes on the right are well spread. Batches of slides vary, with some preparations showing many well-spread metaphases and some none. The cytological map position is assigned from data collected from 10 well-spread chromosomes and the position usually spans a 10–20% interval on the chromosome. Bar-5 μm.

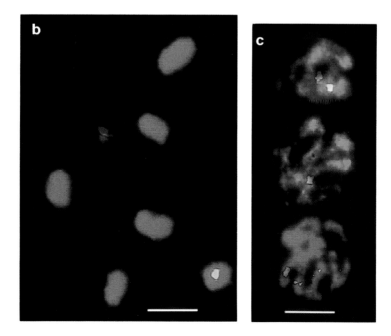

Fig. 3   *(continued)*

V. Probe Labeling

A variety of methods for *in vitro* synthesis of nucleic acids can be used with nucleotides carrying haptens or fluorescent groups. Most DNA or RNA probes have been labeled using modified dUTP or UTP, but more recently, dCTP, modified with either of the cyanine dyes, Cy3 or Cy5, has become available. Both Cy3- and Cy5-labeled dCTP have been successfully incorporated into DNA probes by the nick-translation and random priming procedures outlined below, but have not been tried in the other reactions. Generally, the best probes for DNA *in situ* hybridization are synthesized by nick translation. For RNA *in situ* hybridization, riboprobes synthesized by *in vitro* transcription with SP6 or T7 polymerase have provided the brightest signals.

A. Nick Translation

For hybridization to DNA, the cloned probe is most often labled by *in vitro* nick translation (Rigby *et al.,* 1977) to incorporate the modified nucleotide. Nick translation is useful in this application because the frequency with which nicks are introduced into the probe DNA can be adjusted so that the small pieces of DNA (about 200–400 nucleotides in length), produced on denaturation, are optimal for *in situ* hybridization (Albertson, 1985). The reaction can be difficult to control, however, and the pieces of probe DNA may be too small or snapback DNA can be formed in the reaction that does not hybridize. This will result in weak signal or signal all over the slide, often referred to as a "spotty probe." Failure to label the probe successfully by nick translation is a frequent problem with nonisotopic *in situ* hybridization. The cause is not known, but it appears that the reaction is inhibited by contaminants in the DNA preparation. As the only assay for the quality of the probe is *in situ* hybridization, a method is described for preparing the DNA that ensures that the cloned DNA can be nick translated to incorporate modified nucleotides, such as biotin–dUTP, DIG–dUTP, or nucleotides carrying the fluorescent labels, fluorescein, rhodamine, Cy3, or Cy5 (Fishpool and Albertson, 1992).

1. Preparation of Cosmid DNA

1. Pick single colonies from freshly streaked plates and grow at 37°C for 8 hours or overnight with shaking in 4 ml 2 × TY, plus the appropriate antibiotic.

2. Take 1 ml of the overnight culture and inoculate 100 ml TB (Tartof and Hobbs, 1981) plus the appropriate antibiotic and grow at 37°C with shaking for 8 hours.

3. Collect bacteria by centrifugation in a bench-top centrifuge at 3000 rpm for 15 minutes. The bacteria can be frozen at this time or resuspended in 4 ml of 25 m*M* Tris–HCl, pH 8.0, 10 m*M* ethylenediaminetetraacetic acid (EDTA), 1% glucose.

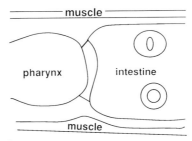

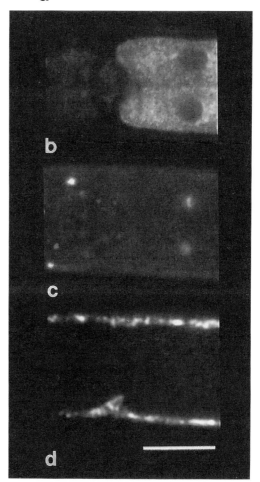

4. Leave pellet on ice for 5 minutes, then add freshly prepared 0.2 *M* NaOH, 1% sodium dodecyl sulfate (SDS), and leave on ice for a further 5 minutes.

5. Add 6 ml "5 *M* potassium acetate" (3 *M* potassium acetate and 2*M* acetic acid) and spin at 10,000 rpm for 20 minutes in a preparative centrifuge.

6. Add 2 vol. of 95% ethanol to the supernatant and leave at room temperature for 2 minutes before spinning at 3000 rpm for 15 minutes in a bench-top centrifuge.

7. Resuspend pellet in 6 ml TE (10 m*M* Tris–HCl, pH 7.4, 0.1 m*M* EDTA) and then add 4.5 ml 5 *M* LiCl. Leave at −20°C for 15 minutes. Spin at 2500 rpm for 10 minutes.

8. Add 25 ml of 95% ethanol to the supernatant, and precipitate at −20°C for 1 hour. Spin at 3000 rpm for 15 minutes, and resuspend the pellet in 10 ml TE.

9. For the final purification of the DNA using a Qiagen-tip 500 column (Diagen), follow the manufacturer's directions for "Maxi Preparations," beginning at step 5.

The yield of cosmid DNA should be 200–800 μg. For the preparation of smaller amounts of plasmid DNA from 3-ml cultures, a modified "miniprep" method omitting the LiCl precipitation step, followed by purification over Qiagen-tip 20 columns, can be used.

TB: Tryptone, 12 g; yeast extract, 24 g; glycerol, 4 g; H_2O, 900 ml. Autoclave and then add 100 ml 0.17 *M* KH_2PO_4, 0.72 *M* K_2HPO_4.

2. Nick Translation

Typically, 1 to 4 μg of cloned DNA is labeled in a 100-μl final volume (Albertson, 1984). In initial experiments, or if required as a marker, a small amount of the ribosomal DNA probe pCe7 (Files and Hirsh, 1981; see also Chapter 22 in this volume) is included.

Fig. 4 Distribution of three RNA species in an optical section from a whole mount of an adult N2. Three probes, nick-translated to incorporate fluorescein–dUTP [probe for *vit-6* mRNA, (b)] Cy3–dCTP [pCe7, ribosomal RNA (c)], and Cy5–dCTP [probe for *unc-54* mRNA (d)] were hybridized to whole animals as described in Section VI,D. The hybridization signals from the three probes were imaged separately from a single optical section with a Bio-Rad MRC600 confocal microscope using a Kr–Ar mixed gas laser. (a) Drawing of a portion of an adult hermaphrodite near the anterior end of the intestine. (b) Hybridization signal from the fluorescein-labeled probe for *vit-6* mRNA is seen in the intestine. The intestinal cell nuclei can be distinguished by the absence of hybridization signal. (c) Hybridization signal from the probe for ribosomal RNA is seen in all cells, with most intense signals from the nucleoli. The signal resulting from hybridization to the nucleoli in the intestinal cell nuclei can be identified by comparing the patterns of hybridization in b and c. (d) Hybridization signal from the Cy5-labeled probe for *unc-54* mRNA can be seen dorsally and ventrally in two body wall muscle quadrants. Bar = 25 μm.

To a 1.5-ml microfuge tube on ice add:

pCe7 DNA, 0.5 μg

Cosmid DNA, 1–4 μg

10× NT buffer I, 10μl

0.5 mM dATP, 2.5 μl

0.5 mM dCTP*, 2.5 μl

0.5 mM dGTP, 2.5 μl

0.5 mM dTTP*, 2.5 μl

0.03 mM biotin–dUTP, 3 μl (*omitting dTTP); or 0.1 mM X–dUTP; 1 μl
(where X is DIG, fluorescein, or rhodamine and *omitting dTTP); or
0.1 mM X–dCTP, 1 μl (where X is Cy3 or Cy5 and *omitting dCTP)

H$_2$O, as required for a final volume of 100 μl

Diluted DNase I, 5 μl

DNA polymerase I, 20 units

Incubate the reaction at 12–13°C for 25 minutes. Stop the reaction by adding
25 μl of 0.1 M EDTA and heat at 65°C for 10 minutes. The probe can be
precipitated at −20°C overnight with 2.5 vol of 95% ethanol after addition of
5 μl of tRNA (10 mg/ml) and 15 μl of 2 M sodium acetate, pH 7.0. Pellet
DNA, wash with 70% ethanol, and air-dry. Typically, if 4 μg of template
DNA has been used in the reaction, then for DNA *in situ* hybridization
the pellet is resuspended in 280 μl of formamide buffer. This will give a final
volume of 400 μl of hybridization mixture after addition of 3 M NaCl and 50%
dextran sulfate at the time of hybridization. For RNA *in situ* hybridization, the
probe is dissolved in 20 μl HS (see Section VI,D,3). The probe can also be
cleaned up using a Qiagen-tip 5 column following the manufacturer's directions
for "DNA Purification after Enzymatic Modifications." Before precipitation with
0.8 vol of isopropanol, add 5 μl 10 mg/ml tRNA and 0.1 vol 4 M Na acetate,
pH 4.8. Pellet the DNA by spinning at 4°C for 1 hour in a microfuge, wash the
pellet twice with 300 μl 70% ethanol, air-dry, and resuspend in 280 μl formamide
buffer or 20 μl HS.

10× NT buffer I: 0.5 M Tris–HCl, pH 7.4, 0.1 M MgCl$_2$, 10 mM dithiothreitol (DTT).

10× NT buffer II: 0.5 M Tris–HCl, pH 7.4, 50 mM MgCl$_2$, 0.1% bovine serum
albumin (BSA).

DNase I: A 1 mg/ml stock solution of DNase I is made up in 20 mM Tris–HCl,
pH 7.4, 50 mM NaCl, 1 mM DTT, 0.01% BSA, and 50% glycerol, and 1-ml
aliquots are stored at −20°C. Just before use, the stock solution is diluted 1 : 400
in 1× NT buffer II.

tRNA: A 10 mg/ml solution of yeast tRNA in water is extracted once with
phenol and stored at −20°C.

Formamide buffer: Formamide (Fluka), 100 μl; 100 mM 1,4-piperazinedie-thanesulfonic acid (Pipes), 10 mM EDTA, pH 7.0, 20 μl; H_2O, 20 μl.

B. Random Priming

In this method, DNA is synthesized *in vitro* from a single-stranded DNA template using random hexanucleotides annealed to the DNA to prime the Klenow fragment of *Escherichia coli* DNA polymerase (Feinberg and Vogelstein, 1984). After hybridization with probes labeled by random priming the background is often high; however, the labeling reaction does not appear to be as sensitive to impurities in the DNA preparation as the nick translation reaction. Random priming has been used to incorporate biotin–dUTP, DIG–dUTP, fluorescein–dUTP, rhodamine–dUTP, Cy3–dCTP, or Cy5–dCTP into a DNA probe.

To a microfuge tube on ice, add: denatured DNA, 0.01–3 μg; hexanucleotide mixture, 2 μl; 10× dNTP–X mixture, 2 μl; H_2O, as required for a final volume of 20 μl; Klenow DNA polymerase, 2 units. The reaction mixture is incubated at 37°C for at least 60 minutes to overnight, and the reaction is stopped by the addition of 2 μl of 0.2 M EDTA. The reaction mixture can then be precipitated with ethanol, and the pellet resuspended in formamide buffer, as described for nick translated probes, or 0.2 to 0.5 μl of the reaction can be diluted directly into formamide buffer just before use.

Hexanucleotide mixture: The random hexanucleotides (Boehringer-Mannheim) are supplied at a concentration of 62.5 A_{260} units/ml in 10× random priming buffer.

10× dNTP–X mixture: 1 mM dATP, 1 mM dCTP, 1 mM dGTP, 0.65 mM dTTP, 0.35 mM X–dUTP (where X is biotin, DIG, fluorescein, or rhodamine). For labeling with Cy3– or Cy5–dCTP, 1 mM fluorescent dCTP is used in place of dCTP. This mixture is made up from a 20× stock solution of the unlabeled nucleotides. This is then diluted to the 10× concentrated mixture by the addition of 1 mM labeled nucleotide (X–dUTP) and water as follows: 20× unlabeled nucleotides, 10 μl; 1 mM X–dUTP, 7 μl; H_2O, 3 μl.

C. Polymerase Chain Reaction

The polymerase chain reaction (Saiki *et al.*, 1988) can be used to synthesize probes for hybridization *in situ* to both DNA (Albertson *et al.*, 1991) and RNA (Birchall, 1993). Deoxynucleotide triphosphates are used at a final concentration of 200 μM, and for labeling the product, 20 to 60% of the dTTP is substituted with biotin–dUTP, DIG–dUTP, or fluorescein–dUTP. In the reaction outlined below, the modified dUTP is added to a final concentration of 40 μM and the dTTP concentration is reduced to 160 μM.

In a 0.5-μl microfuge tube on ice combine the following reagents:

10× PCR buffer, 5 μl

2 mM dATP, dCTP, dGTP, 5 μl

2 m*M* dTTP, 4 μl

1 m*M* X–dUTP, 2 μl (where X is biotin, DIG, or fluorescein)

10 μ*M* forward primer, 5 μl

10 μ*M* reverse primer, 5 μl

Template DNA, 1 ng

H$_2$O, as required for a final volume of 50 μl

Taq polymerase, 5 units

Before adding the enzyme, overlay this mixture with mineral oil and heat at 95°C for 2 minutes. Add the Taq polymerase, centrifuge briefly, and then carry out 30 cycles as follows: 95°C, 0.5 minutes; 55°C, 1.0 minute; 72°C, 1.5 minutes. After a final extension at 72°C for 5 minutes, carefully take the reaction mixture from under the mineral oil. To remove the last few microliters of the reaction mixture from the tube, rinse with 50 μl of 10 m*M* Tris–HCl, 1 m*M* EDTA. Precipitate the DNA at −20°C overnight with 2.5 vol of ethanol, after addition of 12 μl of 4 *M* LiCl and 80 μg of tRNA. Wash the precipitate twice with 95% ethanol to remove any traces of mineral oil and then with 70% ethanol. Air-dry the precipitate and resuspend in 70 μl formamide buffer, as for nick-translated probes. Because a large quantity of DNA is produced in the reaction, these probe mixtures can be diluted a further 10-fold or more for hybridization.

10× PCR buffer: 0.1 *M* Tris–HCl, pH 8.3, 0.5 *M* KCl, 15 m*M* MgCl$_2$, 0.1% gelatin. Autoclave and store aliquots at −20°C.

D. Degenerate Oligonucleotide-Primed Polymerase Chain Reaction

This protocol describes degenerate oligonucleotide primed PCR (DOP-PCR), a method for both general amplification of small quantities of DNA and incorporation of modified nucleotides (Telenius *et al.,* 1992a, b). It has been used to make probes from *C. elegans* DNA cloned in yeast artificial chromosomes (YACs), which have been purified by electrophoresis through low-melting-temperature agarose (Albertson, 1993). First, general amplification of the target DNA is achieved using a partially degenerate primer in the polymerase chain reaction. Initially, low-temperature annealing cycles (program 1) are carried out to promote annealing and extension of the primers at many sites. The molecules synthesized in these first cycles are then amplified in later high-temperature cycles (program 2). An aliquot of this reaction is subsequently labeled using program 2 to incorporate a modified nucleotide in the PCR product.

To a 0.5-μl microfuge tube add:

10× PCR buffer, 5 μl

2 m*M* dNTPs, 5 μl

20 μ*M* primer, 5 μl

Melted gel slice containing YAC DNA, 1 μl

H$_2$O, as required for 50-μl final volume

Taq polymerase, 5 units

Before adding the enzyme and template DNA, overlay the mixture with mineral oil. Incubate the gel slice containing the YAC DNA at 65°C to melt the agarose and add 1 μl to the reaction mixture. Heat at 95°C for 10 minutes. Add 5 units Taq polymerase and carry out five cycles of program 1 and 30 cycles of program 2, followed by a final extension at 72°C for 5 min. A 4-μl aliquot of the reaction can be electrophoresed through a 1.5% agarose gel. Amplification of a YAC will yield a smear of DNA in which 10 to 20 bands can be distinguished. To label the DNA with a modified nucleotide, set up the PCR as described in Section V,C, using 5 μl of the DOP-PCR product as template and 2 μM degenerate primer, and amplify using program 2, followed by a final 5-minute extension at 72°C. For DNA *in situ* hybridization, 0.2 μl of the reaction mixture is added to 14 μl of formamide buffer just before use.

Degenerate primers: Two degenerate primers have been used with *C. elegans,* 6MW (Telenius *et al.,* 1992a, b) and DMW11 (D. G. Albertson, D. M. Williams, and D. Brown, unpublished). The DMW11 primer has the six nucleotides of the *C. elegans* consensus 5' splice acceptor sequence incorporated in the 3' end to promote annealing to *C. elegans* exons.

6MW	5' CCGACTCGAGNNNNNNNATGTGG 3'
DMW11	5' CCGACTCGAGNNNNNNNTTTCAG 3'

Program 1: 94°C, 1.0 minute; 30°C, 1.5 minutes; transition to 72°C, 3.0 minutes; 72°C, 3.0 minutes.

Program 2: 94°C, 1.0 minute; 55°C, 1.0 minute; 72°C, 3.0 minutes, with an addition of 1 s/cycle.

E. Labeling Oligonucleotides with Terminal Deoxynucleotidyl Transferase

Terminal deoxynucleotidyl transferase (TdT) catalyzes the template-independent addition of nucleotides to the 3'-OH ends of DNA and can be used to add modified nucleotides to the 3'-OH ends of oligodeoxynucleotides (Moyzis *et al.,* 1988). The modified nucleotide is used at approximately 200 times the concentration of the 3'-OH ends of oligonucleotide. To compensate for the lower thermal stability of the hybrid formed with the oligonucleotide, the formamide concentration is reduced in the hybridization mixture, or the hybridization may be carried out at a lower temperature.

To a microfuge tube on ice add:

5× tailing buffer, 4 μl

5 mM CoCl$_2$, 6 μl

Oligonucleotide, 7 pmole

1 m*M* X–dUTP, 3 μl (where X is biotin, DIG, or fluorescein)

H₂O, as required for a final volume of 20 μl

TdT, 55 units

Incubate at 37°C for 4 hours. Stop the reaction by adding 10 μl of 0.5 *M* EDTA and precipitate with 2.5 vol of ethanol at −20°C after addition of 2 μl of 4 *M* LiCl, 80 μg tRNA, and 20 μg of glycogen. Resuspend the pellet in 70 μl of formamide buffer as for nick translated probes, except reduce the formamide concentration to 30 to 40%.

  5× Tailing buffer: 125 m*M* Tris–HCl, pH 6.6, 1 *M* potassium cacodylate, 0.125% BSA.

F. *In Vitro* Transcription

  Transcription from a cloned DNA template can be catalyzed by RNA polymerases *in vitro* if the promoter sequence is included 5′ to the cloned sequence (Butler and Chamberlain, 1982). Both SP6 and T7 RNA polymerases have been used to synthesize fluorescently labeled probes for *in situ* hybridization in *C. elegans.* For DNA cloned in a suitable vector (e.g., Stratagene Bluescript KSII or Promega pGEM-4Z), transcription was initiated from the specific promoter sequence included adjacent to the cloning site of the vector. It is also possible to introduce the promoter sequence into the template DNA by means of PCR by including the promoter sequence at the 5′ end of the sequence-specific primers. Typically, two different RNA polymerase promoter sequences are incorporated in opposite orientations, so that both sense and antisense RNA probes can be synthesized *in vitro.* Pyrophosphatase is included in the reaction to eliminate pyrophosphate that accumulates *in vitro* to levels that can inhibit the RNA polymerase by sequestering Mg^{2+} in the form of magnesium pyrophosphate (Cunningham and Ofengard, 1990). In the protocol given below, the modified UTP makes up 70% of the UTP concentration, but the modified nucleotide may replace 20 to 80% of the UTP (Birchall, 1993).

  To a microfuge tube at room temperature add:

5× transcription buffer, 20 μl

100 m*M* DTT, 10 μl

RNasin, 1 unit

10 m*M* ATP, CTP, GTP, 5 μl

10 m*M* UTP, 1.5 μl

10 m*M* X–UTP, 3.5 μl (where X is biotin, DIG, fluorescein, or rhodamine)

Template DNA, >5 μg

pyrophosphatase, 1 unit

H₂O, as required for a final volume of 100 μl

SP6 or T7 RNA polymerase, 60 units

Incubate the reaction at 37°C for 2 hours. Add 1 μl RNase-free DNase I (1 mg/ml) and incubate at 37°C for a further 15 minutes. Stop the reaction by adding 5 μl of 20% SDS. Unincorporated nucleotides are removed using the RNaid kit (Bio-Rad, La Jolla, CA.). Follow the manufacturer's instructions, but wash until no color remains in the supernatant after the labeled RNA is pelleted with the bead matrix. The RNA is eluted with water and used at a final concentration of 1μg/μl.

5× Transcription buffer: 0.4 m*M* 4-(2-hydroxyethyl)-1-piperazineethanesulfonic acid (Hepes)–KOH, pH 7.5, 80 m*M* MgCl$_2$ (for SP6 polymerase) or 60 m*M* MgCl$_2$ (for T7 polymerase), 10 m*M* spermidine, 200 m*M* DTT.

VI. Preparation of Material for Hybridization

A. Metaphase Chromosomes from Embryo Squashes

Embryos are obtained by alkaline hypochlorite lysis of gravid hermaphrodites. Three 5-cm petri plates will yield enough embryos for about five slides.

1. Fixation

1. Collect embryos by alkaline hypochlorite lysis of young gravid adults (see Chapter 1 in this volume), taking care to wash animals off the plates with a gentle stream of water so that pieces of agar that will interfere with the squashing are not dislodged. Older embryos that have already been laid will also remain behind, adhering to the bacterial lawn if this is not disturbed.

2. Pipet 50 to 100-μl aliquots of embryos onto gelatin-subbed slides (see Chapter 16 in this volume). When preparing gelatin-subbed slides for metaphase chromosomes, dissolve the gelatin by heating at 50°C. Commercially available charged slides (Fisher, 15-188-52, or BDH, Polysine, 406/0178/02) can also be used. The drops of embryos should be examined with the dissecting microscope at 25× magnification. Any fragments of glass, for example, or other debris that might interfere with the squashing should be removed, using either a drawn capillary pipet or an eyelash. The volume of buffer should also be adjusted to approximately 10 μl at this time.

3. Overlay embryos with a dust-free 18 × 18-mm coverslip. Invert the slide and carefully place it coverslip side down on a paper tissue. Apply gentle pressure on the back of the slide by placing the thumbs at the edges of the slide, being careful not to push the slide sideways. Place the slide, coverslip side up, on dry ice for 10 minutes to freeze. The appropriate amount of pressure to apply when squashing the embryos can only be determined by practice. Generally, a small amount of liquid will be forced out from under the coverslip and will wet a small area of the tissue. The slide can be examined briefly under the microscope before

freezing. If excess pressure has been applied, or if some material has interfered with the squashing, then air bubbles will appear under the coverslip. Discard these slides.

4. Mark the back of the slide with a diamond pencil to indicate the area where the embryos are located and remove the coverslip (for details, see Chapter 16 in this volume).

5. Immediately fix specimens by immersing the slides in ethanol:acetic acid 3:1 for 30 to 60 minutes.

6. Remove slides from fixative and air-dry. A gentle stream of cool air from a hair dryer can also be used to speed the drying.

7. Rinse slides in 2× SSC and then incubate in boiled ribonuclease (20 μg/ml in 2× SSC) for 60 minutes, at 37°C.

8. Rinse slides in 2× SSC, then dehydrate by passing through two changes each of 70% and 95% ethanol. Air-dry.

2. Denaturing Specimens and Setting up the Hybridization

1. Immerse slides in 0.7 M NaOH (4.2 g/150 ml H$_2$O) for 1.5 minutes.
2. Dehydrate through two changes of 70% and 95% ethanol and air-dry.
3. Add 2 μl of 50% dextran sulfate to 7 μl of probe DNA in formamide buffer. Denature the DNA by heating at 70°C for 10 minutes . Chill on ice and add 0.1 vol 3 M NaCl (1 μl).
4. Apply 10 μl of probe solution to the slide and cover with an 18 × 18-mm coverslip, avoiding air bubbles. Seal the edges of the slide with rubber cement (Carter's).
5. Place slides in a rack and incubate at 37°C overnight in a humidified slide staining jar containing 5 ml of 50% formamide–2× SSC.

3. Posthybridization Washes

1. Carefully peel off rubber cement, so that the coverslip does not move. Immerse slides in 50% formamide–2× SSC and allow the coverslip to float off.
2. Incubate slides for 15 minutes each in two changes of 50% formamide–2× SSC at 37°C.
3. Wash slides for 30 minutes in 1 to 1.5 liters of 2× SSC by suspending the slides in a slide staining rack in a large beaker and stir gently.
4. Wash slides in 1 to 1.5 liters of PBS, as above.
5. Counterstain DNA and mount (see Section VII,B and C).

4. Solutions

Boiled ribonuclease: Dissolve pancreatic ribonuclease in 0.2 M sodium acetate, pH 5.2, at a concentration of 5 mg/ml. Heat at 90°C for 10 minutes. Store at -20°C in 0.6-ml aliquots

20× SSC: 3 *M* NaCl, 0.3 *M* Na citrate, pH 7.

50% Dextran sulfate: Dissolve 50 g dextran in 70 ml H_2O by stirring at 70°C. Store at 4°C.

Phosphate-buffered saline (PBS): 12 m*M* NaCl, 16 m*M* Na_2HPO_4, 8 m*M* NaH_2PO_4.

B. Cut and Flattened Specimens for Hybridization to Meiotic Prophase Nuclei

Nuclei in meiotic prophase can be visualized most easily if the gonad is released from the adult hermaphrodite by cutting the animal with a razor blade near the bend in the gonad or at the vulva. Early meiotic prophase nuclei can be released from the distal arm of the gonad, if this is cut in several places. This protocol yields meiotic chromosome squashes, suitable for characterizing chromosome rearrangements by *in situ* hybridization with cloned probes.

1. Fixation

1. Pick animals from plates into M9 buffer in a watch glass.

2. Using a drawn capillary pipet, transfer worms to charged slides or gelatin-subbed slides (see Section VI,A,1).

3. Cut worms to release intact gonads or pieces of gonad, as required. Use a double-edged razor blade that has been cut in half longitudinally and the end tapered by a diagonal cut. Multiple cuts to the distal arm of the gond will release some of the nuclei in early meiotic prophase.

4. Adjust the volume of buffer to 10 to 20 μl and cover with a 12 × 12-mm coverslip. Examine the slide under the dissecting microscope. The specimens should be flattened between the coverslip and the slide, but should not appear clear and squashed, nor should they be moving under the coverslip.

5. Place the slide on dry ice for 10 minutes, then draw an outline of the coverslip on the back of the slide with a diamond pencil.

6. Remove the coverslip (see Chapter 16 in this volume) and place the slide in ethanol:acetic acid 3:1 fixative for 30 to 60 minutes.

7. Remove slides from fixative and air-dry.

8. Rinse in 2× SSC and incubate at 37°C in ribonuclease (20 μg/ml in 2× SSC) for 60 minutes (see Section VI,A,4).

9. Rinse slides in 2× SSC and dehydrate through two changes of 70% and 95% ethanol. Air-dry.

2. Denaturing Specimens and Setting up the Hybridization

1. Immerse slides in 0.7 *M* NaOH for 1.5 minutes.

2. Dehydrate through two changes of 70% and 95% ethanol and air-dry.

3. Add 4 μl of 50% dextran sulfate to the probe DNA in 14 μl of formamide buffer and denature the DNA by heating at 70°C for 10 minutes. Chill on ice and add 0.1 vol 3 M NaCl (2 μl).

4. Apply the probe mixture to the area of the slide containing the specimens and cover with a square of Parafilm that is just larger than the outline of the coverslip drawn on the back of the slide.

5. Cover the bottom of a petri dish with water and place slides on a raised support, specimen side up, in the covered petri dish at 37°C overnight.

3. Posthybridization Washes

1. Immerse slides in 50% formamide–2× SSC and allow squares of Parafilm to float to the surface.
2. Incubate slides at 37°C in 50% formamide–2× SSC for 30 minutes.
3. Wash in 1 to 1.5 liters of PBS or PBS, 0.1% Tween 20 by suspending the slides in a rack in a large beaker, without agitation.
4. Counterstain DNA and mount (see Section VII,B and C).

4. Solutions

See Section VI,A,4.

C. Whole Mounts for DNA *in Situ* Hybridization

This protocol describes the preparation of material for *in situ* hybridization with DNA probes to visualize the distribution of nucleic acid sequences in three dimensions (Albertson 1984b; Albertson and Thomson, 1993). Whole animals are transferred to glass microscope slides and embryos are obtained by cutting adult hermaphrodites to release the embryos. It is important, when working with whole mounts, that the slides should not be allowed to dry, or the morphology of the specimens will be distorted.

1. Fixation

1. Prepare specimens as in Section VI,B,1, steps 1 to 5, except make only a single cut at the vulva and adjust the volume of buffer under the coverslip so that the specimens are held firmly between the slide and the coverslip, but not squashed. Too much buffer and the specimens will not adhere to the slide when the coverslip is removed. The correct amount of buffer is best determined by practice, for any particular application.

2. After removal of the coverslip (step 6, Section VI,B,1), immediately place the slide in 95% ethanol for 2 minutes. Care should be taken with whole mounts not to drop the slides into the Coplin jars, as this will dislodge the specimens.

3. Fix for 30 to 60 minutes in the following mixture: 95% ethanol, 30 ml; acetic acid, 15 ml; chloroform, 5 ml.

4. Place slides in 95% ethanol, then rehydrate by passing slides through a water–ethanol series in increments of 20% water into two changes of 2× SSC.

5. Incubate slides in boiled ribonuclease (20 μg/ml in 2× SSC) at 37°C for 60 minutes (see Section VI,A,4).

2. Denaturing Specimens and Setting up the Hybridization

1. After ribonuclease treatment, rinse slides in two changes of distilled H_2O.

2. Pass slides through 30% formamide in water, 50% formamide in water, then two changes of 70% formamide in water.

3. Prepare and denature probe DNA (see Section VI,B,2, step 3).

4. After the probe has been incubating at 70°C for 3 to 4 minutes, denature specimens by placing in 70% formamide in water preheated to 80°C and incubate for 3 to 4 minutes at 80°C in a plastic Coplin jar. Denaturation by NaOH treatment cannot be used, because it causes the specimens to fall off the slides.

5. After denaturation, rinse slides in two changes of 50% formamide–2× SSC.

6. Drain excess formamide solution from slides, and proceed as in Section VI,B,2, steps 4 and 5.

3. Posthybridization Washes

See Section VI,B,3.

4. Solutions

See Section VI,A,4.

D. Whole Animals in Suspension for Hybridization to mRNA

In this protocol whole animals are fixed and hybridized in suspension in microfuge tubes (Birchall, 1993). The limits of sensitivity of the method have not been determined, and it may not be possible to visualize very rare messages. It is important that controls be included in each experiment to ensure that the fluorescence is not a fixation artifact. For example, autofluorescence from the specimen often appears similar to the fluorescence emission from fluorescein-labeled probes. The controls should include slides that have been treated with RNase or slides to which no labeled probe was added to the hybridization mixture. During room temperature fixation or pretreatment and posthybridization incubations or washes, the tubes are placed on a rotating mixer of the type used for blood cell suspensions in hematology laboratories. When the tubes are incubated at higher temperatures, the contents of the tubes are mixed by placing them in a hybridization oven with rotating bottles. Stock solutions, except those containing Tris–HCl, may be treated with diethylpyrocarbonate (DEPC) to inactivate ribonucleases by making the solutions 0.1% in DEPC before autoclaving. Buffers containing Tris–HCl are prepared from DEPC-treated ingredients, which are then added to the sterile Tris–HCl buffer, because DEPC reacts with the Tris–HCl.

1. Fixation

1. Collect worms by washing off plates or settling from liquid culture (see Chapter 1 in this volume).

2. Float worms from liquid cultures on sucrose (see Chapter 1).

3. Wash three times in 0.1 M NaCl for 5 minutes on a rotator at room temperature.

4. Wash three times in 0.1 M Hepes–KOH, pH 7.5, 1 mM MgSO$_4$, 2 mM EGTA for 5 minutes at room temperature.

5. For 1 to 2 ml of packed worms, fix in 10 ml of freshly prepared 3.7% formaldehyde, 0.1 M Hepes–KOH, pH 7.5, 1 mM MgSO$_4$, 2 mM EGTA for 6 hours at room temperature. This solution is prepared using 37% formaldehyde solution.

6. To store worms, dehydrate through a series of 20% increments of methanol:fixative into 100% methanol, incubating for 10 minutes with rotation at each change.

7. Store in 100 to 500-μl aliquots of packed worms in 1.5-ml microfuge tubes with 200 to 300 μl methanol at $-20°$C. Aliquots have been stored this way for up to 6 months. Approximately 20 tubes of fixed worms can be prepared from a 500-ml liquid culture. Each tube of fixed worms is sufficient for 10 to 15 hybridizations.

2. Pretreatment

For each step, use 1-ml volumes for the washes, rotating the tubes during the wash, then spin briefly at 5000 rpm in a microfuge between washes. To minimize loss of specimens at each washing step, leave a small volume of liquid covering the pellet at each step.

1. Rehydrate frozen worms through 20% increments of PBST:methanol into PBST, by incubating for 5 minutes at each step at room temperature.

2. Wash three times for 5 minutes in PBST at room temperature.

3. Wash twice for 5 minutes in 5% β-mercaptoethanol in PBST at room temperature.

4. Incubate for 5 minutes in 50 μg/ml proteinase K in PBS at 37°C, rotating tubes by placing them in a 50-ml capped centrifuge tube in a hybridization oven.

5. Fix in freshly prepared 2% paraformaldehyde in PBS for 20 minutes at room temperature.

6. Wash three times in PBST for 10 minutes at room temperature.

PBST: PBS, 0.2% SDS, 0.1% Tween 20.

3. Hybridization

1. Wash 20 minutes in 1 : 1 hybridization solution (HS) : PBST on the rotator at room temperature.

2. Wash 20 to 60 minutes in HS rotating tubes at room temperature.

3. Prehybridize in 1 ml HS for 20 to 60 minutes at 37°C, rotating tubes in a hybridization oven.

4. Microfuge briefly to pellet worms. Remove excess HS, leaving specimens suspended in appropriate volume for the number of hybridization tubes to be set up in step 5.

5. Cut the end off a plastic pipet tip and transfer 18-μl aliquots of packed worms into a 0.5-ml microfuge tube. Add 2 μl of freshly denatured probe (20–100 ng) in HS.

6. Hybridize overnight at 37°C for DNA probes or at 45°C for riboprobes by rotating in a hybridization oven.

HS: 50% deionized formamide, 5× SSC, 0.1 *M* Hepes–KOH, pH 7.5, 80 μg/ml sheared salmon sperm DNA, 0.2% SDS, 0.1% Tween 20.

4. Posthybridization Washes

Use 300-μl volumes for each wash, incubating on a rotator for 20 minutes at room temperature.

HS
HS : PBST 4 : 1
HS : PBST 3 : 2
HS : PBST 2 : 3
HS : PBST 1 : 4
Wash twice in PBST

5. Mounting

Transfer worms into DABCO–glycerol mounting medium (see Section VII,C) by incubating for 10 minutes with rotation in 100-μl volumes of the following dilutions of DABCO–glycerol.

PBST : DABCO–glycerol 4 : 1
PBST : DABCO–glycerol 3 : 2

PBST:DABCO–glycerol 2:3
PBST:DABCO–glycerol 1:4
DABCO–glycerol

Microfuge briefly to pellet worms and mount 5 to 10 μl of worms on a glass microscope slide. Cover with a 22 × 32-mm No. 1.5 coverslip.

VII. Visualization of the Site of Hybridization

The site of hybridization is imaged with either a conventional fluorescence microscope or a confocal laser scanning microscope. It is not necessary to use electronic imaging equipment, except when working with fluorochromes that emit in the infrared, as noted in Table I. For observations on whole mounts, the confocal microscope is used to reduce out-of-focus flare.

A. Detection by Immunofluorescence

For visualization of the site of hybridization of probes labeled with biotin or DIG, detection with antibodies follows the posthybridization washes (see also Chapter 14 in this volume). Fluorescent avidin can also be used for detection of biotin-labeled probes instead of immunofluorescence detection (see, e.g., Pinkel *et al.*, 1986). Further discussion of immunofluorescence methods can be found in Chapter 16 in this volume.

1. Following posthybridization washes, drain PBS from the slide, leaving the specimen area covered.

2. Add 10 μl BSA (10 mg/ml in PBS) to the PBS on the slide.

3. Add one of the following primary antibodies, as appropriate: (a) For biotin labeled probes: rabbit antibiotin (Enzo Diagnostics) diluted 1:10, 2.5 μl; mouse monoclonal antbiotin (British Biotechnology), 1 μl. (b) For DIG-labeled probes: sheep anti-DIG (Boehringer-Mannheim), 1 μl; mouse monoclonal anti-DIG (Boehringer-Mannheim), 1 μl.

4. Cover with an 18 × 18-mm square of Parafilm and incubate in a humid chamber at 37°C for 60 minutes.

5. Float Parafilm off slides by immersing in PBS. Wash in PBS, 0.1% Tween 20 for 10 to 15 minutes.

6. Drain excess PBS from the slide and add 1 to 3 μl of the appropriate fluorochrome-labeled second antibody. Cover with a square of Parafilm and incubate at room temperature in a humid chamber for 20 minutes.

7. Wash for 30 minutes, as in step 5.

8. Counterstain DNA, if required, and mount (see Section VII,B and C).

B. Stains for DNA

When using fluorescent nucleic acids stains, the supplier's cautions and instructions for handling should be read and followed.

DAPI (4′,6-diamidino-2-phenylindole): Make a 10 mg/ml stock solution of DAPI in water and store at 4°C. This solution is diluted 1 : 50 into water to make a working stock solution. Just before use, dilute 10 μl of the working stock solution into 60 ml water. Immerse slides in DAPI solution for 5 minutes, rinse briefly in water, and mount in DABCO mounting medium (see Section VII,C).

Hoechst 33258 (2′-[4-hydroxyphenyl]-5-[4-methyl-1-piperazinyl]-2,5′-bi-1H-benzimidazole): Immerse slides in 1 μg/ml Hoechst 33258 in PBS for 5 minutes. Rinse in PBS and mount in 2% *n*-propyl gallate (Giloh and Sedat, 1982).

Propidium iodide: Propidium iodide is a general nucleic acid stain, but can be used to counterstain nuclei in any protocol that permits the removal of cytoplasmic RNA by incubation in ribonuclease. Immerse slides in 100 μl/ml propidium iodide in PBS for 5 to 10 minutes, rinse briefly in PBS, and mount in DABCO mounting medium (see Section VII,C).

C. Mounting

Pipet a drop of mounting medium onto the area of the slide where the specimens are located. Cover with a 22 × 32-mm No. 1.5 coverslip, avoiding air bubbles. It is not necessary to seal the edges. Store specimens at −20°C in the dark.

DABCO mounting medium: DABCO (1,4-diazabicyclo-[2,2,2]octane) mounting medium (Johnson *et al.,* 1982) is suitable for use with all fluorochromes in Tables I and II, except Hoechst 33258. DABCO is used at a final concentration of 25 g/liter in buffered glycerol: glycerol, 9 parts; PBS, pH 8.6, 1 part. Make PBS pH 8.6 by adding 0.1 *M* NaOH. Dissolve DABCO in glycerol with gentle heating and stirring. Add PBS, and store aliquots in small brown bottles at −20°C.

Acknowledgments

We thank Ian Durrant, Amersham, United Kingdom, for the gift of rhodamine–UTP, and Leslie Gubba, Biological Detection Systems, for the gift of Cy3–dCTP and Cy5–dCTP.

References

Albertson, D. G. (1984a). Localization of the ribosomal genes in *Caenorhabditis elegans* chromosomes by *in situ* hybridization using biotin-labeled probes. *EMBO J.* **3,** 1227–1234.

Albertson, D. G. (1984b). Formation of the first cleavage spindle in nematode embryos. *Dev. Biol.* **101,** 61–72.

Albertson, D. G. (1985). Mapping muscle protein genes by *in situ* hybridization using biotin-labeled probes. *EMBO J.* **4,** 2493–2498.

Albertson, D. G. (1993). Mapping chromosome rearrangement breakpoints to the physical map of *Caenorhabditis elegans* by fluorescent *in situ* hybridization. *Genetics* **134**, 211–219.

Albertson, D. G., Nwaorgu, O. C., and Sulston, J. E. (1979). Chromatin diminution and a chromosomal mechanism for sexual differentiation in *Strongyloides papaillosus*. *Chromosoma* (*Berl.*) **75**, 75–87.

Albertson, D. G., Sherrington, P., and Vaudin, M. (1991). Mapping non-isotopically labeled DNA probes to human chromosome bands by confocal microscopy. *Genomics* **10**, 143–150.

Albertson, D. G., and Thomson, J. N. (1982). The kinetochores of *Caenorhabditis elegans*. *Chromosoma* (*Berl.*) **86**, 409–428.

Albertson, D. G., and Thomson, J. N. (1993). Segregation of holocentric chromosomes at meiosis in the nematode, *Caenorhabditis elegans*. *Chromosomes Res.* **1**, 15–26.

Austin, J. A., and Kimble, J. E. (1987). *glp-1* is required in the germ line for regulation of the decision between mitosis and meiosis in *C. elegans*. *Cell* **51**, 589–599.

Birchall, P. S. (1993). Multicolour fluorescence in *in situ* hybridisation to RNA in whole-mount *Caenorhabditis elegans*. Ph.D Thesis, University of Cambridge, Cambridge, U.K.

Butler, J. E., and Chamberlain, M. (1982). Bacteriophage SP6-specific RNA polymerase. *J. Biol. Chem.* **257**, 5772–5778.

Cunningham, P. R., and Ofengard, J. (1990). Use of inorganic pyrophosphatase to improve the yield of *in vitro* transcription reactions catalyzed by T7 RNA polymerase. *Biotechniques* **9**, 713–714.

Feinberg, P., and Vogelstein, B. (1984). A technique for radiolabeling DNA restriction enzyme fragments to high specific activity. *Anal. Biochem.* **137**, 266–267.

Files, J. G., and Hirsh, D. (1981). Ribosomal DNA of *Caenorhabditis elegans*. *J. Mol. Biol.* **149**, 223–240.

Fishpool, R., and Albertson, D. G. (1992). Gene mapping with the confocal microscope. *In* "Hybridization *in situ méthodes pratiques*" (A. Calas, B. Bloch, J.-G. Fournier, and A. Trembleau, eds.), pp. 87–93. Société Française de Microscopie Electronique, Ivry.

Giloh, H., and Sedat, J. W. (1982). Fluorescence microscopy: Reduced photobleaching of rhodamine and fluorescein protein conjugates by *n*-propyl gallate. *Science* **217**, 1252–1255.

Haugland, R. P. (1994). "Handbook of Fluorescent Probes and Research Chemicals," 5th ed., p. 221. Molecular Probes, Inc., Eugene, Oregon.

Hengartner, M. O., Ellis, R. E., and Horvitz, H. R. (1992). *Caenorhabditis elegans* gene *ced-9* protects cells from programmed cell death. *Nature* **356**, 494–499.

Johnson, G. D., Davidson, R. S., McNamee, K. C., Russell, G., Goodwin, D., and Holborow, E. J. (1982). Fading of immunofluorescence during microscopy: A study of the phenomenon and its remedy. *J. Immunol. Methods.* **55**, 231–242.

Moyzis, R. K., Buckingham, J. M., Cram, L. S., Dani, M., Deaven, L. L., Jones, M. D., Meyne, J., Ratliff, R. L., and Wu, J. R. (1988). A highly conserved repetitive DNA sequence, $(TTAGGG)_n$, present at the telomeres of human chromosomes. *Proc. Natl. Acad. Sci. U.S.A.* **85**, 6622–6626.

Pinkel, D., Straume, T., and Gray, J. W. (1986). Cytogenetic analysis using quantitative, high-sensitivity, fluorescence hybridization. *Proc. Natl. Acad. Sci. U.S.A* **83**, 2934–2938.

Ried, T., Baldini, A., Rand, T. C., and Ward, D. (1992). Simultaneous visualization of seven different DNA probes by *in situ* hybridization using combinatorial fluorescence and digital imaging microscopy. *Proc. Natl. Acad. Sci. U.S.A.* **89**, 1388–1392.

Rigby, P. W. J., Dieckmann, M., Rhodes, C., and Berg, P. (1977). Labeling deoxyribonucleic acid to high specific activity *in vitro* by nick translation with DNA polymerase I. *J. Mol. Biol.* **113**, 237–251.

Saiki, R. K., Gelfand, D. H., Stoffel, S., Scharf, S. J., Higuchi, R., Horn, G. T., Mullis, K. B., and Erlich, H. A. (1988). Primer-directed enzymatic amplification of DNA with a thermostable DNA polymerase. *Science* **239**, 487–494.

Tartof, K., and Hobbs, C. A. (1981). Improved media for growing plasmids and cosmids. *Focus* **3**, 12.

Telenius, H., Carter, N. P., Bebb, C. E., Nordenskjöld, M., Ponder, B. A. J., and Tunnacliffe, A. (1992a). Degenerate oligonucleotide-primed PCR: General amplification of target DNA by a single degenerate primer. *Genomics* **13**, 718–725.

Telenius, H., Pelmear, A. H., Tunnacliffe, A., Carter, N. P., Behmel, A., Ferguson-Smith, M. A., Nordenskjöld, M., Peragner, R., and Ponder, B. A. J. (1992b). Cytogenetic analysis by chromosome painting using DOP-PCR amplified flow-sorted chromosomes. *Genes Chromosom Cancer* **4**, 257–263.

CHAPTER 16

Immunofluorescence Microscopy

David M. Miller[*] and Diane C. Shakes[†,1]

[*] Department of Cell Biology
Vanderbilt University Medical Center
Nashville, Tennessee 37232
[†] Department of Biology
University of Houston
Houston, Texas 77204

I. Introduction

The purpose of this chapter is to provide a practical guide to immunofluorescence microscopy of *Caenorhabditis elegans*. In this method, fixed tissue is stained with a fluorescently labeled antibody and visualized with the light microscope. The antibody ensures that staining is limited to the location of the antigen, and the

[1] Present address: Department of Biology, College of William and Mary, Williamsburg, Virginia 23187.

microscope provides a magnified image of the fluorescent area. Immunofluorescence microscopy is an especially powerful tool for studies of *C. elegans*. The identity of each antibody-stained cell can be determined by reference to detailed knowledge of *C. elegans* anatomy. Because the developmental cell lineage is known, it is also possible to define the timing of antigen expression with great precision. Because of the transparency and small size of the animal, immunofluorescence staining can be clearly observed in whole mounts and does not require sectioning.

Immunofluoresence staining can provide essential information for the analysis of mutant phenotypes. Mutations that alter developmental programs or the expression of particular proteins can be examined *in situ* and described at the level of individual cells or cell lineages (Nonet, 1993; Bowerman *et al.,* 1993). In other cases, immunolocalization of a protein to unanticipated cell types of subcellular structures can sometimes suggest functions not implicated in the original mutant analysis. For instance, the *Drosophila* Tudor protein, which is required for normal germ cell determination, was found not only in polar granules but also in mitochondria (Bardsley *et al.,* 1993); the localization of Notch suggested that it played a role in cell signaling rather than cell adhesion (Fehon *et al.,* 1991); and the *C. elegans* Unc-86 protein was found in many more cells than anticipated (Finney and Ruvkun, 1990). Immunofluorescence can also be used to analyze the detailed patterns of antigen expression even when only limited numbers of mutant animals are available for analysis (Priess *et al.,* 1987; Hresko *et al.,* 1994).

Immunofluorescence microscopy can be used to detect the expression of transgenes in *C. elegans*. Specific epitope tags (e.g., β-galactosidase) can be incorporated into a transgene such that the epitope-tagged protein can be detected with a specific antibody (e.g., anti-β-galactosidase) which does not react with the endogenous protein (Fire, 1992; Miller and Niemeyer, 1995). Epitope tagging is particularly useful for cases in which a null mutation in the endogenous gene is either not available or desirable in the transgenic animal (Soldati and Perriard, 1991).

Immunolocalization complements other molecular studies of gene expression. Unlike Northern blots and RNA *in situ* hybridization studies (see Chapters 14 and 21 in this volume), which provide important information on the transcriptional regulation of particular genes, protein immunofluorescence reveals where the majority of the protein is actually localized and presumably functions. In some cases, striking differences between the two patterns arise from posttranscriptional regulatory mechanisms (Evans *et al.,* 1994) or secretion of the protein product [e.g., yolk proteins are synthesized by the intestine, secreted, and subsequently taken up by oocytes (Sharrock, 1984)].

Immunofluorescence is highly sensitive; antigen-expressing cells can be readily detected against a dark, nonfluorescent background. Until recently, the resolution of immunofluorescent images was inherently limited by stray light from fluorescent objects out of the plane of focus. With the advent of confocal scanning microscopy which uses a laser to precisely scan a single optical section, greatly increased resolution in the z axis eliminates out of focus fluorescence and significantly crisper images of identically prepared specimens are obtained (White *et al.*, 1987). In addition, the attachment of either low-ligh-level video cameras (i.e., SITcam) or cooled CCD cameras to the immunofluorescence microscope further enhances the sensitivity of the technique and can provide a digitized image for manipulation in a desktop computer (Shotten, 1993). These cameras are even more important for observing fluorescently tagged molecules (e.g., green fluorescent protein or GFP; Chalfie *et al.*, 1994) within living organisms, as the low level of exciting light that can be used with these cameras slows bleaching of the fluorescent tag and avoids UV damage to the organism.

In this chapter, we discuss standard immunofluorescence staining methods and the generation of specific antibodies against *C. elegans* proteins, and Figs 1 to 4 are examples of specimens stained by these various techniques. Although not discussed in this chapter, immunohistochemical techniques that rely on enzymatic reactions in lieu of immunofluorescence staining are possible in *C. elegans* (Mackenzie *et al.*, 1978), but their use has been limited largely to the detection of transgene expression (Fire, 1992; Jefferson *et al.*, 1987) and the localization of specific intestinal enzymes (Edgar and McGhee, 1986). Readers should also be reminded that the immunofluorescence methods described in this chapter are designed primarily for the detection of antigens at the cellular level and that when necessary, immuno-electron microscopic methods can provide additional resolution in determining the subcellular localization of antigens (see Chapter 17 in this volume).

II. Preparing Specimens for Immunolocalization Studies

A. General Comments

1. Permeabilization

The principal barriers to antibody penetration are the chitinous eggshell enveloping the embryo and the tough multilayered cuticle surrounding the adult. Several strategies have been devised to permeabilize these structures. In this chapter, we describe the methods most commonly used to permeabilize embryos, larvae, and adults. The extremely tough cuticle of the specialized dauer larvae makes them difficult to stain by any method.

In the freeze-crack procedure for embryos and young larvae, eggshells of embryos affixed to subbed slides (or the cuticles of larvae) are physically broken through the force of quickly popping off a frozen coverslip from the slide (Albertson, 1984; Kemphues *et al.*, 1986). The slide is subsequently submerged in a series of solutions for fixation and antibody staining steps. As an alternative to the freeze-crack method, hypochlorite can be used to dissolve the outer layers of the eggshells in bulk preparations of embryos, followed by treatment with a combination of formaldehyde and methanol to fix and permeabilize the embryos. Lastly, in a whole-mount fixation method for larvae and adults (Finney and Ruvkun, 1990), fixed animals are subjected to a reduction/oxidation reaction to break extensive disulfide bonds between cuticle proteins (Cox *et al.*, 1981). In the last two procedures, permeabilization and staining steps are carried out in microfuge tubes, and low-speed spins are used to pellet the animals between solution changes.

2. Fixation

The choice of fixation method represents a compromise between optimally preserving ultrastructural elements and retaining the ability of the antibody both to penetrate the specimen and to bind to the fixed antigen. Different antibodies vary widely in their ability to react with fixed antigens, and what works well to preserve one antigenic site may abolish the antigenicity of another. The specificity of monoclonal antibodies makes them more finicky in this regard. Fixation solutions are generally health hazards and should be handled in well-covered containers and in chemical fume hoods whenever possible. Commonly used fixatives include organic solvents such as methanol and acetone, which precipitate soluble proteins, or aldehydes such as formaldehyde and glutaraldehyde, which crosslink antigens to prevent diffusion (Osborn and Weber, 1982).

3. Antibody Binding

The goal of these steps is to obtain the brightest possible staining of the antigen-expressing cells while minimizing nonspecific background fluorescence. Although the exact conditions for optimal staining will vary for different antigens and for different antibody preparations, general guidelines for maximizing the signal-to-noise ratio are provided. It is important to use blocking agents such as bovine serum albumin (BSA) or animal serum to prevent nonspecific antibody staining. In the usual case of indirect immunofluorescence staining, the animal serum used for blocking should be from the same species as the secondary fluorescent antibody. In addition, mild nonionic detergents are frequently included to further decrease nonspecific binding and the tendency of worms to stick to each other in bulk preparation methods.

The concentration of antibody can have a significant effect on the quality of the immunofluorescence signal; overly concentrated antibody increases nonspecific background staining, whereas overly diluted antibody fails to produce a strong signal. Optimal incubation times and conditions will vary with the antibody. The optimal concentration of primary antibody used should always be empirically determined by titration as described in Section III. Typical dilutions of primary antibodies are listed in the following table and should be made in either phosphate-buffered saline (PBS) or PBS-blocking solution.

Antibody type	Dilution or final concentration
Polyclonal antiserum	1/50–1/10,000
Purified monoclonals	1–100 µg/ml
Monoclonal	
Ascites fluid, 5–10 mg/ml	1/100–1/10,000
Growth medium, 5–10 µm/ml	1/10–1/50

In our experience, secondary fluorescent antibodies generally work well at a dilution recommended by the supplier. In some instances, however, it is necessary to preadsorb the secondary fluorescent antibody with fixed nematodes to reduce background staining (see Section III).

B. Protocols

1. Freeze-Crack Methods for Permeabilization and Fixation of Embryos and Young Larvae

Caenorhabditis elegans embryos develop within a chitinous shell that hardens shortly after fertilization inside the hermaphrodite parent. Embryos of well-fed hermaphrodites are typically extruded from the uterus at about the 50-cell stage, although later-staged embryos are frequently retained in older or slightly starved hermaphrodites. For the analysis of early development, it is most convenient to obtain the embryos from intact, well-fed, young adult hermaphrodites (Albertson, 1984; Kemphues *et al.*, 1986; H. and R. Schnabel, pers. comm.).

a. Permeabilization by Freeze-Cracking

1. Use a pencil to label the end of a frosted subbed slide (see Section VI) and use a diamond-tipped pen to scratch a small circle on the underside to mark the location of the specimen. Add 5 to 10 µl of distilled water (dH$_2$O) to the top side of the slide over the marked circle. Meanwhile, pick healthy (nonstarved) adult hermaphrodites into a watchglass containing dH$_2$O to rinse off excess bacteria, and then transfer the rinsed worms into the drop on the slide. Use 10 to 20 worms per slide.

2. Cover the worms with a clean 1/4 coverslip, size 18 or 22. While observing under a dissecting microscope, use forceps to press gently on the coverslip directly over the animals until eggs are released from the ruptured vulvas. Alternatively, the hermaphrodite can be cut at the vulva using a 22-gauge syringe needle to extrude the embryos before adding the coverslip.

3. Gently lower the slide into a pool of liquid nitrogen using long forceps (or place horizontally on a block of dry ice). *Note:* Slides can be held frozen in liquid nitrogen, on dry ice, or in a −70°C freezer for several hours. Holding the slides in fixative is not advised, as overfixation may reduce antibody binding (see below). Some brands of slides are less subject to breakage in liquid nitrogen than others; Esco slides (Erie Scientific, Portsmouth, NH) hold up well in our hands.

4. After freezing, wedge the tip of a scalpel blade under one corner of the coverslip and "pop" it off with a quick twist of your wrist. This step must be

done while the slide is still frozen and you should hear an audible "crack." If the embryos are not well permeabilized, try decreasing the liquid volume either in the initial drop or by wicking liquid from the edges of the coverslip before the squash. Once the coverslip is removed, immediately place the slide in fixative (see below).

Variations. R. Schnabel and H. Schnabel (pers. comm.) have developed an alternative method for the small-scale analysis of isolated embryos. In this variation, a small number of early-stage embryos are obtained by cutting gravid adults in a watchglass in water. The released eggs are transferred to polylysine-coated eightwell Teflon-coated slides using glass capillary tubes that have been hand-pulled into micropipets with bores somewhat larger than the eggs. The rubber tubing supplied with the capillary tubes is used for mouth control of embryo transfers. The eggs should stick immediately; if not, you need to make new slides. Shake the slides to remove excess water so that a thin film of water remains in the well and no water is retained between wells. A small micropipet tip cut at an angle can be used to aspirate off any remaining excess water. A coverslip (24 × 60 mm, thickness 1½) is used to cover all eight wells, with about 0.5 cm of the coverslip hanging over the end of the slide for easier removal. The coverslip should not be moved at this point, and the tops of the eggs should touch the coverslip. Freeze the slide on a metal block that is sitting on dry ice. Flick off the coverslip and put the slide in fixative.

This freeze-crack method can also be used to analyze larvae or adults when one is restricted to working with a small number of animals. In general, the method works much better for young larvae than for adults, and for proper freeze-cracking, the animals on a single slide should always be the same age (S. Strome, pers. comm.). In the analysis of older larvae or adults, a small nick on the cuticle with a 22-gauge syringe needle will aid in fixative and antibody penetration. For the analysis of gametogenesis, syringe needle cuts just posterior of the pharynx are excellent for releasing the gonadal arms and for providing a linear timeline view of gametogenesis.

b. Fixation

Methanol/Acetone Fixation. Place the freeze-cracked slides in −20°C methanol for 5 minutes. Transfer to −20°C acetone for 5 minutes. Allow to air-dry on the benchtop or rehydrate at room temperature using either an ethanol or a methanol series (i.e., 2 minutes each in 95, 70, 50, and 30% EtOH followed by 1× PBS). Rehydration using an alcohol series provides better preservation of cellular structures, but air-drying may improve staining with some antibodies. R. Schnabel and H. Schnabel (pers. comm.) suggest a 10-minute fixation in −20°C methanol followed immediately by air-drying and note that air-dried slides can be stored frozen at −70°C. All fixation and rehydration steps should be carried out in solution-filled Coplin jars with side ridges to prevent the vertically held slides from rubbing against each other. For an extremely precious experimentally manipulated animal (e.g., from a laser ablation experiment), some investigators may prefer to lessen the occasional problem of sample loss by keeping the slides in a horizontal position and carrying out each solution change in droplets of liquid as described in the staining protocol below.

Formaldehyde Fixation. Fixation in a solution of 3.7% formaldehyde/75% methanol/0.5X PBS results in optimal preservation of the embryonic cytoskeleton. Typical fixation conditions are either 0.5 hour at room temperature or overnight at 4°C. Alternatively, embryos can be fixed in either 1 to 4% formaldehyde or a combination of 1% formaldehyde and 0.1% glutaraldehyde in an appropriate buffer (usually PBS). Fixation should be for 30 minutes to 1 hour at room temperature. Aldehyde-fixed samples should be thoroughly rinsed by three 10-minute soakings in PBS. Inclusion of 10 mg/ml glycine in one of these rinses will help block remaining covalent aldehyde binding sites which might otherwise increase nonspecific background staining. Formaldehyde-containing solutions should be prepared immediately before use from a fresh 20% formaldehyde stock solution (see Section VI). Detergent and/or a methanol incubation must be included in subsequent steps to permit antibody access to internal sites.

c. Staining

1. Rinse the slides in 1× PBS for 5 minutes in a solution-filled Coplin jar.

2. Use the twisted corner of a Kimwipe or torn piece of filter paper to carefully wick away excess buffer from around the specimen and add enough blocking solution to cover the sample (15–25 μl). Commonly used blocking solutions are 1% BSA or nonimmune animal serum. Serum should be used full strength or diluted 1:10 in PBS. The trick during all of the solution changes is to minimize both solution carryover and the wetting surface without ever letting the sample dry out completely. You really need to firmly dry the area around the specimen so that the small drops of solution saturate the specimen directly and are not diluted by spreading over a large area of the slide. Proper slide labeling prevents you from accidently wiping away your specimen during the solution changing steps.

3. Lay the slides horizontally in a humid chamber (a tightly covered Tupperware container lined with a damp but not dripping paper towel) and incubate for 1 to 2 hours at 4°C.

4. Wick off excess block and cover samples with a drop of optimally diluted primary antibody. Incubate for 1 to 2 hours at 37°C or overnight at 4°C. Optimal incubation conditions will vary depending on the antibody.

5. Transfer the slide to a Coplin jar containing PBS and wash for 10 minutes. Repeat washes two more times.

6. Shake the slide to remove most of the buffer and then wick away the remaining excess buffer from around the sample. Immediately cover the specimen with 10 to 20 μl of appropriately diluted fluorescent secondary antibody. Incubate at 37°C for 1 hour in the dark (or follow the conditions suggested by the supplier).

Note: From this step onward, you should minimize the exposure of the slides to light using foil coverings or lighttight containers.

7. Wash again with three 10-minute changes of PBS in Coplin jars. If desired, add the DNA stain diamidinophenolindole (DAPI) to the first wash. For staining, DAPI should be used at a final concentration of 1 μg/ml. (Alternatively, DAPI can be added to the final mounting medium at 1–2 μg/ml.) A concentrated stock of 1 mg/ml DAPI in double-distilled water (ddH$_2$O) can be kept in a foil wrapped tube at 4°C for long-term storage. Propidium iodide is a frequently used alternative DNA stain which can be viewed in the rhodamine channel.

d. Mounting

1. Carefully wick away as much solution from the specimen as possible without permitting it to dry out.

2. Place a small drop of mounting solution (see Section VI) on the slide. A thin glass rod made from the flame-sealed tip of a Pasteur pipet is dipped into mounting medium and gently touched to the specimen. Cover the specimen with a coverglass and allow it to settle by gravity, being careful not to distort the specimen by any sideways movement of the coverslip.

3. Wick off excess liquid by holding a piece of filter paper to the edge of the coverslip. If the mounting medium is not self-hardening (e.g., glycerol-based solution), seal the edges of the coverslip with clear nail polish. If the mount is too thick, it will be impossible to properly focus the specimen under high-power objectives. Drying slides can be conveniently stored horizontally in cardboard slide trays (Fisher No. 12-587-10) before transferring to traditional slide boxes. An antifade reagent should be included in the mounting medium (see Section VI) to help minimize the loss of fluorescence due to bleaching. Slides should be stored in the dark.

2. Non-Freeze-Crack Method (Hypochlorite Method) for Permeabilizing and Fixing Large–Scale Embryo Preparations

This procedure is a modification of those of Goh and Bogaert (1991) and G. Mullen (pers. comm.). Although not as useful for isolating early one- and two-cell-stage embryos, a non-freeze-crack method has been used to analyze large-scale embryo preparations. The advantages of this preparation are that the solution changes are carried out in centrifuge and microfuge tubes, and the embryos are less prone to mechanical damage.

1. Obtain a large, PBS-rinsed and carcass-free population of eggs using the hypochlorite method described by Lewis and Fleming (see Chapter 1 in this volume).

2. Fix the embryos at room temperature for 5 to 10 minutes in 3% freshly prepared formaldehyde in PBS. Remove the supernatant and chill the tube on ice. Quickly add 2 ml of methanol (−20°C) to the pellet and store at −20°C.

3. Rehydrate embryos through a 75%, 50%, 25%, 0% methanol series and concentrate by gentle centrifugation. Resuspend in PBS (pH 7.2) containing 0.1% Tween 20 and 2% dry milk powder and incubate with appropriately diluted primary antibodies for 2 hours at room temperature or overnight at 4°C.

4. Wash three times in Tween–milk powder–PBS (20 minutes each) and then incubate 1 to 2 hours at room temperature with secondary antibodies.

5. Wash three times in Tween–milk powder–PBS (20 minutes each) and twice with PBS (5-minute washes). Resuspend in PBS and incubate with DAPI (1 μg/ml) for 1 hour at room temperature.

6. Equilibrate embryos through a 20%, 50% glycerol series in PBS (pH 8.0). Mount on slides in 90% glycerol–PBS–antifade reagent (pH 8.0) as described above.

3. Whole-Mount Fixation of Larvae and Adults

This procedure was adapted from that of Finney and Ruvkun (1990).

a. Permeabilization and Fixation

1. Collect worms from an unstarved plate into a 15-ml centrifuge tube using water or buffer (PBS, M9). As an initial cleanup step, the sucrose floatation method can be used to remove debris and bacteria (see Chapter 1 in this volume). Wash over a 1-hour period with several changes of solution in a 1.6-ml microfuge tube or 15-ml conical tube so that bacteria in the gut are excreted. To pellet worms between washes spin microfuge tubes at 3K for 2 minutes or spin 15-ml centrifuge tubes in a clinical centrifuge (e.g., IEC setting 5 for 2 minutes).

2. Transfer the worms from the 15-ml centrifuge tube to a 1.6-ml microfuge tube and pellet again; the pelleted volume should not exceed 0.25 ml. Chill worms on wet ice.

3. Add ice cold 2X Ruvkun fixation buffer (RFB) to a final concentration of 1×. Add 20% formaldehyde to a final concentration of 1 to 2%. The total volume should be about 1 ml. Mix well, and freeze in dry ice/ethanol. If desired, frozen samples may be stored at −80°C.

4. To permeabilize the worms, melt the frozen worm pellet under a stream of tap water until the ice becomes a slurry. You may either proceed with step 5 at this point or repeat the freeze–thaw cycle up to three times if antibody penetration is poor.

5. After the final thaw, incubate on ice with occasional agitation for 10 minutes to 1 hour, depending on the antigen. Optimal fixation times and formaldehyde concentrations should be empirically determined for each antibody preparation, but incubation in 1% formaldehyde for 0.5 hour is a good place to start.

6. Wash the worms twice with Tris–Triton buffer (TTB). To pellet worms between washes, spin in a microfuge at 3K for 2 minutes. To reduce some of

the disulfide linkages and thus permeabilize the highly crosslinked nematode cuticle, resuspend the worms in TTB + 1% β-mercaptoethanol. Incubate for 2 hours to overnight with mild agitation on a rocker platform in a 37°C incubator.

7. To complete the reduction reaction, wash the worms once in 10 to 15 vol of $1\times$ BO$_3$, 0.01% Triton buffer, pellet in the microfuge, then incubate the worms in $1\times$ BO$_3$ buffer + 10 mM dithiothreitol (DTT) + 0.01% Triton for 15 minutes with gentle agitation. Triton is included to keep the worms from sticking to each other.

8. Immediately wash the worms once in 10 to 15 vol of $1\times$ BO$_3$, 0.01% Triton buffer. To oxidize the –SH groups and thereby prevent the re-formation of the disulfide linkages, incubate in $1\times$ BO$_3$ buffer + 0.3% H$_2$O$_2$ + 0.01% Triton for 15 minutes at room temperature. Agitate gently, but keep the tubes upright and secure the lids with Parafilm or else the release of O$_2$ may cause the lids to pop open.

9. Wash once with $1\times$ BO$_3$ buffer + 0.01% Triton and once for at least 15 minutes with AbB buffer (see Section VI). Store worms at 4°C in AbA buffer. The worms are good for at least a month in this buffer if 0.05% azide is included to inhibit bacterial growth.

Notes. This method is very effective and is considerably less expensive than permeabilization by treatment with collagenase (Ruvkun and Guisto, 1989). This method also works well for staining embryos. Although most antibodies work on these preparations, certain epitopes may be inactivated. In particular, epitopes that depend on disulfide bonds are destroyed during the reduction reactions. Cysteine- and methionine-centered epitopes may be destroyed during the oxidization reactions.

b. Staining

1. Transfer an aliquot (25 μl) of fixed worms to a 1.6-ml microfuge tube (To reduce potentially damaging shear forces, clip the end of the micropipet tip with a razor blade to widen the bore.)

2. Add an appropriate dilution of antibody in AbA buffer to bring the total volume to 100 to 200 μl. (Smaller volumes can be used for precious antibodies.) Incubate the worms in antibody buffer solution overnight at room temperature (RT) or in the cold room depending on the antibody. Use a rocker to provide gentle agitation.

3. Pellet fixed worms (3K for 2 minutes). (It is possible to reuse the supernatant to stain another sample.) Wash with several changes of AbB over the next 15 minutes. Resuspend with AbB and rock gently for 2 hours to overnight at RT or at 4°C.

4. Rinse once with AbA and then add an appropriate dilution of fluorescently tagged secondary antibody in 100 to 200 μl of AbA. Wrap in aluminum foil to protect from light. Incubate at RT for 2 hours to overnight with gentle shaking.

5. Pellet worms and wash with AbB as above.

c. Mounting

Prepare a pad of 2% agarose in PBS. Mix equal volumes (e.g., 5 μl) of fixed worms and 2× mounting medium in a 0.6-ml microfuge tube and transfer 5 μl of the worm suspension to the agarose pad. [DAPI can be included in the mounting medium to stain the DNA (see Section VI).] Apply the coverslip. The agar pad prevents the coverslip from crushing the animals (for agar pad protocol see Fig. 8 in Chapter 10 of this volume).

C. Controls, Tips, and Troubleshooting

1. Suggested Antibody Controls

1. Omit the first antibody to check for nonspecific binding of the secondary antibody.

2. For monoclonal antibodies, stain with more than one antibody to confirm that results accurately reflect localization of whole antigen and not just that of a given epitope.

3. Include purified antigen during the primary antibody incubation of a control specimen. If the primary antibody is specific, preincubation with purified antigen should eliminate staining.

4. A null mutation in the antigen encoding gene is an especially useful negative control for specific staining (Miller et al., 1983; Rogalski et al., 1993).

5. Use other methods such as in situ hybridization (Evans et al., 1994; see Chapter 14 in this volume) or a lacZ reporter gene to confirm antibody staining pattern (Fire, 1992; see Chapter 19 in this volume).

6. Omit both the primary and secondary antibodies to check for autofluorescence. In C. elegans, intestinal granules are strongly autofluorescent when irradiated with 300- to 400-nm light and may pose a problem when using UV filter sets (e.g., DAPI staining). On the other hand, these autofluorescent intestinal granules can serve as a useful marker of intestinal cell differentiation in early embryos (Laufer et al., 1980).

7. Use a previously characterized antibody to confirm that negative results are not due to technical or reagent-related problems such as poor permeabilization or problems related to the secondary antibody.

2. Other Antibody Staining Methods

Special methods are required for cases in which the specimen is stained with more than one antibody. Fluorophores with different excitation and emission maxima should be used to provide separate signals from each antibody (see Section III). For indirect immunofluorescence staining, the primary antibodies should be of different isotypes or derived from different species to prevent cross-reaction by the secondary fluorescent antibodies (see double staining of embryonic GLP-1 and P-granules in Fig. 1, see color plate). For cases in which this solution is not possible (e.g., all primary antibodies are mouse IgGs), fluorescently labeled primary antibodies can be used. A simple method for conjugating either fluorescein or rhodamine B isothiocyanate (FITC or RITC) to a mouse monoclonal antibody is described in Section III,C. An example of double direct immunofluorescence staining of *unc-54* and myosin A is shown in Fig. 2, see color plate. It is also possible to use a combination indirect/direct labeling scheme for primary antibodies from the same species by adding antibodies in the sequence given in the following example: mouse monoclonal; fluorescein-conjugated goat anti-mouse; nonimmune mouse IgG (to block unoccupied goat anti-mouse sites); mouse monoclonal coupled to rhodamine (see Osborn and Weber, 1982; Miller *et al.,* 1983; Epstein *et al.,* 1993).

For low-abundance antigens, it may be necessary to use more elaborate staining strategies to enhance the signal. For example, GLP-1 expression in *C. elegans* embryos was detected with a biotinylated secondary antibody in combination with fluorescein-labeled avidin (Evans *et al.,* 1994).

3. Troubleshooting Guide

a. High Background Staining

1. The primary or secondary antibody may be too concentrated.

2. The secondary fluorescent antibody should be immunoadsorbed with fixed nematodes (see Section III) to remove contaminating antibodies.

3. Try a different blocking method, include blocking agents with the diluted antibodies or add a second blocking step before adding the secondary antibody.

4. Include a mild nonionic detergent such as 0.1% Tween 20 in the antibody incubation solutions.

5. After formaldehyde fixation, residual aldehydes may covalently bind to immunoreagents. Preincubation with either 0.2 M glycine for 5 minutes or protein blocking agents such as BSA or pre-immune serum should eliminate this problem.

Fig. 1 *In situ* localization of GLP-1 and other early embryonic markers using a modified freeze-crack method for specimen preparation. Time series of early embryogenesis shows changes in the protein distribution. *Left column:* Embryos stained for GLP-1, using rat polyclonal antibodies against GLP-1 peptides and an FITC-labeled anti-rat secondary antibody. In the bottom photo, the anti-GLP-1 antibody has been preincubated with GLP-1 fusion peptide to confirm the specificity of antibody binding. *Middle column:* The same embryos stained for actin, DNA, and P-granules using specific monoclonal antibodies and a rhodamine-labeled anti-mouse secondary antibody. Antiactin antibody (from ICN) marks the surface of all blastomeres and helps outline cell boundaries; anti-DNA antibody (MAb 030, Chemicon) marks cell nuclei; anti-P granule staining (from S. Strome) identifies the posterior blastomeres P1, P2, P3, and P4. *Right column:* Diagrams of embryos in which the AB descendants are crosshatched, showing that GLP-1 is expressed in these cells. Courtesy of Sarah Crittendon. Reprinted with permission from Evans *et al.* (1994).

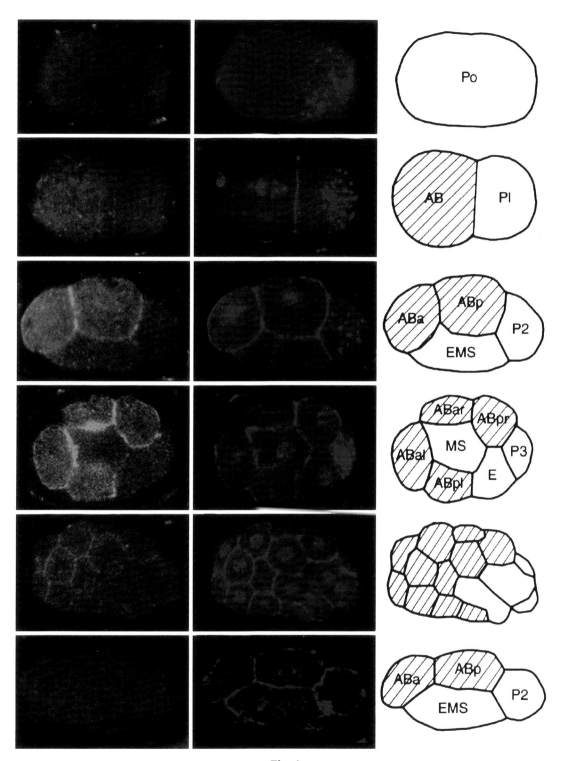

Fig. 1

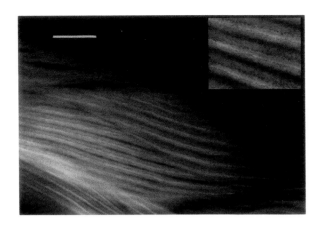

Fig. 2

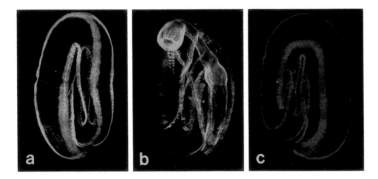

Fig. 3

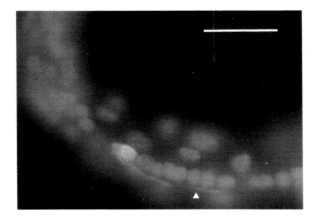

Fig. 4

b. Too Little Immunolabeling

1. Use other methods such as immunoblotting or reaction with tissue from another species to confirm that the primary antibody does in fact react with the antigen.

2. Too little signal can be due to overfixation. Try alternate fixatives or decrease fixation time.

3. Blurred signals can be due to diffusion from underfixation. Try alternative fixatives or increase fixation time. When using mixed aldehyde fixes, note that formaldehyde fixes faster, whereas glutaraldehyde creates stronger crosslinks.

4. Blurred signals can also result from improper specimen preparation. Shear forces generated by accidental sliding of the coverslip during the final mounting will seriously distort cellular structures. Extra thick mounts due to too much mounting solution or extra thick agar pads will also result in blurred images.

5. Antigens can also be physically masked. For whole-mount adults and older larvae, a partial dissection of the animal can ensure that antibody reaches internal structures such as the pharynx and gonad.

6. Poor permealization will prevent the antibody from reaching internal antigenic sites. Try acetone permeabilization or detergent treatment for 5 to 30

Fig. 2 Body wall muscle stained with antimyosin monoclonal antibodies (mAbs). mAb 5-6 ascites fluid was directly labeled with RITC and mAb 5-8 ascites fluid was labeled with FITC as described in the text. Animals were fixed using the method of Finney and Ruvkun (1990). mAb 5-6 reacts specifically with myosin heavy chain A (red) and mAb 5-8 reacts with *unc-54* myosin heavy chain (green) to demonstrate that these MHC isoforms are differentially localized in the muscle sarcomere (see Miller *et al.*, 1983). Bar = 10 μm. The inset is 3× further enlarged. (Photographed in Nikon Microphot, 100×, 1.25 NA. The original photograph was digitized on a flat bed scanner and the contrast was enhanced using Adobe Photoshop 3.0.)

Fig. 3 *In situ* localization of proteins encoded by the *unc-52* (perlecan) gene in late stage (3-fold) wild-type embryos. Embryos were prepared by the non-freeze-crack large-scale embryo method, and the slides were examined by laser scanning confocal microscopy. Perlecan, basement membrane proteoglycan, is differentially spliced to give rise to a number of distinct isoforms. (a) Localization pattern of polyclonal GM2 which was raised against a fusion protein containing exons 14, 15, and 18. Stained with FITC-labeled anti-mouse secondary antibody. (b) Localization pattern of polyclonal GM1, which was raised against a fusion protein containing exons 9 and 10. (c) Embryo stained with MH2, a monoclonal antibody against exon 19, and a rhodamine-labeled anti-mouse secondary antibody. Courtesy of Greg Mullen.

Fig. 4 Motor neuron labeled with a *lacZ* reporter gene. View of the tail region (posterior to left) of a late L1 larva expressing an *unc-4–lacZ* transgene in the VA11 motor neuron (Miller and Niemeyer, 1995). Note the axon (arrowhead) projecting beneath cell nuclei (light blue) of other motor neurons in the ventral nerve cord. Fixed according to Finney and Ruvkun (1990). Stained with anti-β-galactosidase monoclonal antibody (Promega) and RITC-labeled antimouse secondary antibody (Sigma). Counterstained with DAPI to show nuclei (blue). Bar = 10 μm. (Photographed in Nikon Microphot, 100×, 1.25 NA.)

minutes at room temperature immediately after fixation but before beginning the immunolabeling. Typical detergents and concentrations (in buffer) include Triton X-100 (0.05–1%) and Tween 20 (0.05–2%). This technique is especially applicable to aldehyde-based fixation methods.

7. Improper freeze-cracking prevents antibody access. Wick away more liquid before freezing the slide. Remove the coverslip faster from the frozen slide to give an audible crack.

8. Alter the incubation times with the antibodies. Try decreasing the temperature (e.g., 4°C) and increasing the time of incubation.

9. Include sodium azide (0.05%) in all storage solutions as well as long-term incubation solutions to prevent bacteria-related degradation of the antibody and specimens. *Caution:* Sodium azide is a toxic substance.

10. Improperly stored antibodies can degrade rapidly. Antibodies should be aliquoted rather than subjected to repeated freezing and thawing. Store diluted antibodies at 4°C rather than freezing them and include a high concentration (10 mg/ml) of "inert" protein such as BSA to prevent nonspecific binding to the storage vessel. Some monoclonal antibodies are inactivated by freezing at any concentration.

III. Preparation of Antibodies to Nematode Antigens

A. Antigens

Because of the small size of the organism, it is generally difficult to purify endogenous antigens from *C. elegans* in sufficient quantities for immunization. The exceptions are muscle contractile proteins (Schachat *et al.,* 1978; Gossett *et al.,* 1982), the major sperm protein (Klass and Hirsch, 1981), and the vitellogenins (Sharrock, 1984), which are highly abundant and have been used successfully to raise specific antibodies. One solution to this problem is to prepare monoclonal antibodies that can be obtained from immunizations with heterogeneous preparations. Success with this approach, however, requires an antigen-specific assay for screening hybridoma lines. As many *C. elegans* genes are cloned on the basis of mutant phenotypes before the corresponding proteins are known, antibodies are frequently raised against recombinant proteins expressed in bacteria (Krause *et al.,* 1990; Finney and Ruvkun, 1990; Nonet *et al.,* 1993). Lastly, antibodies can be raised to synthetic peptides designed on the basis of known peptide sequences or from nucleotide coding sequences.

B. Monoclonal versus Polyclonal Antibodies

Both monoclonal and conventional polyclonal antibodies to *C. elegans* antigens have been prepared. The choice of method depends on several factors. As mentioned earlier, the option of preparing monoclonal antibodies is especially useful for low-abundance proteins or antigens that cannot be readily purified. Banks of monoclonals can be screened to identify interesting antigens based solely on the staining pattern of the corresponding antibody (e.g., tissue-specific antibodies: Okamato and Thomson, 1985; Francis and Waterston, 1985). Furthermore, once a clonal hybridoma cell line is established, unlimited quantities of the secreted antibody can be generated. In cases in which the immunogen is highly purified, such as a recombinant fusion protein, the conventional approach of generating polyclonal antibodies may be a better option, particularly if the investigator does not have ready access to cell culture facilities. With careful preparation and appropriate controls, both polyclonal and monoclonal antibody preparations can yield highly specific and reproducible patterns of immunofluorescence staining in *C. elegans* (Fig. 3, see color plate). Special methods that apply to each of these approaches are discussed below.

1. Monoclonal Antibodies

Methods for preparing monoclonal antibodies are described in detail elsewhere (Harlow and Lane, 1988) and are not discussed here. It is important, however, to emphasize that cell fusions should not be undertaken until antiserum from an immunized mouse shows an immune response to the desired antigen. Indeed, the immunoassay that is employed at this stage is critically important later when it is typically necessary to screen large numbers of separate hybridoma cell lines. Immunoassays that have been used for this purpose include enzyme-linked immunosorbent assay and Western blotting (Miller *et al.,* 1983) and large-scale immunofluorescence screens of embryos or worms (Francis and Waterston, 1985; Okamoto and Thomson, 1985; Sithigorngul *et al.,* 1989).

It is generally desirable to obtain more than one monoclonal antibody to a particular antigen because of the homogeneous binding specificity of each separate monoclonal antibody. By definition, a given monoclonal antibody reacts with an epitope that encompasses a small fraction of the total immunogenic surface of a given antigen. Epitopes may correspond to short sequences of amino acids or to segments of polysaccharide chains, for example. Any one of these antibody combining sites may not be accessible *in situ* or may be altered to an unreactive state by fixation. Steric effects or fixation artifacts probably account for the general observation that some monoclonals that are reactive on Western blots or by ELISA may not work well for immunofluorescence staining. Thus, it may be necessary to screen a battery of monoclonal antibodies to identify one that yields a strong immunofluorescence signal. This problem is obviated, of course, in cases in which immunofluorescence is used as a primary screen for monoclonal producing hybridoma clones.

It is also important to appreciate the possibility that a particular epitope or similar structure may be present in more than one antigen and thus could result in a misleading antibody staining pattern. This consideration is especially important for studies of closely related proteins which may be expressed in different cells or located in distinct subcellular structures but which may nonetheless share immunogenic epitopes. Most of the monoclonal antibodies raised to purified *C. elegans* myosin, for example, recognize epitopes that are present in more than one of the four muscle myosin heavy-chain isoforms (Miller *et al.*, 1986). Monoclonal antibodies that show preferential reaction with one of the myosins also produce detectable reactions with other myosin isoforms at high antibody concentrations. These weaker interactions are presumably due to the presence of related amino acid epitopes in the cross-reactive myosins (Miller *et al.*, 1983). Thus, a general rule for immunofluorescence staining is to employ the lowest concentration of antibody that yields a detectable signal. Where possible, direct titration of the monoclonal antibody either on Western blots or *in situ* should be undertaken to test for cross-reaction. A particularly useful control is the absence of staining in a null mutant for the antigen of interest. A variant of this strategy is to test for predictable changes in staining in mutants that would be expected to alter the expression or distribution of the antigen (Nonet *et al.*, 1993).

2. Polyclonal Antibodies

Polyclonal antisera have also been used to obtain specific immunofluorescence staining in *C. elegans*. In this case, the immunogen should be highly purified, if possible, to reduce the immune response to contaminants. A general strategy is to obtain nucleotide coding sequence for the protein of interest and then to immunize with either a fusion protein purified from bacteria or with a synthetic peptide derived from the inferred amino acid sequence. Even in these cases, however, it is usually necessary to immunoadsorb the antiserum to remove unwanted antibodies which may be generated by low levels of impurities in the immunogen (see below).

In some instances, preimmune serum produces specific staining and may be indicative of exposure to nematode antigens before immunization. This problem is not trivial because the laboratory animals that are used to produce antibodies are susceptible to common parasitic nematode infections and thus could be mounting a powerful immune response against unrelated nematode antigens. Animal care personnel should carefully check the animals for nematode infections before immunization, and must be informed that recently "dewormed" animals are not acceptable for your studies.

The best approach around this problem is to immunize more than one rabbit and then to compare staining patterns obtained with each separate antiserum. Alternatively, the primary antibody can be selectively adsorbed onto a column matrix of purified antigen and subsequently eluted to produce an affinity-purified reagent (see next section). Unwanted cross-reaction with related epitopes in other antigens can be reduced by titrating to find the lowest concentration of antibody that yields a bright signal. As mentioned earlier, commercially prepared fluorochrome-labeled secondary antibodies may produce high backgrounds or, in some cases, specific staining patterns (e.g., anti-P-granule antibodies; Strome and Wood, 1982). These contaminating antibodies can be easily removed by immunoadsorption with fixed nematodes (see next section).

C. Methods

Procedures for generating and purifying bacterial fusion proteins are described in several references and are not included here (Finney and Ruvkun, 1990; Krause et al., 1990; Bowerman et al., 1993; Nonet et al., 1993). Special methods for purifying antisera to nematode antigens are described below.

1. Preparation of Bacterial Acetone Powder and Immunoadsorption of Polyclonal Antiserum

This simple procedure (Harlow and Lane, 1988) can be used to remove unwanted antibodies to contaminating bacterial proteins from polyclonal antisera raised against bacterial fusion proteins. To make the acetone powder, use a bacterial culture that is not expressing the fusion protein. To remove antibodies against the vector-encoded portion of the fusion protein, make the acetone powder from induced bacteria that have been transformed with the expression vector alone.

a. Preparation of Acetone Powder
1. Harvest bacteria by centrifugation and resuspend pellet in 0.9% NaCl.
2. Freeze suspension on dry ice and thaw on wet ice.
3. Submit thawed suspension to 5×30 second pulses with probe sonicator. Keep sonicate on water–ice slurry during sonication.
4. Transfer sonicate to a glass centrifuge tube and add approximately 5 vol of acetone (precooled to $-20°C$). Incubate on water–ice slurry for 30 minutes, mixing periodically.
5. Centrifuge at 9000g for 20 minutes at 4°C.
6. Remove supernatant and resuspend pellet in 5 vol of $-20°C$ acetone. Incubate on water–ice slurry for additional 10 to 15 minutes with occasional shaking.
7. Repeat centrifugation in step 5 and discard supernatant.
8. Put filter paper disk on glass plate. Use spatula to spread damp pellet on filter paper to dry. Recover dry powder by scraping the filter with a razor blade. The powder can be stored for several months at room temperature in a sealed vial.

b. Adsorption of Antisera with Bacterial Acetone Powder
1. Dilute antiserum into AbA (see Section VI) in a 1.6-ml microfuge tube.
2. Add 25 mg powder/ml of antiserum and rock gently at RT for 1 hour.
3. Spin at top speed in a microfuge for 5 minutes and transfer supernatant to a fresh tube for storage.

4. Check adsorbed antiserum for residual contaminating activity on Western blots or by *in situ* immunofluorescence.

2. Preparation of Acetone-Fixed *C. Elegans* for Adsorption of Antiserum

Acetone-fixed *C. elegans* can also be made using the same procedure described above for the preparation of a bacterial acetone powder. We have used acetone-fixed worms to remove antibodies against nematode antigens from fluorescent secondary antibodies (e.g., rhodamine–goat anti-mouse, Sigma T-5393, diluted 1/100 in AbA). In cases in which a null mutation exists for a particular antigen, it may be very helpful to adsorb primary antiserum with acetone-fixed mutant nematodes. Secondary antibodies can also be cleaned up by preadsorption with worms or embryos that have been fixed for antibody staining by one of the methods described above.

3. Direct Affinity Purification of Antiserum

This procedure is especially useful for cases in which the immunoadsorption methods described above do not eliminate contaminating antibody reactivity (Ruvkun and Giusto, 1989).

a. Coupling Purified Fusion Protein to Affigel–10 Matrix

1. Swirl bottle of Affigel-10 matrix (Bio-Rad No. 153-6099) to make a homogenous suspension and transfer 5 ml to a 15-ml plastic centrifuge tube.

2. Pellet matrix in a tabletop centrifuge. Wash pellet several times with ice-cold dH_2O.

3. Add 2.5 ml of purified fusion protein (6 mg/ml) in Mops buffer (see Section VI) to matrix and allow to couple overnight. Use a rocker to gently mix in a 15-ml capped tube at 4°C.

4. Add 1 ml of 1 *M* ethanolamine, pH 8, to fusion protein–matrix mixture and incubate for 1 hour at 4°C. (This step blocks unoccupied coupling sites on Affigel matrix.)

5. Wash matrix with Mops + 2 *M* NaCl in a tabletop centrifuge. Repeat three times.

6. Use a Bradford assay (Bio-Rad No. 500-0002) to measure the protein concentration in each wash and to calculate fusion protein coupling efficiency (should be 60–70%). For precise measurements, IgG makes a better standard than BSA because of the different responses of the two proteins in Bradford assays.

Notes. This procedure should be preceded by adsorption against an acetone powder of bacterial carrying the expression vector alone to avoid immunopurifying antibodies to the vector-encoded portion of the fusion protein.

4. Immunoadsorption of Antiserum to Fusion Protein–Affigel-10 Matrix

1. Add 10 ml antiserum to fusion protein–Affigel matrix (~3.5 ml settled volume) and incubate overnight in capped tube on vertical rotating platform at 4°C.

2. Pour slurry into column (Bio-Rad No. 732-1010) and wash with 25 ml Mops buffer.

3. Elute antibody with 0.5-ml aliquots of 2 M guanidine–HCl, pH 5.4. (It may be necessary to use harsher treatments such as 100 mM glycine, pH 2.5, or 0.1 M Na borate, pH 10, to elute antibody. If acidic or alkaline elution is used, preload the receiving tube with 50 to 100 μl of 1 M Tris, pH 8, to bring the antibody solution to neutral pH immediately after elution.)

4. Dialyze peak fractions against Mops at 4°C and assay for activity. Concentrate antibody fractions, if necessary, by precipitation with 50% ammonium sulfate at 4°C.

5. Directly Labeling Monoclonal Antibodies for Immunofluorescence

This procedure has been used to label purified monoclonal antibodies (Miller *et al.*, 1983; Epstein *et al.*, 1993) as well as monoclonal antibody-containing ascites fluids (Fire and Waterston, 1989) with either RITC (Sigma R-1755) or FITC (Isomer I, Sigma F-7250).

1. Dialyze the monoclonal antibody solution against 0.15 M NaCl, 0.1 M sodium carbonate, pH 9.5, overnight at 4°C.

2. Remove the antibody solution from the dialysis bag and use a Bradford assay to measure the protein concentration.

3. Prepare fresh stocks of RITC, 5 mg/ml in dimethyl sulfoxide. Protect from light.

4. In a darkened room, add 25 μg of RITC stock/mg monoclonal antibody or about 12.5 μg of RITC stock/mg ascites protein (typical reaction volume: 200 μl ascites fluid at 13 mg/ml total protein).

5. Cover the reaction tube with foil and rock for 1 to 2 hours at RT.

6. Stop the reaction by adding ammonium acetate to a final concentration of 50 mM.

7. Separate unreacted RITC from labeled protein by gel filtration over Sephadex G-25 Medium (Pharmacia). Swell beads as described by manufacturer and fill column (Bio-Rad No. 732-1010) to a volume approximately 20× the volume of the sample. Wash column with PBS. Add 1/5 vol of loading buffer [0.25% bromophenol blue, 25% Ficoll (type 400)] to the sample and allow to settle on top of the column matrix beneath overlying PBS. It is usually convenient to collect samples by hand in microfuge tubes. The labeled antibody will elute first as a colored band (red for RITC or yellow for FITC) that is well separated from

the unreacted fluorescent label and from the bromophenol blue tracking dye that are retarded by passage through the gel matrix.

8. Use a Bradford assay to determine the protein concentration of the labeled eluate and stain at dilutions that work well for indirect immunofluorescence with the unlabeled monoclonal antibody.

Notes. Some monoclonal antibodies may be inactivated by the reaction presumably due to modification of amino acid side chains in the antibody combining site. If this happens, try labeling a different monoclonal antibody.

High staining backgrounds can result from overlabeling the antibody. Try shorter reaction times or reduce the label/antibody ratio. It may be necessary to chromatograph the antibody conjugates on an ion-exchange column (Harlow and Lane, 1988) and then empirically test different fractions for specific staining.

IV. Microscopy: Necessary Equipment and Photomicrography Tips

The basic requirement is a compound microscope equipped for epifluorescence illumination and photography. High-resolution objective lenses (60× or 100×, NA > 1.25) are essential because of the small size of the *C. elegans* embryo (~40 μm in diameter) and of most cell nuclei (1–2 μm in diameter). These objectives should also transmit UV light for DAPI excitation (e.g., Zeiss 100× Plan Neofluar, NA 1.3, or Nikon 60 × Plan Apo, NA 1.4). DAPI stains all cell nuclei, which is frequently useful for establishing the exact location and thus identity of the immunofluorescent cells (Fig. 4, see color plate). Ideally, the microscope should also have high-resolution differential interference contrast (Nomarski) optics to allow crisp optical sectioning that is oftentimes essential for the reliable identification of stained cells.

The two most frequently used immunofluorescent compounds are FITC and RITC (Figs. 2 and 3). FITC (green) is typically brighter but also fades faster than RITC (red). In addition, the DAPI emission peak overlaps the FITC excitation spectrum and thus tends to bleach the FITC signal. (This problem can be avoided by viewing the DAPI image after photographing the FITC image.)

A minimum of two separate fluorescence filter sets for DAPI and for either RITC or FITC are recommended. For black and white photographs of double-labeled samples in which it is important to obtain separate images of each antibody stain, special bandpass filter sets are used to prevent the RITC signal from leaking into the FITC channel. The recently developed dye Texas red requires a third type of filter set, but is an excellent alternative to RITC for double-labeling experiments with FITC; the excitation/emission spectrum of Texas red is shifted toward longer wavelengths and thus exhibits less overlap with FITC (Haugland, 1992). High-quality, low-cost fluorescence filter sets can be purchased from Chroma Technology (Brattleboro, VT).

The photography system for the microscope can be as simple as a 35-mm SLR camera equipped with a built-in light meter. These can be attached to most upright microscopes with a standard phototube and appropriate relay lens. The major disadvantage of this setup is vibration from the mechanical shutter in the SLR camera, although typical fluorescence exposures are for several seconds and are thus not noticeably affected. More sophisticated photography systems offered by microscope manufacturers avoid this problem and also may allow spot metering and memory functions which are essential for setting exposures of small, bright off-center fluorescent objects in dark backgrounds (e.g., GLP-1 or P-granules in early embryos). The ability to take double exposures is also a useful feature for photomicroscopy.

For black and white photography, Kodak Tmax-400 is sufficiently sensitive for most images, but if you have a very bright image such as DAPI-stained nuclei which can be shot at ASA 125, the highest-resolution film is Kodak Technical Pan. Color print or Ektachrome slide film, ASA 200-400 (Fuji, Kodak), is especially convenient if automatic film processing is available. In our experience, most photo laboratories can reliably process color slide film but have a harder time getting both the reds and greens correct on print film. Higher ASA color print films (i.e., ASA 800, ASA 1600) are more sensitive but are also unacceptably grainy and effectively diminish the resolution of the image. Because of cost factors, reliability, and processing times, many laboratories choose to shoot color slide film and then print only the slides that will be used for publication.

For faint images, it is possible to alter developing conditions to "push" lower ASA black and white films (e.g., develop Kodak Technical Pan in HC110 developer diluted 1:10 for 6 minutes). Long exposure times can be reduced by setting the camera sensitivity to a higher ASA than indicated on the film. For example, Ektachrome 200 shot at ASA 400 or 800 usually gives a good exposure (R. Schnabel and H. Schnabel, pers. comm.).

Another method that will probably expand in use in the future is to digitize 35-mm slide images in a high-resolution slide scanner (Nikon Coolscan) for computer enhancement using digital "darkroom" software such as NIH Image or Adobe Photoshop. Clarity can be significantly improved by digital filtering algorithms and images can also be conveniently cropped and sized, (Fig. 2). Pictures can be imported into either Quark Express (Eficolor) or Aldus Freehand as TIFF-files to apply labels or to combine with text. The final figure can then be printed on a dye sublimation printer (Tektronix Phaser IISDS or Sony UDP7000D) or, in some cases, submitted directly to the journal on disk for publication.

Low-light-level video cameras (SIT) or cooled CCD cameras are excellent alternatives to conventional film photography, especially when analyzing living organisms or rapidly quenching specimens that cannot be viewed with high-intensity UV light. Although photographic film affords higher-resolution images, these cameras are substantially more sensitive than film and the output can be processed in a desktop computer to enhance contrast and effective resolution

386 David M. Miller and Diane C. Shakes

(Shotten, 1993). One particularly promising application will be to use either SIT cameras or cooled CCD cameras to capture images of transgene protein chimeras containing the newly described green fluorescent protein (GFP) (Chalfie *et al.,* 1994). This technique should enable investigators to record the expression of GFP-labeled proteins in live animals. SIT cameras are generally more sensitive than cooled CCD cameras and are therefore preferable for rapidly moving or weakly fluorescent objects. On the other hand, CCD camera output is considerably less noisy than the SIT camera signal and therefore will yield a cleaner image of a stationary fluorescent object. (See Shotten, 1993, for a comparison of SIT camera and cooled CCD camera performance.)

As mentioned earlier, confocal microscopy is an especially useful technique for enhancing the effective resolution of immunofluorescent images. Detailed descriptions of confocal microscopy are available in several recent articles and are not included here (White *et al.,* 1987; Paddock, 1994).

V. Concluding Remarks

The goal of this chapter is to provide a practical guide to immunofluorescence analysis methods in *C. elegans.* Because of space limitations, we have restricted our discussion to the techniques that are routinely used in our laboratories. Alternative fixation and staining protocols that have been used successfully by others are described in the following references (Priess and Thompson, 1987; Ardizzi and Epstein, 1987; Ruvkun and Giusto, 1989; Li and Chalfie, 1990; McIntire *et al.,* 1992; Nonet *et al.,* 1993; Evans *et al.,* 1994). Further details on the use of particular antibodies are found in the references included in Table I.

The recent introduction of the green fluorescent protein (GFP) provides an exciting alternative to immunofluorescence staining for some applications; cells expressing chimeric GFP-transgenes can be detected in live animals using a standard FITC epifluorescence filter set (Chalfie *et al.,* 1994). This approach should prove to be particularly useful for pinpointing the precise time and place of GFP expression since cell lineages can be simultaneously observed using DIC imaging. Using somewhat more complicated constructs, this technique could potentially provide a powerful method for analyzing temporal changes in antigen localization as well. This technique, however, will always be limited to proteins for which gene regulatory regions have been sufficiently well characterized for the construction of chimeric GFP transgenes. In addition, the use of GFP transgenes will never supplant the use of conventional immunofluorescence staining, as it will always be necessary to confirm that the pattern of expression of the GFP-chimeric protein matches that of the endogenous protein.

Recent studies that demonstrate a striking difference between GLP-1 RNA and protein expression patterns reinforce the importance of comparing RNA *in situ* hybridization results with protein immunofluorescence staining (Evans *et al.,* 1994). Obvious differences between transcriptional and translational regulation should be detectable using GFP constructs; however, because the GFP fusion could conceivably alter the distribution of the labeled protein in the cell, antibodies to specific antigens will continue to provide the most reliable method for analyzing the subcellular localization of particular proteins using either the immunofluorescence techniques described in this chapter or the immuno-electron microscopy techniques described by Hall in Chapter 17.

In this chapter, we have emphasized methods for fixing and staining *C. elegans* animals for immunofluorescence microscopy. These techniques are well established. The analysis of fluorescent images is rapidly evolving, however, as conventional photography is supplanted by digital microscopy. In the future, the reliance on confocal microscopy as well as low-light-level video cameras for image collection and digital darkroom software for image processing will dramatically expand the amount of information that can be extracted from immunofluorescent samples.

Table I
Useful *Caenorhabditis elegans* Antibodies and Other Staining Methods

Antigen	Antibody or method	Reference
Early Embryonic		
GLP-1 (AB derived)		Evans *et al.*, 1994
SKN-1 (specifies EMS)	Anti-SKN-1	Bowerman *et al.*, 1993
α-Tubulin (spindles)	Antitubulin	Piperno and Fuller, 1985
β-Tubulin (spindles)	E7	NICHD-Ab Bank
P-granules	K76	Strome and Wood, 1983
Actin capping	C4 actin	Monoclonal available from ICN
	Polyclonal	For pattern, see Waddle *et al.*, 1994
Stage Specific		
LIN-14 (stage specific)		Ruvkun and Giusto, 1989
Subtractive polyclonals		Cox *et al.*, 1980; Politz *et al.*, 1987
Dauer cuticle	CUT-1	Sebastiano *et al.*, 1991
Body Wall Muscle		
Actin	Phalloidin	Embryos, Hill and Strome, 1988
		Worms, Priess and Hirsh, 1986
α-Actinin	MH35, MH40	Francis and Waterston, 1985
Myosin HC A	5-6	Miller *et al.*, 1983, 1986
Myosin HC B (unc-54)	5-8, 28.2	Miller *et al.*, 1983, 1986
paramyosin (unc-15)	5-23	Epstein *et al.*, 1982, 1985
	MH1, MH16	Waterston, 1988
Twitchin (unc-22)	R11-3 (p)	Moerman *et al.*, 1988
I-bands	MH7	Waterston, 1988
Vinculin	MH23, MH24	Francis and Waterston, 1985
		Barstead and Waterston, 1989
Blast cells	CeMyoD	Krause *et al.*, 1990

(*continues*)

Table I (Continued)

Antigen	Antibody or method	Reference
Pharynx		
Myosin HC C	9.2.1, 5-11	Epstein *et al.*, 1982; Miller *et al.*, 1986
Myosin HC D	5-17	Epstein *et al.*, 1982; Ardizzi and Epstein, 1987
Early marker (400 min)	3NB12	Priess and Thomson, 1987
21/34 pharyngeal muscles		
2 intestinal and 2 neural cells		
Intermediate filaments (marginal, hypodermal)	Anti-IFA	Pruss *et al.*, 1981
I-bands and intermediate filaments	MH20	Francis and Waterston, 1985
Germ line		
P-granules	K76	Strome and Wood, 1983
Major sperm protein	SP56	Ward *et al.*, 1986
GLP-1 (mitotic cells)	Anti-GLP-1	Evans *et al.*, 1994
Intestine		
Gut granules	Polarized light autofluorescence	Laufer *et al.*, 1980
62-, 64-, 68-kDa proteins	MH33	Francis and Waterston, 1985
GES-1	Histochemical	Edgar and McGhee, 1986
Acid phosphatase	Histochemical	Beh *et al.*, 1991
Neurons		
All neurons	Antibody	Hekimi, 1990
Multiple neurons	Anti-UNC-86	Finney and Ruvkun, 1990
	Antitubulin	Siddiqui *et al.*, 1989
	Anti-horseradish peroxidase	Siddiqui and Culotti, 1991
	Synaptotagmin	Nonet *et al.*, 1993
Various neurons	FMRFamide	Schinkman and Li, 1992; Atkinson *et al.*, 1988
Neuronal subset		
Strong (ADL, ASH, ASJ, ASK, PHA, PHB)		
Weak (AWB, ASI)	DiI and DiO	C. Bargmann[a]
Chemosensory		
(ADF, ASH, ASI, ASJ, ASK, ADL, PHA, PHB)	FITC filling	Hedgecock *et al.*, 1985
Sensory socket and sheath cells, IL2 neuron	Di4ANEPPS, RH421	C. Bargmann[a]
Dopaminergic	Formaldehyde-induced fluorescence	Sulston *et al.*, 1975
Serotonin		Desai *et al.*, 1988
GABA		McIntire *et al.*, 1992
CAN neurons	P-substance	C. Bargmann[a]
Touch cells	Anti-MEC-7	Hamelin *et al.*, 1992
Motor neurons	Anti-UNC-18	Gengyo-Ando *et al.*, 1993
Others		
Band desmosomes	MH22, MH27	Francis and Waterston, 1985
300-kDa protein (pharyngeal and hypodermal hemidesmosomes)	MH5	Francis and Waterston, 1985

(continues)

Table I (*Continued*)

Antigen	Antibody or method	Reference
Integrin	MH25	Francis and Waterston, 1985
Mixed (intestinal, sperm, IL2 neuron, CEM cells, pharyngeal gland, valve, and sensory process in male tail	ICB4 (also 2CB7)	Okamato and Thomson, 1985; Bowerman *et al.,* 1992
Mixed (neuron, intestinal, hypodermal)	MH38	Francis and Waterston, 1985
Mixed (pharyngeal precursors, ventral cord, and some neural precursors	48C7	Granato *et al.,* 1994
Excretory cell	MH26	Francis and Waterston, 1985
Copulatory bursa and vulva		Link *et al.,* 1988
Cell cycle related		Hecht *et al.,* 1987
Body seams	NE2/1B4-14	R. Schnabel and H. Schnabel[a]
Perlecan (produced in muscle, located in basement membrane)	MH2, MH3	Francis and Waterston, 1991; Rogalski *et al.,* 1993

[a] Personal communication.

VI. Recipes

Subbed Polylysine Slides. Heat 200 ml of dH$_2$O to 60°C in a 1-liter flask. Add 0.4 g gelatin, mix, and cool to 40°C. Add 0.02 g chromium potassium sulfate 1,2-hydrate. Add this solution to a second 1-liter flask containing 0.2 g of poly-D-lysine. Stir to mix. Subbing solution can be stored at 4°C in an amber bottle for 1 week, but should be reheated to 40°C before using to melt the gelatin.

While wearing gloves, briefly dip the dry, acid-washed glass slides into the subbing solution. Allow the slides to dry in a location where they will not pick up dust. Repeat for a second coat. Subbed slides that have been stored in slide boxes at 4°C will keep for months.

Following are two alternative methods for making polylysine slides:

1. One alternative method, which is essential when working with eight-well Teflon-coated slides, was developed by R. Schnabel and H. Schnabel (pers. comm.). Slides are heated to 80°C on a metal block. A polylysine solution of 0.25 mg/ml (in ddH$_2$O) is applied to the slides by dipping a rubber policeman into drop of this solution and then spreading the liquid across the hot slide. Repeat three times and follow by baking the slide another 5 minutes on the metal block. Cool the slides to room temperature before use.

2. A quick method for making polylysine slides is to add one drop of 1% polylysine (in ddH$_2$O) directly to a dry ethanol-washed slide and to subsequently spread it using an ethanol-cleaned Pasteur pipet bulb. Allow the slides to air-dry and use immediately.

20% Buffered Formaldehyde. Weigh out about 250 mg of paraformaldehyde into a 15-ml plastic centrifuge tube. Multiply weight in milligrams of paraformal-

MOPS Buffer.   1 mM phenylmethylsulfonyl fluoride (PMSF), 0.1 M NaCl, 0.1 M 4-morpholinepropanesulfonic acid (Mops), pH 7.5. Combine 10 ml 0.1 M PMSF, 20.93 g Mops, 5.84 g NaCl, and 900 ml distilled H$_2$O. Adjust to pH 7.5 with NaOH. Add dH$_2$O to 1000 ml. *Note:* PMSF (Sigma P-7626) is a protease inhibitor and highly toxic. Dissolve 0.435 g PMSF in 25 ml of 100% ethanol. Store in the dark at RT.

PBS.   Combine 7.31 g NaCl, 2.36 g Na$_2$HPO$_4$, and 1.31 g NaH$_2$PO$_4$·2H$_2$O. Adjust the pH to 7.0 to 7.2 and adjust final volume to 1 liter.

PBS from Harlow and Lane (1988).   Combine 8.0 g NaCl, 0.2 g KCl, 1.44 g Na$_2$HPO$_4$, and 0.24 g KH$_2$PO$_4$. Dissolve in 800 ml dH$_2$O. Adjust to pH 7.2. Sterilize by autoclaving.

2× Ruvkun Fixation Buffer (RFB).   Combine 160 mM KCl, 40 mM NaCl, 20 mM disodium ethylene glycol bis (β-aminoethyl ether)-*N,N'*-tetraacetic acid (Na$_2$EGTA), 10 mM spermidine–HCl, 30 mM Na 1,4-piperazinediethanesulfonic acid (Pipes), pH 7.4, and 50% methanol.

Tris–Triton buffer (TTB).   100 mM Tris–HCl, pH 7.4, 1% Triton X-100 or Nonidet P-40, and 1 mM ethylenediaminetetraacetic acid (EDTA).

20× BO$_3$ Buffer.   1 M H$_3$BO$_3$, 0.5 M NaOH.

1× BO$_3$ Buffer.   Make fresh and adjust to pH 9.5 with NaOH.

Antibody Buffer A (AbA).   1× PBS, 1% bovine serum albumin, 0.5% Triton X-100 or Nonidet P-40, 0.05% sodium azide (highly toxic powder, use extreme caution), and 1 mM EDTA.

Antibody Buffer B (AbB).   AbA with 0.1% BSA.

Glycerol-Based (Non-Self-Hardening) Mounting Media.   DAPI (2 μg/ml) can be added to the mounting media. Three media are available:

20 mM Tris–HCl, pH 8.0, 0.2 M 1,4-diazabicyclo-2,2,2-octane (DABCO), 90% glycerol (keep at 4°C). Premixed reagent is available from Molecular Probes as SlowFade.

1 mg/ml *p*-phenylenediamine, 10% PBS, 90% glyerol adjusted to pH 8 with 1 N NaOH. Aliquot and store in the dark at −70°C (Johnson and Nogueira Araujo, 1981).

50 mM Tris–HCl, pH 8.8, 10% glycerol, 0.5 mg/ml *p*-phenylenediamine (Johnson *et al.*, 1982).

Self-Hardening Mounting Medium (Gelutol, Monsanto).   To make 1× gelutol, add 1.2 g of gelutol to 3.0 g of glycerol in a 15-ml tube. Stir well with a glass rod. Add 3 ml of dH$_2$O. Stir and leave at room temperature for 4 hours. Add 6 ml of 0.1 M Tris, pH 8.5, and heat tube in a 50°C water bath for 10 minutes with stirring. Centrifuge at 3000 rpm to clear the reagent. This can be stored at 4°C in a capped 15-ml disposable centrifuge tube. *Note:* 2× gelutol solutions can be mixed with concentrated antifade solutions such as SlowFade (Molecular Probes).

References

Albertson, D. G. (1984). Formation of the first cleavage spindle in nematode embryos. *Dev. Biol.* **101**, 61–72.

Ardizzi, J. P., and Epstein, H. F. (1987). Immunochemical localization of myosin heavy chain isoforms and paramyosin in developmentally and structurally diverse muscle cell types of the nematode *Caenorhabditis elegans. J. Cell Biol.* **105,** 2763–2770.

Atkinson, H. J., Issac, R. E., Harris, P. D., and Sharpe, C. M. (1988). FMRFamide-like immunoreactivity within the nervous system of the nematodes *Pangrellus redivivus, Caenorhabditis elegans,* and *Heterodera glycines. J. Zool.* **216,** 663–671.

Barstead, R. J., and Waterston, R. H. (1989). The basal component of the nematode dense-body is vinculin. *J. Biol. Chem.* **264,** 10177–10185.

Bardsley, A., McDonald, K., and Boswell, R. E. (1993). Distribution of tudor protein in the Drosophila embryo suggest separation of functions based on site of localization. *Development* **119**(1), 207–219.

Beh, C. T., Ferrari, D. D., Chung, M. A., and McGhee, J. D. (1991). An acid phosphatase as a biochemical marker for intestinal development in the nematode *Caenorhabditis elegans. Dev. Biol.* **147,** 133–143.

Bowerman, B., Eaton, B. A., and Priess, J. R. (1992). *skn-1,* a maternally expressed gene required to specify the fate of ventral blastomers in the early *C. elegans* embryo. *Cell* **68,** 1061–1075.

Bowerman, D., Draper, B. W., Mello, C. C., and Priess, J. R. (1993). The maternal gene *skn-1* encodes a protein that is distributed unequally in early *C. elegans* embryos. *Cell* **74,** 443–452.

Chalfie, M., Tu, Y., Euskirchen, G., Ward, W. W., and Prasher, D. C. (1994). Green fluorescent protein as a marker for gene expression. *Science* **263,** 802–805.

Cox, G. N., Laufer, J. S., Kusch, M., and Edgar, R. S. (1980). Genetic and phenotypic characterization of roller mutants of *C. elegans. Genetics* **95,** 317–339.

Cox, G. N., Kusch, M., and Edgar, R. S. (1981). Cuticle of *C. elegans:* Its isolation and partial characterization. *J. Cell Biol.* **90,** 7–17.

Desai, C., Garriga, G., McIntire, S., and Horvitz, R. (1988). A genetic pathway for the development of the *Caenorhabditis elegans* HSN motor neurons. *Nature* **336,** 638–646.

Edgar, L. G., and McGhee, J. D. (1986). Cell cycle control by the nucleo-cytoplasmic ratio in early Drosophila development. *Cell* **44,** 365–372.

Epstein, H. F., Miller, D. M., Grosset, L. A., and Hecht, R. M. (1982). Immunological studies of myosin isoforms in nematode embryos. *In* "Muscle Development: Molecular and Cellular Control" (M. L. Pearson and H. F. Epstein, eds.), pp. 7–14. Cold Spring Harbor Laboratory, Cold Spring Harbor, New York.

Epstein, H. F., Miller, D. M., III, Ortiz, I., and Berliner, G. C. (1985). Myosin and paramyosin are organized about a newly identified core structure. *J. Cell. Biol.* **100,** 904–915.

Epstein, H. F., Casey, D. L., and Ortiz, I. (1993). Myosin and paramyosin of *Caenorhabditis elegans* embryos assemble into nascent structures distinct from thick filaments and multi-filament assemblages. *J. Cell Biol.* **122,** 845–858.

Evans, T. C., Crittenden, S. L., Kodoyianni, V., and Kimble, J. (1994). Translational control of maternal *glp-1* mRNA establishes an asymmetry in the *C. elegans* embryo. *Cell* **77,** 183–194.

Fehon, R. G., Johansen, K., Rebay, I., and Artavanis-Tsakonas, S. (1991). Complex cellular and subcellular regulation of notch expression during embryonic and imaginal development of Drosophila: Implications for notch function. *J. Cell Biol.* **113,** 657–669.

Finney, M., and Ruvkun, G. B. (1990). The unc-86 gene product couples cell lineage and cell identity in *C. elegans. Cell* **63,** 895–905.

Fire, A. (1992). Histochemical techniques for locating *Escherichia coli* beta-galactosidase activity in transgenic organisms. *Genet. Anal. Tech. Appl.* **9,** 152–160.

Fire, A., and Waterston, R. H. (1988). Proper expression of myosin genes in transgenic nematodes. *EMBO J.* **8,** 3419–3428.

Francis, G. R., and Waterston, R. H. (1985). Muscle organization in *C. elegans:* Localization of proteins implicated in thin filaments attachment and I-band organization. *J. Cell Biol.* **101,** 1532–1549.

Gengyo-Ando, K., Kamiya, Y., Yamakawa, A., Kodaira, K., Nishiwaki, K., Miwa, J., Hori, I., and Hosono, R. (1993). The *C. elegans unc-18* gene encodes a protein expressed in motor neurons. *Neuron* **11,** 703–711.

Goh, P., and Bogaert, T. (1991). Positioning and maintenance of embryonic body wall muscle attachments in *C. elegans* requires the mup-1 gene. *Development* **111,** 667–681.

Gossett, L. A., Hecht, R. M., and Epstein, H. F. (1982). Muscle differentiation in normal and cleavage-arrested mutant embryos of *C. elegans*. *Cell* **30,** 193–204.

Granato, M., Schnabel, H., and Schnabel, R. (1994). Genesis of an organism: Molecular analysis of the *pha-1* gene. *Development* **120,** 3005–3017.

Hamelin, M., Scott, I. M., Way, J. C., and Culotti, J. G. (1992). The *mec-7* beta-tubulin gene of *Caenorhabditis elegans* is expressed primarily in the touch receptor neurons. *EMBO J.* **11,** 2885–2893.

Harlow, E., and Lane, D. (1988). "Antibodies: A Laboratory Manual" Cold Spring Harbor Laboratory, Cold Spring Harbor, New York.

Haughland, R. P. (1992). "Handbook of Fluorescent Probes and Research Chemicals" Molecular Probes, Eugene, Oregon.

Hecht, R. M., Berg-Zabelshasky, M., Rao, P. N., and Davis, F. M. (1987). Conditioned absence of mitosis-specific antigens in a temperature-sensitive embryonic arrest mutant of *C. elegans*. *J. Cell Sci.* **87,** 305–314.

Hedgecock, E. M., Culotti, J. G., Thomson, J. N., and Perkins, L. A. (1985). Axonal guidance mutants of *Caenorhabditis elegans* identified by filling sensory neurons with fluorescein dyes. *Dev. Biol.* **111,** 158–170.

Hekimi, S. (1990). A neuron-specific antigen in *C. elegans* allows visualization of the entire nervous system. *Neuron* **4,** 855–865.

Hill, D. P., and Strome, S. (1988). An analysis of the role of microfilaments in the establishment and maintenance of asymmetry in *Caenorhabditis elegans* zygotes. *Dev. Biol.* **125,** 75–84.

Hresko, M. C., Williams, B. D., and Waterston, R. H. (1994). Assembly of body wall muscle and muscle cell attachment structures in *Caenorhabditis elegans*. *J. Cell Biol.* **124,** 491–506.

Jefferson, R. A., Klass, M., Wolf, N., and Hirsh, D. (1987). Expression of chimeric genes in *Caenorhabditis elegans*. *J. Mol. Biol.* **193,** 41–46.

Johnson, B. D., and Nogueira Araujo, G. M. de C. (1981). A simple method of reducing the fading of immunofluorescence during microscopy. *J. Immunol. Methods* **43,** 349–350.

Johnson, G. D., Davidson, R. S., McNamee, K. C., Russell, G., Goodwin, D., and Holborow, E. J. (1982). Fading of immunofluorescence during microscopy: A study of the phenomenon and its remedy. *J. Immunol. Methods* **55,** 231–242.

Kemphues, K. J., Wolf, N., Wood, W. B., and Hirsch, D. (1986). Two loci required for cytoplasmic organization in early embryos of *Caenorhabditis elegans*. *Dev. Biol.* **113,** 449–460.

Klass, M. R., and Hirsh, D. I. (1981). Sperm isolation and biochemical analysis of the major sperm protein from *C. elegans*. *Dev. Biol.* **84,** 299–312.

Krause, M., Fire, A., Harrison, S. W., Priess, J., and Weintraub, H. (1990). CeMyoD accumulation defines the body wall muscle cell fate during *C. elegans* embryogenesis. *Cell* **63,** 907–919.

Laufer, J. S., Bazzicalupo, P., and Wood, W. B. (1980). Segregation of developmental potential in early embryos of *Caenorhabditis elegans*. *Cell* **19,** 569–577.

Li, C., and Chalfie, M. (1990). Organogenesis in *C. elegans:* Positioning of neurons and muscles in the egg-laying system. *Neuron* **4,** 681–695.

Link, C. D., Ehrenfels, C. W., and Wood, W. B. (1988). Mutant expression of male copulatory bursa surface markers in *Caenorhabditis elegans*. *Development* **103,** 485–495.

MacKenzie, J. M., Schachat, F. H., and Epstein, H. F. (1978). Immunocytochemical localization of two myosins within the same muscle cells in *C. elegans*. *Cell* **15,** 413–420.

McIntire, S. L., Garriga, G., White, J. G., Jacobson, D. M., and Horvitz, H. R. (1992). Genes necessary for directed axonal elongation for fasciculation in *C. elegans*. *Neuron* **8,** 307–322.

Miller, D. M., Ortiz, I., Berliner, G. C., and Epstein, H. F. (1983). Differential localization of two myosins within nematode thick filaments. *Cell* **34,** 477–490.

Miller, D. M., Stockdale, F. E., and Karn, J. (1986). Immunological identification of the genes encoding the four myosin heavy chain isoforms of *Caenorhabditis elegans*. *Proc. Natl. Acad. Sci. U.S.A.* **83,** 2305–2309.

Miller, D. M., III, and Niemeyer, C. J. (1995). Expression of the UNC-4 homeoprotein in *C. elegans* motor neurons specifies presynaptic input. *Development,* in press.

Moerman, D. G., Benian, G. M., Barstead, R. J., Schriefer, L. A., and Waterston, R. H. (1988). Identification and intracellular localization of the unc-22 gene product of *Caenorhabditis elegans*. *Genes Dev.* **2,** 93–105.

Nonet, M. L., Grundahl, K., Meyer, B. J., and Rand, J. B. (1993). Synaptic function is impaired but not eliminated in *C. elegans* mutants lacking synaptotagmin. *Cell* **73,** 1291–1305.

Okamoto, H., and Thompson, J. N. (1985). Monoclonal antibodies which distinguish certain classes of neuronal and supporting cells in the nervous tissue of the nematode *Caenorhabditis elegans*. *J. Neurosci.* **5,** 643–653.

Osborn, M., and Weber, K. (1982). Immunofluorescence and immunocytochemical procedures with affinity purified antibodies: Tubulin-containing structures. *Methods Enzymol.* **24,** 97–127.

Paddock, S. W. (1994). To boldly glow . . . Applications of laser scanning confocal microscopy in developmental biology. *Bioessays* **16,** 357–365.

Piperno, G., and Fuller, M. T. (1985). Monoclonal antibodies specific for an acetylated form of alpha-tubulin recognize the antigen in cilia and flagella from a variety of organisms. *J. Cell Biol.* **101,** 2085–2094.

Politz, S. M., Chin, K. J., and Herman, D. L. (1987). Genetic analysis of adult-specific surface antigens differences between varieties of the nematode *C. elegans*. *Genetics* **117,** 467–476.

Priess, J. R., and Hirsh, D. I. (1986). *Caenorhabditis elegans* morphogenesis: The role of the cytoskeleton in elongation of the embryo. *Dev. Biol.* **117,** 156–173.

Priess, J. R., and Thomson, J. N. (1987). Cellular interactions in early *C. elegans* embryos. *Cell* **48,** 241–250.

Pruss, R. M., Mirsky, R., Raff, M. C., Thorpe, R., Dowding, A. J., and Anderton, B. H. (1981). All classes of intermediate filaments share a common antigenic determinant defined by a monoclonal antibody. *Cell* **27,** 419–428.

Rogalski, T. M., Williams, B. D., Mullen, G. P., and Moerman, D. G. (1993). Products of the *unc-52* gene in *Caenorhabditis elegans* are homologous to the core proteins of the mammalian basement membrane heparan sulfate proteoglycan. *Genes Dev.* **7,** 1471–1484.

Ruvkun, G. B., and Giusto, J. (1989). The *Caenorhabditis elegans* heterochronic gene *lin-14* encodes a nuclear protein that forms a temporal developmental switch. *Nature* **338,** 313–319.

Schachat, F., Garcea, R. L., and Epstein, H. F. (1978). Myosins exist as homodimers of heavy chains: Demonstration with specific antibodies purified by nematode mutant myosin affinity chromatography. *Cell* **15,** 405–411.

Schinkmann, K., and Li, C. (1992). Localization of FMRFamide-like peptides in *Caenorhabditis elegans* *J. Comp. Neurol.* **316,** 251–260.

Sebastiano, M., Lassandro, F., and Bazzicalupo, P. (1991). *cut-1*, a *Caenorhabditis elegans* gene coding for a dauer-specific noncollagenous component of the cuticle. *Dev. Biol.* **146,** 519–530.

Sharrock, W. J. (1984). Cleavage of two yolk proteins from a precursor in *Caenorhabditis elegans*. *J. Mol. Biol.* **174,** 419–431.

Shotten, D. M. (1993). An introduction to the electronic acquisition of light microscope images. *In* "Electronic Light Microscopy: The Principles and Practice of Video-Enhanced Contrast Digital Intensified Fluorescence, and Confocal Scanning Light Microsopy" (D. M. Shotten, ed.), pp. 1–38. Wiley-Liss, New York.

Siddiqui, S. S., Aamodt, E., Rastinejad, F., and Culotti, J. (1989). Anti-tublin monoclonals antibodies that bind to specific neurons in *Caenorhabditis elegans*. *J. Neurosci.* **9,** 2963–2972.

Siddiqui, S. S., and Culotti, J. G. (1991). Examination of neurons in wild type and mutants of *Caenorhabditis elegans* using antibodies to horseradish peroxidase. *J. Neurogenet.* **7,** 193–211.

Sithigorngul, P., Cowden, C., Guastella, J., and Stretton, A. O. W. (1989). Generation of monoclonal antibodies against a nematode peptide extract: Another approach for identifying unknown neuropeptides. *J. Comp. Neurol.* **284,** 389–397.

Soldati, T., and Perriard, J. C. (1991). Intracompartmental sorting of essential myosin light chains: Molecular dissection and in vivo monitoring by epitope tagging. *Cell* **66,** 277–289.

Strome, S., and Wood, W. B. (1983). Generation of asymmetry and segregation of germ-line granules in early *C. elegans* embryos. *Cell* **35,** 15–25.

Sulston, J., Dew, M., and Brenner, S. (1975). Dopaminergic neurons in the nematode *C. elegans*. *J. Comp. Neurol.* **163,** 215–226.

Waddle, J. A., Cooper, J. A., and Waterston, R. H. (1994). Transient localized accumulation of actin in Caenorhabditis elegans blastomeres with oriented asymmetric divisions. *Development* **120,** 2317–2328.

Ward, S., Roberts, T. M., Strome, S., Pavalko, F. M., and Hogan, E. (1986). Monoclonal antibodies that recognize a polypeptide antigenic determinant shared by multiple *Caenorhabditis* sperm-specific proteins. *J. Cell Biol.* **102,** 1778–1786.

Waterston, R. H. (1988). Muscle. *In* "The Nematode *Caenorhabditis elegans*" (W. B. Wood, ed.), pp. 281–335. Cold Spring Harbor, New York.

White, J. G., Amos, W. B., and Fordham, M. (1987). An evaluation of confocal versus conventional imaging of biological structures by fluorescence light microscopy. *J. Cell Biol.* **105,** 41–48.

CHAPTER 17

Electron Microscopy and Three-Dimensional Image Reconstruction

David H. Hall

Department of Neuroscience
Albert Einstein College of Medicine
Bronx, New York 10461

I. Introduction

Although *Caenorhabditis elegans* was originally chosen as a model organism for cell biology with serial section electron microscopy (EM) methods in mind, these methods have remained a daunting challenge. There is an apocryphal story that Nichol Thomson originally advised Sydney Brenner that *C. elegans* was unsuitable for electron microscopy and that Brenner should choose another species. Other experienced microscopists have probably shared similar dark thoughts from time to time. Nonetheless, the worm's very small size, simple organization, and cablelike nervous system have permitted Brenner's colleagues to characterize every cell and cell contract in the wild-type animal, potentiating the genetic characterization of cellular development in remarkable detail.

We attempt to provide an adequate background for anyone to initiate EM studies of *C. elegans*. Two decades ago, as the first of Brenner's postdoctoral fellows left his laboratory to establish new worm laboratories, it was standard practice to include an EM component in their studies. Their combined efforts to characterize the adult animal's cell types and the essential steps in its development helped to erect a lovely scaffold of key manuscripts, capped by the description of the "Mind of the Worm" in some 600 micrographs and 175 drawings (White *et al.,* 1986). Many of these works required technical heroics or suffered long delays before publication. Most people later chose to leave electron microscopy behind in pursuit of molecular quarry. The fruits of their molecular and genetic studies should soon stimulate a renewed flowering of electron microscopy. We hope to smooth your entry or reentry into these techniques.

We also summarize our methods for three-dimensional (3D) image reconstruction, based largely on film techniques introduced by John White and Randle Ware. Digital imaging techniques seem poised to make 3D reconstruction more accessible, and may simplify the exchange of morphological data between laboratories. We discuss several computer systems that the *C. elegans* community could adopt for high-resolution studies of structure and function. In addition, we briefly cover several specialized specimen preparation techniques for electron microscopy, including freeze fracture and electron microscopic immunocytochemistry.

II. Fixation and Embedding for Electron Microscopy

Your quarry is a small slippery worm, wrapped in an impenetrable cuticle.

A. Anesthesia

Use of an anesthetic straightens animals prior to and during fixation. Without this step, specimens may be bent or kinked when finally embedded. Straightened animals are easily oriented and sectioned at precise angles; a bent animal is not. Nematodes show remarkable powers of activity during fixation. Without anesthesia, they often thrash actively for minutes, and continue slower bending motions for at least half an hour.

1-Phenoxy-2-propanol is an effective anesthetic as a 1% solution in buffer, but prolonged exposure may cause ultrastructural damage. Ethanol works well, and we often use an 8% solution in M9 buffer as a preliminary treatment. Sodium azide also has anesthetic properties, but has not been used for electron microscopy to date.

B. Fixatives

For most EM projects, a primary fixative should contain buffered aldehydes to preserve proteins, followed by a secondary fixative containing osmium tetroxide to preserve lipids. A sample protocol is shown in Table I. Stock solutions are given in Section VIII,B. In early efforts to reconstruct the adult nervous system of *C. elegans* (Ward *et al.*, 1975; Ware *et al.*, 1975; White *et al.*, 1976; Hall, 1977), aldehyde fixatives were not used. By use of a single primary osmium

Table I
Standard Electron Microscopy Protocol (Summary)

1. Rinse twice in M9 buffer, then M9 + anesthetic for 3–5 minutes.
2. Fix in aldehyde at room temperature for 1–2 hours; cut open immediately.
3. Rinse 5 times in buffer to remove all traces of aldehydes.
4. Stain with osmium tetroxide at room temperature for 1 hour.
5. Rinse 3 times in buffer.
6. Stain en block with uranyl acetate (buffered) at room temperature for 1 hour.
7. Rinse 3 times in buffer.
8. Embed in agarose.
9. Dehydrate 5 minutes each in 30, 50, 75, and 95% ethanol.
10. Dehydrate 10 minutes each in three changes of 100% ethanol.
11. Infiltrate 10 minutes each in three changes of either 100% acetone or 100% propylene oxide.
12. Infiltrate 1–3 hours in 1:2 mixture of resin and solvent (acetone or propylene oxide).
13. Infiltrate 3–12 hours in 2:1 mixture of resin and solvent.
14. Infiltrate in multiple changes in pure resin over 12–36 hours.
15. Cure in oven for 2–3 days at 60°C.

fixation, protein components were extracted prior to embedment, leaving individual nerve processes looking empty but highly contrasted and easy to trace. This washed out appearance is not informative regarding cytoplasmic details, and is not generally acceptable for publication purposes. One can also combine glutaraldehyde and osmium in the primary fixative, followed by a second fix in osmium alone (E. Jorgensen and E. Hartwieg, pers. comm.).

A variety of buffers can be used to control the working pH of these solutions: 4-(2-hydroxyethyl)-1-piperazineethanesulfonic acid (Hepes), cacodylate, and phosphate have been used successfully. The time and temperature of fixation steps do not appear to be critical; 1 hour at 4°C or at room temperature works well, but longer fixations are not harmful.

Two aspects seem to be critical to success. First, each animal should be cut open very soon after entry into the primary fixative (within a few minutes) to improve access to tissues inside the cuticle. The cut(s) should be near the area of interest. One must assume that during the time that an intact animal continues thrashing in fixative, general degradation of ultrastructural features can continue until aldehydes infiltrate the tissue. Formaldehyde is expected to invade faster than glutaraldehyde, but probably does not fix proteins as firmly as the latter. Second, there must be efficient wash steps between aldehyde and osmium fixations, as even faint traces of aldehydes can block the osmication.

Osmium, aldehydes, and cacodylate buffer (arsenic-based) are extremely hazardous substances, and special precautions are mandatory in handling all fixative solutions, including safe waste disposal. Because osmium solutions emit dangerous vapors at working temperature, they should be handled in a fume hood.

C. Methods for Handling Small Pieces

Centrifugation can be used to pellet live worms and wash them in M9 buffer, before and immediately after anesthesia. It is, however, necessary to move the animals to a dish to cut them into pieces in the primary fix.

Moving small cut pieces of *C. elegans* through a protocol of 20 solution changes is difficult to achieve without losing many specimens along the way. Initial steps can be carried out in a clear watchglass or multiwell glass slide with hemispherical depressions. Animals are observed in the dissecting microscope and cut open with a curved scalpel blade. Finer dissections are best carried out with 22-gauge needles. Fixatives and buffer solutions can be changed carefully by Pasteur pipet from the top of the well, allowing specimens to settle by gravity between solution changes.

After osmication and buffer washes, fixed pieces are positioned onto a thin agar pad, generally placing several animals in close proximity in parallel; then a second thin layer of agar is poured to sandwich the animals together. SeaPlaque agarose 2.5% (FMC BioProducts) is dissolved in buffer or in water and cooled to 31 to 35°C just before application. This low-temperature agarose gels at 30°C, minimizing the heat pulse to the specimens, which is especially important for immunocytochemistry procedures. For routine electron microscopy, Difco Bac-toagar or another agar could be used instead. After the agar is hardened at 4°C for several hours or overnight, each small group of specimens is cut out separately as an agar cube of roughly $3 \times 2 \times 2$ mm. These agar cubes are treated together in snap cap glass vials, one vial per treatment group. Alternately, the cubes will serve to hold small specimens inside the basket enclosures of an automated tissue processor (Leica). The cubes can also be marked on the corner with India ink (via syringe needle) to help in visualization during solution changes.

This preembedding method is very helpful during staining and dehydration steps, and becomes essential during final resin embedding steps, where individual cut animals will no longer settle out of solution. The small agar blocks are easily handled even in viscous resins. The grouping of several specimens in very close proximity allows the simultaneous sectioning of several animals (Fig. 1), provid-

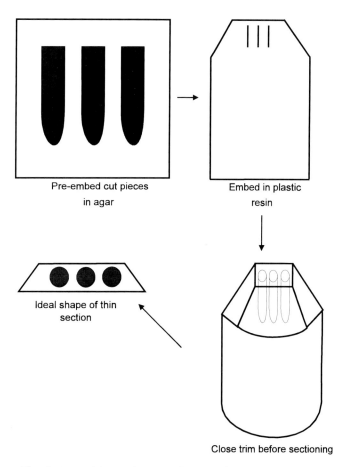

Pre-embed cut pieces
in agar

Embed in plastic
resin

Ideal shape of thin
section

Close trim before sectioning

Fig. 1 Essential steps in embedding and trimming small pieces.

ing a quick means to replicate a result and reducing the labor required to section multiple specimens.

Helpful Hints. A thin piece of filter paper is helpful to wick away excess buffer around each group of animals just before applying the top layer of agar; this brings the pieces into close contact. An eyelash attached to a toothpick makes a useful tool for manipulating animals into final alignment. To prevent animals from scattering, agar is applied dropwise directly over each group of pieces. Agar blocks must be of a size too large to be sucked up into a Pasteur pipet, but small enough to fit easily into the slot of an embedding mold or capsule. Cutting out the agar blocks is done very carefully with a scalpel or spatula blade, so as not to tear the agar while it is soft. After dehydration, the agar becomes much more durable. Smaller, flatter "cubes" ($1 \times 2.5 \times 2.5$ mm) are advisable if one later intends to orient the cube into the tip of a BEEM capsule for resin embedment.

D. Stains to Increase Contrast

We often include a buffered uranyl acetate (UAc) stain to enhance tissue contrast. This step stains the outer leaflet of cell membranes to produce a trilaminar appearance; otherwise, membranes are often seen as a single dense band. Buffered UAc requires an acidic pH ($0.1 M$ sodium acetate, pH 5.2). This stain is applied for 1 hour at room temperature or at $4°C$.

Uranyl acetate can also be applied to the thin sections as a postembedding stain to increase contrast (see below), but it cannot preserve the outer membrane leaflet at that stage. Poststaining UAc solutions are generally alcohol based.

Pitfalls. Buffered UAc can sometimes function as a negative stain, infiltrating into narrow openings and precipitating out of solution before the unbound solute can be washed out. This effect can be seen as a dense extracellular staining of the amphid channel, leaving individual cilia silhouetted against the background stain. Therefore, this step should be avoided for studies of cilia morphology. A similar effect can sometimes be seen when the stain invades between closely apposed membranes, where it may precipitate out around tight junctions and septate junctions.

This staining solution should always be filtered prior to use to reduce the chance of precipitates forming a negative stain.

E. Dehydration

As most embedding resins are immiscible in water or alcohol, it is necessary to dehydrate tissue prior to embedment. A typical dehydration schedule is shown in Table I, steps 9–13. It is important to keep the solvents and resins well sealed and free of water. This schedule can be carried out at room temperature, or in the cold for immuno-electron microscopy protocols.

F. Embedding

Following dehydration through alcohols and a resin solvent, resin infiltration should use four or five changes in pure resin mixture over a 12- to 36-hour period, during which the specimens should be held in sealed containers and placed on a rotator at very slow speed to allow mixing of the viscous solution. Some workers omit the accelerator during early steps in infiltration to promote infiltration; we find that the 1:2 and 2:1 solvent:resin steps mentioned in Table I accomplish the same goal. When infiltration is complete, individual specimens are positioned carefully in flat embedding molds or in BEEM capsules in fresh resin and cured in the oven for 2 to 3 days at 60°C. Small paper labels may be embedded with each specimen to provide an identification code. See Section VIII,C regarding the choice of embedding resins.

Orientation of the specimen within the final block is often critical to obtain sections either orthogonal or parallel to the body axis (see below). Orientation should be rechecked just prior to curing the plastic resin.

G. Troubleshooting

Diagnosis of a poor initial result is a common step in electron microscopy. These protocols include a large number of steps with seemingly arbitrary choices of temperature, concentrations, times, and components. Prior to investing any effort to serially section a specimen, one is well advised to cut a few test sections to evaluate the success or failure of the fixation and embedment.

Poorly fixed tissue may reflect poor access (failure to cut open promptly in primary fixative), use of a bad lot or expired lot of fixative, or an unwanted interaction between the primary and secondary fixatives. If the specimens look uniformly washed out or low in contrast, the osmium fix may have failed. Even in well-stained animals sectioned at oblique angles, cell membranes may be difficult to discern; test sections should be transverse to the body axis.

Poorly embedded tissue often shows differential compression of the specimen versus the surrounding plastic matrix. The tissue may sag or tear away from the pure plastic portions of the section, leaving holes. If water remains in smaller pockets within the tissue, this may leave microscopic soft spots or holes within the tissue. In worst cases, a solvent barrier can develop as a visible whitish rind between the tissue and the plastic resin that prevents infiltration of resin into the tissue. Slow rotation of the specimen throughout the embedding process helps promote an even infiltration.

III. Sectioning Methods

"Have a little patience."   —*Guns and Roses*

Actually, a restful sleep and some mood music sets the stage for success here.

A. Block Trimming

Proper trimming prior to sectioning is essential to obtaining good thin sections. A poorly trimmed block will rarely deliver any useful sections and will never permit serial sections. A person with steady hands will probably be able to learn trimming with the use of a simple block holder. A variety of trimming helpers are described in Section VII,E.

Inspect the untrimmed block to locate the specimen(s) within the plastic resin and choose the preferred plane of sectioning (see discussion on preferred orientation below). Mark the block with a few ink dots to indicate where the specimen is located, as it may not be easily visible during early stages of trimming. Tighten the block firmly in a microtome chuck and place the chuck into a holder vertically under a dissecting microscope (or vertically on the microtome platform). Trim away excess plastic from the sides and top of the block, using smooth downward strokes to cut thin slivers off the block with a razor blade. The blade is firmly held in two hands, and each downstroke must avoid any backlash that would restrike the block and dull the knife. No sawing motions are needed. One must not undercut the specimen, and in general no vertical cuts are needed, as this will also tend to undercut the specimen. In this manner, a better view of the specimen is obtained within a small pyramid of plastic. Some patience is demanded to make these many thin trimming cuts, as larger attacks on the block are prone to damage the whole block or to trim away the specimen inadvertently. The pyramidal shape is required to firmly support the final specimen, so that it does not bend or break during thin sectioning.

As the specimen becomes directly visible through the sides and top of the block, reexamine and recalculate the best orientation (perhaps orthogonal to the body axis). Use a trimming blade to make a new top face. When this top face is satisfactory, one can make the final trim of the sides as follows. Using a fresh blade, two opposing sides of the specimen should be trimmed very tightly to create exactly parallel faces. The two parallel faces will become the top and bottom edges of each thin section during microtomy; if they are not exactly parallel, the strip of thin sections will not be straight. The more narrowly spaced one can trim these two faces, the more thin sections can be fit into a single strip on a microscope grid. The other faces are retrimmed to form a parallelogram as shown in Fig. 1. It is not advisable to make these other faces too close together, or the entire block will be weakened and one will obtain a very narrow strip of sections, which can cause problems during section pickup (see Section C). As shown, the longer parallel edge will become the bottom edge during microtomy, while the shorter edge will become the top.

Helpful Hints. Dull or scratched blades leave dull facets on the plastic. Ideally, one should be able to see clearly into each newly cut facet. In the worst case scenario, a block may become completely opaque due to poor trimming: this may be the result of taking random chips, perhaps on the backswing, rather than smooth downward cuts. As one gets closer to the specimen, continue shifting to fresh portions of the blade's edge and use a fresh blade for the final trim.

Try to trim the parallel edges to almost touch the specimen. Sometimes the specimen may be lost in the effort, but the best series usually results from a very close trim. More conservative trimming may allow only 5 to 10 sections per grid, while a tight trim may allow 25 or more sections per grid.

If the trimmed block does not have a good top face, that is, orientation to the body axis is wrong, you may be forced to change approach angle on the microtome (see below). Any change in approach angle will knock the parallel edges out of alignment and produce a curving strip of sections during microtomy.

B. Cutting Serial Thin Sections

1. Aligning Block and Knife Edge

Fasten the block to the microtome arm, positioning the bottom face of the block to be exactly horizontal. Examine from the sides to ascertain the exact alignment of the specimen within the plastic resin. If the specimen is angled upward or downward, the microtome chuck should be readjusted to bring the animal's body axis into a horizontal orientation (assuming that transverse sections are desired). The diamond knife is now installed in its holder, and the knife angle is adjusted to position the specimen exactly orthogonal to the knife edge. If the animal is somewhat bent within the resin block, one may need to readjust the knife angle occasionally during sectioning to obtain transverse sections continuously. It is imperative to cut sections exactly transverse to the body axis to obtain the clearest images of cell membranes for those cell types with longitudinal orientations within the body.

2. Approaching the Knife Edge

Reset the microtome advance mechanism, then manually bring the knife close to the block, stopping short of the block face by 10 to 20 μm. Recheck the alignment, ensuring that the bottom edge of the block face is exactly horizontal. Tighten all knife and block fittings; the knife and specimen must be held securely. Watch several test sweeps of the microtome arm, which is still too distant to cut a section, to ensure that the arm sweep slows well above the knife edge and remains slow until the specimen has passed the knife edge.

Fill the knife boat with distilled water. The knife edge is sometimes difficult to keep wet at first; overfill the boat before withdrawing some water to achieve a slightly concave surface. If the water draws away from the edge, use a sharpened toothpick to rewet the edge without poking the knife itself.

Using the manual advance, bring the specimen closer to the knife by 1 μm and take a test sweep of the microtome arm. Continue carefully until a partial section is cut. Set the section thickness setting to 150 nm and cut another section. Check the cutting action to ensure that the entire bottom edge of the block face is reaching the knife edge simultaneously. If the specimen still lies a few micrometers deeper in the block, continue cutting 150-nm sections, then reset the section thickness to collect 50 to 70-nm thin sections. Section thickness is easier to judge by color than by microtome settings. (While floating on the knife boat, 50-nm sections appear silver to gray in color; 60-nm sections are a bright silver color; and 70-nm sections are pale gold color.)

Position an antistatic device very close to the knife edge (Fig. 2). Sections should float on the surface of the water in the knife boat. Unwanted test sections can be discarded by wicking them off the surface with a Kimwipe. If the water level is too low, sections may not be visible. If the water level is too high, water droplets may be transferred onto the blockface during the sweep of the microtome

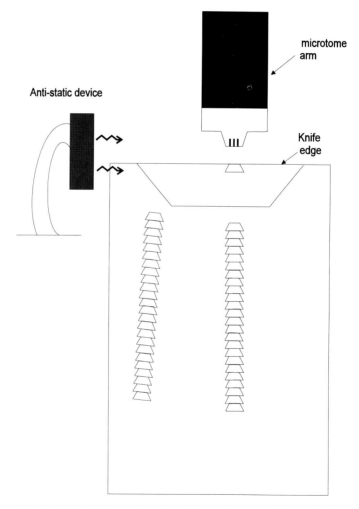

Fig. 2   Strips of thin sections float in boat adjacent to diamond knife.

arm, wetting the block and causing sections to sink below the surface of the boat or to be sucked back onto the blockface as the water droplet expands. Ideally, the water level should be very slightly concave in the boat. In some circumstances, discussed below, one may need to lower the water level to promote better sectioning.

3. Cutting Serial Thin Sections

As sectioning proceeds from cutting blank sections to sections containing a cross-sectioned worm, a slight dimple will become evident in each section silhouetting the worm's profile. This dimple may be visible for only 10 seconds after cutting. If every thin section is desired from this point, the microtome should be set on automatic advance, and serial sections collected as strips of floating sections, adhering to the knife edge.

If one wishes to reach a particular region of the animal, one can collect the first few thin sections on a specimen grid (see Section C), and view the dried sections by EM. To enhance the contrast before viewing, it is advised to poststain the grid with uranyl acetate and/or lead citrate (see Section D and Section VIII below). If the orientation fieldmarks are especially obvious, one may be able to view the test sections without poststaining. Perhaps on viewing the test sections, the desired landmark is not yet achieved: then a judicious number of thick sections (1 μm thick or less) can be cut before resuming thin sectioning. This careful approach may require several hours to reach the region. We often do the approach on one day, then leave the specimen on the microtome overnight before cutting all the serial sections during the following workday. Arriving fully rested is often a help in success in the next step. There are two caveats. First, you must have permission to tie up the microtome for a second day; it would generally be unwise to remove the specimen or the knife, as one might damage the specimen during reapproach. Second, the trimmed block may slowly deform and lose its carefully trimmed shape if left too long; do not wait more than a few days to resume sectioning.

Finally, thin sections are cutting completely through the specimen, and sticking together to form a strip of sections (see Fig. 2). Although the initial sections may have shown a rainbow of colors, every section now should be rather uniform in color, representative of the desired section thickness. Each time the operator makes a motion near the knife edge, slight changes in section thickness may occur for one or two sections, probably due to temporary heating effects. Thus the operator will do best to let the machine cut on automatic motor drive, keeping hands off except when necessary to manipulate strips of sections.

When a strip of sections is long enough to fit the slot on an electron microscope grid (approx 2 mm), a sharpened toothpick or an eyelash is used to detach the strip from the knife. If done delicately, one can detach a strip while allowing the microtome to continue operation; several strips can float in the boat at once. Do not try to detach the section directly on the knife edge, as one could easily scratch the knife. Instead, poke the corner of the second section and pull the strip away from the first section. By counting the sections in each strip, one can identify them individually. When four or five strips are floating on the boat, it is time to stop the microtome and collect the sections onto grids.

When all sections are picked up (except for one or two sections still adhering to the knife edge), the surface of the boat water can be cleaned by drawing a Kimwipe quickly across it to remove any debris. Readjust the water level if necessary and resume microtome action. As cutting was suspended for several minutes to pick up sections, the block will have cooled slightly and shrunk back from the knife edge. No section is likely to appear on the first pass of the knife, or if the block is still very near, the last section may be dragged back over the knife edge by the blockface as it sweeps past (which we call "suckback"). If a longer period has transpired, several sweeps may occur in reapproaching the knife edge, before a suckback event takes away the last section. To avoid this loss of an occasional section, we use the "BYPASS" feature on the Sorvall microtome to make one or more sham advances toward the knife without allowing the block to touch the knife. With practice, one can learn to advance the knife just close enough to cut a thin section on the first pass after each pause to collect sections. Early in a session, bypass one to three advances before allowing the knife to touch the specimen; after 3 hours of sectioning, one may need to bypass five to seven advances to obtain the same result. Of course, bypassing too many times may lead to getting a thick section on the first pass.

This procedure is not terribly difficult, but requires a few days of practice to get everything working well. If good sections are not obtained, the fault must lie in one of the steps outlined above regarding specimen embedment, trimming, or microtome operation.

Troubleshooting

1. Alternating colors in sections and complete misses on every other section are characteristics of an unstable block. Either a fitting on the microtome is loose, allowing the specimen chuck to wobble, or the block is very soft or fractured, allowing the specimen to deflect when hitting the knife.

2. If sections show parallel stripes of thick and thin "chatter" parallel to the knife edge, there may be serious vibrations of the entire microtome platform or a loose fitting of the knife holder.

3. Partial suckback of sections is a common problem, which may relate to static charges, poor trimming (sticky bottom edge of blockface), or a wet blockface. Each section may drag the preceding section partway over the knife edge, so that sections become choppy or overlaid with fragments of previous sections. Lower the water level slightly (it must be somewhat concave) and dry the blockface with a Kimwipe. If suckback problems persist, one can take more drastic action by lowering the water level to an extreme concave level, so that the knife edge is just barely kept wetted. This condition does not allow good visibility of

the resulting section strips, so section counting can be difficult, but even a poorly trimmed block can sometimes be forced to yield serial sections in this manner.

4. Failure of sections to stick together in strips is a result of poor trimming or poor alignment of the block with the knife edge. If the edges of the block face are not cleanly trimmed, a ragged interface between successive sections will result, and the sections will break apart from each other. If the bottom edge of the blockface does not strike the knife edge cleanly across its entire length, the leading corner of the block may push away the preceding section before the next section can adhere to it. The best solution is to realign or retrim as necessary. If this is not possible, one temporary solution is to apply a small amount of adhesive to the top face of the block. We have used a drop of acetone to dissolve the glue from Scotch Tape (3M Company), then spread a small amount of glue onto the block with a toothpick. This will sometimes give strips of sections even when poorly trimmed.

5. Curling strips of sections result from poor trimming. Top and bottom edges are not quite parallel.

6. Partial sections are expected during the initial approach of the knife to a freshly trimmed block. Once the cutting action involves the whole blockface, complete sections should result with each sweep. Ragged, uneven sectioning or partial sections of uneven thickness can result when the plastic resin is poorly cured or the specimen is poorly embedded.

7. For alternative methods to collect serial thin sections, consult Fahrenbach (1984), Meyer and Domanico (1993), Stevens et al. (1980), or Reider (1981).

4. Decompression of the Sections

The cutting action compresses the specimen due to the force of the knife, which results in the sections being foreshortened. A transverse section of the roundworm will look elliptical. This compression can be reversed by briefly exposing the floating sections to a cotton swab soaked in chloroform. Before trying to pick up the sections onto grids, hold the swab above the sections for 5 to 10 seconds at a distance of 2 to 3 in. above the boat.

5. Counteracting Static Charges

Static charges are a common enemy of collecting thin sections. Their influence is highly variable from day to day, but can sometimes cause the sections to fly away from the knife edge (when cutting on a dry knife, as in frozen thin sections), to stick tightly to the face of the specimen, jumping out of the boat and over the knife edge, or to sail crazily across the surface of the boat water, evading capture by the copper grid.

After the first thin sections have begun to cut successfully each day, we position a Staticmaster cartridge (see Section VII) as close to the cutting region as possible.

It may have to be pushed aside during section pickup, but should be immediately repositioned before resuming sectioning.

6. Retrimming during Serial Sections

As the ideal block is a well-trimmed pyramid, the average cross-sectional area will increase as one sections further into a block, and the number of sections that will fit per grid will diminish. A very tightly trimmed adult worm, sectioned transversely, may give 30 sections per grid at first. After cutting perhaps 500 to 700 sections, one may be getting only 10 to 15 sections on a grid. The block can be removed to the trimming stand and retrimmed as before to give a tightly trimmed blockface. Remount onto the microtome arm, reapproach the knife edge carefully, and resume sectioning.

Helpful Hints. This episode of retrimming and resuming sectioning is the prime time for accidents to happen, and often can lead to a break in serial sections. Do not stop to retrim more often than necessary.

As one sections further into the block, the animal may also undergo slight bends which require changes in section angle to maintain a transverse orientation. Establish new top and bottom edges to keep them parallel under the new approach angle.

C. Picking up Sections onto Grids

Two primary types of specimen grids are available for EM: mesh grids and slot grids. For conventional transmission EM (TEM), one will generally use copper grids; nickel grids are recommended for immuno-EM. Mesh grids are somewhat easier to use in picking up sections, but some sections will be obscured by tissue falling over a grid bar. Mesh grids are also thinner and less rugged during section staining. Slot grids potentially allow the recovery of every serial section without obscuring grid bars, but require more skill to pick up the sections.

1. Mesh Grids

We recommend using 200- or 300-mesh copper grids, with a Formvar coating on one side to support the edges of the sections. Carbon coating of the Formvar is not absolutely needed, but can help to stabilize the Formvar film. Position the desired strip of sections in the boat well away from the knife edge with an eyelash or sharpened toothpick. Hold the mesh grid over the sections with a forceps (No. 5 Dumont), Formvar side down, and press the grid against the sections from above. As you lift the grid away from the surface of the water, the sections will adhere to the Formvar. Still holding the grid in the forceps, gently blot away excess liquid from the edge of the grid with filter paper, then set aside the grid to dry before placing it into a grid box. Take care to record the section numbers for each strip as you place them into the grid box.

Helpful Hints.   Never touch the knife edge with a grid or forceps! Mesh grids are thin and easily bent or dropped from the forceps during drying. Self-closing forceps are useful to keep from dropping grids, but are expensive. We make closing rings to hold standard forceps shut, so that a forceps holding a grid can be set aside to dry without dropping the grid. An O-ring ($5/16 \times 1/16$, Thomas Scientific) fits onto the forceps nicely for this purpose; it can close the forceps securely by sliding the O-ring toward the specimen, and can be released by sliding the O-ring toward the base of the handle.

2. Slot Grids

Electron microscope grids are available in a variety of sizes and shapes. Although round-hole grids may seem easier to use, we recommend slot grids. Grids should be precoated on the dull side with Formvar and carbon (see Section VIII) and stored in a dustproof container until ready to use. The plastic sections will readily stick to either the copper grid or the Formvar coating, so precautions are necessary to lessen the chances of a strip of sections hitting the copper. Each grid is detergent treated just prior to use, making the copper more hydrophobic.

Position a strip of sections away from the knife edge, using an eyelash or sharpened toothpick. Pick up a coated slot grid in a forceps (No. 5 Dumont) and dip the grid into 0.1% Triton X for a few seconds, remove, and briefly rinse the grid in two beakers of distilled water to remove excess detergent. Blot away liquid from the forceps and grid with a tissue. Plunge the grid into the boat, holding the grid almost vertically, until the top of the slot is even with the surface of the boat water. The shiny side of the grid should face the sections. Move the grid horizontally toward the desired strip of sections, then away, and repeat until the sections align with the top of the slot (Fig. 3). Continue this motion until the strip lies *directly against the slot,* making sure that the boat water just covers the top edge of the slot. Lift the grid out of the boat, and a droplet of water containing the sections will cover the slot, while the copper grid will remain dry due to the detergent treatment. If sections do lie on the copper, immediately dip the grid back into the boat to refloat them if possible; otherwise, the sections will be irreversibly stuck to the copper.

Blot the grid and the forceps with a Kimwipe, taking care not to let the tissue touch more than the extreme edge of the grid, then set aside the grid to dry while still held by the forceps. Use self-closing forceps or make forceps with O-ring closures as described above. By using four or five forceps, several successive strips can be picked up and dried as a set before resuming sectioning. Carefully inspect each dry grid to count the sections, and place securely in a grid box, recording the order and number of sections contained on each grid.

With practice, it is possible to collect several short strips per slot grid, which may be necessary if the strips break into smaller pieces during pickup. Narrow slots (No. GC42S, Ted Pella) are inherently less likely to suffer a catastrophic break in the Formvar than are the wide slots (No. GC12H). Therefore, narrow

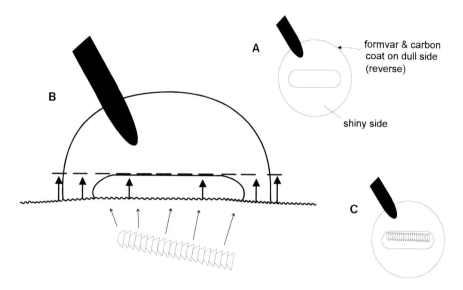

Fig. 3 Collecting sections onto specimen grid from underneath. (A) Formvar-coated copper grid held in forceps (black). (B) After detergent treatment, grid is dipped into boat water until water level (jagged line) reaches top edge of slot (dashed line). Horizontal motions bring strip into alignment (thin arrows) with top of slot. Lift grid out of water. (C) Sections adhere to Formvar on the slot. Blot forceps and back of grid with filter paper or Kimwipe.

straight strips of sections are usually collected on narrow slots, whereas wide or curving strips are put onto wide slots.

Helpful Hints. The forceps must not grip too close to the slot on the grid (Fig. 3), or a liquid pathway may be established between the slot and the forceps which could drag sections onto the forceps during drying. The blotting step just after detergent treatment is required to reduce the chance for such a liquid pathway to form. It is essential to blot the forceps to remove any liquid held between the points, especially before replacing grid into grid box; otherwise, a water droplet can pull the grid onto the forceps and possibly break the Formvar.

Never touch the knife edge with the grid or forceps!

Slot grids are rugged, but the Formvar coating is very fragile. A break or tear, or a set of holes, can lead to breakage and loss of sections. Although the carbon coating minimizes breaks in the Formvar, it lessens the contrast obtained during electron microscopy.

The ideal strip of sections is roughly two-thirds the width of the narrow slot; wider strips may not fit well, and narrower strips can crumple during drying.

After using 20 to 50 grids, detergent buildup can occur in the boat. The boat water should be exchanged for fresh distilled water. Detergent can form a scummy surface that seems to repel the sections during pickup, so that sections run away from the grid. In addition, debris should be cleared from the surface of the boat with a Kimwipe after every 5 to 10 grids.

If the detergent solution is too weak, or if grids are washed too thoroughly, the bare surface of the copper grid will be wet, that is, too hydrophilic, during section pickup.

D. Poststaining Methods

Sections must be stained to enhance contrast before EM study. As we are dealing with hundreds or thousands of sections, held on many grids, the process of staining each grid sequentially would be very laborious. Although staining machines are available through Reichert and others, they are too expensive for most of us to consider. Stevens *et al.* (1980) have described a special grid holder for collecting, staining, and examining serial thin sections, but it requires two people to smoothly collect the sections and a large number of these grid holders in which to process the grids. The Hiraoka grid-holding device (Bio-Rad, Electron Microscopy Sciences) can be flexed to allow many grids to be inserted, then unflexed to hold the grids securely. The whole device can then be dipped into stains and wash solutions. Another device (Ladd) holds grids inside a flow-through container. The SynapTek "Grid Stick" is sold through several vendors (Stevens and Trogadis, 1984). We use Randle Ware's version of the grid stick to hold our grids during staining. We use a razor blade to cut out a thin strip of dental wax which will fit into a 15-cc test tube, and incise rows of narrow indentations into the wax that will hold grids securely. (This device works best for copper slot grids; mesh grids are very fragile and bend while securing them on the holder.)

1. Staining Conventional Thin Sections

The most common contrasting agents are lead and uranium salts, which may be used in either aqueous or alcoholic solutions at widely varying concentrations and staining times. Nematode tissues lack inherent contrast, and the use of carbon-coated Formvar reduces contrast even further. Thus we recommend using two sequential poststains to boost contrast. When working at high magnifications to visualize small structures inside the worm, however, overstaining can easily cause staining artifacts that may obscure these features. Study of serial sections is even more demanding, as staining artifacts on just a few grids can break up data continuity. As a result, the recommended poststains (Table II) for *C. elegans* may seem quirky to microscopists with experience in other tissues. Each stain is followed by immediate destaining and washes to reduce the chance of creating artifacts.

2. Staining Thin Sections Following Immunocytochemistry

Single mesh grids can be stained sequentially in aqueous uranyl acetate solution, followed by two brief washes in distilled water. Blot grids on filter paper at the extreme edge, then allow grids to dry several minutes before replacing in

Table II
Poststaining Thin Sections for Electron Microscopy

1. Alcoholic uranyl acetate stain
    a. Stain 15 min at room temperature.
    b. Rinse twice in 100% ethanol, 30 seconds, with gentle agitation.
    c. Rinse once in 95% ethanol, 15 seconds.
    d. Rinse once in 50% ethanol, 15 seconds.
    e. Rinse once in 30% ethanol, 15 seconds.
    f. Rinse four times in distilled water, 15 seconds each.

Leave grids in holder and continue with second poststain.

2. Aqueous *dilute* Reynolds lead citrate stain
    a. Stain 5 min at room temperature.
    b. Rinse twice in 0.02 M NaOH, 60 seconds, with gentle agitation.
    c. Rinse five times in distilled water, 15 seconds each.

Blot excess water from grid stick row by row and replace grids in grid box. Allow grids to continue drying in open grid box for 10 minutes before closing box.

grid box. Resulting specimens will still have low inherent contrast; examine at 40 kV on an electron microscope to increase contrast.

IV. Basic Electron Microscopy of *Caenorhabditis elegans*

It is not our purpose here to describe detailed features of the many tissues that will be encountered in thin sections. As most available texts and articles show very limited views of a few features at high magnification, leaving the reader unsure of basic relationships between nearby structures, here we try to give enough information to identify dorsal versus ventral, left versus right, anterior versus posterior, and so on, in transverse and longitudinal sections. These are not always trivial to distinguish because of the worm's high degree of symmetry. We have even suffered the ignominy of confusing head versus tail at first glance in a newly sectioned worm.

The general anatomy of the head and tail have been described in several previous publications (Ware *et al.,* 1975; White *et al.,* 1976, 1986; Hall, 1977; Hall and Russell, 1991; Wood, 1987), so we will give more attention to the general features of the midbody.

A. Orientation Landmarks in Transverse Sections

Figure 4 shows schematic views through select positions along the length of the body. Take special note that sections may be left/right inverted depending

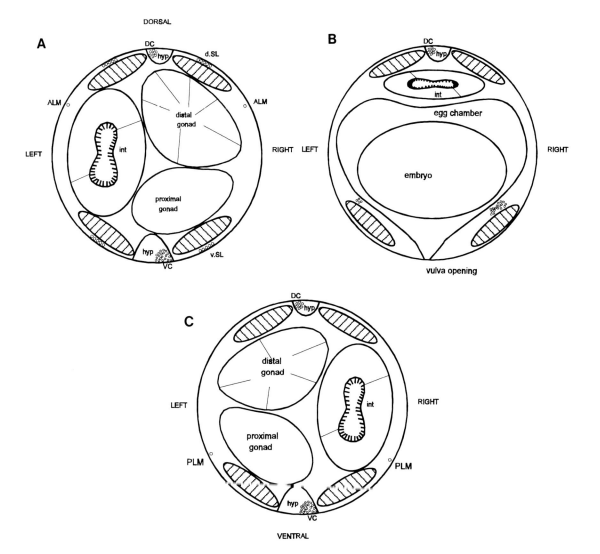

Fig. 4 Key landmarks for transverse sections of midbody region. (A) Anterior to the vulva. Ventral nerve cord is larger than dorsal nerve cord; thus, dorsal/ventral axis can be established. Anterior midbody is distinguished by the presence of sublateral nerves (d.SL and v.SL) and ALM touch dendrites, which lie dorsolaterally and contain distinctive large-caliber microtubules. Regardless of section handling, dorsal nerve lies slightly toward the true left and ventral nerve lies slightly toward the true right of the associated hypodermal cord (hyp); thus left/right axis can be established. Distal gonad lies dorsally and contains a cluster of oocytes joined by a central rachis, while ventral gonad may hold single embryos and/or sperm and specialized tissues associated with the ovary. Left/right orientation of gonad arms versus intestine (int) is not always reproducible. Body muscles are shown as stippled profiles. (B) Vulval region. Ventral nerve cord is split into two ventrolateral fascicles that depart from midline. Smaller dorsal nerve cord remains at dorsal midline, slightly toward true left. Fertilized embryo (often multicellular) lies within egg chamber. Additional specialized vulval muscles lie obliquely (not shown). Intestine is squeezed toward dorsal midline. (C) Posterior to the vulva. Dorsal/ventral axis can be determined as above. Posterior midbody is distinguished by PLM touch dendrites containing large microtubules, and lacks any sublateral nerves except very near the vulva. Left/right axis can again be distinguished best according to the relative position of nerve cords and their associated hypodermal cords.

on the direction of sectioning, the handling of the sections between microtome and microscope, and the optical characteristics of the electron microscope. Fortunately, most left-versus-right asymmetries within the body of *C. elegans* are extremely consistent (Wood and Kershaw, 1991) and can be used to quickly ascertain the true orientation of almost any section through the animal. There are some features that are switched in certain mutant backgrounds; for example, gonad outgrowth in *unc-5* and *unc-6* can show reverse handedness or dorsal/ventral wanderings (Hedgecock *et al.*, 1990); however, the handedness of dorsal and ventral nerve cords and the presence or absence of touch dendrites and sublateral nerves are very robust indicators.

B. Orientation Landmarks in Longitudinal Sections

Figure 5 shows a schematic view of a longitudinal section, emphasizing the general order of tissues to be encountered as a section passes through the body of the worm. As the relative angle of sectioning is difficult to control relative to the body's rotation about its central axis, a great variety of nonstandard views are possible. Plasma membranes may seem blurred or absent in this orientation, but most tissues are still distinctive in their cytoplasmic detail.

C. Strategies for Examining Serial Thin Sections

Deciding how to examine a good set of serial sections is not trivial, as one's potential data set is held within a very fragile group of electron microscope grids which could be damaged during inspection. A related problem is the decision

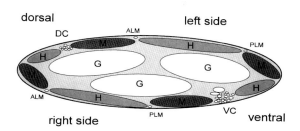

Fig. 5 Landmarks for longitudinal or oblique section through midbody. Individual tissues may look distorted or different at oblique angles, and any tissue may lie toward acute margin of the cross section; however, their general order along the body wall remains distinctive. Dorsal/ventral axis can be determined by relative size of nerve cords; ventral cord is larger and is associated with several neuron cell bodies in any given section. In addition, ventral hypodermal cord (H) is larger in profile than the dorsal hypodermal cord. ALM touch dendrites occur in anterior sections, while PLM dendrites occur in posterior sections. Dorsal nerve cord lies toward true left side of dorsal hypodermal cord, while ventral nerve cord lies toward true right side. Relative positions of gut (G) and gonad (G) are not as instructive. Lateral hypodermis is larger than dorsal or ventral hypodermis. Body muscle, M.

on what magnification(s) will best display the data without losing detail or dropping out data from the periphery. Finally, one must make a conscious decision on how many micrographs need to be collected per specimen and how many sections can be skipped between photographs without losing continuity. We cannot answer all of these questions regarding your project, but can make a few suggestions that can reduce costs and maximize efficiency.

During section collection, we recommend collecting every possible group of sections, without pausing to screen for the exact region of interest. This is slightly more work than collecting intermittent sections, but gives much more security that the correct region is included within the series. This strategy also provides occasional grids throughout the series that may hold just a few sections each. These grids are the place to begin a general survey to look for (1) the quality of the fixation, embedment, and thin sections; (2) the true region of interest within the series; and (3) the magnification(s) that will display the whole region and the smaller features of prime interest.

It is difficult to resolve fine details on the electron microscope viewing screen, so during this survey one should collect micrographs of sample sections on each survey grid. This is a good time to select one or two standard magnifications; then each section should be photographed at standard settings. As a grid is most likely to suffer damage during insertion or removal from the electron microscope, take micrographs during this inspection; there may not be a second chance later. If a grid shows a hole or Formvar defect, be even more careful to photograph as many sections as possible. Make prints from the test micrographs and inspect closely. If one intends to make a three-dimensional reconstruction, the easiest approach is to collect all micrographs for the reconstruction at one magnification. It is hoped the entire region of interest will fit into one field of view at this magnification. The most important criterion is that the details of interest be visible at the chosen magnification.

If the region of interest cannot be adequately defined from grids holding one or two sections, select another single grid containing a potentially good set of sections and follow the same strategy. Assume that the first look is the last chance, and photograph at least every third section now.

If one is trying to reconstruct the outlines of a relatively large cell, perhaps a muscle or intestinal cell, it may be sufficient to photograph every 20th or 50th section at approximately $2500\times$ without losing continuity. Following thinner muscle arms as they extend toward the nerve cord will require photographing every 3rd to 5th section at a higher magnification ($5000\times$). To record synaptic interactions between neuronal processes may require photographing every section (or at least every third section) at about $10,000\times$.

V. Three-Dimensional Reconstruction Methods

Many investigators have been intrigued by the possibility of producing three-dimensional renderings of cells from serial sections. Nematode neurons were being traced and reconstructed from thick sections almost 100 years ago (Goldschmidt, 1909). Attempts to accomplish this task from electron micrographs of *C. elegans* have been frustrated by the expense and effort required to deal with so much film, especially to make a prealigned movie before entering data into a computer, and also by the high level of human intervention required to interpret the EM image during the tracing of data into the computer. Despite the dramatic cost reductions available in microcomputer data handling, these obstacles remain substantial. Newer confocal light microscopes often come bundled with reconstruction software and it is relatively simple to collect self-aligned focus through series of digital images. Most transmission electron microscopes still do not have high-quality digital image capabilities, which would be a first step in finally making serial reconstruction a cheap and efficient procedure for thin-section data.

We describe here some of the methods used to reconstruct *C. elegans* neurons and muscles in serial sections. We anticipate that digital image techniques (Russ, 1990) may soon supplant the use of film and will certainly supplant the use of cinematography. At present screen resolutions, however, a film image (2 × 2 in. or 35 mm) contains far more information than a 1024 × 1024 array of pixels. Cheaper video cameras may deliver only 200 to 300 lines of resolution, even in a field containing 400+ scan lines.

A. Cinematographic Reconstruction from Negatives

We have outlined the methods making it feasible to collect hundreds of micrographs of cells or cell processes from a serially sectioned nematode. After assembling an ordered collection of negatives, all produced at one magnification, one desires to view them sequentially in a well-aligned "movie" through the specimen. One can quickly comprehend and trace the continuity of individual processes as they course through a nerve bundle from a movie, even when the registration of profiles from print to print is difficult to discern.

The "image combiner," instrumentation for the production of a 35-mm film from electron micrographs, was designed by Randle Ware (Ware *et al.,* 1975). Micrographs are aligned sequentially and rephotographed onto movie film. This film can be viewed directly or projected onto a data tablet from which the operator can trace cell outlines into a computer. Alternately, the operator can mark the identities of reconstructed cell profiles onto a series of EM prints from selected sections within the series. Similar image combiners may be available in other laboratories that have specialized in serial reconstructions (cf. White, 1974; Macagno *et al.,* 1979; Stevens and Trogadis, 1984).

Internal features are used as fiducial markers for alignment from section to section. This is required to avoid gradual drift or twisting of the image from section to section (Ware and LoPresti, 1972; Hubbard *et al.,* 1993).

Pitfalls.   Individual thin sections will suffer from differential compression, wrinkles, and local defects that can obscure the image and make alignment of the series difficult. Stevens and Trogadis (1984) described a computerized system to compensate for compression and distortion during the transfer of serial images onto the filmstrip.

B. Manual Reconstruction from Prints

Cinematography and computerized reconstruction are very labor intensive. Manual methods can be quite satisfactory to quickly draw an image of a reconstructed cell (Ware and LoPresti, 1972). To optimize this procedure one should (1) collect micrographs at a standard magnification as before, and (2) print each micrograph in a prealigned fashion so that the body axes are consistent from one print to the next. Unless the alignment of the specimen's body axis has been controlled on the microscope stage (cf. Stevens *et al.,* 1980; Stevens and Trogadis, 1984), the initial micrographs will be a jumble of rotated images. While working in the darkroom, however, one should print every image in a standard format. The resulting stack of prints can be easily flipped through to view each section from a standard orientation.

Once a good set of prints has been made, one can begin to follow individual cell profiles through the stack, marking cell identities on the prints with colored markers. Use a marker that can be erased with alcohol; this will not damage the print and allows mistakes to be easily corrected.

C. Computerized Serial Reconstruction Systems

Efforts to marry the computer and the two-dimensional photos or drawings from anatomical sections to represent tissues in three dimensions have been ongoing for many years (Lindsay, 1977; Turner, 1981; Capowski, 1989). The early systems ran on mainframe computers and stretched the bounds of computer graphics, memory storage, and laboratory budgets. Some of these individually customized systems may still be available in various university departments, and might be adaptable to *C. elegans* data sets (Johnson and Capowski, 1983; Harris and Stevens, 1988; Young *et al.,* 1987). Many promising generic computer programs are now available to run on microcomputers or on graphics workstations (Huijsmans *et al.,* 1986), but no single program has emerged as the standard for the *C. elegans* community. There is currently no convenient interface to allow simultaneous display of a thin-section reconstruction and a confocal image reconstruction. This could become a very useful means to compare images produced through different modalities. We first describe a system that we have found useful in our laboratory and then briefly describe several other available systems. The theoretical basis for image digitization and analysis has been reviewed elsewhere (see Hubbard *et al.,* 1993; Macagno *et al.,* 1979; Russ, 1990; Turner, 1981).

1. The RECON Program

This vector-based graphics package from Eutectic Electronics (Raleigh, NC) requires several pieces of customized hardware in addition to a standard PC.

Data are entered from a data tablet as wire-frame outlines of the cells of interest, with seven colors available for the simultaneous display of different cells. After two-dimensional outlines from a stack of prints or from a movie projected onto the data tablet are entered, a three-dimensional representation can be displayed on a vector graphics terminal and rotated about any axis to choose an ideal viewpoint. Multiple objects can be traced in simultaneously, displayed in different colors on the terminal, and ported to a multipen plotter or laser printer. In the final image, one can select which objects are to be displayed, or images from several files can be added together. The program allows the deletion of hidden lines from the back side of the figure.

Figure 6 shows wire-frame reconstructions of a *C. elegans* excretory cell and a body muscle cell from a wild-type animal. Each cell was manually traced from about 50 prints into the RECON program. Aspects of the body wall and pharynx were used as fiducial markers to align the individual cross sections during tracing into the computer. The excretory cell data file was produced by entering data from every 25th thin section spanning 1200 sections. The muscle cell data file includes tracings from every 20th section spanning 1040 sections, except for the thinner muscle arms surrounding the nerve ring, which were traced from every 6th section. In one display, a few tracings of the cuticle (faint lines) are shown to emphasize the close apposition of muscle to the body wall.

One strength of this system for *C. elegans* tissues is the unlimited number of sections that can be entered into a data file. Other systems may be limited to a small number of sections, some accepting as few as 20. The speed of real-time rotation of a 3D file on the vector display monitor is instantaneous, and the display angle is easily controlled by the cursor on the digitizing tablet. The RECON manual is simple to follow, and the program has useful tools for measuring cross-sectional areas, perimeters, and cell volumes. Data can be easily reedited during data entry, and there are useful programs to readjust or smooth the data before final display, including rotation and realignment of individual sections or objects within a section.

Drawbacks of This System. Data entry is entirely operator dependent and time consuming. There is a restriction on the number of data points (1000) per block of data from a single section, although complex images can be subdivided to span multiple blocks. Complex images can overload the vector graphics display if too many vectors are in the display file, but the vector terminal is still useful in viewing subsets of large files to choose desirable viewing angles. Computer processing times for each new perspective vary widely; generation of an image such as that in Fig. 6A takes only seconds, whereas generation of complex hidden line files as in Fig. 6B or 6C may take an hour or more. No surface renderings are available from these data sets.

2. The STERECON Program

The Wadsworth Center's Biological Microscopy and Image Reconstruction Facility in Albany, New York, is a National Biotechnology Resource funded

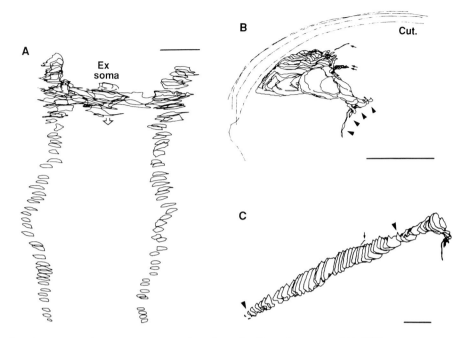

Fig. 6 Sample wire-frame reconstructions from the Eutectics system. (A) Wild-type excretory canal cell is displayed in part (posterior canals are truncated just behind the soma). Anterior canals extend along lateral body wall from a soma centered along ventral midline. Contents of each canal lumen are collected centrally in the soma and excreted via the excretory pore on ventral surface (open arrowhead). The perspective is tilted to show anteriormost sections toward the bottom; this perspective causes the canals to be foreshortened by 35%. Complete tracings of each profile are shown, so that lines hiding behind another structure are visible, making a rather noisy display. The canals are not completely straight, even after rigorous efforts to align each section versus the rest of the set. Most of this relative drift in lateral position is real, but subtle changes may also result from differential compression of individual sections. (B, C) Wild type muscle cell in the head is shown from two perspectives, with hidden lines removed; these provide good representations of cell surfaces facing the viewer. (B) Muscle cell shown from a perspective almost transverse to the body axis, emphasizing close apposition of the cell's contractile zone to cuticle (Cut), and a thick muscle arm extending centrally to the nerve ring (arrowheads indicate sites of synaptic input from nerve ring; nerve ring is in foreground, looking anteriorly). A very thin process (small arrow) sticks out medially to touch a neighboring muscle cell. A double arrow indicates the distant anterior end of the cell. From this perspective, contractile zone is foreshortened by 90%. (C) Same cell as in B shown from an oblique side view at lower magnification, with nose to lower right edge and nerve ring on far right edge. Contractile portion of the cell extends between arrowheads. Small arrow indicates the thin medial muscle arm as in B. Apparent length of contractile zone is foreshortened by 33% from this perspective. Bar = 5 μm in each panel.

through the National Institutes of Health (NIH). The director of the facility is Dr. Conly Rieder. The STERECON computer program operates there on a Sun workstation. The system can recognize structures semiautomatically in 2D, before stacking these images into 3D image files, with stereoscopic viewing capabilities.

Image enhancement routines are also available. Both wire-frame and surface renderings can be used for the display of cell reconstructions (Marko *et al.,* 1988). The facility also operates a high-voltage electron microscope (HVEM), which opens the possibility of imaging structures in a few serial thick sections rather than in many serial thin sections. The facility also offers equipment and software techniques devoted to cryo-EM, X-ray microanalysis EM, and analysis of macro-molecular structures. A mail-in service is available for HVEM studies of thick-section samples.

3. The CARTOS Program

CARTOS is a semiautomated reconstruction system based on an Iris Indigo workstation at Columbia University. Dr. Eduardo Macagno is the director of this facility, which can be made available to outside users by arrangement. Routines for the automated recognition of cell outlines have been described (Macagno *et al.,* 1979; Allen and Levinthal, 1990). New routines allow volume renderings and surface renderings to be projected as well as wire-frame views. A portable version of the CARTOS software is under development.

4. The IMAGE Program

This is a public domain software package available through the NIH (via Internet from zippy.nimh.nih.gov[128.231.98.32] or through National Technical Information Service, Springfield, VA) which runs on a Macintosh computer with at least 4 MB of memory (8 MB or more recommended). This is a versatile package, allowing data to be imported through digitizers, frame grabbers, or flatbed scanners and output can be directed to laser or color printers. A variety of image enhancement techniques are offered, and automated measurements can be made. Two-dimensional images can be edited with MacPaint-like commands at eight levels of magnification. These images can be assembled into 3D "stacks." These stacks can be animated or resliced at 90° angles to display the data from new aspects. User support is not available by telephone, but an active on-line user group communicates on the Internet.

One experienced user of the IMAGE package in the *C. elegans* community is the Integrated Microscopy Resource at the University of Wisconsin, which is now directed by Dr. John White. The facility also hosts an HVEM and cryo-EM equipment.

VI. Other Electron Microscopy Methods

A. Freeze–Fracture and Freeze–Etching of *Caenorhabditis elegans*

Freeze-fracture (FF) and freeze-etching (FE) are related techniques. FF provides a high-magnification view of the physical relationships between membrane components, for example, the clustering of ion channels. FE is useful in studying the relationships between cytoskeletal elements. Both techniques require access to a freeze-etch device, made by Balzers, Cressington, or JEOL, as well as a conventional transmission electron microscope in which to view the metal replicas produced. The replicas represent detailed topographic maps of the fractured samples. Brief reports using FF in *C. elegans* have detailed the distribution of intracellular junctions (Hall, 1987) and compared the cuticles of adults and dauer larvae (Peixoto and De Souza, 1994). FF has previously been used in other nematode species to study a variety of cell junctions (Burghardt, 1980; Davidson, 1983; Wright *et al.*, 1985), membrane fusion events (Burghardt and Foor, 1978), and cuticular specializations (Martinez-Paloma, 1978; Lee *et al.*, 1984, 1986).

1. Freeze-Fracture Protocol

Animals are fixed for 2 hours in 2% glutaraldehyde in 0.1 *M* cacodylate buffer, pH 7.2, rinsed, and stored in buffer in the cold for 0 to 5 days until the day of fracture. Longer fixation times tend to ruin the fracture process, so it is preferable to store fixed tissue in buffer than to allow the tissue to soak overnight in fix. Samples are soaked for 90 minutes in 30% glycerol just before FF. The glycerol infiltration is essential to prevent the formation of ice crystals during the freezing process. We have used the plunge-freeze technique, employing liquid isopentane (or ethane or Freon) in a small metal cup chilled by liquid nitrogen. Animals in glycerol are pipetted onto a small gold disk, the excess liquid is wicked away, and a second disk is placed on top, sandwiching the animals between the disks. Stout forceps are used to clamp the sandwiched disks together as they are plunged into isopentane for 30 seconds. Samples are then loaded into a prechilled double replica holder and transferred into the freeze-etch device. Under high vacuum within the device (10^{-6} Torr, $-110°C$), the gold disks are pulled apart, fracturing the animals preferentially between intramembrane leaflets. Immediately after fracture, the samples are shadowed at an angle (or rotary shadowed) with platinum and then shadowed from above with an even coat of carbon.

The disks are removed from the device and soaked for 1 hour in fresh Chlorox bleach. The replicas float away from the tissue, which dissolves in the bleach. Replica pieces are easily transferred from solution to solution in a multiwell ceramic dish using a small platinum wire loop. After a second wash in bleach and a wash in 50% bleach (1 hour each), the replicas are rinsed four or five times in distilled water and collected on electron microscope grids. We prefer to collect onto carbon-coated Formvar slot grids, so that the entire replica can be examined in the transmission electron microscope.

By clustering about 100 animals per gold disk, a substantial number can be fractured per sample. One can fracture 6 to 10 samples per day in modern freeze-etch devices, which yields a very large number of fractured animals to inspect.

Helpful Hints. Avoid looking too long at any replicas dominated by ice artifacts. A variety of other artifacts are also possible (Rash and Hudson, 1979).

Ice artifacts are formed if there is any delay between fracture and shadowing, as water vapor released during fracture can immediately refreeze onto the exposed surfaces. Be sure that the vacuum is low enough compared with the fracturing temperature to favor etching conditions rather than crystallization. Always use fresh bleach; old bleach will fail to digest tissue, leaving dull gray deposits masking the metal replica.

2. Freeze–Etch Protocol

Animals can be fixed and stored in buffer as for FF, but *do not use glycerol,* as this will not etch away. Specimens are fast frozen as above and loaded into the freeze-etch device. After fracture at 10^{-6} Torr and $-100°C$, the samples are held under high vacuum for an additional few minutes to "etch" away water from the surface of the fractured specimen before metal shadowing. Replicas are removed from the device and floated onto bleach and prepared as for FF. By varying the length of etching time and/or the temperature, one can vary the speed and depth of the etching process to reveal details of the cytoskeleton. A rotary shadowing attachment on the freeze-etch device is useful for good FE replicas.

3. Landmarks for Recognizing Tissues

As the fixed animals all tend to be oriented to lie within the plane of fracture, fracture planes will run lengthwise. Glancing fractures may invade only the cuticle layers, revealing striated layers of collagen in extracellular space (Fig. 7). Mild etching conditions were used to accentuate these extracellular fibrils. Fracturing slightly deeper, hypodermal and body muscle membranes will appear. Hypodermis is distinguished by deep parallel infoldings in the face opposing the cuticle ("canals": Zuckerman *et al.,* 1973) and gap junctions in membranes where two hypodermal cells are apposed (Hall, 1987). Muscle membranes in *C. elegans* have distinctive orderly arrays of large depressions and rectilinear arrays of intramembrane particles that match those found in other nematode species (Wright *et al.,* 1985; Lee *et al.,* 1986). Cross-fractures or etching will also reveal thick muscle filament arrays within the muscle cytoplasm. Longitudinal and circumferential nerves are often visible, and particle arrays underlying synaptic contacts are sometimes evident (Fig. 8). Deep fractures into the body cavity are rare. As most fracture planes preferentially cleave within cell membranes, few views of cytoplasm within cells should be expected.

The two sides of the plasma membrane show different characteristics when cleaved (Branton, 1971; Rash and Hudson, 1979). The extracellular leaflet is exposed as the "E-face" and is relatively free of intramembrane particles (IMPs), except for some forms of channel proteins that span the entire membrane (e.g., gap junction connexons; see Fig. 8). The cytoplasmic leaflet, or "P-face," is very particle rich, and various types of IMPs have characteristic sizes and spacing.

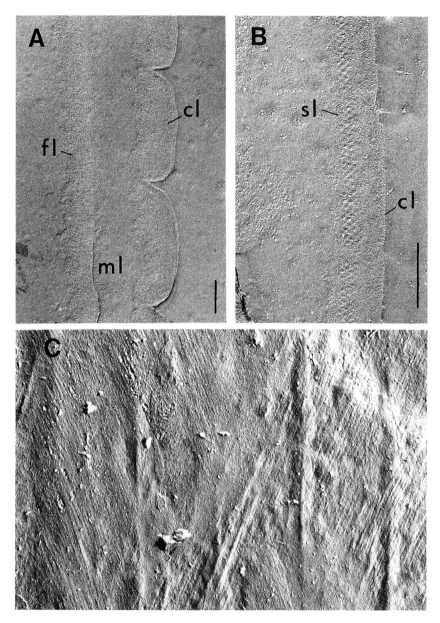

Fig. 7 Freeze-etch images of basal layer in wild-type cuticle. (A) Longitudinal fracture of adult cuticle shows annuli in outer cortical layer (cl), an empty medial layer (ml), and diffuse fibrous material (collagen) in basal layer (fl) (compare with Cox *et al.*, 1981). (B) Longitudinal fracture of juvenile cuticle shows no distant annuli in cortical layer (cl). Striated layer (sl) shows a striking meshlike organization. (C) Glancing longitudinal fracture of adult cuticle shows basal fibrous layer en face. Annuli are visible as widely spaced indentations running vertically; body axis runs left to right. Layers of fibrils are oriented at a 70° angle to body axis, but in opposite handedness to each other; each layer apparently runs in helical fashion along body wall. Bars in A and B = 0.5 μm.

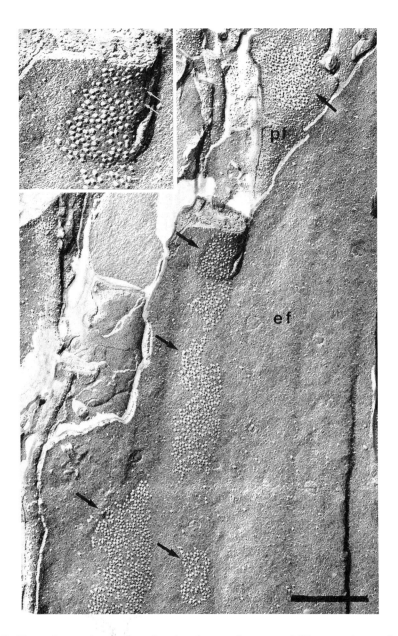

Fig. 8 Freeze-fracture image of gap junctions in ventral nerve cord. Electron micrograph shows freeze-fracture replica through ventral nerve cord membranes. Large intramembrane particles (IMPs) are clustered at gap junctions (large arrows) between closely apposed neuronal processes. A large E-face membrane (ef) shows long parallel ridges running vertically where four neighboring axons press against it; three of these are involved in en passant synapses. The fracture runs longitudinally near ventral margin of body (cuticle was cross-fractured to reveal consecutive annuli just to the right of region shown). The large number of axons within nerve bundle (not shown) identified this as ventral cord. As cells are unlabeled, one cannot identify individual axons with certainty. The arrangement is similar to known wiring diagram for the interactions of VD1, VD2 and DD1 (see White *et al.,* 1986; p. 337). Inset shows one gap junction at higher magnification. Shallow pits (white arrows) are interspersed in this E-face membrane between IMPs. Neuronal gap junctions in *C. elegans* contain about 50% IMPs and 50% pits on each face (Hall, 1987). In this replica most pits are difficult to see; the favorable angle of shadowing in this small area reveals more pits than elsewhere. This replica was made with a fixed-angle Pt gun; rotary shadowing would have provided somewhat finer detail. Bar = 0.5 μm.

B. Electron Microscopic Immunocytochemistry of *Caenorhabditis elegans*

1. Choosing the Best Fixative and Resin Combination

Although immunochemical methods are commonly used to localize proteins in the nematode using light microscopy or confocal microscopy, experience with EM methods is still quite limited. Methods that offer striking views at the light microscope level will generally look terrible when magnified under EM. The very light degree of fixation required to preserve antigenicity leads to the total loss of ultrastructural detail. Although Okamoto and Thomson (1985) reported success in *C. elegans* tissues using postembedding labeling on Epon thin sections, Epon is not a very accessible plastic for most antigen labeling without etching (see Mar and Wight, 1988). LR White resin is very popular for immuno-EM of many vertebrate tissues, but we have found that *C. elegans* tissues shrink severely in this resin. LR Gold resin is preferable for postembedding methods with nematode tissues (Selkirk *et al.*, 1991). Lowicryls might also work for postembedding. An alternate "preembedding" approach is to fast-freeze worms after light fixation (or *no* fixation), collect frozen thin sections, and treat these thin sections with immunochemical reagents before embedment, following the techniques of Toku-yasu (1986, 1989). Stirling (1990) reviewed these possibilities in more detail.

2. Postembedding Methods Using LR Gold Resin

a. Fixation

The proper degree of fixation is highly dependent on the antibody and the antigen to be localized; some are easily degraded by any exposure to glutaraldehyde, or by moderate amounts of formaldehyde, or by ethanol and other solvents, whereas others are fairly robust. The proper fixative needs to be pretested for each antibody by conventional immunochemical procedures at the light microscope level before embarking on immuno-EM procedures. As the worm is protected by a thick cuticle, it is again helpful to cut open the animals while in fix to aid in penetration. Compare several test fixes with light microscope immuno-methods:

1. 2% formaldehyde in buffer for 60 minutes
2. 2% formaldehyde, 0.1% glutaraldehyde in buffer for 20 minutes, followed by 2% formaldehyde in buffer for an additional 20 minutes
3. 2% formaldehyde, 0.5% glutaraldehyde in buffer for 60 minutes

Ideally one should use the most fixation possible before antigenicity appears to fall off. *All steps must be carried out on ice.* No osmium can be used.

b. Embedding

Fixed animals are rinsed in buffer and pre-embedded in SeaPlaque agarose as described in Section II,C. The 2.5% agarose solution should be precooled to 32°C before embedment to limit heating of the specimens. We recommend that animals be grouped in large aggregates, perhaps in parallel arrays, or embedded as large pellets. Agarose blocks are then cooled back to 4°C in 50% methanol and dehydrated stepwise in 70, 90, and 100% methanol at −25°C. Stepwise embedment into LR Gold begins with 30 minutes in 1:1 methanol:LR Gold with 0.1% BME, then 60 minutes in 3:7 methanol:LR Gold/BME, then several changes over 72 hours in 100% LR Gold/BME; each step is carried out at −25°C (Selkirk *et al.,* 1991). Samples are transferred into gelatin capsules in fresh resin and cured under UV at −25°C. Take care to match the proper accelerator to the light source: 0.1% benzoin methyl ether (BME) is used for curing by UV, whereas 0.1% benzil is supposed to work well for curing under blue light. For embedding lightly fixed tissue into LR Gold, 20% poly (vinyl pyrrolidone) (PVP) can be added to dehydration steps and early infiltration steps to minimize osmotic damage.

LR Gold blocks are trimmed and sectioned by conventional procedures, mounting the thin sections on Formvar-coated nickel-mesh grids (200 or 300 mesh). As no heavy metal stains are used prior to immuno-EM procedures, the embedded animals are practically transparent and orientation and trimming are problematic. By combining many animals into a large array or pellet in one block, one hopes to section important regions of many animals within the same thin sections, maximizing the chance to apply antibody solutions to appropriate targets. Sample grids should contain as many sections as will fit, again to maximize the tissue being treated with antibody. A few sample grids from a series can be screened by EM at this time to choose which grids contain the region of interest. Grids may be viewed at 40 kV to enhance contrast, or stained briefly in aqueous uranyl acetate (these stained grids should not be used for immuno-EM afterward).

c. Immunocytochemistry

Primary antibody (or preimmune serum) is placed in 5-μl aliquots on Parafilm in a covered petri dish. A wet piece of filter paper is used *under* the Parafilm to humidify the petri dish. Grids are prerinsed in five changes of 0.01 M glycine in phosphate buffer (PB), blocked for 15 minutes in 0.2% gelatin, 0.01 M glycine, 0.1% nonfat dry milk in PB at 37°C, rinsed in warmed 0.01 M glycine in PB, then placed section side down over the primary antibody in 0.2% gelatin in PB for 60 minutes at room temperature. Grids are rinsed again 6 × 5 minutes in PB, then placed onto a 10-μl droplet of the colloidal gold-labeled secondary antibody (Ab) for 60 minutes. (Secondary Ab is diluted in PB plus 0.2% gelatin; exact dilution may vary from 1:20 to 1:100 depending on the secondary Ab.) Again, the grids are rinsed five times in PB, then immersed for 5 minutes in 2% glutaraldehyde in PB. Next the grids are rinsed twice in distilled H_2O, blotted dry, and stored in a grid box. Prior to viewing by EM, the grids should be post-stained with aqueous uranyl acetate.

Several dilutions of primary antibody should be tested. The best dilution for light microscopy can be used as a starting point, but the best dilution for EM may be different. At limiting dilutions, background label should be practically absent while specific label lying on regions of interest is retained. Necessary controls should be (1) preimmune serum instead of primary Ab, (2) no primary Ab, (3) primary Ab preabsorbed with excess immunogen, and (4) a different, reliable primary Ab as a positive control.

Helpful Hints. If LR Gold embedding is poor, or if resin fails to harden, consult the supplier for advice. Test that the mixture of LR Gold plus accelerator by itself will harden adequately in a gelatin capsule.

An alternate blocking solution might include nonimmune serum from the host animal of the secondary Ab if necessary.

Tissue will not look especially nice under mild fixation. Cut pieces of worms should improve access by fixatives. Contrast of tissue will also be quite low, as no osmium is used. It is generally preferable not to carbon-coat the grids, as this will further lower section contrast.

Specificity of the primary antibody may prove less obvious under immuno-EM than by light microscopy techniques. True antigenicity may be masked by the resin, or destroyed altogether by exposure to ethanol during processing. If either result is encountered, try a preembedding technique as an alternative approach.

Immunoperoxidase methods are generally more difficult to intepret than colloidal gold methods at the electron microscope level. There is probably little advantage to using gold-enhancing techniques for immuno-EM, although they may be useful in screening antigen/antibody interactions at the light microscope level.

3. Preembedding Methods Using Frozen Thin Sections

This technique is potentially useful for *C. elegans* tissues, although we are not aware that any laboratory has put the method into general use. A freezing ultramicrotome is required to collect the sections.

a. Tissue Preparation

Live or lightly fixed animals should be rinsed in M9 buffer and cryoprotected in either 2.3 M sucrose or in sucrose plus 20% PVP for 30 to 90 minutes. Allow the animals to settle in a centrifuge tube to produce a thick slurry of animals. Place a droplet of the sample onto the tip of a metal stub and wick away excess fluid with a strip of filter paper. Plunge the stub into liquid nitrogen to fast-freeze the animals, and store the metal stubs under liquid nitrogen until sectioning (a plunge into liquid isopentane may be necessary to fast-freeze samples in sucrose/PVP). The stub is transferred to the precooled microtome arm (−80°C) and trimmed if necessary while in place. Sectioning proceeds on a precooled dry knife (glass or diamond), also at −80°C. (Good ultrathin sections may cut in the range between −80 and −110°C; sucrose/PVP samples will cut best at −114°C.) Cutting speed should be slow (0.4 mm/s). Best sections should look green/gold or pink. Frozen thin sections are assembled on the knife edge with an eyelash, as flat as possible, and transferred onto a platinum wire loop containing a droplet of 2.3 M sucrose by bringing the loop close to the sections. The sections will jump to the loop and melt onto the sucrose drop; these are transferred onto a nickel-mesh grid coated with Formvar and carbon. (Grids may need to be deionized prior to use in a glow discharge chamber.) Grids should be stored briefly in the cold until one is prepared to carry out immunochemical procedures.

b. Immunocytochemistry

Each grid is inverted onto successive drops of 0.01 M glycine in PB to wash, then onto blocking solution (see above) before exposing to the primary antibody. Invert the grid directly onto a 5-μl droplet of primary antibody solution in 0.2% gelatin in PB on a Parafilm strip in a humidified covered petri dish at room temperature. The incubation time should be brief for unfixed tissue (10 minutes), but can be longer (60 minutes) for fixed tissue. Then the grid is rinsed in PB and exposed to the colloidal gold-labeled secondary antibody. Now fix the grid in 2% glutaraldehyde in PB for 5 minutes; rinse once in PB and five times in dH$_2$O. One can fix again with osmium tetroxide, if desired. Finally the grid is stained and embedded in one step in 0.2% acidic uranyl acetate plus 3% polyvinyl alcohol (Tokuyasu, 1989).

Pitfalls.   This technique is technically difficult, as there are no reasonable means to preselect sections for orientation nor even for specific regions of interest and no likelihood of examining any region in true serial sections. Sections tend to fly off the knife edge due to static forces; use an antistatic device to reduce this effect. The one-step embedding technique is also problematic and requires some practice to achieve the right amount of liquid on the embedding loop. As no resin and little fixative are used prior to antibody interactions, antigenicity should be excellent; however, tissue degradation will proceed after thawing if no prefixation is used.

VII. Equipment

A. Ultramicrotomes

Several models are suitable for collecting thin sections, but for serial sections one is advised to look for models featuring a mechanical rather than a thermal advance mechanism. The Reichert Ultracut series is excellent; some models can be upgraded to allow frozen thin sectioning for immuno-EM as well. The RMC MT 7000 (Research and Manufacturing Company, Tucson, AZ) is also a good choice. The Sorvall MT2-B was a very reliable model but is no longer marketed; working instruments may still be available secondhand. Modern microtomes have better lighting than the Sorvall to help in initial alignment and close approach of the specimen to the knife. RMC offers service and upgrades for Sorvall microtomes, including retrofits for cryosectioning.

A microtome bench can minimize vibrations which induce section chatter. The microtome should be installed in a quiet corner of the laboratory, enclosed by a curtain or plastic shield to minimize air currents that might blow floating sections or cause thermal gradients. If building vibration is noticeable, a move to the basement is advisable. One may also shut down ventilation equipment during sectioning or work at night to avoid daytime vibrations.

B. Diamond Knives

A diamond knife is essential for cutting serial thin sections, as glass knives become dull after 10 successive sections. A 2.0-mm knife is priced at about $1000 to $2000 depending on the supplier (Diatome, Delaware, Edgecraft, etc.). Longer knives are more expensive, but cheaper per millimeter of useful cutting edge. Sapphire knives are even cheaper, but are not as scratch resistant as diamond. Diamond knives can usually be resharpened for 30 to 70% of the price of a new knife.

One must take care not to scratch the diamond's cutting edge and to keep the edge free of dried plastic sections before storage. With proper care, a diamond can last years before resharpening is required. Knives can be cleaned immediately after use with a clean styrofoam rod soaked in ethanol, pushing section debris away with lateral motions along the knife edge. The extreme lateral edges of the knife are generally used for cutting thicker sections and for cutting test sections. High-quality thin sections can be collected from the central portion. Over months of use, one can map out any serious scratches as they develop and avoid them when cutting thin-section series.

C. Antistatic Devices

Static charges can cause major difficulties in section collection for both plastic sections and frozen sections. Several devices are available to defuse static. The Staticmaster (NRD Inc., Grand Island, NY) consists of a cartridge holding a radioactive strip of polonium which can be positioned close to the knife edge; a metal stand with a flexible arm is available from NRD to position the cartridge. The cartridge loses effectiveness after 6 months. The Zerostat (EMS) antistatic gun also seems to be effective. The Static-Line Ionizer II (Diatome) is a variable-voltage device that is supposed to be helpful in cryo-thin sectioning.

D. Evaporators

The Denton DV-502A evaporator (Denton Vacuum, Cherry Hill, NJ) is used for the production of carbon films over newly cast Formvar grids. Instructions for use are available from the manufacturer. Unless the machine is equipped with a quartz-crystal monitor, there is no simple way in which to judge the thickness of the film produced. A liquid nitrogen cold trap is useful in quickly achieving a high vacuum.

Evaporators are also available through Ladd, EMS, and Bio-Rad.

E. Trimming Devices and Blades

Most microtome vendors offer special trimming block holders that fit onto the microtome platform or as free-standing pedestals that can be positioned under a dissecting microscope. These hold the block in a standard microtome chuck at a useful angle for trimming by hand under good illumination. The Reichert TM60 and the LKB Pyramitome are more elaborate solutions to the task; each can hold and illuminate the block, hold the trimming knife securely, and perform the individual cuts at precise angles.

Double-edged stainless-steel blades are the best tool for trimming the block. There are many vendors of similar products, but there is a remarkable variety in quality. We recommend the Wilkinson Sword Blade for its extreme sharpness and durability. Carefully break the Wilkinson blade into halves to yield two single-edged blades. Other brands may require a precleaning in 100% alcohol to remove an oily coating prior to use.

═══════ VIII. Materials

A. Making Formvar-Coated Grids

Formvar-coated grids are easily prepared in the laboratory, but special equipment is necessary to shadow them with carbon. Bare Formvar is not very strong, although sufficient to coat mesh grids for some purposes. In this state, Formvar-coated grids should be used within a few days or discarded. Formvar can be stabilized with a thin layer of carbon to become much more resilient. We have been able to reexamine carbon-coated grids in the electron microscope even 15 years after collecting the thin sections. The carbon should be added within 2 days of preparing the Formvar, so that the Formvar does not sag or break. Once coated, such grids can be used to collect sections up to a year later. Other possible support films include Collodion and Parlodian.

Some vendors sell precoated Formvar grids, but we have not been very satisfied with the quality of the samples we have examined. Formvar can be purchased as a powder or in solution in ethylene dichloride. We buy a prepared 1% solution and hold it tightly stoppered until use. The solution should be poured into a clean wide-mouth bottle or Coplin jar for use.

Glass microscope slides are rinsed in toluene, cleaned with a Kimwipe until very clean and dry, then dipped into the Formvar solution. As the slide is withdrawn, use a clean No. 3 forceps to hold the slide just above the surface for 45 seconds so that the solvent vapors bathe the slide; this gives a thinner film because excess solution drains back into the bottle before drying. After drying for a minute, use a razor blade to score the top and bottom edges of the Formvar film on each side of the slide. Breathe gently on the slide to fog the slide, which loosens the Formvar film, then vertically dip the slide slowly into a large crystallizing dish full of distilled water. A Formvar film should float off each side of the slide onto the surface of the water. Using a No. 5 forceps, place grids onto the floating Formvar film, dull side down, avoiding any portion of the film that shows wrinkles, holes, or bright colors. Clean another glass slide with ethanol, and let the slide dry. Carefully lower the slide onto the floating film from above, then lift away from the water. Allow the slide to dry thoroughly in a petri dish and keep covered until ready to carbon coat.

Specialized equipment is needed to do the carbon coating; we use a Denton evaporator. Place the glass slides with Formvar and grids into the chamber and follow manufacturer's instructions to produce a very light coating of carbon on top of the Formvar film. This step is difficult to calibrate exactly, as methods for seeing a visible carbon coating on a white ceramic marker, for instance, produce too much carbon (a visible carbon film is already too thick). We evaporate from a carbon point in ten short bursts (2–4 seconds each), or in one 20-second burst, at a 22-A reading on the Denton current gauge. With this amount of carbon shadow, the Formvar film becomes slightly brittle when poked with a forceps. Store grids in a covered dish until ready to use. To pick up an individual grid from the slide, it is best to scratch with the forceps around the circumference of the grid, so that the film does not tear off the grid.

Pitfalls. Formvar solutions can become contaminated (probably by water) to make holey films that are unsuitable for EM. Discard old solutions and keep new solutions tightly capped. Too much carbon will make the grids less electron opaque and reduce the final contrast of electron microscope images. Be very careful not to poke a hole in the Formvar once the grids are coated; a single hole or tear is likely to propagate across the entire slot and doom the grid.

B. Stock Solutions for Conventional Electron Microscopy

1. Aldehydes

"EM-grade" glutaraldehyde should be purchased in sealed ampules as a 25% solution. Paraformaldehyde is also available in sealed ampules as a 20% solution. Ampules should be stored at 4°C until use. Use only until expiration date. Making up formaldehyde solutions from paraformaldehyde powder is possible, but more difficult. *Avoid* any aldehyde stock that contains methanol as a stabilizer.

Buffered aldehyde working solutions should be made up fresh on the day of use. A good working solution is 2.5% glutaraldehyde, 1% formaldehyde in 0.05 M sodium cacodylate, 0.2 M sucrose, 1 mM MgCl, pH 7.2. Buffer rinses should use 0.2 M cacodylate to maintain equivalent osmolarity.

2. OsO$_4$

A 2 or 4% solution in distilled water can be stored at 4°C for months. The solution is good as long as it retains faint yellow color. This is extremely toxic;

store and handle carefully. Buffered osmium working solutions should be made up just before use. Waste osmium solutions can be neutralized by adding sodium borate. A good working solution is 1% OsO₄ in 0.1 M cacodylate buffer, pH 7.2.

3. Ethanolic Uranyl Acetate

Saturated solution (20% in 100% ethanol) can be stored in a brown bottle at 4°C for up to a year. Stain should be filtered before use (0.2-μm filter; PTFE filter only, other filters do not withstand the alcohol well). Use at room temperature. Stain can be recycled into stock bottle and reused.

4. Modified Reynolds Lead Citrate

Make up according to standard method (Reynolds, 1963), but dilute the stain by 1000-fold in 0.01 M NaOH and store in a sealed brown bottle at 4°C. Stain is OK to use for 3 to 6 months. Stain from each use can be recycled into stock bottle and reused. Filter this solution just before use (0.2-μm filter) and centrifuge to remove precipitates. Use at room temperature.

5. Aqueous Uranyl Acetate

A solution of 2% UAc in distilled water can be stored in a brown bottle at 4°C for months. Filter before use (0.2-μm filter). Add one drop of stain to one drop of absolute ethanol and allow to stand on clean surface in closed chamber. Place inverted grid onto stain solution for 1 minute, then remove with forceps and rinse briefly in distilled water. Staining drop can be reused over the period of an hour.

6. Buffered Uranyl Acetate

For en bloc staining, prepare a 1.0% UAc solution in 0.1 M sodium acetate, pH 5.2. This solution can be stored in a brown bottle in the cold for up to 6 months. Filter before use. Be certain to prerinse the tissue in sodium acetate buffer before beginning the staining procedure. Staining can be done at room temperature for 1 hour; then do more buffer rinses.

C. Embedding Resins

1. Epon Substitutes

Epon 812 plastic resin and Epon–Araldite mixtures were the favorite choices for EM until Epon was banned from production because of its carcinogenicity. During the past 25 years, a variety of products have been introduced by different suppliers that nearly match Epon's hardness, cutting properties, moderate shrinkage, and electron opacity. Some of these substitutes may appear slightly grainy under the electron beam. Modern products include Medcast (Ted Pella), Poly/Bed 812 (Polysciences), and EMbed-812 (Electron Microscopy Sciences). Several Araldite formulations are still widely available. Exact formulations to mix these resins with extenders, crosslinkers, and accelerators are available from each vendor to produce resin mixtures of the appropriate hardness. A typical mixture using Medcast is

45 ml Medcast + 30 ml DDSA + 25 ml NMA

where DDSA is dodecenyl succinic anhydride, NMA is nadic methyl anhydride, and DMP-30 is 2,4,6-tri[dimethylaminomethyl] phenol.

Measure these components by volume (or by weight) into a predried disposable beaker and stir slowly using a dry wooden applicator or a stirring bar. Then add 1 ml DMP-30 accelerator and stir again for 3 minutes, minimizing the introduction of air vapor into the resin mixture. To keep the resin mixture dry, degas the solution under a vacuum and store in a desiccator until use. It is also feasible to freeze aliquots of the prepared mixture for days in sealed disposable syringes until use. At room temperature, the mixture will become very viscous over a 36-hour period. Resin components are allergenic to some people and possibly toxic; we recommend use of gloves and a fume hood to minimize exposure when mixing or using the resin.

2. LR Gold

The use of methacrylate resins predated the use of Epon for electron microscopy, but they suffer from greater shrinkage and are sometimes difficult to cure evenly. Modern resins LR Gold and LR White (London Resin Company, available through several vendors in the United States) have gained new acceptance particularly for postembedding immuno-EM protocols. They produce a more hydrophilic thin section which probably provides greater access to antigens than an Epon section. In our experience, LR White is not suitable for use with *C. elegans* because of a severe shrinkage problem, but LR Gold appears to work well and produces a block of suitable hardness for good thin sections.

LR Gold is provided with two different accelerators, one for curing with UV (benzoin methyl ether) and another for curing with blue light (benzil). The resin is shipped under refrigeration to prevent premature hardening, and all infiltration steps must be conducted in the cold. The resin is miscible with alcohol, so the number of dehydration steps is reduced.

Individual specimens are placed into predried gelatin capsules filled with fresh resin, excluding air from the capsule as far as possible (residual air or water vapor can inhibit hardening). Curing LR Gold is highly exothermic and requires special handling to obtain a hard block. An insulated container with a UV lamp mounted in the lid is available from Ted Pella for this purpose. Specimens are loaded in gelatin capsules and placed into the device with a load of dry ice to chill them to about $-35°C$ during curing overnight. A more elaborate set of devices (CS-Auto and CS-UV) available from Reichert hold individual capsules in a chilled metal block to conduct heat away from the samples during UV irradiation.

3. Lowicryl

Two low-temperature embedding resins, Lowicryl K4M and Lowicryl K11M (Polysciences or EMS), are useful for immuno-EM protocols. We do not have personal experience with these for *C. elegans,* but they may prove suitable. Curing again involves irradiation by UV in the cold, and a controlled temperature device is recommended as discussed above.

Acknowledgments

Richard Russell first kindled my interest in *C. elegans,* as he did for many others. Randle Ware taught me the fine points of thin sectioning and reconstruction. I also thank Sarah Wurzelmann, Christine Roy, Erika Hartweig, and Ed Hedgecock for their advice, and Laura Hall for help in preparing the figures.

References

Allen, B. A., and Levinthal, C. (1990). CARTOS II semi-automated nerve tracing: Three dimensional reconstruction from serial section micrographs. *Comput. Med. Imaging Graph.* **14,** 319–329.

Branton, D. (1971). Freeze-etching studies of membrane structure. *Philos. Trans. R. Soc. Lond.* **261,** 133–138.

Burghardt, R. C. (1980). Intercellular junctions and exocytosis in the vas deferens of *Ascaris. J. Ultrastr. Res.* **71,** 162–172.

Burghardt, R. C., and Foor, W. E. (1978). Membrane fusion during spermiogenesis in *Ascaris. J. Ultrastr. Res.* **62,** 190–202.

Capowski, J. J. (1989). "Computer Techniques in Neuroanatomy". Plenum Press, New York.

Cox, G. N., Staprans, S., and Edgar, R. S. (1981). The cuticle of *Caenorhabditis elegans.* II. Stage-specific changes in ultrastructure and protein composition during postembryonic development. *Dev. Biol.* **86,** 456–470.

Davidson, L. A. (1983). A freeze fracture and thin section study of intestinal cell membranes and intracellular junctions of a nematode, *Ascaris. Tissue Cell* **15,** 27–37.

Fahrenbach, W. H. (1984). Continuous serial thin sectioning for electron microscopy. *J. Electron Microsc. Tech.* **1,** 387–398.

Goldschmidt, R. (1909). Das nervensystem von *Ascaris lumbricoides* und *megalocephala. Zeitschr. Wiss. Zool.* **92,** 306–357.

Hall, D. H. (1977). The posterior nervous system of the nematode *Caenorhabditis elegans.* Ph.D. Thesis. California Institute of Technology, Pasadena.

Hall, D. H. (1987). Freeze fracture and freeze etch studies of the nematode, *Caenorhabditis elegans. N.Y. Acad. Sci.* **494,** 215–217.

Hall, D. H., and Russell, R. L. (1991). The posterior nervous system of the nematode *Caenorhabditis elegans:* Serial reconstruction of identified neurons and complete pattern of synaptic interactions. *J. Neurosci.* **11,** 1–22.

Harris, K. M., and Stevens, J. K. (1988). Dendritic spines of rat cerebellar Purkinje cells: Serial electron microscopy with reference to their biophysical characteristics. *J. Neurosci.* **8,** 4455–4469.

Hedgecock, E. M., Culotti, J. G., and Hall, D. H. (1990). The *unc-5, unc-6,* and *unc-40* genes guide circumferential migrations of pioneer axons and mesodermal cells on the epidermis in C. elegans. *Neuron* **4,** 61–85.

Hubbard, L. S., Grothe, R. A. Jr., Arnicar-Sulze, T. L., Dovey-Hartman, B. J., and Page, R. B. (1993). Computerized three-dimensional reconstruction of median-eminence capillary modules: Image alignment and correlation. *J. Microsc.* **171,** 39–56.

Huijsmans, D. P., Lamers, W. H., Los, J. A., and Strackee, J. (1986). Towards computerized morphometric facilities: A review of 58 software packages for computer-aided three-dimensional reconstruction, quantification, and picture generation from parallel serial sections. *Anat. Rec.* **216,** 449–470.

Johnson, E. M., and Capowski, J. J. (1983). A system for the three-dimensional reconstruction of biological structures. *Comput. Biomed. Res.* **16,** 79–87.

Lee, D. L., Wright, K. A., and Shivers, R. R. (1984). A freeze-fracture study of the surface of the infective-stage larva of the nematode *Trichinella. Tissue Cell* **16,** 819–828.

Lee, D. L., Wright, K. A., and Shivers, R. R. (1986). A freeze-fracture study of the body wall of adult, *in utero* larvae and infective-stage larvae of *Trichinella* (Nematoda). *Tissue Cell* **18,** 219–230.

Lindsay, R. D. (1977). "Computer Analysis of Neuronal Structures" Plenum Press, New York.

Macagno, E. R., Levinthal, C., and Sobel, I. (1979). Three-dimensional computer reconstruction of neurons and neuronal assemblies. *Annu. Rev. Biophys. Bioeng.* **8,** 323–351.

Mar, H., and Wight, T. N. (1988). Colloidal gold immunostaining on deplasticized ultra-thin sections. *J. Histochem. Cytochem.* **36,** 1387–1395.

Marko, M., Leith, A., and Parsons, D. (1988). Three-dimensional reconstruction of cells from serial thin sections and whole-cell mounts using multilevel contouring of stereo micrographs. *J. Electron Microsc. Tech.* **9,** 395–411.

Martinez-Paloma, A. (1978). Ultrastructural characterization of the cuticle of *Onchocerca volvulus* microfilaria. *J. Parasitol.* **64,** 127–136.

Meyer, E. P., and Domanico, V. J. (1993). A device for picking up serial thin sections. *J. Microsc.* **172,** 153–156.

Okamoto, H., and Thomson, J. N. (1985). Monoclonal antibodies which distinguish certain classes of neuronal and support cells in the nervous tissue of the nematode *Caenorhabditis elegans. J. Neurosci.* **5,** 643–653.

Peixoto, C. A., and De Souza, W. (1994). Freeze-fracture characterization of the cuticle of adult and dauer forms of *Caenorhabditis elegans. Parasitol. Res.* **80,** 53–57.

Rash, J. E., and Hudson, C. S. (1979). "Freeze Fracture: Methods, Artifacts and Interpretations". Raven Press, New York.

Reynolds, E. S. (1963). The use of lead citrate at high pH as an electron-opaque stain in electron microscopy. *J. Cell Biol.* **7,** 208.

Rieder, C. L. (1981). Thick and thin serial sectioning for the three-dimensional reconstruction of biological ultrastructure. *In* "Methods in Cell Biology" (J. N. Turner, ed.), vol. 22. pp. 215–250. Academic Press, New York.

Russ, J. C. (1990). "Computer-Assisted Microscopy: The Measurement and Analysis of Images" Plenum Press, New York.

Selkirk, M. E., Yazdanbaksh, M., Freedman, D., Blaxter, M. L., Cookson, E., Jenkins, R. E., and Williams, S. A. (1991). A proline-rich structural protein of the surface sheath of larval *Brugia* filarial nematode parasites. *J. Biol. Chem.* **266,** 11002–11008.

Stevens, J. K., Davis, T. L., Friedman, N., and Sterling, P. (1980). A systematic approach to reconstructing microcircuitry by electron microscopy of serial sections. *Brain Res. Rev.* **2,** 265–293.

Stevens, J. K., and Trogadis, J. (1984). Computer-assisted reconstruction from serial electron micrographs: A tool for the systematic study of neuronal form and function. *Adv. Cell. Neurobiol.* **5,** 341–369.

Stirling, J. W. (1990). Immuno- and affinity probes for electron microscopy: A review of labeling and preparation techniques. *J. Histochem. Cytochem.* **38,** 145–157.

Tokuyasu, K. T. (1986). Application of cryoultramicrotomy to immunocytochemistry. *J. Microsc.* **143,** 139–149.

Tokuyasu, K. T. (1989). Use of poly(vinylpyrrolidone) and poly(vinyl alcohol) for cryoultramicrotomy. *Histochem. J.* **21,** 163–171.

Turner, J. N. (1981). Three Dimensional Ultrastructure in Biology. *In* "Methods in Cell Biology" (J. N. Turner, ed.), Vol. 22. Academic Press, New York.

Ward, S., Thomson, J. N., White, J. G., and Brenner, S. (1975). Electron microscopical reconstruction of the anterior sensory anatomy of the nematode *Caenorhabditis elegans. J. Comp. Neurol.* **160,** 313–337.

Ware, R. W., Clark, D., Crossland, K., and Russell, R. L. (1975). The nerve ring of the nematode *Caenorhabditis elegans:* Sensory input and motor output. *J. Comp. Neurol.* **162,** 71–110.

Ware, R. W., and LoPresti, V. (1972). Three-dimensional reconstruction from serial sections. *Int. Rev. Cytol.* **40,** 325–440.

White, J. G. (1974). Computer aided reconstruction of the nervous system of *C. elegans.* Ph.D. Thesis. University of Cambridge.

White, J. G., Southgate, E., Thomson, J. N., and Brenner, S. (1976). The structure of the ventral nerve cord of *Caenorhabditis elegans. Phil. Trans. R. Soc. Lond. [Biol.]* **275,** 327–348.

White, J. G., Southgate, E., Thomson, J. N. and Brenner, S. (1986). The structure of the nervous system of *Caenorhabditis elegans. Philos. Trans. R. Soc. Lond. [Biol.]* **314,** 1–340.

Wood, W. B. (1987). "The Nematode *Caenorhabditis elegans*" Cold Spring Harbor Laboratory, Cold Spring Harbor, New York.

Wood, W. B., and Kershaw, D. (1991). Handed symmetry, handedness reversal and mechanisms of cell fate determination in nematode embryos. *Ciba Found. Symp.* **162,** 143–164.

Wright, K. A., Lee, D. L., and Shivers, R. R. (1985). A freeze-fracture study of the digestive tract of the parasitic nematode *Trichinella. Tissue Cell* **17,** 189–198.

Young, S. J., Royer, S. M., Groves, P. M., and Kinnamon, J. C. (1987). Three-dimensional reconstruction from serial micrographs using the IBM PC. *J. Electron Microsc. Tech.* **6,** 207–217.

Zuckerman, B. M., Himmelhoch, S., and Kisiel, M. (1973). Fine structure changes in the cuticle of adult *Caenorhabditis briggsae* with age. *Nematologica* **19,** 109–112.

CHAPTER 18

Proteins and Protein Assemblies

Henry F. Epstein and Feizhou Liu

Departments of Neurology, Biochemistry, and Cell Biology
Baylor College of Medicine
Houston, Texas 77030

I. Introduction: Approaches to Subcellular Fractionation and Biochemical Purification

The ultimate goal of subcellular fractionation and biochemical purification is to better understand the relationships between structure and function of proteins and protein assemblies. Examples of such relationships with respect to specific gene products include the formation of stable complexes, elucidation of catalytic activities, and subcellular localization at the organellar and supramolecular levels. The detailed aspects of such relationships are not always readily predictable from genetic or molecular studies of the gene products or from their cellular localization by immunological methods. Subcellular fractionation and biochemical purification are generally prerequisites to experimental analysis of biochemical mechanisms underlying a biological phenomenon. These approaches can mutually enhance and interact with parallel cellular, genetic, and molecular analyses.

To achieve such goals, methods for isolating proteins and protein assemblies must preserve both structural integrity and biological activity. Ideally, both objectives should be met; practically, it may be critical to know which of these conditions is true. In general, specific protocols must be designed for the optimal isolation, purification, and characterization of each specific protein of interest. Additionally, one wishes to achieve as high a yield as possible; however, each step in protein purification generally produces some reduction in yield.

A variety of proteins and protein assemblies have been isolated and purified from *Caenorhabditis elegans.* Enzymes such as isocitrate lyase, RNA polymerase, and cathepsin D (Rothstein and Mayoh, 1964; Sanford *et al.,* 1983; Sarkis *et al.,* 1988) have been isolated and purified as catalytically active species. Proteins involved in cell motility and the cytoskeleton such as actin, tubulin, myosin, troponin, and tropomyosin (Harris and Epstein, 1977; Harris *et al.,* 1977; Aamodt and Culotti, 1986) have been purified and shown to exhibit biologically specific interactions. Transcriptionally active nuclei, respiring mitochondria, and ATP-sensitive thick and thin myofilaments (Honda and Epstein, 1990; Patel and Mc-Fadden, 1977; Harris *et al.,* 1977) have been isolated at various levels of purity.

II. Inhibition of Proteolysis and Proteases

Many investigators believe that the addition of particular inhibitors of specific proteases is sufficient to prevent proteolysis. Experienced biochemists have learned that proper handling of biological material from the living state all the way through to the final purification steps is critically important. Special care must be taken to preserve the structural integrity of tissues, cells, and organelles as long as possible and to regulate the actual temperature of samples appropriately. Some of these views have been variously heeded and ignored in various applications in the nematode field.

Broken cell preparations and especially frozen and thawed materials are highly prone to proteolysis regardless of the inhibitors present. Freezing for biochemical purposes should be as rapid as possible, ideally using liquid nitrogen. The addition of cryoprotectants or antifreeze compounds when larger volumes of nematode slurries are frozen (greater than milliliters) can prevent disruption and permits fractionation following cryosectioning. Alternatively, smaller volumes of nematodes can be frozen as pellets which are suitable for analysis of total protein.

Temperature is a much abused concept. For example, most cold rooms are at least 8°C; most ordinary freezers are rarely lower than -12°C. Neither may provide appropriate temperatures for particular applications. Self-defrosting freezers may thaw samples. A sample on ice is never colder than 4°C. A liquid sample must equilibrate for some time with an ice–water mixture to be at 0°C. The two temperatures are not equivalent because the physical properties of water change significantly in this region. Liquid nitrogen is significantly colder ($-196°C$) and more reliable than ultracold freezers (usually no colder than $-75°C$), which are subject to electrical or mechanical failures.

The issue of what proteolytic inhibitors to use should be pursued in conjunction with optimization of fractionation and temperature. Selection of the appropriate inhibitor or set of inhibitors for isolation of a particular protein or protein assembly is best performed empirically. Qualitative and quantitative criteria for how much proteolysis of a specific protein is acceptable should be kept in mind as one proceeds. For example, the sensitivity of detection of proteolytic breakdown products of myosin heavy chain increases from Coomassie blue staining to silver staining to enzyme-linked immunostaining of blot transfers of sodium dodecyl sulfate–polyacrylamide gel electrophoresis (SDS–PAGE) separations (see relevant chapters in Deutscher, 1990). Both the levels and the detectability of breakdown products may increase with additional purification. It is very unlikely that all proteolysis (greater than 99%) of large muscle proteins such as myosin heavy chain, paramyosin, and twitchin can be eliminated except in total homogenates involving minimal manipulation and storage of fresh worms.

A. Protocols for Homogenates

The most important generality to be made about protocols regarding the isolation, purification, or characterization of proteins or protein assemblies is that each process and step may have to be extensively modified for any specific application. This caveat applies even to SDS–PAGE and immunoblotting. For example, intrinsic membrane proteins may aggregate under the standard boiling or high-temperature protocols for SDS–PAGE (Fung and Hubbell, 1978), whereas only in specific cases has boiling been shown to be required for disaggregation (Jorgensen and Jones, 1986). We recommend that even SDS–PAGE be optimized for each type of protein sample. Conversely, some protein mixtures can be proteolyzed by the same procedure (Kim *et al.*, 1985). *No protocol can be optimal for all or even the vast majority of cases.* For these reasons, relevant sections of several protocols are provided only as examples of the modification/ optimization approach, but no general protocols are provided. Various techniques for homogenization are compared in Table I. Figure 1 shows the difference in proteolysis of the glyoxylate cycle protein (Liu *et al.*, 1995) between homogenization by freezing and thawing and homogenization by sectioning with a cryostat.

1. Minimal Proteolysis of Myosin Heavy Chain in Homogenates

See Miller *et al.* (1983). Fresh worms are washed off an NGM plate with M9 buffer (Sulston and Brenner, 1974), permitted to settle, and collected. The worms are immediately resuspended in complete gel buffer and boiled for 3 to 5 minutes. After minimal cooling (the solution is still warm), the sample is loaded and run on already prepared SDS–PAGE. Any storage or waiting leads to proteolysis

Table I
Comparison of Homogenization Techniques

Method	Positives	Negatives
Boiling and sodium dodecyl sulfate–polyacrylamide gel electrophoresis	Proteolysis minimized; quick; cheap	Useful only for evaluating homogenates; must be done fresh
Freeze and thaw	Solubilizes many proteins efficiently	Major proteolysis due to lysis of membranes, mixing, and inherent temperature problem
Sonication	Quick; cold temperature may be maintained	Useful only for small samples; care must be taken about heating; mixing of compartments
French press	Useful for large volumes; cold temperature maintained; degree of breakage can be controlled	Mixing of compartments; initial investment of about $6900
Cryostat and Dounce	Minimal disruption of compartments and structures; limited proteolysis and mixing; cold temperature maintained	Labor intensive; primarily for small volumes; initial investment of $13,000 (new automated version)

detectable by immunoblotting with monoclonal antibody specific to myosin heavy chain B! No protease inhibitors are added. Attention to the details of handling is what prevents proteolysis.

2. High Yield of Myosin Heavy Chain in Homogenates

See Zengel and Epstein (1980). Fresh worms are harvested, freed of bacteria, and resuspended in 62.3 mM Tris–HCl, pH 6.8, at 4°C. The worms are disrupted by sonication with four 11-second pulses at output 5 on a Branson sonifier with 3 to 4 seconds between pulses. During sonication, the suspensions are in Brinkmann microfuge tubes surrounded by ice. After sonication, equal volumes of the gel sample buffer are added, and the mixtures are heated in a heating block at 90°C for 5 minutes. The samples are then run immediately on SDS–PAGE. Note that 90°C is different from boiling and leads to different results.

B. Antiprotease Recipes for Isolation of Different Proteins and Assemblies

Remember that these recipes are examples. For your application, specific inhibitors may have to be added or deleted, or their concentrations increased or decreased. Only the details of each protocol relevant to the problem of inhibiting proteolysis are presented. The complete protocols are published.

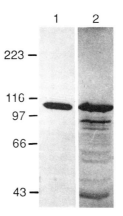

Fig. 1 Effects of homogenization technique on proteolysis. (1) Sample was homogenized by the cryostat and Dounce method, then immunoprecipitated, run on sodium dodecyl sulfate–polyacrylamide gel electrophoresis (SDS–PAGE), and immunoblotted. (2) Sample was frozen in liquid N_2, then thawed and homogenized with the French press, run on SDS–PAGE, and immunoblotted. Both immunoprecipitation and immunoblotting were performed with monoclonal antibody F-11, which is specific to the *C. elegans* glyoxylate cycle protein (Liu *et al.*, 1995). Both samples were prepared with the same mixture of antiprotease agents according to Epstein *et al.* (1988).

1. Purified Contractile Proteins with Significant Proteolysis of Paramyosin

Harris and Epstein (1977). One millimolar phenylmethylsulfonyl fluoride (PMSF) and 1.0 mM ethylenediamine tetraacetic acid (EDTA) are used in all aqueous solutions of this purification. PMSF is insoluble in water and hydrolyzed in alkaline solutions. Our stock PMSF solutions are 100 mM in dimethyl sulfoxide. They are then diluted in final buffers. The concentration of PMSF may be critical; however, the compound is not soluble in aqueous buffers at much above 2 mM. Other serine protease inhibitors may have to be used to alleviate proteolysis. On disruption of thick filament structure, essentially all paramyosin is proteolytically cleaved, resulting in a selective loss of about 5 to 10 kDa as detected by SDS–PAGE. Myosin prepared by this method has between 1 and 5% proteolytic breakdown products, which are very noticeable by immunoblotting (Miller *et al.*, 1983). Thus, PMSF and EDTA (at 4°C), although necessary inhibitors for many isolations, are not sufficient to prevent significant proteolysis of key muscle proteins.

2. Purified Tubulin and Associated Proteins, Highest Yields

Aamodt and Culotti (1986) performed a detailed study of the requirements for specific protease inhibitor compounds; however, they also froze slowly, stored, and thawed their worms and then disrupted by sonication before embarking on a significant purification. It is perhaps likely that lower concentrations of the inhibitors would work if different approaches to the handling of the worms are tried. Homogenization is performed in the presence of 80 μg/ml leupeptin, 80 μg/ml pepstatin, and 1.0 mg/ml p-toluidinyl sulfonyl-1-arginine methyl ester (TAME) at 4°C. For other details of the purification, see protocols for purification of cytoskeleton in Section III,C.

3. Purified Muscle Thick Filaments (Thin filaments, ribosomes), Minimal Proteolysis of Paramyosin

See Epstein *et al.* (1988). The introduction of specific protease inhibitor compounds prevents paramyosin proteolysis on its dissociation from thick filaments. PMSF (1 mM) and 1 μg/ml each of soybean trypsin inhibitor, leupeptin, chymostatin, pepstatin, N-benzoyl-L-arginine ethyl ester (BAEE), and TAME (Sigma) are added to all buffers of the procedure. For other details see purification of cytoskeleton in Section III,C.

4. Purified Paramyosin, Minimal Proteolysis

See Schrieffer and Waterston (1989). Paramyosin is prepared in bulk from disrupted nematodes without loss of its N or C terminals as determined by CNBr-cleaved peptides and amino acid analysis and sequencing. For *in vitro* phosphorylation studies, sucrose-cleaned worms (Sulston and Brenner, 1974) are broken in a French press as described below in 10 vol of 40 mM NaCl, 6.7 mM potassium phosphate, pH 6.0, 1 mM ethylene glycol bis(β-aminoethyl ether)-N,N'-tetraacetic acid (EGTA), 2 mM dithiothreitol (DTT), 1 mM PMSF, 80 μg/ml pepstatin, 80 μg/ml leupeptin, and 1.0 mg/ml TAME. The broken worms are spun at 10,000g for 10 minutes at 4°C. The resulting pellet is resuspended in a solution suitable for protein kinase assays (see Schrieffer and Waterston, 1989, for these details) and, after incubation, repelleted. The pellet is solubilized directly in 6.0 M guanidine, 0.01 M Tris–HCl, pH 7.5, 2 mM EDTA, 1 mM DTT, and the above combination of protease inhibitors. For determination of endogenous protein phosphate, the worms are directly broken in 6.0 M guanidine, 0.01 M Tris–HCl, pH 7.5, 1 mM DTT, 2 mM EDTA, and the inhibitors as above.

III. Fractionation and Isolation of Cell Constituents

Three major sources of constituents are considered: organelles, cytosol, and the cytoskeleton. For such constituent structures, two methods of homogenization have proved most useful: the French press and the combination of cryostat sectioning and the handheld Dounce glass homogenizer. Both of these methods can be used while maintaining the temperature of the sample between 0 and 4°C.

In general, the French press technique will at least partially disrupt organelles and the cytoskeleton. It is most useful for the purification of individual proteins and oligomeric protein complexes in high yields from any of the locations, particularly the cytosol. Because it necessarily involves mixing otherwise cell type-specific compartmentalized molecules, such as extensive disruption technique increases the possibility of proteolysis and loss of activity. Nevertheless, this technique has proved useful for the isolation of many kinds of proteins, including RNA polymerase II, tubulin, and the muscle contractile and regulatory proteins (Sanford *et al.*, 1983; Aamodt and Culotti, 1986; Harris and Epstin, 1977; Harris *et al.*, 1977). It has also been suitable for the isolation of DNA for hybridization analysis (Sulston and Brenner, 1974). Note that a considerable range of pressures may be developed in the French press. There is no optimal pressure at which to break worms. Although more worms and worm fragments are homogenized at higher pressures, there is also more breakage of organelles, cytoskeletal filaments, membranes, and chromatin. Lipids and DNA from the latter structures can contaminate and interfere with many isolations. The probability that proteases, nucleases, and other classes of enzymes will be released from one compartment and catalyze unwanted reactions with components of other compartments is enhanced with increased homogenization.

The cryostat sectioning of worms frozen after treatment with the cryoprotectant OCT compound (Miles, Diagnostic Division, Elkhart, IN) followed by gentle hand homogenization in appropriate buffer solutions with the Dounce glass apparatus maintains the structural integrity of fragile organelles with greater structural integrity and a minimum of either nucleolysis or proteolysis (Fig. 2). This technique has been useful in the isolation of transcriptionally active nuclei and native thick filaments from body wall muscle (Epstein *et al.*, 1988; Honda and Epstein, 1990).

A. Protocol for Use of French Press

The French press and high-pressure cells (invented by Vernon French, late Director of the Carnegie Institution Department of Plant Biology at Stanford) are manufactured by American Instrument, (AMINCO, Travenol Laboratories, Silver Springs, MD). It is important to check all internal gaskets and the Teflon ball within the cell before using. All of these deteriorate with use and time. In our laboratory, the cell is routinely cooled in ice–water for at least one-half hour before use instead of merely refrigerating it or storing it in the cold room. For different amounts of material, a 3.6-ml cell, a 40-ml cell, and a continuous loading device with the 40-ml cell may be used. The release pressure may be continuously varied from hundreds of psi to more than 10,000 psi. About 8000 psi was used in the isolation of contractile proteins from whole nematodes (Harris and Epstein, 1977), whereas 2000 psi was used to homogenize cryostat-sectioned material for the isolation of thick filament fragments (Mackenzie and Epstein, 1980). Care must be taken, especially at higher pressures, to release pressure and liquid slowly, as this is the key to proper homogenization. A second run through the press is usually performed. Plastic tubing of appropriate diameter and composi-

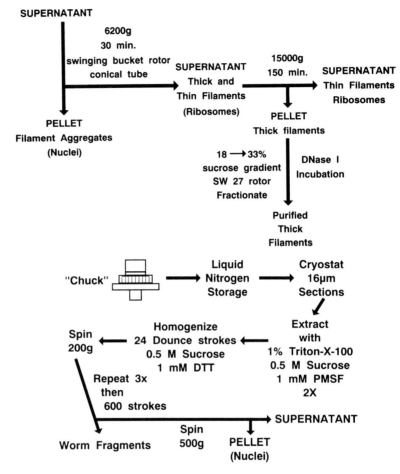

Fig. 2 Scheme of organelle isolation and consequent purification of thick filaments from *C. elegans* according to Deitiker and Epstein (1993).

tion is attached to the exit spigot of the cell so as to avoid splattering and to permit convenient collection in a vessel on ice or in ice–water.

B. Protocol for Freezing and Cryostat Technique

The following protocol outlined in Fig. 2 is currently used in our laboratory and is based on published procedures (Mackenzie and Epstein, 1980; Epstein *et al.*, 1986, 1988). This procedure is designed primarily for the isolation of organelles but is also suitable for the isolation of proteins with minimal proteolysis. For each gram of packed worms, 2.0 ml of OCT is added and mixed well. The mixture is taken up into 50-ml plastic syringes (convenient for marking volumes and handling slurry) and frozen in the vapor over the liquid N_2 using a Biological Freezer accessory (preferred) or at $-75°C$ in the Revco (necessitated for larger volumes) and stored in liquid N_2. Desired quantities are cut off with a jeweler's saw and incubated for 30 minutes at $-20°C$ in a precooled cryostat (International Equipment, Needham Heights, MA). The equilibrated "chunk" is sectioned at the coarsest setting (equivalent to 16-μm sections). The sections are collected in appropriate buffer and kept at the desired temperature for each application. An automated cryostat is more convenient than the manual device for quantities greater than several grams.

C. Protocol for Differential Isolation of Cytosol, Nuclei, and Cytoskeleton

The maintenance of intact nuclei is critical to the isolation of other structures and even smaller, soluble components. Broken or disrupted nuclei imply release of chromatin or DNA, both of which can bind or trap many other molecular and structural components. Because of this problem, many classic isolation procedures involved long overnight incubations at elevated temperatures for autolysis (hopefully nucleolysis, but likely proteolysis as well) or precipitation of nucleic acids by addition of streptomycin. Inclusion of 0.5 M sucrose or osmotically equivalent solutes in homogenization solutions can limit disruption of nuclei. Note that limiting disruption does not mean preventing all of it. All aqueous solutions should be made using glass-distilled water.

For isolation of transcriptionally active nuclei (Honda and Epstein, 1990), cryostat sections are thawed in 0.5 M sucrose, 50 mM Tris–HCl, pH 8.0, 1.0 mM EDTA, 1.0 mM EGTA, 25 mM KCl, 1.5 mM spermidine, 0.15 mM spermine, 1.0 mM 2-mercaptoethanol (isolation buffer) at 0°C. The fragments are washed five times in 20 ml of isolation buffer per gram and collected by sedimentation at 230g for 4 minutes. The resulting pellets are resuspended in 1% Triton X-100 in isolation buffer, and nuclei are released by 20 to 50 strokes in a 7.0-ml Dounce glass homogenizer (Wheaton Instruments, Millville, NJ) incubated at 4°C for 10 minutes and rehomogenized. The second homogenate is filtered through 5-μm Nitex (Tetko, Elmsford, NY) and residual fragments are removed by sedimentation at 100g for 3 minutes. The nuclei-containing supernatant is layered onto 5 ml of 1.8 M sucrose in isolation buffer in a 30-ml Corex tube. The nuclei are pelleted at 8000g for 15 minutes and washed in modified isolation buffer (EDTA and EGTA reduced to 0.1 mM each). The nuclear pellets are resuspended in 50% (v/v) glycerol, 20 mM Tris–HCl, pH 8.9, 75 mM NaCl, 0.5 mM EDTA, 0.85 mM DTT, 0.125 mM PMSF and stored in 20-μl aliquots for up to 3 months.

For isolation of cytoskeletal and contractile structures (Epstein *et al.,* 1988), nematode sections are suspended in 10 ml/g in 100 mM KCl, 10 mM MgCl$_2$, 1 mM Na$_2$EDTA, 6.7 mM potassium phosphate, 1 mM DTT, 5 mM ATP, and the protease inhibitor mixture described above, all at pH 6.34 and 0°C. The sections are washed twice by sedimentation in 50-ml conical centrifuge tubes (Corning Glass Works, Corning, NY) in an IEC clinical centrifuge at set-ting 4 for 4 minutes. The pellet is resuspended in 10 ml of the pH 6.34 buf-fer and 1.0 ml of 10% (v/v) Triton X-100. Triton solubilizes much but not all of the membrane lipids as small micelles which both releases many membrane-associated molecules and prevents association of membrane vesicles with the cytoskeleton. The mixture is incubated at 0°C for 30 minutes with gentle inversion at each 10-minute interval. The sections are repelleted, reincubated, and then collected by sedimentation. The Triton-treated sections are resuspended in the pH 6.34 buffer, 0.5 M sucrose, and 0.5% Triton X-100 and incubated for 10 minutes in an ice–water bath at 0°C. The suspension is homogenized using the glass Dounce homogenizer described above with a type A glass pestle (Wheaton Instruments). The number of strokes can be varied. Material liberated by the first 50 strokes is enriched for nuclei (see above); material liberated after 100 strokes or multiples of 100 strokes become progressively more enriched for cytoskeletal structures (Deitiker and Epstein, 1993). By both biochemical and morphological examination, ribosomes are the major contaminant, and there are still nuclear contaminants.

True cytosolic fractions are most conveniently obtained from bulk nematodes, either fresh or frozen. For the purification of RNA polymerase II (Stanford *et al.,* 1983), 8 g of fresh worms is harvested from liquid culture, washed four times with distilled water, and incubated in water with proper aeration for 1 hour to clear their guts of undigested food. The worms are collected and resuspended in 16 ml of 0.05 M Tris–HCl, pH 7.9, 25% (v/v) glycerol, 0.1 mM EDTA, 6.5 mM DTT, 0.32 M NH$_4$SO$_4$, and 1.5 mM PMSF at 4°C. The worms are disrupted by ten 15-second bursts with a Heat Systems W-375 sonifier at the maximum setting for the microprobe. Ninety to ninety-five percent of worms are disrupted; more disruption leads to loss of RNA polymerase activity. The extract is centrifuged at 160,000g for 1 hour at 2°C, and the supernatant is filtered through Miracloth (CalBiochem) to produce cytosol suitable for further purification of active RNA polymerase II.

Alternatively, the following protocol for isolating cytosol was devised for the purification of tubulin and associated proteins (Aamodt and Culotti, 1986). Thawed worms, previously frozen by storage at −80°C, are mixed with 2 vol of 0.05 M 1,4-piperazine diethanesulfonic acid (Pipes), 1.0 mM EGTA, 1.0 mM MgSO$_4$, 0.5 M mannitol, 80 μg/ml leupeptin, 80 μg/ml pepstatin, 1.0 mg/ml TAME, 2.0 mM DTT, pH 6.6. The mixture is homogenized at 12,000 psi in the French press and centrifuged at 40,000g, and the supernatant is recentrifuged at 140,000g. The final supernatant represents the cytosolic fraction.

IV. Additional Purification Techniques

A multitude of different techniques for purification of proteins exists (see Deutscher, 1990, for an up-to-date compendium). Classic techniques are based on solubility and molecular size, shape, and charge. Newer neoclassic methods involve affinity, hydrophobicity, and polarity. High-performance liquid chromatography and related techniques improve on both classic and neoclassic methods by providing faster separations but not necessarily, as commonly believed, better resolutions of proteins.

The differential solubility of proteins can be exploited using pH, ionic strength, and the binding of salts such as ammonium sulfate. Heat steps were also used in many classic procedures and should be very useful in heat-stable proteins that are already at least partially purified, but this approach is rarely used today because of possible increases in denaturation and proteolysis. The advantages of these approaches are speed and applicability to crude fractions early in a purification scheme. Their proper application can be critical to the overall success of a purification.

Differences in molecular size and shape can be exploited by gel filtration chromatography for single polypeptide and oligomeric proteins. Sedimentation velocity in gradients of density and viscosity (glycerol, sucrose) can separate larger polymeric complexes and smaller organelles in the ultracentrifuge. Larger organelles can be separated by lower centrifugal forces in ordinary buffers on the basis of size or in the presence of concentrated solutes, such as sucrose and Ficoll, on the basis of density.

Most protein separations on the basis of molecular charge have used some version of ion-exchange chromatography. Precipitation of a protein at its isoelectric point is a special application of pH-mediated solubility, which may be the method most exquisitely sensitive to molecular charge. These methods require great care in the equilibration of both samples and column matrices with respect to both pH and ionic strength, the avoidance of overloading, and sensitivity to nonspecific interactions with other proteins, nucleic acids, and complex carbohydrates. Optimization of gradients in pH and/or ionic strength is often necessary to obtain useful separations.

The newer approaches such as affinity, polarity, and other specialized chromatography techniques are most useful in the final steps of a purification scheme, where interference from components present in cruder fractions has been minimized. These approaches are not universally useful. For example, despite the rational definition of affinity purification based on binding by specific antibody or ligand, its actual application may be dominated by empirical considerations. The release of many proteins from either antibody or ligand affinity matrices requires strong conditions such as extreme pH and denaturants instead of competition with free ligands. Some proteins may not regain activity after such treatments.

V. A Model Protein: Myosin

The complete details of this scheme for the purification of myosin and paramyosin are in Harris and Epstein (1977). The related protocols for the purification of actin and tropomyosin are in Harris *et al.* (1977). The following is a discussion and explanation of the approach used.

The critical step in this purification was the separation of myosin and paramyosin under native conditions. This step is very difficult to achieve by standard methods because both myosin and paramyosin are homologous proteins with very similar chemical and physical properties and tightly interact with one another in thick filaments. Its success is dependent on the specific affinity of actin filaments and myosin molecules in the absence of ATP under conditions of high ionic strength and pH (0.6 *M* KCl, pH 8.0). Under these conditions, myosin and paramyosin molecules and actin filaments and tropomyosin molecules dissociate from one another. The myosin–actin filament complexes (equivalent to actomyosin under rigor conditions) are then pelleted by high-speed sedimentation, while molecular paramyosin and tropomyosin remain in the supernatant.

VI. A Model Assembly: The Thick Filament

The complete protocols for the purification of thick filaments are in Epstein *et al.* (1988) and Deitiker and Epstein (1993). The following is a discussion and explanation of the approach used.

The three critical steps in this purification are minimizing the disruption of thick filaments during isolation, preventing irreversible contamination of thick filaments by chromatin fragments and membrane-derived lipids, and separating thick filaments from ribosomes and thin filaments.

It has not been possible to extract thick filaments of uniformly native length from *C. elegans.* The best preparations contain a population with a mean length of about 7.4 μm, instead of the *in situ* length of about 9.7 μm. This comparison may be flawed in that L4 larvae are preferred for thick filament isolation, whereas the most precise determination of *in situ* length was in adult worms (Mackenzie and Epstein, 1980). To obtain these filaments, the worms are sectioned using the freezing and cryostat procedure above, and then the structures are released using the Dounce glass homogenizer and pestle procedure. Procedures using the French press or sonication are not as successful because the thick filaments are more heavily sheared and are complexed with chromatin and membrane fragments.

The prevention of contamination and chromatin and membranes has been discussed above. The chromatin arises from the disruption of nuclei as the result of both mechanical and osmotic factors. Inclusion of 0.5 *M* sucrose minimizes osmotic shock of nuclei, and use of a Dounce homogenizer reduces mechanical breakage. The contamination with membrane vesicles is reduced or prevented by homogenization in the presence of 1% Triton X-100.

Separation of thick filaments from contaminating ribosomes and thin filaments (troponin tropomyosin–actin filaments) is achieved by velocity sedimentation on concentration gradients of either glycerol or sucrose in swinging-bucket rotors in the ultracentrifuge. Fractions markedly enriched in thick filaments and diminished in ribosomes and thin filaments are obtained. Further purification to about 93% homogeneity can be achieved by rebanding the thick filament-enriched fractions. Gradient sedimentation is also useful for the purification of oligomeric enzymes such as RNA polymerase II (Sanford *et al.*, 1985).

References

Aamodt, E. J., and Culotti, J. G. (1986). Microtubules and microtubule-associated proteins from the nematode *Caenorhabditis elegans:* Periodic cross-links connect microtubules in vitro. *J. Cell Biol.* **103**, 23–31.

Deitiker, P. R., and Epstein, H. F. (1993). Thick filament substructures in *Caenorhabditis elegans:* Evidence for two populations of paramyosin. *J. Cell Biol.* **123**, 303–311.

Deutscher, M. P. (ed.) (1990). Guide to protein purification. *In* "Methods in Enzymology" Vol. 182, p. 894. Academic Press, San Diego.

Epstein, H. F., Berliner, G. C., Casey, D. L., and Ortiz, I. (1988). Purified thick filaments from the nematode *Caenorhabditis elegans:* Evidence for multiple proteins associated with core structures. *J. Cell Biol.* **106**, 1985–1995.

Epstein, H. F., Ortiz, I., and Traeger Mackinnon, L. A. (1986). The alteration of myosin isoform compartmentation in specific mutants of *Caenorhabditis elegans. J. Cell Biol.* **103**, 985–993.

Fung, B. K-K., and Hubbell, W. L. (1978). Organization of rhodopsin in photoreceptor membranes. *Biochemistry* **17**, 4396–4402.

Harris, H. E., and Epstein, H. F. (1977). Myosin and paramyosin of *Caenorhabditis elegans:* Biochemical and structural properties of wild-type and mutant proteins. *Cell* **10**, 709–719.

Harris, H. E., Tso, M-Y. W., and Epstein, H. F. (1977). Actin and myosin-linked calcium regulation in the nematode *Caenorhabditis elegans:* Biochemical and structural properties of native filaments and purified proteins. *Biochemistry* **16**, 859–865.

Honda, S., and Epstein, H. F. (1990). Modulation of muscle gene expression in *Caenorhabditis elegans:* Differential levels of transcripts, mRNAs, and polypeptides for thick filament proteins during nematode development. *Proc. Natl. Acad. Sci. U.S.A.* **87**, 876–880.

Jorgenson, A. O., and Jones, L. R. (1986). Localization of phospholamban in slow but not fast canine skeletal muscle fibers: An immunocytochemical study. *J. Biol. Chem.* **261**, 3775–3781.

Khan, F. R., and McFadden, B. A. (1980). Embryogenesis and glyoxylate cycle. *FEBS Lett.* **115**, 312–314.

Kim, K., Rhee, S. G., and Stadtman, E. R. (1985). Nonenzymatic cleavage of proteins by reactive oxygen species generated by dithithreitol and iron. *J. Biol. Chem.* **260**, 15394–15397.

Liu, F., Thatcher, J. D., Barral, J. M., and Epstein, H. F. (1995). Bifunctional glyoxylate cycle protein of *Caenorhabditis elegans:* A developmentally regulated protein of intestine and muscle. *Dev. Biol.,* **169**, 399–414.

Mackenzie, J. M., and Epstein, H. F. (1980). Paramyosin is necessary for determination of nematode thick filament length in vivo. *Cell* **22**, 747–755.

Miller, D. M., Ortiz, I., Berliner, G. C., and Epstein, H. F. (1983). Differential localization of two myosins within nematode thick filaments. *Cell* **34**, 747–757.

Patel, T. R., and McFadden, B. A. (1977). Particulate isocitrate lyase and malate synthase in *Caenorhabditis elegans. Arch. Biochem. Biophys.* **183**, 24–30.

Rothstein, M., and Mayoh, H. (1964). Nematode biochemistry. IV. On isocitrate lyase in *Caenorhabditis briggsae. Arch. Biochem. Biophys.* **108**, 348–353.

Sanford, T., Golomb, M., and Riddle, D. L. (1983). RNA polymerase II from wild-type and α-amanatin-resistant strains of *Caenorhabditis elegans. J. Biol. Chem.* **258**, 12804–12809.

Sanford, T., Prenger, J. P., and Golomb, M. (1985). Purification and immunological analysis of RNA polymerase II from *Caenorhabditis elegans. J. Biol. Chem.* **260**, 8064–8069.

Sarkis, G. J., Kurpiewski, M. R., Ashcom, J. D., Jen-Jacobson, L., and Jacobson, L. A. (1988). Proteases of the nematode *Caenorhabditis elegans*. *Archiv. Biochem. Biophys.* **261,** 80–90.

Schrieffer, L., and Waterston, R. H. (1989). Phosphorylation of the N-terminal region of *Caenorhabditis elegans* paramyosin. *J. Mol. Biol.* **207,** 451–454.

Sulston, J., and Brenner, S. (1974). The DNA of *Caenorhabditis elegans*. *Genetics* **77,** 95–104.

Zengel, J. M., and Epstein, H. F. (1980). Mutants altering coordinate synthesis of specific myosins during nematode muscle development. *Proc. Natl. Acad. Sci. U.S.A.* **77,** 852–856.

CHAPTER 19

DNA Transformation

Craig Mello* and Andrew Fire[†]

* University of Massachusetts Cancer Center
Biotech II
Worcester, Massachusetts 01605
[†] Department of Embryology
Carnegie Institution of Washington
Baltimore, Maryland 21210

I. Introduction

DNA transformation assays in a whole organism provide experimental links between molecular structure and phenotype. Experiments with transgenic *Caenorhabditis elegans* start in general with the injection of DNA into the adult gonad. Effects on phenotype or gene expression patterns can be analyzed either in F1 progeny derived from the injected animals or in derived transgenic lines.

Microinjection of *C. elegans* was first carried out by Kimble *et al.* (1982). Stinchcomb *et al.* (1985) then showed that injected DNA could be maintained for several generations in transgenic lines. The first selective methods for producing and maintaining transgenic lines were reported in 1986 (Fire, 1986). These methods have been considerably improved since then (Mello *et al.*, 1991), so that assays involving DNA transformation are now a standard part of the experimental repertoire for *C. elegans*.

II. Microinjection Techniques for *Caenorhabditis elegans*

A. Background

The *C. elegans* hermaphrodite gonad consists of two arms, each of which is reflexed into a U-shape (Fig. 1). In the adult ovary, thousands of germ-like nuclei surround a common core of cytoplasm. The distalmost nuclei are mitotic, while the more proximal nuclei are arrested in meiosis. Near the bend in the gonad, plasma membranes begin to fully encompass individual oocyte nuclei, incorporating portions of the core cytoplasm as individual oocytes are formed.

Germ-line transformation has been achieved by microinjection of DNA directly into oocyte nuclei (Fire, 1986) or by microinjection of DNA into the cytoplasm of the hermaphrodite syncytial gonad (Stinchcomb *et al.*, 1985; Mello *et al.*, 1991). Three forms of heritable DNA transformation have been observed in *C. elegans:* (1) extrachromosomal transformation, (2) nonhomologous integration, and (3) homologous integration. Spontaneous homologous insertions of injected DNA are extremely rare, but have been observed in at least three cases in two different laboratories (Broverman *et al.*, 1993, Harrison and Fire, unpublished). Extrachromosomal transformants and nonhomologous integrants are considerably more straightforward to obtain, using protocols described below.

B. Equipment

Setting up microinjection in a laboratory already equipped for *C. elegans* genetics and molecular biology requires a modest investment in space and money. A small free-standing heavy office desk (positioned away from air currents and strong vibrations) will generally be sufficient as a working surface for the injection microscope. Minimal costs for essential equipment (injection microscope, manipulator, needle puller, and pressure system) range from $20,000 to $25,000.

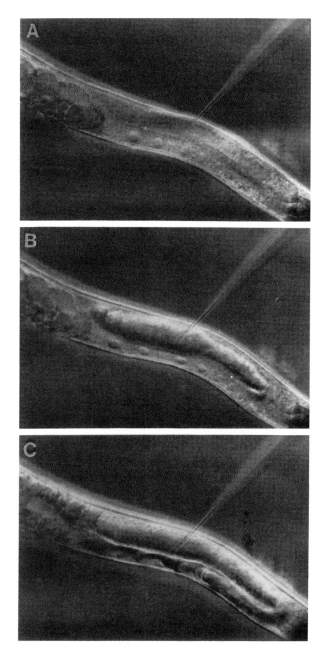

Fig. 1 Injection of DNA into the cytoplasmic syncytium of the *C. elegans* gonad. Top: Needle has been inserted into the gonad at the widest point in the gonad syncytium. Middle: Fluid is expelled from the needle with moderate pressure; the gonad swells up around the point of injection. Bottom: Fluid filling continues in both directions. The needle is removed before the gonad bursts. Reprinted with permission from Mello *et al.* (1991).

1. Microscope

A dissecting microscope with diffused illumination from below is used for preparation and recovery of injected animals. A high-resolution inverted microscope such as the Zeiss Axiovert or equivalent Nikon or Olympus microscope is used for microinjection. The injection microscope should be equipped with a flat, free-sliding glide stage with centered rotation, differential interference contrast (DIC) optics, and objectives of approximately 2.5×, 10×, and 40×. A basic video camera setup with monitor is a useful accessory (cost ~$1500) for demonstrating microinjection.

2. Micromanipulator

The needle is held and brought into position using a micromanipulator mounted on the microscope or on a separate stand. Suitable manipulators are available from several sources including Leitz, Narashige, and Zeiss.

3. Needle Puller

Properly shaped and freely flowing needles are a critical requirement for facile microinjection. A variety of commercially available microelectrode pullers can be used to produce appropriate needles. Because needles can be pulled in large batches and stored (apparently indefinitely), a "multiuser" needle puller can be shared by several laboratories or a department.

4. Mounting and Pressurization of the Needle

The needle is held in an instrument collar that forms a tight seal around the needle. This is connected via plastic tubing to a controllable pressure source. Connectors and valves for pressurizing the needle via a nitrogen tank are described in Mello *et al.* (1991); this system allows pressure to be applied and relieved rapidly using a hand-operated valve. A convenient footpedal-operated system is marketed by Tritech (Los Angeles, CA).

C. Materials

1. Preparation of DNA Samples

A variety of vectors have been used successfully as sources of DNA for microinjection into worms. These include bacterial plasmids, phage, cosmids, and yeast artificial chromosomes (YACs). In each case, a choice of standardized protocols exists for preparing material of sufficient purity for microinjection. DNA samples can be injected into the distal gonad cytoplasm in standard DNA storage buffer [TE: 10 mM Tris–Cl pII 7.5, 1 mM ethylenediaminetetraacetic acid (EDTA)]. An alternative sample buffer (20 mM KPO$_4$, 3 mM K citrate, 2% polyethylene glycol (PEG) 6000, pH 7.5) may be beneficial when samples are to be injected directly into nuclei.

The specific clone (or clones) to be tested for function is injected at concentrations ranging from 1 to 100 μg/ml. In some cases, a second DNA molecule such as a plasmid is added to raise the overall DNA concentration. For high-efficiency transformation with minimal toxicity, we generally strive for a total DNA concentration between 100 and 200 μg/ml. It is often convenient to include a well-defined scoreable or selectable marker in the injection solution. Injected sequences incorporated into heritably transformed lines undergo a high frequency of homologous recombination. Therefore, if the molecule to be tested for function and the coinjected scoreable marker share homology (e.g., if they have similar vector backbones), then transformed lines identified by scoring for the visible marker will amost always contain the homologous coinjected sequence (Mello *et al.*, 1991).

a. Plasmid and Cosmid DNA Preparation

Standard alkaline lysis DNA preparations of bacteria contain contaminants that are toxic when microinjected into worms (even if diluted considerably). Therefore, it is necessary to further purify plasmid and cosmid DNA preps. Purification of DNA over a CsCl gradient, although sufficient, incurs unnecessary work and expense. We have found that standard alkaline-lysis minipreps that have been further cleaned up by PEG or hexadecyltrimethylammonium bromide (CTAB) precipitation (or by LiCl precipitation followed by RNase and protease treatments) yield suitable DNA for injection. [Commercial kits for plasmid preparation (e.g., Qiagen) have been used in many laboratories, although we have found that these preparations contain varying levels of contaminants which interfere with transformation.]

The following yields a suitable DNA preparation for microinjection, subcloning, and sequencing (modified by S. Xu and B. Harfe from standard protocols). All manipulations are in 1.5-ml microfuge tubes.

1. Centrifuge 1.5 ml of bacterial culture (14,000 rpm, 2 minutes) and decant supernatant.
2. Resuspend pellet in 125 μl of GTE (50 mM glucose, 25 mM Tris, pH 8, 10 mM EDTA) (2 μl of 5 mg/ml RNase A can also be added at this stage).
3. Add 200 μl 0.2 M NaOH, 1% sodium dodecyl sulfate (SDS). Mix by gentle inversion. Keep at room temperature (RT) 5 minutes.
4. Add 185 μl of KoAc [3 M K acetate (Ac), 2 M HAc]. Mix gently.
5. Place tubes in ice–water bath for 5 minutes. Centrifuge 10 minutes.
6. To a new tube, add as much supernatant as can be cleanly removed with a transfer pipet.
7. Add 50 μl of 5% CTAB (5% CTAB precipitates at RT, so warm to 37°C (Sigma No. H-6269) before use).

8. Centrifuge 10 minutes; discard supernatant (a pellet may or may not be visible).

9. Add 400 μl of 1 M MH$_4$Ac, 10 mM EDTA, and 1 ml of ethanol. Mix and centrifuge 10 minutes.

10. Wash pellet with 0.5 ml of EtOH; air-dry and resuspend in 50 μl TE, pH 7.4.

11. Approximate DNA concentration is determined by resolving a restriction digest on a gel adjacent to DNA markers of known concentration.

b. Preparation of Phage DNA

PEG precipitation protocols yield phage DNA that requires no further purification prior to microinjection (Maniatis *et al.*, 1982). Note that when phage clones are coinjected with plasmid clones, the resulting transformants will not always contain both types of molecules. Presumably this is because these sequences lack homology and therefore recombine less frequently after injection.

c. Preparation of YAC DNA

YAC sequences must be purified away from the endogenous yeast chromosomes prior to injection. The objective is to obtain sequences enriched for the YAC DNA and to remove contaminants or genomic sequences that suppress transformation. Isolation of YAC DNA is most easily accomplished using pulsed field electrophoresis. Once electrophoresis conditions are identified that resolve the YAC from the yeast chromosomes, one or more preparative gels are run. Commercially available kits such as Gelase (Epicentre Technologies, Madison, WI) can be used to recover the YAC sequences from the gel slice. Typical yields are less than 100 ng. YAC DNA at a concentration of 1 to 10 μg/ml is mixed with a concentrated solution of a marker plasmid to raise the total DNA concentration to 100 to 200 μg/ml (without diluting the YAC sequences). Concentrations of YAC DNA greater than 10 μg/ml are probably optimal (much lower concentrations of YAC DNA, e.g., $< \mu$g/ml, are suboptimal, but may be sufficient to yield a fraction of transformed lines carrying the YAC sequences). Transformants are usually identified by scoring for the coinjected marker gene; transformed lines are then tested for expression of genes on the YAC. Because the YAC sequences are present at low concentration in the injection solution, not all transformed lines will incorporate YAC sequences. Therefore, negative results should be checked by assaying the transformed lines for the presence of the YAC sequences.

2. Microinjection Needles

Microinjection needles are produced from glass capillaries with a fine glass filament adhered to the internal wall (available from several electrophysiology suppliers including World Precision Instruments, Sarasota, FL, and Clark Electromedical Instruments, Reading, England); the filament has the distinct advantage of efficiently filling the tip with any liquid applied along the length of the barrel.

We use standard-thickness borosilicate glass capillaries with an outer diameter of 1.2 mm.

The settings to use for preparing needles are determined in large part by trial and error and, to a lesser extent, by consulting the operating manual for the needle puller. A desirable needle will taper quickly to a sharp open point (see Fig. 1). The novice injector will form an opinion as to the optimal needle shape after limited practice in injecting with needles of different shapes. In particular, the needle should be stiff enough to allow penetration of the animal's cuticle without bending, but narrow enough at the tip so as not to cause the animal to hemorrhage after withdrawal. Once settings have been determined for production of optimal needles, a large number can be pulled and stored (dry) for an indefinite period in a large petri plate. Double-stick tape or clay can be used to prevent the needles from rolling into each other.

Certain microelectrode puller settings produce needles that are closed at the tip; if this is the case, then needle tips must be broken or opened before they will flow. A well-shaped needle will break acceptably upon being inserted into the first worm or upon touching the agar pad.

Microinjection needles are loaded on the day of use and stored in a humidified microinjection chamber (a 150-mm petri plate with wetted Kimwipes in one corner and a clay barrier in the center on which the needles are placed crosswise to immobilize them). To reduce the frequency of clogging, it is best to routinely spin the DNA solution in a microcentrifuge before loading. DNA is put into the needles by placing a small volume of liquid inside of the needle (just before the drawn-out tip) using a loading pipet (the loading pipet is a hand-drawn narrow capillary). To prepare the loading pipet, flame the center of a 100-μl glass capillary until it begins to melt, then remove from the heat while pulling on both ends (this takes practice . . . the object is to obtain a section of 6–8 in. in which the diameter of the capillary is 0.2–0.4 mm). Break the drawn-out portion in the center and save both halves. Place the tip of the loading pipet in contact with the DNA solution and allow capillary action to draw a small quantity into the tip ($\sim$1 μl). Insert the loading pipet down the back of the needle until the front end of the loading pipet reaches the tip of the needle. The DNA solution is expelled from the loading pipet using a mouthpiece connected to the loading pipet by a length of rubber tubing or a small mechanical handheld pipetman.

3. Injection Pads

Worms move in the wild by swimming in a layer of moisture located between their body and the substrate. Injection pads containing a very thin layer of dried agarose (Fire, 1986) immobilize worms by depriving them of this layer of moisture. Injection pads are prepared as follows: One to four drops ($\sim$50 μl) of boiling 2% agarose in water is placed along the center of a 50 $\times$ 22-mm coverslip and a second coverslip is applied to evenly flatten the agarose solution. The agarose drops should spread into one another, almost covering the entire coverslip. After the agarose solidifies, the top coverslip is removed (by gently sliding laterally) and the remaining coverslip-pad is baked in a vacuum oven at 80°C for 1 hour (or overnight). It is very important to thoroughly bake the injection pads or the worms will not stick. Agarose pads can be stored indefinitely in a dry, covered petri dish, and can be rebaked if necessary. The optimal thickness of the injection pads depends somewhat on the animals to be injected: older (larger) animals dehydrate more slowly, and can optimally be injected using somewhat thicker injection pads, whereas smaller (younger) animals can require much thinner injection pads.

4. Additional Materials

Young to middle-aged adult hermaphrodites should be grown under well-fed conditions. Worms are transferred to the injection pad using a flat sharpened platinum "worm pick" mounted in a broken-off Pasteur pipet. Series 700 halocarbon oil (Halocarbon Products, River Edge, NJ) or Heavy Paraffin Oil (BDH Chemicals, Poole, England; Gallard Schlesinger, Carle Place NY) is used; as noted below, the mounting protocol is slightly different for the two oils. Several 0.5-ml aliquots of sterile M9 buffer (see Chapter 1 in this volume) are used for recovery of worms after injection.

D. Injection Protocol

1. Place the loaded needle into the collar of the instrument holder, and mount the assembly on the micromanipulator.

2. Deposit several large drops of oil on an injection pad.

3. Touch a worm pick to the surface of the oil. Working under a dissecting microscope use the oil droplet on the pick to pick up and transfer several animals to the injection pad. Animals should be picked from areas of the plate away from the bacterial lawn (to avoid transferring large amounts of bacteria to the injection pad). A plate with no bacteria can be used as an intermediate transfer plate to obtain animals free of bacteria.

Paraffin oil procedure: Place individual worms directly onto agarose pad in a row. Each worm is placed down by allowing a single part of the worm to contact the pad and then gently withdrawing the pick. The worm will then situate itself on the pad after a few minutes of writhing. Worms should be placed at approximately 1-mm intervals.

Halocarbon oil procedure: After animals are deposited in the oil above the pad, flame the pick to remove residual moisture or bacteria. Use the clean pick to orient a worm with the ventral side facing away from the future direction of injection. Gently push with the pick to move the worm into contact with the pad. If a worm is oriented incorrectly under halocarbon oil, it can usually be removed with the pick and repositioned. Water droplets or bacteria that adhere to the worm may prevent it from remaining immobilized; therefore, it is often necessary to rub the body of the worm with the pick several times until these droplets are removed. This process is repeated, forming a row or column of worms.

4. For most people, mounting worms for injection is the most difficult and time consuming part of the injection procedure. While mounted, the worms will slowly desiccate, which can reduce their viability. Therefore beginners should expect to inject only one or two animals at a time. With practice, one can mount and inject about 20 worms before the worms on the pad become overly desiccated. When injecting large numbers of animals it is convenient to align animals across the short axis of the pad, with individuals separated by about one-half of a worm body length. This spacing facilitates movement from one animal to the next while working at high magnification. Orienting the animals in rows instead of columns conserves space if the pad is to be reused (see below).

5. Transfer the slide to the inverted microscope and bring the animals and the needle into focus while using the 2.5× or 10× objective. While the needle is away from the worms, apply pressure briefly to ensure that the needle is flowing properly. Bring the needle in close proximity to the first animal. Make sure that the worm and the needle tip are both in focus and are centered in the field of view; then switch to the 40× objective.

6. Position the needle at the center of the field of view. Move the stage until a clearly visible portion of the distal gonad cytoplasm is lined up adjacent to the needle tip. Once the target and the needle are both in focus (under the 40× objective), the stage is moved to push the worm into contact with the needle. Most often it will be apparent at this point that the needle tip is depressing the external cuticle of the worm and/or the membranes surrounding the gonad without actually penetrating the gonad. When the needle tip is positioned in the apparent center of the gonad cytoplasm, a gentle tap is applied to the back of the micromanipulator, causing the needle tip to penetrate. Pressure is then applied to the needle, causing the DNA solution to infiltrate the gonad cytoplasm in both directions from the point of insertion (see Fig. 1). After injection, remove the needle by moving the stage and turn off the pressure. Reposition the stage to inject the second gonad arm or move to the next worm and repeat the process.

7. Breaking needles: Needles frequently become clogged during injection. In some cases flow can be restored by simply increasing the nitrogen pressure (however, it is important to know the pressure tolerance of the pressure system being used; pressures greater than 80–100 psi can blow gaskets or launch the needle out of its holder). If the offending particle remains lodged near the tip of the needle, first repair the pressure seals, then begin pushing the pressurized needle (gently at first) into dust particles embedded in the injection pad. Stop when a sustained flow resumes. Breaking the needle tip will often generate a sharp needle with a large but serviceable opening. Test the broken needle on a few animals, if the animals are not overtly ruptured by inserting and removing

the needle then they will probably yield transformed progeny. If the needle is too large or too blunt, discard it and load a second needle. Chronic needle clogging is often a sign that the injection solution contains impurities such as dust and bacteria. If needles continue to become clogged, consider preparing fresh DNA samples.

8. After injecting all of the mounted animals, return to the dissecting scope to recover the injected animals. Two recovery protocols are presented. The "quick recovery" protocol should be appropriate for injection of DNA into the distal gonad cytoplasm of adult hermaphrodites. The "gentle recovery" protocol may be useful in more delicate injection procedures, in particular for the injection of younger animals or injection of oocyte nuclei (which requires slightly desiccated recipients: Fire, 1986).

Quick recovery: Use a drawn-out capillary with a wide opening to deposit a small drop of sterile M9 solution on the pad around the injected animals. In most cases, the animals will immediately come free of the pad and resume swimming. If necessary, gently nudge the animals with the pipet to free them and transfer them in groups of one to five to a fresh culture plate. If the worms are not active immediately after removing them from the pad, they often recover after a few minutes.

Gentle recovery: An isotonic recovery buffer used in this protocol allows recovery of animals even after considerable desiccation. A single drop of the recovery buffer [0.1% salmon sperm DNA (for viscosity), 4% glucose, 2.4 mM KCl, 66 mM NaCl, 3 mM CaCl$_2$, 3 mM 4-(2-hydroxyethyl)-1-piperazineethane sulfonic acid (Hepes), pH 7.2] is added after microinjection. After several hours, M9 buffer is added dropwise (20 drops over the course of 1 hour) to slowly reduce osmotic strength. The worms are transferred to seeded NGM plates using a standard worm pick.

E. Troubleshooting the Injection Protocol

1. The Injected Worm Died and . . .

a. The Body Was Severely Ruptured at One or More Points.
Likely cause.   Injection with an overly large needle tip or ripping of the cuticle during injection.
Solution.   Practice with injections should help with this; also, it is important to experiment with a variety of needle tapers. If you must inject with a large needle (e.g., because of clogging problems), inject in only one gonad arm and inject more animals.

b. The Body Is Stiff and Unmoving after Removal from the Pad.
Likely Cause.   Desiccation. The animal was on the pad too long or the agarose layer on the pad was too thick.
Solution.   Place fewer animals on the pad in each injection session and/or make thinner pads. In addition, try the gentle recovery method (above).

2. The Animals Stick at First but Quickly Work Themselves Free.

Likely Cause. The pads were too thin or need to be baked longer, or the culture plates that animals were taken from are too wet.

Solution. Bake the pads again. If necessary, make new pads. In some climates it may be necessary to bake the pads before each use or to remove the lid from the worm culture plate for 30 minutes to 1 hour prior to injection.

3. The Worms Desiccate Very Quickly.

Likely Cause. The agarose pads are too thick or the culture plates are too dry.

Solution. Make new pads using fresh 2% agarose. Transfer the worms to fresh moist culture plates for several hours before injecting.

Note. Pad problems are very common; if reproducible pads are difficult to obtain, then it is possible to reuse a pad that performs well. After recovering the first row of injected worms, remove excess M9 from the pad and apply the next row of worms to a dry portion of the pad. This allows a single good injection pad to be reused several times.

4. There Are No Transformed Progeny and . . .

a. The Injection Process Does Not Look like the Example in Fig. 1.

Likely cause. The needle is not positioned inside the gonad, there is inadequate flow from the needle, or the animals are unhealthy and have an atrophied gonad cytoplasm.

Solution. Practice tapping the manipulator to ensure penetration of the needle tip into the gonad cytoplasm. If the needle is inside the gonad but does not flow sufficiently, try breaking the needle or increasing the pressure until adequate flow is obtained. In starved animals, the core cytoplasm is smaller and difficult to see; therefore, injections will be difficult and will not result in the characteristic ballooning shown in Fig. 1. This can be addressed by growing a healthier population of animals, injecting a different strain, or injecting oocyte nuclei.

b. There Are No Transformed Progeny and the Injections Looked Good.

Likely Cause. One of the DNA preparations injected is toxic (generally due to impurity in the prep).

Solution. Make a new DNA prep or purify the prep being used.

Note. This problem is very common. If both gonad arms were injected you may notice that the injected animals lay few if any viable eggs for about 1 to 2 days after injection.

5. There Are F1 Transformants but No Transmitting Lines.

Likely Cause. A DNA sequence present in the injection mixture is not tolerated in high-copy-number arrays (e.g., a poison gene).

Solution. Dilute the suspected poison sequence to 1 to 5 µg/ml while keeping the marker gene concentration at greater than 100 µg/ml. This will permit the assembly of arrays carrying one or a few copies of the poison gene.

Note. Many transformants in such an experiment will have zero copies of the "poison" gene; this makes it critical to test several transformed lines with each combination of injected DNAs.

III. Identification and Inheritance Properties of Transformed Animals

A. Markers for Identifying and Selecting Transformed Lines

A separate easily scoreable marker gene to identify transformed animals can be extremely useful in a variety of injection experiments. As noted above, the propensity for injected DNA molecules to recombine with each other generally allows one to coinject the selectable marker with a DNA segment to be tested for activity. The desired properties of the marker plasmid depend on the details of the experimental assay. Several concerns should be kept in mind. First, the marker should be easily scored in the genetic background in which the experiment is performed. Second, the possibility that the marker phenotype (e.g., rolling or twitching) might interfere with the scoring of the experimental phenotype should be considered. Third, the possibility that sequences in the marker DNA could interact *in cis* with sequences in the coinjected experimental plasmid to affect expression must be considered.

1. *rol-6*

Perhaps the most convenient visible marker for identifying transformed animals is a plasmid called pRF4 that carries the dominant collagen mutation, *rol-6(su1006)* (Kramer *et al.,* 1990). The mutant collagen gene encoded by *rol-6(su1006))* causes animals to roll and move in circles, a behavior easily recognized using a dissecting microscope. The *rol-6* marker can be used in a variety of genetic backgrounds, but is best used with strains that are not dumpy and that have wild-type motility. Many dumpy mutations suppress the roller phenotype completely, while mutations that cause severely reduced motility necessitate a very close inspection of animals to identify rollers.

There are some applications for which the *rol-6* marker is not appropriate. The twisted cuticle of roller transformants can in some cases complicate the task of identifying or following cell types in roller larvae and adults. A second potential problem is the failure of certain roller males to mate. Where possible, it is easiest to perform crosses by mating roller hermaphrodites with males heterozygous for a marker to be introduced. These crosses often require an excess of males, because of difficulty in copulating with a rolling target. If it is necessary to use roller males for a cross, it is generally possible to find individuals that roll only occasionally. These males can sometimes mate with an efficiency comparable to that of wild-type males.

Although we do not have extensive data on interactions between the *rol-6* gene and coinjected DNA constructs incorporated into the same array, these interactions may be significant. In particular, *rol-6* may contain both temporal and tissue-specific expression signals. This might either activate or suppress expression of other adjacent genes in mixed arrays. In this context, it is worth noting that some constructs have diminished expression in late larvae and adults when cotransformed with *rol-6* (Krause *et al.*, 1994).

2. *unc-22* Antisense (Twitcher) Constructs

unc-22 encodes a large muscle filament protein that is required for sustained muscle contraction (Moerman *et al.*, 1988). Disruption of *unc-22* function by mutation or antisense RNA production leads to a distinctive twitching phenotype and to resistant behavior in the presence of a variety of drugs including levamisole and nicotine. Constructs expression *unc-22* antisense RNA can thus be used as selectable markers to isolate transgenic lines. We have most frequently used a plasmid pPD10.46, in which *unc-22* antisense RNA is expressed from control signals normally responsible for myosin heavy-chain gene expression. This DNA has transformation and heritability properties similar to those of the *rol-6(su1006)* plasmid pRF4, with the only difference being a considerably lower frequency of transient transformation with pPD10.46. This can be an advantage in deriving transgenic lines, in that about half of the strongly twitching worms resulting in the F1 from injection of pPD10.46 give rise to transformed lines.

The twitching phenotype in the transgenic lines carrying these constructs is somewhat less obvious than the rolling phenotype of pRF4 transformed animals. With some practice, however, the twitching phenotype can readily be scored in all but the most highly paralyzed genetic backgrounds. As with *rol-6*, the twitching phenotype can interfere with male mating ability (although weakly twitching males can often mate) and with scoring certain subtle phenotypes.

A major feature to take into account in using the *unc-22* antisense construct is the presence of a strong body muscle-specific transcriptional enhancer in the construct. This enhancer is capable of acting at considerable distances in extrachromosomal arrays. Although somewhat less of a concern in experiments with cosmid, YAC, or phage DNAs used for coinjection, the occurrence of body wall muscle expression in constructs cotransformed with pPD10.46 must always first be assumed to result from signals in the marker plasmid.

3. Other Visible and Selectable Markers

It is possible to use any of the lethal and visible mutations that can be rescued by injection of the corresponding wild-type gene to select for transformed animals and lines. These experiments require that transformation be performed in a balanced or conditional mutant genetic background. The choice of marker and recipient strain then depends on the precise details of the experimental assay, keeping in mind the concerns discussed above. Two markers that have been relatively convenient to date are *unc-4* (Miller *et al.*, 1992), which allows rescue of a visible but healthy uncoordinated phenotype, and *spe-26* (J. Varkey and S. Ward, pers. comm.), which allows rescue of a temperature-sensitive sterile mutation.

B. Expression and Metabolism of DNA Following Injection

1. Probable Fate of Injected Sequences

In planning DNA transformation experiments, it is important to consider the behavior and fate of injected sequences. Our current view of this is summarized in Fig. 2. Frequently, the injected DNA construct is expressed in the first generation following microinjection, but not carried through the F1 germ line to the next generation. These F1-expressing animals are often mosaic (expressing in only a fraction of cells in a given tissue); this suggests that F1 expression could result from the simple partitioning of the injected DNA among the cells of the F1 embryo.

In a fraction of F1 progeny, the newly injected sequences are substrates for a set of highly efficient recombination reactions, including homologous recombination between injected DNAs (Stinchcomb *et al.*, 1985; Mello *et al.*, 1991). If the DNA is injected directly into the oocyte nucleus (Fire, 1986), integration of the DNA into chromosomes can occur during this reactive period. The frequency of spontaneous integration after cytoplasmic injection is much lower; this may reflect the timing of events: sequences injected into the cytoplasm may remain compartmentalized away from the chromosomes during the initial recombinogenic phase.

If the DNA concentration in the injection solution is sufficient (>100 μg/ml), then the recombining sequences can assemble into large arrays. Arrays that attain a size greater than approximately 700 kb become heritable as extrachromosomal elements, whereas smaller arrays appear to be maintained only if integrated into an existing chromosome (Mello *et al.*, 1991). Once assembled into heritable arrays, the transforming sequences are not an active target for intraarray recombination (Stinchcomb *et al.*, 1985; Mello *et al.*, 1991), and will rarely integrate into chromosomes unless recombination is induced by irradiating the animals (Fire *et al.*, 1991; Krause *et al.*, 1990; see section D for a description of the irradiation protocol).

2. Effect of Double-Stranded Breaks on Recombination

Homologous recombination between coinjected molecules is stimulated in *C. elegans* (as in other organisms) by appropriately placed double-stranded breaks

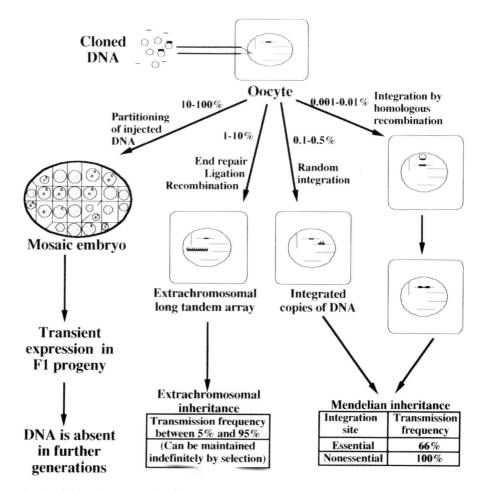

Fig. 2 Schematic diagram describing fates of DNA injected into the *C. elegans* germ line. This cartoon describes our current understanding of the fate of DNA injected into oocyte nuclei. In a large fraction of the animals from injection, DNA is retained in the F1 to produce transient expression, with no retention in the germ line (e.g., Fire and Waterston, 1989). At low frequency, the injected DNA can form extrachromosomal tandem arrays, which are inherited by a fraction of progeny at each subsequent generation (Stinchcomb *et al.,* 1985). Random integration of injected DNA can also occur (Fire, 1986), albeit at a lower frequency, generating stably inherited Mendelian transgenes. At very low frequencies, the injected DNA can recombine homologously with endogenous chromosomal sequences (Broverman *et al.,* 1993; A. Fire and S. Harrison, unpublished). Injection of DNA into the gonadal syncytium (Mello *et al.,* 1991) gives both transient expression and extrachromosomal transformation, but produces few direct integration events (see text).

(Orr-Weaver *et al.,* 1981; Kucherlapati *et al.,* 1984; Lin *et al.,* 1984). In *C. elegans,* molecules that cannot be joined by homologous recombination appear to intersperse in arrays with a lower efficiency. Overhanging sequences at the ends of linear molecules are often lost during array assembly in *C. elegans* (A. Fire and C. Mello, unpublished observations).

In some cases, the properties of injected linear DNA have been used as a tool for rough mapping of a functional gene. Digesting DNA with a restriction enzyme that cuts within a gene prior to injection causes the resulting arrays to contain fewer functional copies of the gene (Kim and Horvitz 1990; C. Mello, unpublished observations). In interpreting these experiments, it is important to realize that for some genes, one or a few functional copies within an array is sufficient for function (or even advantageous in recovering healthy transformed animals). Therefore, before conducting this type of experiment, it is important to first determine a threshold at which reducing the DNA concentration of the gene of interest begins to reduce the frequency of transformed lines that express that gene.

C. Extrachromosomal Arrays

Extrachromosomal arrays are the predominant form in which a nontoxic DNA can be inherited beyond the F1 generation (Stinchcomb *et al.*, 1985). Derivation of array-containing lines can routinely be carried out by picking F1 transformed animals clonally or in small groups and surveying in the next generation for F2 transformants. An alternative is to allow plates derived from the initial injected animals to starve, followed by direct selection of F2 or F3 transformants (in this case, only one line from each initially starved plate should be kept).

Extrachromosomal arrays appear to behave very much like fragments of the endogenous worm chromosomes called free duplications (see Chapter 6 in this volume). Like free duplications, independently established arrays have characteristic levels of inheritance ranging from ~10% to ~90%, with an average of about 50% inheritance in each generation. Each array can include hundreds of linked copies of the injected DNA molecules (Stinchcomb *et al.*, 1985; Mello *et al.*, 1991; Hope, 1991). A related question is how many copies of each array are carried in each nucleus. It appears that only one or a few copies of the complete array are present in each nucleus of the transformed lines (D. Albertson, pers. comm.; Mello *et al.*, 1991). The differing levels of heritability associated with different arrays probably reflect a simple size difference between arrays: larger molecules may be replicated or segregated more efficiently than smaller ones.

In attempts to obtain smaller autonomous replicons in *C. elegans,* several defined sequences from *C. elegans* or yeast (including yeast centromeres, telomeres, and origins) have been tested for their effects on segregation; these do not appear to increase heritability or the frequency of DNA transformation in *C. elegans* (Stinchcomb *et al.*, 1985; C. Mello, unpublished observations).

D. Integrated Lines

Integrated transgenes can contain the injected DNA at copy numbers of one to several hundred. The first techniques for generating integrated transgenes involved the use of a selectable marker gene (*sup-7*) that causes toxic effects at high copy number, thereby selecting against high-copy-number extrachromosomal arrays (Fire, 1986). Injection of *sup-7*-containing constructs into oocytes of appropriately marked strains could be used to generate integrated transgenes in a single step (Fire, 1986). Unfortunately the oocyte injections are technically more difficult than the syncytial injection techniques described in this article (Mello *et al.*, 1991). Below, we describe two newer methods that allow the isolation of integrated transgenes using syncytial injection.

1. Gamma Ray-Induced Integration of Extrachromosomal Arrays

(C. Kari, G. Seydoux, S. White Harrison, A. Fire, and R. Herman)

Overview. The most straightforward method for generating an integrated transformed line is to gamma-irradiate a population carrying an extrachromosomal array. After nonselective growth for several generations, several hundred individuals still expressing the transgene marker are cloned and their progeny examined to test homozygosity for the transforming sequences.

1. Generate a few extrachromosomal transgenic lines using standard injection protocols. For the purposes of this description it will be assumed that the *rol-6* dominant marker has been used. If possible, integration should be tried on two or three independent lines, since some arrays integrate more readily than others. In choosing among several array-containing lines, we recommend starting with lines that exhibit a transmission frequency of 0.25 to 0.35 from generation to generation (very low frequencies of transmission will make subsequent collection of F2 rollers more difficult, whereas high frequencies will negate the enrichment that is obtained below by picking rollers in the F3).

2. Gamma-irradiate plates containing 100 to 200 roller L4 animals with 2000 to 4000 rad from a ^{137}Cs source. We have not tried any other radiation source for this, but X rays might work equivalently.

3. Pick four or five irradiated animals each on 25 to 50 seeded (6-cm) NGM plates.

4. Let the population of worms grow on each plate until starvation (10–14 days at 20°C). The animals remaining on the plate are now presumably F2 larvae derived from the irradiated animals.

5. Transfer a chunk from each starved plate to a separate seeded 9-cm plate. After 2 to 3 days, pick roller animals from each of the new plates onto individual 6-cm seeded plates (15–20 animals from each of the chunked plates, keeping track of the parent plate to confirm independence of different integrated lines).

6. Check after several days for segregation of only rollers in the population. To rule out possible new roller mutations appearing in the strain (not generally a problem), we make sure that any putative integrated locus is dominant or semidominant and causes rolling with the same handedness as *rol-6*. Once a

putative integrated roller strain is identified, it should be propagated an extra generation to confirm stable integration. Occasionally, very high frequency lines arise that still have some nonroller progeny. This can occur for two reasons: (i) The array may be integrated but may be expressed somewhat more weakly, so that only a fraction of the animals are actually rolling. Or (ii) the array has been partially stabilized but is still extrachromosomal. To distinguish these possibilities, a few nonrollers as well as rollers should be cloned from plates with very high fractions of rolling animals.

7. Strains should be outcrossed to confirm that no major translocations or unlinked mutations have occurred as a result of the radiation treatment (Rosenbluth *et al.*, 1985).

2. Obtaining Integrated Arrays Following Cytoplasmic Injections in the Presence of a Single-Stranded Oligonucleotide

Mello *et al.* (1991) describe the use of a single-stranded oligonucleotide included in the injection mixture to stimulate nonhomologous integration of DNA injected into the syncytial gonad cytoplasm. Although it is not known how the oligonucleotide stimulates integration, this procedure can be used to isolate an integrated transgene in a single step.

The injection mixture should contain 50 to 100 μg/ml double-stranded sequence to be integrated and 1 mg/ml of the oligonucleotide. (The sequence of the oligonucleotide does not appear to be important; a sequence that has been used by C.M. is 5'-GGAACCGCTTCCAACCGTGTGAGATGTCAACAATATGGAGGAT-ATGGAGC-3'.) The presence of the oligonucleotide reduces the frequency of extrachromosomal transformation at least tenfold. The experienced injector will need to inject between 50 and 100 animals. These injections should yield one or two F1 transformants per injected animal (both arms) and a total of 5 to 10 heritably transformed lines. Typically, one or two of these lines will prove to be integrated. This procedure usually results in 1 to 10 tandem copies of the double-stranded sequence integrated at apparently random chromosomal sites.

IV. Assays for Function of Native *Caenorhabditis elegans* Genes

A. Mutant Rescue Assays

The most conceptually straightforward assay for injected DNA is to introduce DNA containing the wild-type copy of a gene into a mutant genetic background, using rescue of the mutant phenotype as an assay for function of the injected DNA. In the simplest case, this can be done by injecting the DNA into mutant parents, followed by screening for rescued progeny. In many cases, however, more subtle concerns must be taken into account.

In principle, any mutation that can be suppressed by a wild-type copy of the corresponding gene could be used in the recipient strain. Given a choice of alleles, a viable recessive allele with a distinctive phenotype would be preferred.

In some cases, dominant or semidominant alleles could also be used (if their effect can be mitigated or enhanced by the wild-type gene); in these cases, the resulting phenotype may be particularly dependent on the expression level for the reintroduced gene, so that partial function of the reintroduced DNA might be difficult to reproducibly detect.

For genes with lethal, sterile, or generally scrawny mutant phenotypes, it is not feasible to introduce the rescuing DNA directly into a homozygous mutant background. Two options should be considered in these cases. First, the DNA could be introduced into mutant heterozygotes. Second, the DNA could be introduced into a wild-type strain, with the relevant mutation subsequently introduced by genetic crosses. In either case, genetic markers linked to the mutation can be useful in eventually identifying animals homozygous for the mutant chromosomal allele. Even if these markers are closely linked, the possibility of recombination should be taken into account; indeed, anecdotal evidence from several different groups suggests that recombination rates may be modestly increased on microinjection (increases in mutation rates have also been observed: Fire *et al.*, 1991).

The degree of phenotypic rescue depends very much on the gene used. In many cases, F1 expression, extrachromosomal arrays, and integrated copies of a locus each produce complete rescue of a chromosomal mutation to a wild-type phenotype. In other cases, rescue is partial by any or all of these methods. Partial rescue can manifest either as incomplete rescue of the mutant phenotype or as relatively complete suppression occurring in only a fraction of transformed animals. Mosaic inheritance of the introduced DNA is one possible cause for incomplete rescue, although partial rescue has also been observed in lines carrying an integrated transgene.

Dominant effects of injected DNA can also complicate the analysis of transformed animals. This is most frequently a concern in situations where a long tandem array containing multiple copies of an introduced gene has been created. The observed dominant effects can apparently result from a variety of causes; these include titration of critical DNA binding factors, production of complementary (antisense) RNAs, product overexpression, and production of aberrant proteins. In many cases these effects are sufficiently deleterious to prevent the derivation of transgenic lines from animals injected with a specific DNA. Because transiently expressing animals in the first generation following microinjection contain relatively few copies of the transforming DNA, the appearance of transformed phenotypes in the F1 generation is usually unaffected. The few animals in the F1 generation carrying high-copy-number arrays might be affected in such a way that they die amongst the usual casualties of the microinjection process. This results in a situation in which transient expression of injected DNA (either the selectable marker or gene to be tested) might be observed, but transgenic lines cannot be obtained. In such cases, dominant effects can often be avoided by using a lower concentration of the offending DNA molecule, while keeping the total DNA concentration in the injection mix approximately constant; this is normally performed by adding a nondeleterious DNA such as Bluescript or by increasing the concentration of the marker DNA used for selection.

B. Rescue as an Assay in Cloning Mutationally Defined Genes

Despite the potential complications, rescue of mutant phenotypes can often be used as an assay for cloning genes and analyzing expression. As a first approach, we recommend the following generalized strategy for cloning by microinjection rescue.

1. Physical and genetic map data are initially compared to narrow down the position of the gene. A critical first step in this process is always to telephone or e-mail individuals whose names are associated with (i.e., appear beneath) clones on the physical map; this will provide the latest information on characterization of specific genes and potential probes for restriction fragment length polymorphisms (RFLPs) in the area. Genetic mapping of polymorphisms with respect to the gene of interest is the most reliable and straightforward way of narrowing the physical region to be tested to a manageable size. There is a trade-off between the amount of effort expended in genetic mapping and the number of clones that will need to be injected. The decision of how far to pursue physical/genetic mapping before starting microinjection depends on several factors, including the nature of the physical map in a given region and the ease with which a microinjection rescue assay can be performed.

2. Once the interval is reduced to a manageable size (usually 5 to 20 cosmid lengths depending on the factors noted above), the cosmid and/or YAC clones spanning the delineated region can be obtained from the genome project. In a region well covered by cosmids, these should be tested first for rescue activity. Cosmids are preferred over YACs at present because YAC DNA is more difficult to prepare and analyze, and because YAC rescue must eventually be followed up by growing and injecting the corresponding cosmids. For both cosmids and YACs, several overlapping clones covering each segment analyzed should be tested, if available. This will increase the chances of obtaining an appropriate clone in cases where one or a few cosmid or YAC clones are difficult to grow or have an evident or subtle deletion or rearrangement.

3. Overlapping cosmid clones are pooled in groups of 5 to 10. These pools are then injected into an appropriately marked mutant strain with a dominant selectable marker (such as the *rol-6*-containing plasmid pRF4). As a starting point, each cosmid could be included in the injection mix at a concentration of 10 to 50 μg/ml. If roller lines cannot be obtained from a given cosmid mix, then

subpools of the relevant cosmid group should be injected, while at the same time testing the initial mix of cosmids at a lower concentration (e.g., injecting the cosmid at 1 μg/ml while keeping the total concentration greater than 100 μg/ml). Several independent transgenic lines should be tested for each region analyzed; this increases the probability that at least one will contain the DNA of interest.

4. Once a positive rescue signal has been obtained for a given pool, subpools should be tested with the goal of eventually obtaining a single clone sufficient for rescue. If no single clone is sufficient for rescue, then the gene may reside on two overlapping cloned fragments. (Because of the high frequency of recombination between injected sequences, coinjected overlapping clones might be expected to rescue the corresponding mutation.)

5. If initial attempts at rescue are unsuccessful, then three possibilities should be considered. First, the injected clones might not contain an intact copy of the relevant gene. Second, presence of the wild-type gene in an extrachromosomal array might be insufficient to rescue the mutation (as noted below, this may be particularly significant for genes that must be expressed in the germ line). Third, errors in the physical and genetic maps might have resulted in choice of an incorrect set of clones.

If the experimenter is confident that the gene lies within a region covered by clones that have been injected, several experimental approaches may be useful. A subtle examination of phenotype in transformed lines should be performed to identify partially rescued lines. If available, a different set of cosmid and YAC clones spanning the same region should be grown to address the possibility of a fortuitous rearrangement in the clones used for the initial assays. If there are gaps in the cosmid coverage of the region, then several YAC clones that bridge these gaps should be carefully characterized and injected.

In all of the cases discussed above, refinements in the correlated physical and genetic maps in the region can be critical in eventually cloning the gene. Clones that have been prepared for injection can readily be used as probes for continued efforts to identify and map RFLPs. Generating new types of alleles such as small deficiencies and transposon-induced mutations can likewise be useful in generating polymorphisms directly in the gene of interest. It may also be possible to improve the correlation between physical and genetic maps by rescuing genes that map close to the gene of interest.

V. Use of Chimeric "Reporter" Constructs to Analyze Gene Expression

Once a gene has been cloned, a proximal goal is to determine its expression pattern during development. The definitive means for determining expression patterns involve *in situ* hybridization and immunostaining with antibody probes specifically directed at the products of the gene (see Chapters 14 and 15 in this volume). Reporter fusions, although not a definitive means to determine expression pattern, can be useful in many cases. The assumptions that come into interpretation of the reporter expression pattern are (1) that the transforming construct contains all relevant *cis*-acting control sequences, and (2) that neither the reporter construct nor the novel context of the transforming DNA has a profound effect on the expression pattern of the gene. These assumptions have often proven acceptable for genes expressed in specific patterns of somatic tissues. Unfortunately, expression of many reporter constructs (including all *lacZ* fusion constructions tried to date) seems to be blocked in the germ line. In addition, expression of some ubiquitous "housekeeping" genes may not be faithfully reproduced in transgenic animals containing reporter constructions (A. Fire, unpublished; D. Bird, pers. comm.). In general, we view the use of reporter constructs to be most valuable in analyses of expression patterns that have already been confirmed by independent means (e.g., *in situ* hybridization or antibody staining). In these cases, the transgene reporter systems can provide means for detailed temporal and spatial characterization of the expression pattern and for precise definition of factors responsible for setting up the expression pattern.

Available reporter vectors (Fire *et al.*, 1990; Chalfie *et al.*, 1994) permit a variety of strategies for constructing reporter fusions. As a first step, a fragment spanning the 5' end of the gene can be used to construct a translational fusion. Only limited experience in mapping control regions is available for *C. elegans*, but in general, 3 to 4 kb of upstream sequence has been sufficient to contain upstream signals. Expression signals are also frequently found within the transcribed region, particularly in larger intron sequences. (Many *C. elegans* introns are smaller than 100 bp; longer introns near the 5' end of a gene are candidates for containing control sequences, including enhancers.)

Expression of transgene constructs also depends on signals in the 3' region downstream of the transgene. A set of standard expression vectors contain 3' flanking sequences from the *unc-54* gene in this position. These sequences are sufficient to allow high-level expression in most (probably all) somatic tissues. In several cases, however, translational regulation acting through the 3' end of a specific mRNA has been shown to be involved in specifying temporal and spacial patterns of gene expression (Wightman *et al.*, 1993; Goodwin *et al.*, 1993; Evans *et al.*, 1994). Vectors containing a 3' multiple cloning site for insertion of potential 3' regulatory sequences are available for these constructs (e.g., pPD16.43: Fire *et al.*, 1990).

Several different reporter molecules have been used for *C. elegans*, with the most widely used being the *Escherichia coli* gene *lacZ*, encoding β-galactosidase. When stained at neutral pH, *C. elegans* shows no background of endogenous β-galactosidase. The localization of transgene products can thus be easily determined in fixed animals using a sensitive chromogenic stain (Fire, 1992). A second *E. coli* enzyme, β-glucuronidase (the product of the *E. coli uidA* gene) has also been used as a reporter in *C. elegans* (Jefferson *et al.*, 1987). In this case, a slight background of endogenous staining is seen in nontransformed animals [this can be avoided using mutations that lack the endogenous enzyme as hosts for microinjection (Sebastiano *et al.*, 1986; Jefferson *et al.*, 1987)]. In our experience, the β-glucuronidase assays are somewhat less sensitive than equivalent assays for β-galactosidase (Okkema *et al.*, 1993).

One disadvantage of the use of hydrolytic enzymes as reporters is that appropriate chromogenic substrates cannot in general diffuse through the cuticle into live animals. Thus it is not possible to use these enzymes to analyze expression patterns in live animals. It has, however, been possible to perform staining for β-galactosidase or β-glucuronidase in adult animals that have been permeabilized to substrate but that retain live eggs in the uterus (Sebastiano *et al.*, 1986; Fire, 1992; Zie, Jia, and Aamodt, pers. comm.).

Recently Chalfie *et al.* (1994) described the use of gene encoding an intrinsically fluorescent protein for reporter experiments in *C. elegans*. This reporter can be used to track gene expression in living animals and should be a remarkable tool.

In some cases, it is advisable for the reporter to have a minimal effect on the function and localization of the transgene product. In these cases, an alternate strategy of peptide tagging can be used: the cloned endogenous gene is marked by insertion of a short segment encoding a defined (nonworm) epitope that can be recognized by a well-characterized and available monoclonal antibody. An epitope from hemagglutinin (Field *et al.*, 1988) has been used successfully for this purpose with the genes *unc-76* and *unc-6* (L. Bloom and H. R. Horvitz, pers. comm.; W. Wadsworth, pers. comm.). This approach can be particularly informative if the tagged molecule can rescue mutations in the corresponding chromosomal gene, thus demonstrating at least some correspondence between the expression pattern of the transgene and biological requirements for the activity.

VI. Directed Expression of Coding Regions and Antisense RNAs

A. Directed Expression Vectors

A set of modular vectors has been constructed that are intended to allow production of an RNA or protein product in well-defined cells and/or temporal patterns. The general structure of the vectors is shown in Fig. 3. The design is modular, with an abundance of restriction sites in defined positions to facilitate transfer of equivalent cassettes between vectors. The vectors are related to the modular *lacZ* fusion vectors (Fire *et al.*, 1990), so that cassettes can often be exchanged between the two vector sets.

The "canonical" vector pPD49.26 has just two signals: a synthetic intron and the 3' region from the *unc-54* gene. These signals are interspersed between three consecutive MCS (polylinker) segments:

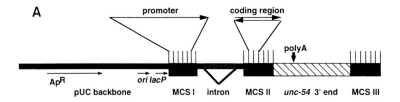

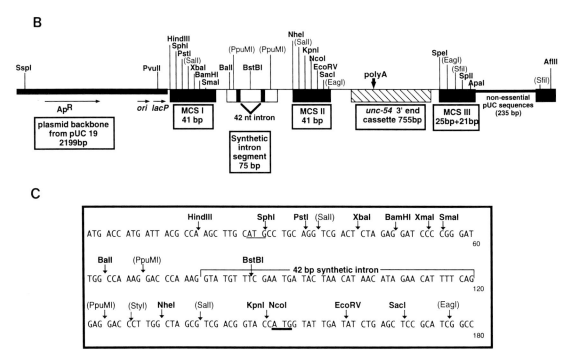

Fig. 3 Vectors for ectopic expression. (A) Overall scheme for producing vectors. MCS, multiple cloning site (polylinker). Ap^R, *ori,* and *lacP* are the β-lactamase gene, replication origin, and *lacZ* promoter from pUC19. (B) Structure of the basic vector pPD49.26. The synthetic intron segment and the inversion of pUC sequences are described in Fire *et al.* (1990). (C) Sequence of the 5' region of the parent vector pPD49.26.

I. For insertion of promoter elements (also enhancers if needed)

II. For insertion of the segment to be expressed

III. Distal to the *unc-54* 3' terminus

The construction of new expression vectors with defined promoter sequences requires an appropriate restriction fragment containing the 5' flanking region of the gene. Since this set of vectors is designed to produce proteins beginning precisely at the start codons of the inserted sequences, promoter sequences are taken to end just upstream of the ATG. Alternatively, promoter sequences just downstream of the ATG can be included, with the ATG mutated to prevent its use as a translational initiator. If a convenient restriction site just upstream of the ATG exists, then this is used; otherwise, a polymerase chain reaction (PCR) product is produced using (1) a standard sense primer approximately 3 kb upstream and (2) an antisense oligonucleotide primer starting several nucleotides downstream of the ATG and having a point change to eliminate the ATG. These primers each should contain extra 5' base pairs to form restriction sites that allow directed insertion into MCS-I of pPD49.26 (e.g., *Pst*I upstream and *Bam*HI downstream).

Ectopic expression vectors produced by S. White-Harrison and A. Fire using a set of characterized *C. elegans* promoters are summarized in Table I (vectors, detailed restriction maps, and sequence information are available on request from A. Fire). These vectors have been used to express RNA both as mRNA for eventual translation (e.g., Perry *et al.*, 1993) and as antisense RNA to inhibit expression of cloned genes (e.g., Fire *et al.*, 1991). For many applications, an initial goal is to produce optimal levels of a protein product in specific tissues. Either cDNA or genomic sequence could in principle be expressed. cDNA expression has the advantages of a shorter insert and should avoid any regulatory sequences within the coding region to be expressed. Genomic expression is

Table I
Vectors for Directed Expression of Specified cDNAs[a]

Promoter	Vector	Promoter analysis	Expression pattern
myo-2	pPD30.69	Okkema *et al.*, 1993	Pharyngeal muscle
unc-54	pPD30.38	Okkema *et al.*, 1993	Body muscle
hlh-1	pPD52.99	Krause *et al.*, 1994	Body wall muscle and clonal precursors
mec-3	pPD57.56	Way *et al.*, 1991	Touch neurons (expression begins just after birth of these cells)
mec-7	pPD52.102	Hamelin *et al.*, 1992	Touch neurons (expression begins slightly later than *mec-3*)
hsp16-2	pPD49.78	Stringham *et al.*, 1992	Heat-induced expression; strongest activity neural, hypodermal
hsp16-41	pPD49.83	Stringham *et al.*, 1992	Heat-induced expression; strongest activity in gut
mtl-1	pPD52.37	Freedman *et al.*, 1993	Gut (heavy metal inducible) + pharynx
mtl-2	pPD54.01	Freedman *et al.*, 1993	Gut (heavy metal inducible)
glp-1	pPD50.30	Fire and Priess, unpub	Rare somatic expression with a *lacZ* reporter; this construct has been useful as a basal promoter for assaying enhancer function

[a] All vectors were initially tested by insertion of *lacZ* followed by F1 injection/stain assays to localize expression. In addition, the *unc-54, hlh-1, mec-7, hsp16-2,* and *hsp16-41* promoter vectors have been tested by insertion of the *hlh-1* cDNA, production of transgenic lines, and detection by antibody staining of the transgene-expressed HLH-1 protein (S. White Harrison, M. Krause, and A. Fire, unpublished). These vectors can be obtained by request from A. Fire.

advantageous if natural introns promote expression or if cDNA clones are unavailable.

B. Interpreting Ectopic Expression Experiments

By allowing the experimenter to choose which proteins are to be made in which cells, ectopic expression vectors provide a remarkable tool. Nonetheless, these experiments have to be interpreted with caution, and the literature is full of analogous experiments in other systems that are insufficiently controlled. We recommend (if possible) three controls to be carried out to confirm any biological conclusions:

1. If expression of a protein creates a phenotypic effect, then a mutation creating a frameshift or stop codon should be assayed and shown to be nonfunctional. [This is particularly important for experiments in which an expression construct designed to produce a putative regulatory factor is coinjected with a reporter construct (e.g., a construct ectopically producing a putative regulatory factor coinjected with a *lacZ* reporter construct, with the endpoint assay being for ectopic expression of the *lacZ* reporter). Because extensive recombination occurs between injected DNAs, this experiment will often lead to expression of the reporter construct by proximity to expression signals in the expression vector construct. The observation could be misinterpreted as *trans*-activation, when the true effect is actually *cis*-activation dependent on the expression construct but not on the putative "regulator" product.]

2. If possible, the expression pattern for a given ectopic expression construct should be confirmed directly (by showing that the RNA and/or protein product of the inserted coding sequence is indeed expressed in the expected pattern of tissues). Different inserts or modes of transformation (e.g., transient versus extrachromosomal arrays) could affect the pattern of expression; it is important in each case to test the assumption that true expression patterns reflect the expected activity of the expression vector.

3. If the expressed product is proposed to interact specifically with the product of an endogenous gene, then any available mutations in that gene should be used as a critical test for the nature of the observed effects.

VII. Possible Sources for Inefficient or Inappropriate Expression

A. Level and Pattern of Expression

Frequently, a reintroduced transgene construct will express in precisely the pattern and level expected from the constituent elements used to produce the injected recombinant DNA. In other cases, however, the observed expression pattern of the transgene can exhibit discrepancies either qualitatively or quantatively from the expected pattern. Several types of discrepancies have been observed.

The method by which the DNA is introduced into the animals could affect the expression pattern. Some expression signals appear to function well in low-copy-number integrated transformation and/or transient expression but poorly in transgenic lines carrying extrachromosomal arrays (Okkema *et al.,* 1993). Other constructs appear to function most efficiently when present at high copy number in transgene arrays (e.g., the antisense *unc-22* construct pPD10.46 described in Fire *et al.,* 1991). High transgene copy number (e.g., several hundred tandem copies of the injected DNA) might be expected to lead to dramatic increases in the level of expression; in some cases, this overexpression is observed, although the actual expression level might not be a linear function of copy number (e.g., Fire and Waterston, 1989; Macmorris, *et al.,* 1994). In many cases, expression levels seem to be limited, so that a high copy number of injected construct does not lead to dramatically increased expression (Macmorris *et al.,* 1995; M. Krause and A. Fire, unpublished).

Chimeric DNA constructs can express at unexpectedly low levels due to several circumstances. If a simple 5′ flanking fragment has been used as a "promoter" segment, then internal control elements might be absent from the expression vector. [We found such an element for the *unc-54* gene; placing this element 5′ to the *unc-54* promoter in an expression vector resulted in higher-level and more robust expression (Okkema *et al.,* 1993).] Conversely, signals within the inserted segment could activate or interfere with expression from the promoter. Although we have not in general observed such effects for *lacZ* or *gfp* insertions, endogenous nematode coding regions might reasonably be expected in some cases to retain control signals influencing promoter activity.

Other features of chimeric mRNAs may affect processing and or translation activity in *C. elegans.* Aberrant processing signals could be present in an RNA to be ectopically expressed or could be generated in chimeric fusions. In designing chimeric constructs, particular care should be taken at junctions to avoid creating exons of less than 50 bp (such exons might be poorly recognized by the splicing apparatus). ATGs upstream of the real start codon should also be noted, as these could inhibit translation. (In particular it should be remembered that *NcoI* and *SphI* sites in some expression vectors contain an ATG.) In some cases, natural upstream ATGs could be involved in modulation of translation. Because the effects of upstream ATGs could be dependent on RNA secondary structure, it is conceivable that these effects would be either diminished or amplified in the chimeric expression vector constructs.

Physiological regulatory sequences have been found in the 3′ UTRs of several *C. elegans* genes (Wightman *et al.,* 1993; Goodwin *et al.,* 1993; Evans *et al.,* 1994). In general, these act by suppressing translation in specific circumstances. Although many of the available vectors use "generic" 3′ UTR signals (e.g., from *unc-54*), alternate vectors are available that allow insertion of 3′ UTR sequences from a gene of choice (Fire *et al.,* 1990; Chalfie *et al.,* 1994).

B. Mosaic Expression

An endogenous gene will in general exhibit an identical expression program in all animals. In contrast, expression of individual transgenes has frequently been found to vary between otherwise identical transformed animals (e.g., Okkema *et al.,* 1993; Krause *et al.,* 1994).

This variation is in part due to mosaicism for the presence of the injected DNA. This is expected in F1 animals transiently expressing an injected DNA: some cells will contain injected sequences, whereas others will not. Similarly, exogenous DNA carried in extrachromosomal arrays can be lost in mitotic division, leading to animals that are effectively mosaic for the presence of the transforming DNA. The rate of mitotic loss in transgenic lines appears to be at least in part correlated to the observed transmission rate from one generation to the next. Lines with low transmission frequencies tend to exhibit higher rates of mitotic loss.

Not all mosaicism in expression is accounted for by loss of the transforming DNA. Mosaicism at the DNA level can be factored out by using transgenic lines in which the DNA has been integrated into a chromosome. Surprisingly, these strains can still exhibit mosaic expression, expressing in variable and apparently random sets of cells in a tissue in which the construct is active. In some cases, these patterns appear to follow lineal boundaries (Krause *et al.,* 1994). The level of mosaicism apparently depends on several variables including the promoter and expression signals, the reporter, and the copy number of the transforming DNA.

The molecular basis for mosaic expression is still under investigation. Regardless of the mechanisms, the possibility of mosaic expression should be taken into account in planning experiments that require complete and uniform transgene expression.

C. Expression in Inappropriate Tissues

In a fraction of cases, transgene expression has been observed in tissues that were unexpected given the expression patterns of the endogenous *C. elegans* gene(s) from which the construct was derived (e.g., Aamodt *et al.,* 1991; Krause *et al.,* 1994). In such cases, the context of the transforming DNA (e.g., proximity to plasmid vector sequences) or the lack of negative regulatory sequences could produce the unexpected expression pattern. For the *ges-1* and *hlh-1* genes, the inclusion of larger promoter fragments (>3 kb in the case of *hlh-1*) can overcome the inappropriate expression (Aamodt *et al.,* 1991; Krause *et al.,* 1994). Certain tissues may be particularly prone to express injected DNA (particularly constructs with deleted promoters) inappropriately; these include the posterior cells in the intestine of young animals (Krause *et al.,* 1994), as well as several different types of cells in the pharynx (Hope, 1991; Aamodt *et al.,* 1991; Krause *et al.,* 1994).

VIII. Other Applications of Transformation Technology

A. Promoter/Gene Trap Screens

For many purposes, it is useful to identify developmentally critical genes based on their expression patterns. The details of the *C. elegans* transformation system facilitate this type of screen by allowing several hundred *lacZ* fusions to be incorporated into a single extrachromosomal array (Hope, 1991). A library of plasmid constructs with the *lacZ* coding sequence fused to random genomic segments is constructed in bacteria. Pools of cloned DNAs from the library are injected with a selectable marker such as *rol-6* to generate transgenic lines, each of which contains many different potential *lacZ* fusions. Lines are then stained to determine the expression pattern of *lacZ*. The responsible clone can in general be isolated by successive expression assays of subpools from the original DNA population. This scheme has been used to isolate chromosomal segments with a variety of defined promoter activities (Hope, 1991; G. Seydoux and A. Fire, unpublished).

B. Screens for Altered Expression Pattern

Transgenic lines expressing specific reporter molecules can be a starting point in a mutagenic analysis of *cis-* and *trans-*acting regulatory signals. A strain exhibiting a defined expression pattern is mutagenized and allowed to grow for one to three generations depending on the nature of the mutation to be isolated. Animals are then screened for altered expression patterns. In screens for viable mutant animals, this could be done either by using a marker visible in live animals (Chalfie *et al.*, 1994) or by fixing adult animals with retention of live embryos in the uterus (Sebastiano *et al.*, 1986; Fire, 1992; Xie, Jia, and Aamodt, pers. comm.). Screens for lethal or sterile mutants would also be possible, using a scheme incorporating cloning of individual mutagenized animals or sib selection.

The precise properties of the transgenic line used in the initial mutagenesis are critical in determining the facility with which a screen for altered expression can be carried out. In particular, any mosaicism or incomplete staining may make the isolation of strains with decreased or lost aspects of the expression pattern difficult. The converse screen, looking for strains exhibiting extra or ectopic expression, should be practical even with a modest degree of mosaicism in the original transgenic lines.

C. Reverse Genetics

Many molecular approaches to developmental questions lead to the identification of genes for which no preexisting genetic data are available. At present, the best schemes for determining loss-of-function phenotypes are labor-intensive chemical and transposon mutagenesis strategies (Waterston, 1986; Barstead and

Waterston, 1991; Zwaal *et al.,* 1993). Alternatively, antisense expression can give a strong suggestion of hypomorph or loss-of-function phenotype (Fire *et al.,* 1991; Greenstein and Ruvkun, pers. comm.); in considering an antisense approach, however, it should be understood that antisense can never be used as a definitive assessment of gene knockout, since the possibility of residual expression of the endogenous gene remains, even with a vast excess of the antisense transcript.

Analysis of gene function in *C. elegans* is likely to be facilitated by future developments in DNA transformation technology. In particular, recent demonstrations of (rare) homologous recombination events between transgenes and their chromosomal counterparts (Plasterk and Groenen, 1992; Broverman *et al.,* 1993; S. Harrison and A. Fire, unpublished; S. Kim, pers. comm.) indicate that we should eventually be able to modify endogenous genes at will.

Acknowledgments

We thank the worm community for sharing their observations on DNA transformation, and L. Bloom, J. Kramer, M. Montgomery, J. Priess, G. Seydoux, and D. Shakes for comments on the manuscript. Work in the authors' laboratories is supported by the National Institutes of Health. A. F. is a Rita Allen Foundation Scholar.

References

Aamodt, E. J., Chung, M. A., and McGhee, J. A. (1991). Spatial control of a gut-specific esterase during *Caenorhabditis elegans* development. *Science* **252,** 579–582.

Barstead, R. J., and Waterston, R. H. (1991). Vinculin is essential for muscle function in the namatode. *J. Cell Biol.* **114,** 715–724.

Broverman, S., MacMorris, M., and Blumenthal, T. (1993). Alteration of *Caenorhabditis elegans* gene expression by targeted transformation. *Proc. Natl. Acad. Sci. U.S.A.* **90,** 4359–4363.

Chalfie, M., Tu, Y., Euskirchen, G., Ward, W., and Prasher, D. (1994). Green fluorescent protein as a marker for gene expression. *Science* **263,** 802–805.

Evans, T. C., Crittenden, S. L., Kodoyaianni, V., and Kimble, J. (1994). Translational control of maternal glp-1 mRNA establishes an asymmetry in the *C. elegans* embryo. *Cell* **77,** 183–194.

Field, J., Nikawa, J.-I., Broek, D., MacDonald, B., Rodgers, L., Wilson, I., Lerner, R., and Wigler, M. (1988). Purification of a RAS-responsive adenylyl cyclase complex from *Sacchromyces cerevisae* by use of an epitope addition method. *Mol. Cell. Biol.* **8,** 2159–2165.

Fire, A. (1986). Integrative transformation of *Caenorhabditis elegans. EMBO J.,* **5,** 2673–2680.

Fire, A. (1992). Histochemical techniques for locating *Escherichia coli* β-galactosidase activity in transgenic organisms. *Genet. Anal. Tech. Appl.* **9,** 152–160.

Fire, A. and Waterston, R. (1989). Proper expression of myosin genes in transgenic nematodes. *EMBO J.* **8,** 3419–3428.

Fire, A., Harrison, S., and Dixon, D. (1990). A modular set of *lacZ* fusion vectors for studying gene expression in *Caenorhabditis elegans. Gene* **93,** 189–198.

Fire, A., Kondo, K., and Waterston, R. (1990). Vectors for low copy transformation of *C. elegans. Nucleic Acids Res.* **18,** 4269–4270.

Fire, A., Albertson, D., Harrison, S. W., and Moerman, D. G. (1991). Production of antisense RNA leads to effective and specific inhibition of gene expression in *C. elegans* muscle. *Development* **113,** 503–514.

Freedman, J., Slice, L., Dixon, D., Fire, A., and Rubin, C. (1993). The novel metallothionein genes of *Cuenorhabditis elegans.* Structural organization and cell-specific transcription. *J. Biol. Chem.* **268,** 2554–2564.

Goodwin, E. B., Okkema, P. G., Evans, T. C., and Kimble, J. (1993). Translational regulation of tra-2 by its 3′ untranslated region controls sexual identity in *C. elegans*. *Cell* **75**, 329–339.

Hamelin, M., Scott, I. M., Way, J. C., and Culotti, J. G. (1992). The *mec-7* beta-tubulin gene of *Caenorhabditis elegans* is expressed primarily in the touch receptor neurons. *EMBO J.* **11**, 2885–2893.

Hamelin, M., Zhou, Y., Su, M., Scott, J., and Culotti, J. (1993). Expression of the UNC-5 guidance receptor in the touch neurons of C. elegans steers their axons dorsally. *Nature* **364**, 327–330.

Hope, I. A. (1991). "Promoter trapping" in *Caenorhabditis elegans*. *Development* **113**, 399–408.

Jefferson, R. A., Klass, M., Wolf, N., and Hirsh, D. (1987). Expression of chimeric genes in *Caenorhabditis elegans*. *J. Mol. Biol.* **193**, 41–46.

Kennedy, B. P., Aamodt, E. J., Allen, F. L., Chung, M. A., Heschl, M. F., and McGhee, J. D. (1993). The gut esterase gene from the nematodes *Caenorhabditis elegans* and *Caenorhabditis briggsae*. *J. Mol. Biol.* **229**, 890–908.

Kim, S. K., and Horvitz, H. R. (1990). The Caenorhabditis elegans gene lin-10 is broadly expressed while required specifically for the determination of vulval cell fates. *Genes Dev.* **4**, 357–371.

Kimble, J., Hodgkin, J., Smith, T., and Smith, J. (1982). Suppression of an amber mutation by microinjection of suppressor tRNA in C. elegans. *Nature* **299**, 456–458.

Kramer, J., French, R. P., Park, E., and Johnson, J. J. (1990). The *Caenorhabditis elegans* rol-6 gene, which interacts with the *sqt-1* collagen gene to determine organismal morphology, encodes a collagen. *Mol. Cell. Biol.* **10**, 2081–2090.

Krause, M., Fire, A., Harrison, S. W., Priess, J., and Weintraub, H. (1990). CeMyoD accumulation defines the body wall muscle cell fate during *C. elegans* embryogenesis. *Cell* **63**, 907–919.

Krause, M., White Harrison, S., Xu, S., Chen, L., and Fire, A. (1994). Elements regulating cell and stage-specific expression of the *C. elegans* MyoD homolog *hlh-1*. *Dev. Biol.* **166**, 133–148.

Kucherlapati, R. S., Eves, E. M., Song, K. Y., Morse, B. S., and Smithies, O. (1984). Homologous recombination between plasmids in mammalian cells can be enhanced by treatment of input DNA. *Proc. Natl. Acad. Sci. U.S.A.* **80**, 3153–3157.

Lin, F.-L., Sperle, K., and Sternberg, N. (1984). Model for homologous recombination during transfer of DNA into mouse L cells: Role for DNA ends in the recombination process. *Mol. Cell. Biol.* **4**, 1020–1034.

Macmorris, M., and Blumenthal, T. (1993). In situ analysis of *C. elegans* vitellogenin fusion gene expression in integrated transgenic strains-effects of promoter mutations on RNA localization. *Gene Expression* **3**, 27–36.

Macmorris, M., Spieth, J., Madej, C., Lea, K., and Blumenthal, T. (1994). Analysis of the VPE sequences in the *Caenorhabditis elegans* vit-2 promoter with extrachromosomal tandem array-containing transgenic strains. *Mol. Cell. Biol.* **14**, 484–491.

Maniatis, T., Fritsch, E. F., and Sambrook, J. (1982). "Molecular cloning, A Laboratory Manual" Cold Spring Harbor Press, Cold Spring Harbor, New York.

Mello, C. C., Kramer, J. M., Stinchcomb, D., and Ambros, V. (1991). Efficient gene transfer in *C. elegans*: Extrachromosomal maintenance and integration of transforming sequences. *EMBO J.* **10**, 3959–3970.

Miller, D. M., Shen, M. M., Shamu, C. E., Burglin, T. R., Ruvkun, G., Dubois, M. L., Ghee, M., and Wilson, L. (1992). C. elegans unc-4 gene encodes a homeodomain protein that determines the pattern of synaptic input to specific motor neurons. *Nature* **355**, 841–845.

Moerman, D., Benian, G., Barstead, R., Schriefer, L., and Waterston, R. (1988). Identification and intracellular localization of the unc-22 gene product of C. elegans. *Genes Dev.* **2**, 93–105.

Okkema, P., White-Harrison, S., Plunger, V., Aryana, A., and Fire, A. (1993). Sequence requirements for myosin gene expression and regulation in C. elegans. *Genetics*, **135**, 385–404.

Orr-Weaver, T. L., Szostak, J. W., and Rothstein, R. J. (1981). Yeast transformation: A model system for the study of recombination. *Proc. Natl. Acad. Sci. U.S.A.* **78**, 6354–6358.

Perry, M., Li, W., Trent, C., Robertson, B., Fire, A., Hageman, J., and Wood, W. (1993). Molecular characterization of the *her-1* gene suggests a direct role in cell signaling during *Caenorhabditis elegans* sex determination. *Genes Dev.* **7**, 216–228.

Plasterk, R., and Groenen, J. (1992). Targeted alterations of the *Caenorhabditis elegans* genome by transgene instructed DNA double strand break repair following Tc1 excision. *EMBO J.* **11**, 287–290.

Rosenbluth, R. E., Cuddeford, C., and Baillie, D. L. (1985). Mutagenesis in *Caenorhabditis elegans*. II. A spectrum of mutational events induced with 1500 R of gamma-radiation. *Genetics* **109**, 493–511.

Rushforth, A. M., Saari, B., and Anderson, P. (1993). Site-selected insertion of the transposon Tc1 into a *Caenorhabditis elegans* myosin light chain gene. *Mol. Cell. Biol.* **13**, 902–910.

Sebastiano, M., D'Alessio, M., and Bazzicalupo, P. (1986). Beta Glucuronidase mutants in the nematode *Caenorhabditis elegans*. *Genetics* **112**, 459–468.

Stinchcomb, D. T., Shaw, J. E., Carr, S. H., and Hirsh, D. (1985). Extrachromosomal DNA transformation of *Caenorhabditis elegans*. *Mol. Cell. Biol.* **5**, 3484–3496.

Stringham, E. G., Dixon, D. K., Jones, D., and Candido, E. P. M. (1992). Temporal and spatial expression patterns of the small heat-shock (HSP16) genes in transgenic *Caenorhabditis elegans*. *Mol. Biol. Cell* **3**, 221–233.

van Luenen, H. G., Colloms, S. D., and Plasterk, R. H. (1993). Mobilization of quiet, endogenous Tc3 transposons of *Caenorhabditis elegans* by forced expression of Tc3 transposase. *EMBO J.* **12**, 2513–2520.

Way, J. C., Wang, L., Run, J. Q., and Wang, A. (1991). The *mec-3* gene contains cis-acting elements mediating positive and negative regulation in cells produced by asymmetric cell division in *Caenorhabditis elegans*. *Genes Dev.* **5**, 2199–2211.

Wightman, B., Ha, I., and Ruvkun, G. (1993). Posttranscriptional regulation of the heterochronic gene *lin-14*, by *lin-4* mediates temporal pattern formation in *C. elegans*. *Cell* **75**, 855–862.

Zwaal, R. R., Broeks, A., van Meurs, J., Groenen, J. T., and Plasterk, R. H. (1993). Target-selected gene inactivation in *Caenorhabditis elegans* by using a frozen transposon insertion mutant bank. *Proc. Natl. Acad. Sci. U.S.A.* **90**, 7431–7435.

CHAPTER 20

Transcription and Translation

Michael Krause

Laboratory of Molecular Biology
National Institute of Diabetes, Digestive, and Kidney Diseases
National Institutes of Health
Bethesda, Maryland 20892

I. Introduction

The genetics of *Caenorhabditis elegans* provides a convenient experimental entry point into many developmental processes and a powerful tool that can be exploited to characterize interactions among a set of genes regulating a particular pathway. Eventually, though, the study of developmental processes becomes a molecular study of gene regulation. At this level, the determination of the on/ off state of a gene requires an understanding of not only its transcriptional state, but also post-transcriptional, translational, and post-translational control mechanisms.

Although the vertebrate literature is rich in details of factors that influence these regulatory processes, relatively few of the factors responsible for gene expression in the nematode *C. elegans* have been characterized. This lag in knowledge reflects both the relatively recent arrival of *C. elegans* on the list of experimental systems, as well as its general unsuitability for biochemistry. There are no tissue culture cell lines established from *C. elegans,* and it is difficult to isolate, in large amounts, any homogeneous cell type. Moreover, the impermeable eggshell encasing the embryo and the cuticle encasing the worm make pharmacological studies in intact animals difficult and tedious.

Grim as this sounds, progress has been made in *C. elegans* in the field of gene expression. The sensitivity of techniques has improved and the available molecular tool kit has expanded. The study of individual genes has provided descriptions of several regulatory processes, some general and some gene specific. Our current level of understanding of gene regulation is sufficient to say that *C. elegans* appears, in general, to be a typical eukaryote. As such, *C. elegans* is amenable to many of the standard analytical approaches used in other developmental systems. The purpose of this chapter is to review our current state of knowledge of transcription and translation in *C. elegans* (for a review of embryonic transcription, see also McGhee and Mains, 1992).

II. Transcription

A. General Information

Transcription in eukaryotes is accomplished by three RNA polymerases, each transcribing a particular type of RNA; RNA polymerase I transcribes ribosomal RNA, RNA polymerase II transcribes mRNAs and snRNAs, and RNA polymerase III transcribes tRNAs and other low-molecular-weight RNAs. Genes transcribed by RNA polymerases I and III have been cloned from the nematode and their organization and sequence suggest they behave like those of other eukaryotes. Beyond this, not much is known about the biochemistry of their function or the details of the subsequent processing of the transcripts. The discussion in this chapter therefore focuses on RNA polymerase II transcription.

B. Embryonic Transcription

Historically, the nematode has been presented as a prime example of "mosaic" development in which maternally provided determinants are segregated during embryogenesis in a stereotypical and invariant fashion, resulting in the autonomous execution of cell fates. An early demonstration of such development in *C. elegans* came from embryos that were able to express cell-specific markers in lineal precursors after cleavage arrest at various stages of embryogenesis (Laufer *et al.,* 1980; Cowan and McIntosh, 1985; Edgar and McGhee, 1986). The importance of maternal factors is evident from many genetic studies over the years that show that most of embryogenesis is dependent and directed by factors present in the oocyte; maternal effect lethals often die late in embryogenesis and zygotic lethals tend to die after hatching (see, e.g., Kemphues *et al.,* 1988; Storfer-Glazer and Wood, 1994). Yet, as the events in early embryogenesis become dissected in more detail, it becomes evident that zygotic gene activity, minor as it may be, most likely plays a critical role in early embryogenesis.

Studies in some developmental systems, such as *Drosophila* and *Xenopus,* show there are discrete times in development when embryonic transcription of mRNA begins. For flies, bulk zygotic transcription begins at a transition from the syncytial blastoderm stage to cellularization (Edgar and Schubiger, 1986). In frogs, zygotic transcription is initiated at the midblastula transition (MBT) and occurs about 8 hours after fertilization, when there are greater than 4000 cells (Newport and Kirshner, 1982a,b). For both of these organisms, this transitional point signals a conversion from a dependence on maternally encoded products to those produced by the embryonic genome. These precedents, coupled with the early molecular and genetic evidence in favor of a maternally directed, ''mosaic'' pattern of development in the early embryo, suggested that a similar transitional stage might exist during *C. elegans* embryogenesis.

As the techniques and probes available to address this question in the worm have increased in sensitivity, the time of the earliest observed zygotic transcription has been pushed closer to the beginning of embryonic development. The data now support the notion that at least some zygotic transcription occurs as early as the four-cell embryo. Therefore, in *C. elegans* there may not be a sharp transition from maternal to zygotic transcription analogous to MBT. Instead, zygotic transcription, of at least a few genes, starts shortly after fertilization, reminiscent of mammalian (Clegg and Piko, 1983) and ascidian (Meedel and Whittaker, 1978) development. In *C. elegans,* this early expression presumably serves to augment the more substantial maternal contributions, and together these gene products direct development.

Several molecular studies in the nematode have focused on identifying the earliest stage of detectable zygotic transcription. Hecht *et al.* (1981) used *in situ* hybridization to detect poly(A)-containing RNAs in squashed embryos. They showed that *C. elegans* embryonic nuclei could be labeled (inferring novel transcription) at the 90- to 100-cell stage of embryogenesis.

Subsequent studies by Edgar and McGhee (1986, 1988) on gut-specific gene expression corroborated these results and suggested that a much earlier onset of zygotic transcription might occur. Schauer and Wood (1990), using nuclear run-on transcription assays, showed that this was indeed the case; zygotic message is present prior to the 30-cell stage of embryogenesis. Somewhat surprisingly, quantitation of transcription suggested that from about the 30-cell stage and beyond, the rate of transcription per nucleus is constant and at its maximal level.

The earliest detectable zygotic transcription in these experiments, estimated to involve 20 to 30 genes, occurred in approximately 8-cell embryos. The inability to collect perfectly synchronized embryos, however, made it difficult to determine the exact cell number of embryos actively transcribing.

More recent experiments have yielded the same results by assaying the incorporation of radiolabeled nucleotides in cultured embryos that have been stripped of their eggshell. Because individual embryos can be assayed by this approach, it provides a more exact correlation between label incorporation, cell number, and localization of incorporated counts. The earliest detected zygotic transcription in these permeabilized embryos occurs between the 8- and 16-cell stages, in which label is seen uniformly over the nuclei of all cells of the embryo (Edgar *et al.*, 1994).

With time, several maternally and zygotically active genes have been cloned, allowing one to study specific, rather than general, transcriptional initiation. One example relevant to early zygotic expression is the *skn-1* gene. Antibodies raised against the *skn-1* gene product have localized this maternal product in nuclei of the embryo from the one- to the four-cell stages, during which time it becomes localized to the two posterior blastomeres (Bowerman *et al.*, 1993). By the eight-cell stage, SKN-1 is no longer detectable in any blastomere; SKN-1 is expressed again later in development. The *skn-1* gene encodes a protein resembling bZIP transcription factors and is known to affect determination of the EMS blastomere in the four-cell embryo (Bowerman *et al.*, 1992). By the time it disappears at the eight-cell stage it has presumably already exerted its effects on its target genes. Assuming SKN-1 is acting as a positive transcription factor, this result implies that zygotic expression of SKN-1 targets must occur at, or before, the four-cell stage of embryogenesis, when SKN-1 is last detected.

Analyses of individual zygotic transcription units have become possible with the development of gene fusion assays and improved *in situ* hybridization protocols (see Chapters 14 and 15 in this volume). Several of these studies demonstrate an early onset of zygotic transcription. For example, a *hlh-1::lacZ* reporter gene faithfully reproduces the endogenous *hlh-1* expression pattern, including a transient period of expression beginning just prior to the 28-cell stage. Because this pattern of expression is observed when the reporter gene is donated by the male to cross-progeny, zygotic transcription of this transgene must begin prior to the 28-cell stage (Chen *et al.*, 1992; L. Edgar, pers. comm.).

Seydoux and Fire have used both gene fusions assays and *in situ* hybridization to detect expression of several genes prior to the 28-cell stage of embryogenesis, such as the histone H1 gene and *lin-19*. The earliest detectable transcription begins in the four-cell embryo; hybridization with a probe to *pes-10* (a gene of unknown function as yet) yields a signal in the nuclei of the three somatic cells of the embryo (Seydoux and Fire, 1994). Because the hybridization signal in these cases is localized to the nucleus, and is absent at earlier stages, one assumes that zygotic transcription is responsible for the signal.

C. Postembryonic Transcription

The postembryonic transcription pattern of several genes of *C. elegans* has been studied in some detail (Honda and Epstein, 1990; Kramer *et al.*, 1985; Spieth *et al.*, 1988; Austin and Kimble, 1989). Although there are good examples of stage-, tissue-, and sex-specific expression, for most of these genes the elements regulating their respective patterns of transcription have yet to define general rules governing postembryonic transcription in the nematode. (Specific elements and post-transcriptional regulatory mechanisms are discussed later.) For example, the collagen gene family consists of about 150 genes in *C. elegans* that are combinatorially expressed to give rise to the fluctuating cuticular repertoire of the animal during development (Kramer *et al.*, 1982; Cox and Hirsh, 1985; Cox *et al.*, 1984); however, even this large and dynamically expressed set of genes has failed to provide any molecular clues as to the factors responsible for the temporal specificity of transcription of these genes. Similarly, the well-characterized vitellogenin gene promoters have not yet led to the identification of the transcription factors responsible for tissue- or sex-specific expression (Spieth *et al.*, 1985).

What has emerged from these studies, in combination with embryonic expression studies, are a couple of developmental themes regarding transcription in the nematode. First, the same gene may be expressed at different times of development to affect widely different developmental processes. This multiuse phenomenon for a single gene product is not novel; it is commonly seen with many genes in *Drosophila* development, exemplified by segmentation genes such as *engrailed* (Lawrence and Morata, 1976; Lawrence and Struhl, 1982; Brower, 1986) and *fushi tarazu* (Carroll and Scott, 1985). In *C. elegans*, the *glp-1* gene provides the clearest example of a gene that serves different functions at different stages of development. The *glp-1* gene encodes a protein that is related to the Notch family of transmembrane receptor proteins. Not surprisingly, the *glp-1* product is involved in several cell–cell interactions throughout development. *glp-1* mediates inductive interactions in the early embryo important for pharyngeal development (Priess *et al.*, 1987) and controls germ cell proliferation in the adult (Austin and Kimble, 1987). An additional level of redundancy of *glp-1* function is provided by its close relative, *lin-12*, which also mediates many cell–cell interactions (Yochem *et al.*, 1988; Yochem and Greenwald, 1989). Double mutants in both *glp-1* and *lin-12* demonstrated that these homologous genes share overlapping functions and can compensate for one another in certain developmental processes (Lambie and Kimble, 1991).

A second general theme to emerge from the study of postembryonic transcription is that gene expression is influenced by positional information in the animal. The examples to date indicate the existence of an anteroposterior positional signaling mechanism; other axial cues may also exist but have yet to be identified.

The most overt example of positional expression comes from a set of homeotic genes in the nematode. Like *Drosophila* and the vertebrates, *C. elegans* contains a cluster of *antennapedia* class homeotic genes that are expressed in certain domains along the anteroposterior axis of the animal (Bürglin *et al.,* 1991; Wang *et al.,* 1993). As yet, the mechanisms that establish the anteroposterior pattern of expression for these genes is unknown, but the pattern presumably reflects the action of some sort of positional signaling system. Furthermore, these homeotic genes are presumably influencing the expression of several target genes that consequently are also expressed in a position-dependent manner.

Two other lines of evidence support a role for position-dependent influences on expression. Vitellogenin gene transcription in the gut of intersex mosaic animals was shown by *in situ* hybridization often to be graded. Higher levels of *vit* gene expression were seen in the posterior cells of the intestine as compared with the anterior cells, suggesting that sex determination in the intestine is influenced by anteroposterior position (Schedin *et al.,* 1991). Second, screens for enhancer sequences active in body wall muscle cells have turned up several enhancer elements which preferentially activate transcription in the anterior or posterior of the animal (A. Fire and S. Xu, pers. comm.). Regardless of their biological relevance to normal expression, the properties of these enhancer elements demonstrate that anterior–posterior positional cues are active in the body wall muscles.

D. Germ-Line Expression

Although artificial, several transgenic studies have shown that gene expression in the germ line is regulated differently from that of somatic cells (discussed in greater detail in Chapter 19). Genes that are known to be expressed and function in the germ line frequently are not expressed when fused to the β-galactosidase reporter gene. For example, *glp-1* is expressed in germ cells to regulate their proliferative (Austin and Kimble, 1987); however, *glp-1::lacZ* transgenes fail to be expressed in either the germ line or the early embryo (J. Priess and A. Fire, pers. comm.). It is not clear if this is primarily a problem of transcription, translation, or a combination of both. Whatever the cause, the lack of reporter gene expression in the germ line demonstrates that the mechanisms regulating germ-line expression are different from those of the somatic tissue, where numerous reporter gene constructs have been used successfully (Fire *et al.,* 1990).

A difference between germ-line and somatic expression might also be responsible for the early embryonic pattern of expression of *lin-19* and *pes-10* seen by Seydoux and Fire (1994). These genes are transcribed in the early somatic lineages but not in the germ-line progenitor blastomeres P1 through P4. These authors suggest the possibility that the germ-line progenitor blastomeres suppress expression of these genes that are otherwise ubiquitously expressed in the early lineages (Seydoux and Fire, 1994).

E. Chromatin Structure and Expression

In higher eukaryotes, the role of nucleosomes and higher-order chromatin structure are beginning to be defined at the molecular level. For example, methylation, histone acetylation, nucleosome positioning, and chromatin domain boundaries are all known to be involved in the regulation of transcription for many genes (Felsenfeld and McGhee, 1982; Wittig and Wittig, 1982; Forrester *et al.*, 1987; Felsenfeld, 1992; Lee *et al.*, 1994; Chung *et al.*, 1993).

Caenorhabditis elegans has typical eukaryotic histone genes, including H1, suggesting a general organization of chromatin analogous to that of other eukaryotes (Roberts *et al.*, 1989; Sanicola *et al.*, 1990). Histone acetylation may play a role in gene expression in the nematode as it does in other systems. Recent studies with antisera specific for each of the four monoacetylated isoforms of histone H4 have demonstrated unique staining patterns in *C. elegans*. For example, antiserum to one form of acetylated H4 stains only the nuclei of early spermatocytes, whereas antisera specific for two other H4 isoforms stain the nuclei of all cells at all developmental stages. Antiserum to the remaining H4 isoform uniquely stains the nucleoli of all cells (Sussel and Meyer, pers. comm.). The relationship between these staining patterns and gene expression is, at present, unknown. Methylation of cytosine residues does not appear to occur in *C. elegans* eliminating it from playing a role in gene expression (Simpson *et al.*, 1986).

To date there has been only a single study of chromatin structure and specific gene expression. Dixon, Jones, and Candido (1990) investigated changes in chromatin structure of heat shock genes before and after induction by assaying DNAseI hypersensitive sites and micrococcal nuclease sensitivity in isolated nuclei. They showed that nuclease sensitive sites did change upon heat shock suggesting an alteration in chromatin configuration accompanies induction of these heat shock genes.

On a more global scale, two proteins have been identified in *C. elegans* that appear to play a role in chromatin structure. Nishiwaki *et al.*, (1993) have shown that the embryonic lethal gene *emb-5* encodes a protein present in all interphase nuclei of the embryo. The predicted EMB-5 protein is similar to a nuclear protein in yeast that is thought to play a role in chromatin assembly or modification (Swanson *et al.*, 1990). A second protein, that is encoded by the dosage compensation gene *dpy-27*, has been shown to be a homolog of a chromosome condensation protein (Chuang *et al.*, 1994). In *C. elegans,* dosage compensation reduces the X chromosome expression in hermaphrodite nuclei (XX) to the level of expression from the single X chromosome in male nuclei (XO) (Meyer and Casson, 1986). In hermaphrodite nuclei, the DPY-27 protein is localized specifically to the two X chromosomes whereas in male nuclei DPY-27 appears distributed throughout the nucleus. This strongly suggests that the down regulation of X chromosome expression in hermaphrodites is a consequence of DPY-27 induced alterations in the chromatin structure of the X chromosomes (Chuang *et al.*, 1994).

Two other lines of evidence reflect a critical role for chromatin structure in *C. elegans* gene expression. Edgar and McGhee (1988) demonstrated that a specific round of DNA replication was necessary to express certain gut cell marker genes, suggesting that an alteration in chromatin structure might be required to convert these genes from silent to potentially active states. A second piece of evidence linking chromatin structure and gene expression in *C. elegans* comes from studies of transgenic animals that show mosaic patterns of transgene expression when the transgene is integrated into the genome. For the genes *ges-1, vit-2,* and *hlh-1,* certain gene sequences promote expression in transgenic animals in a mosaic pattern. These mosaic patterns of expression frequently follow lineal boundaries and are stable over several cell divisions (Aamodt *et al.,* 1991; MacMorris *et al.,* 1994; Krause *et al.,* 1994). Because different animals from the same transgenic strain show different patterns of expression, the expression of the transgene in any given lineage appears to be stochastic. Since all cells contain the DNA in an integrated transgenic line, the ability to express the gene must reflect an ability of each expressing cell to exceed some threshold for assembly of a stable transcription complex. These stochastic expression patterns could be explained with models that invoke chromatin structure alterations as a critical event in the establishment and inheritance of stable transcription complexes (Felsenfeld, 1992).

F. Transcriptional Regulatory Elements and Factors

The *C. elegans* gene for the large subunit of RNA polymerase II has been cloned and shown to encode a protein that resembles its vertebrate counterparts (Bird and Riddle, 1989). For most polymerase II transcribed genes in *C. elegans,* one can find a sequence fitting the consensus TATA element about 30 bp upstream of the transcriptional start site. Recently, a cDNA encoding the TATA box binding protein, or TBP subunit of TFIID, has been identified in the nematode. This protein shows extended regions of sequence similarity to vertebrate TBP, binds to a TATA box sequence, and can substitute for vertebrate TFIID basal activity in *in vitro* extracts (Lichtsteiner and Tjian, 1993). These results illustrate, as expected, a high degree of evolutionary conservation in the basic transcription machinery. It is likely that most of the vertebrate basal transcription factors exist in *C. elegans* and will be uncovered in directed searches or through the genome sequencing project.

In addition to these general features, gene-specific control elements (such as enhancers) have been defined for several *C. elegans* genes. These elements are often identified through a combination of approaches that together suggest they play a role in the normal pattern of expression. One of these approaches is a systematic functional assay using transgenic strains harboring reporter genes fused to the promoter of interest (Fire *et al.,* 1990; see Chapter 19 in this volume). Important control regions can be delineated by serial deletions or enhancer assays in which gene segments are tested for their ability to drive correct cell type expression of "naive" promoters (Aamodt *et al.,* 1991; Okkema *et al.,* 1993; Krause *et al.,* 1994).

A second approach to identifying gene control elements involves sequence comparisons between *C. elegans* and more distantly related nematode species such as *C. briggsae* and *C. vulgaris* (Snutch *et al.,* 1988; Zucker-Aprison and

Blumenthal, 1989; Heschl and Baillie, 1990; Kennedy *et al.*, 1993; Lee *et al.*, 1993; Krause *et al.*, 1994). Functional regulatory elements in noncoding regions of the gene will show a much higher degree of conservation than the flanking nonfunctional sequences. Sequence motifs identified in interspecific comparisons can then be assayed for function in transgenic strains.

Some of the control elements defined to date look remarkably similar to their vertebrate counterparts. The heat shock genes of *C. elegans* have been well characterized (Jones *et al.*, 1986; Kay *et al.*, 1987; Dixon *et al.*, 1990). Their function depends on a consensus eukaryotic heat shock element that binds heat shock protein. The evolutionary conservation of these elements is sufficient enough to allow the nematode sequences to function in vertebrate cells (Kay *et al.*, 1986).

Analysis of the vitellogenin gene promoters of *C. elegans* also reveals an evolutionarily conserved regulatory mechanism. The *vit* genes in the nematode are expressed only in the intestinal cells of L4 and adult hermaphrodites and are positively regulated, in part, by GATA box elements (Spieth *et al.*, 1988; MacMorris *et al.*, 1992). In vertebrates, GATA box-binding transcription factors play a role in the expression of many erythroid-specific genes. At least two GATA-like proteins have been identified in *C. elegans,* although their developmental roles have yet to be determined (Spieth *et al.*, 1991; J. McGhee, personal communication). Their presence, however, does suggest that the GATA system of endodermal gene regulation has ancient roots.

In addition to the heat shock and *vit* genes, a number of other examples of transcription factors from the nematode underscore the high degree of conservation, in both sequence and function, of transcription factors through evolution. Most of the transcription factor families defined in other eukaryotes have relatives in *C. elegans*. A partial compilation of these genes is shown in Table I.

G. Message 3' End Processing

Message maturation in mammals includes cleavage and polyadenylation at specific 3' end sites of the primary transcript (for review, see Wahle and Keller, 1992). These reactions are catalyzed by a complex of several proteins that recognize the poly(A) signal sequence, AAUAAA, and a second, undefined sequence element downstream (Irniger and Braus, 1994). The message is cleaved 10 to 35 nucleotides downstream of the poly(A) signal sequence, and a second enzymatic activity in the complex carries out the polyadenylation reaction, resulting in 50 to 250 adenosine residues attached to the 3' end of the mature message.

In *C. elegans* 3' end message maturation seems to follow a similar pathway. A recent analysis of 1300 cDNA clone sequences shows that polyadenylation usually begins about 13 nucleotides downstream of a sequence matching the AAUAAA consensus (T. Blumenthal, O. White, and C. Fields, pers. comm.). Some variations on this six-nucleotide consensus sequence are tolerated, most notably in the first position (22% have bases other than A) and the fourth position

Table I

Transcription Factor Genes Identified in *Caenorhabditis elegans*

Family	Gene	Product	Function	Reference[a]
Homeodomain				
POU class	*unc-86*	UNC-86	Neurogenesis	1
	ceh-6	CEH-6	Neurogenesis	2
	ceh-18	CEH-18	Hypodermis/molting	3
HOM-C class	*egl-5*	EGL-5	Posterior body	4, 5
	lin-39	LIN-39	Middle body	4, 5
	mab-5	MAB-5	Mid-posterior body	4, 5
	mab-18	MAB-18	Anterior body	6
Other	*vab-7*	VAB-7	Posterior body	7
	mec-3	MEC-3	Neurogenesis	8
	ceh-10	CEH-10	Neurogenesis?	9
	ceh-22	CEH-22	Pharyngeal muscle	10
	unc-30	UNC-30	Neurogenesis	11
Zinc finger				
GATA class	*elt-1*	ELT-1	Intestine?	12
	elt-2	ELT-2	Intestine?	13
Other	*tra-1*	TRA-1	Sex determination	14
	sdc-1	SDC-1	Sex determination dosage compensation	15
	sdc-3	SDC-3	Sex determination dosage compensation	16
	egl-43	EGL-43	HSN migrations	17
	lin-26	LIN-26	Hypodermis/germ line	18
	lin-29	LIN-29	Seam cell differentiation	19
Helix–loop–helix				
	hlh-1	CeMyoD	Body wall myogenesis	20
	hlh-2	CeE12/47	Ubiquitous HLH protein?	21
	hlh-3	HLH-3	Neurogenesis?	22
	hlh-4	HLH-4	Neurogenesis?	22
	lin-32	LIN-32	Neurogenesis (ray development)	23
Steroid receptor				
	daf-12	DAF-12	Dauer formation	24
	crf-1	CRF-1	Unknown	25
	crf-2	CRF-2	Posterior body	26
Fork head/HNF-3				
	lin-31	LIN-31	Vulval cell fate	27
	fkh-1	Cefkh-1	Intestine	28
	pes-1	PES-1	Early embryo	29
Miscellaneous				
(b-ZIP?)	*skn-1*	SKN-1	EMS blastomere specification	30
(CSD/Y-box)	*cey-1*	CEY-1	Body wall muscle?	31
(ETS domain)	*lin-1*	LIN-1	Vulval induction	32
(MADS box)	X	CeMef-2	Myogenesis/neurogenesis?	33

[a] 1. Finney *et al.*, 1988
2. Bürglin *et al.*, 1989
3. D. Greenstein and G. Ruvkun, pers. comm.
4. Wang *et al.*, 1993
5. Bürglin *et al.*, 1991

20. Krause *et al.*, 1990
21. A. Fire, G. Seydoux, and M. Krause, unpublished
22. J. Yuan, I. Greenwald, and M. Cole, pers. comm.
23. C. Zhao and S. Emmons, pers. comm.
24. P. Larsen, W.-H. Yeh, and D. Riddle, pers. comm.

(continues)

Table I (*Continued*)

6. Y. Zhang and S. Emmons, pers. comm.	25. R. Eagen, A. Purac, P. Davison, and B. Honda, pers. comm.
7. J. Ahringer, pers. comm.	26. A. Sluder and G. Ruvkun, pers. comm.
8. Way and Chalfie, 1989	27. Miller *et al.*, 1993
9. P. Svendsen and J. McGhee, pers. comm.	28. M. Azzaria, B. Goszczynski, and J. McGhee, pers. comm.
10. Okkema and Fire, 1994	
11. Y. Jin, R. Hoskins, and R. Horvitz, pers. comm.	29. Hope, 1994
12. Spieth *et al.*, 1991	30. Bowerman *et al.*, 1992
13. J. McGhee, pers. comm.	31. V. Jantsch-Plunger, W. Kelly, and A. Fire, pers. comm.
14. Zarkower and Hodgkin, 1992	
15. Nonet and Meyer, 1991	32. G. Beitel, X. Lu, and R. Horvitz, pers. comm.
16. Klein and Meyer, 1993	33. D. Dichoso and M. Krause, unpublished
17. Garriga *et al.*, 1993	
18. M. Labouesse, pers. comm.	
19. J. Bettinger, K. Mansanares, and A. Rougvie, pers. comm.	

(13% have G). Utilization of the consensus sequence and variants at positions 1 and 4 accounts for about 94% of the sequenced clones; another 6% of clones have no identifiable poly(A) signal sequence.

H. *cis*-splicing

Caenorhabditis elegans, like most eukaryotes, has genes composed of exons separated by introns, the latter being removed as part of message maturation. The splicing of conventional introns in the nematode appears to be very similar to eukaryotic splicing, involving a snRNP-containing spliceosome complex. The genes encoding the standard eukaryotic snRNP RNAs (U1, U2, U4, U5, and U6) have been cloned from the nematode and are of expected structure and sequence (Thomas *et al.*, 1990).

Introns in *C. elegans* genes are smaller in general than those of other eukaryotes; a compilation of introns for cloned genes suggests an average intron length of about 50 bp (Blumenthal and Thomas, 1988). Larger introns also exist; for example, the *act-4* gene contains a 2081-bp intron (Krause *et al.*, 1989) and introns larger than 1 kb are commonly encountered as the list of sequenced genes expands (e.g., see Krause *et al.*, 1990; Kennedy *et al.*, 1993).

The most obvious features of intron sequences are the boundary splice site sequences. Like other eukaryotes, the nematode fits the GT/AG rule; that is, intron sequences in genes begin with the residues GT and end with the residues AG (Tables II and III). The splice site consensus sequences for *C. elegans* genes can be further extended with gene donor sites usually fitting the sequence **GT**RART (where R is a purine) and acceptor sites usually fitting the sequence TTTC**AG** (Fields, 1990). This extended 3' consensus splice sequence is not typical for higher eukaryotes and has been shown to be poorly used when introduced into mammalian cells (Kay *et al.*, 1987; Ogg *et al.*, 1990). The pyrimidines in this

Table II
5′ Intron Splice Donor Sites[a]

	−3	−2	−1		1	2	3	4	5	6	7
A	78	112	29		0	0	116	140	24	38	48
C	49	36	9		0	0	1	15	4	14	14
G	41	12	128		192	0	50	16	148	11	23
U	24	32	26		0	192	25	21	16	129	107
Consensus	N	A	G		**G**	**U**	**A**	**A**	**G**	**U**	**U**

[a] Raw data compiled by, and courtesy of, Phil Green.

sequence have been experimentally determined to influence splice site choice in *C. elegans in vivo* (Conrad *et al.*, 1993). A second departure from mammalian splicing is that intron branch sites have not been identified in the nematode, even though U2 snRNP genes exist in the nematode and contain an exact match to the U2 sequence that recognizes the intron branch site in vertebrate splicing reactions. These features of nematode introns, along with their high A/U sequence content, suggest they may be more closely related to plant introns than to vertebrate introns (Fields, 1990).

Recently, exceptions (albeit unnatural) to the GT/AG rule have been reported for intron splicing in *C. elegans.* For two genes, *let-23* and *dpy-10,* there are reduction-of-function mutations that alter the 3′ AG dinucleotide of a short intron (53 nucleotides and 48 nucleotides, respectively) to AA. Although in both cases this change results in aberrant splicing products, there is also frequent use of the AA dinucleotide as the 3′ splice site (Aroian *et al.*, 1993). A different allele of *let-23,* in which the AG at the 3′ end of a 316-nucleotide intron was altered to AA, showed exclusive use of this 3′ AA splice site. These results demonstrate that the 3′ AG dinucleotide is not necessarily required for 3′ splice site selection in *C. elegans.*

I. *Trans*-splicing

One of the surprising phenomena to emerge from the study of nematode genes is *trans*-splicing. *Trans*-splicing is defined as the ligation of exon sequences

Table III
3′ Intron Splice Acceptor Sites[a]

	−7	−6	−5	−4	−3	−2	−1		1	2	3
A	53	12	0	14	4	192	0		61	62	59
C	21	6	1	32	157	0	0		25	40	43
G	8	3	0	18	1	0	192		88	22	39
U	110	171	191	128	30	0	0		18	68	51
Consensus	U	U	U	U	C	**A**	**G**		R	N	N

[a] Raw data compiled by, and courtesy of, Phil Green.

originating in independently transcribed RNAs. This contrasts with conventional eukaryotic *cis*-splicing, described above, in which intervening RNA sequences are removed from a single primary transcript during message maturation. Although the process of *trans*-splicing had been previously described in trypanosomes (Van der Ploeg *et al.,* 1982; Nelson *et al.,* 1983; Kooter *et al.,* 1984; Sutton and Boothroyd, 1986; Murphy *et al.,* 1986), it was unexpected in a prototypical metazoan like the nematode, particularly because conventional introns had previously been identified. The nematode is, to date, the only animal that combines both *cis*- and *trans*-splicing mechanisms during the maturation of a single message.

The discovery of *trans*-splicing in *C. elegans* came from a routine characterization of the actin genes. In an attempt to resolve conflicting results obtained in determining the transcriptional intitiation site for some of the actin genes, it was found (by direct RNA sequencing) that the 5′-most 22 nucleotides of these RNA were not encoded by the actin genes themselves (Krause, 1986). Instead, these 22 nucleotides originate as part of a novel, small RNA. This RNA is transcribed principally from the 1-kb repeat that also contains the 5 S ribosomal RNA genes. The 5 S ribosomal repeat is present in the genome of *C. elegans* at about 110 copies (Nelson and Honda, 1985). The novel small RNA, known now as spliced leader RNA or SL1 RNA, donates its 5′-most 22 nucleotides (nt) (SL1) to the actin messages by a splicing reaction *in trans* (Krause and Hirsh, 1987; Bektesh *et al.,* 1988; Thomas *et al.,* 1988). As each actin gene also contains conventional introns, maturation of these actin mRNAs involves both *cis*- and *trans*-splicing.

Subsequent work has shown that a large fraction (perhaps greater than 40%) of messages in *C. elegans* are *trans*-spliced to the 22-nt SL1 leader sequence (Spieth *et al.,* 1993). The requirements for the recipient message to acquire the SL sequence appear to be relatively simple. The 5′ UTR region of a gene need have only a 3′ splice acceptor lacking an upstream 5′ splice donor site to be a substrate for *trans*-splicing (Conrad *et al.,* 1991, 1993). Such a gene segment has been termed an *outron* to distinguish it from conventional *cis*-spliced introns. More subtle features of outrons, such as sequence composition, may be important for splicing but are difficult to identify.

Conventional eukaryotic *cis*-splicing has been well characterized and the mechanism is understood in some detail (for review, see Moore *et al.,* 1993). *Cis*-splicing occurs in a complex known as a spliceosome that consists of proteins and small nuclear ribonucleoprotein particles, or snRNPs, that catalyze the splicing reaction. The spliceosomal snRNPs (U1, U2, U4, U5, and U6) each play specific roles in splice site and branch site selection and often involve a base pairing intermediate between the message and a region of the RNA of the particular snRNP.

SL1 RNA can also assemble as a snRNP. SL1 RNA has a trimethylguanosine cap at its 5′ end, can adopt a secondary structure similar to the splicing snRNP RNAs, and associates with SM, a protein that is characteristic of splicing snRNPs (Bruzik *et al.,* 1988; Thomas *et al.,* 1988; Van Doren and Hirsh, 1988). The *trans*-splicing reaction is catalyzed by most of the same snRNPs that participate in *cis*-

splicing (Thomas *et al.*, 1990; Hannon *et al.*, 1991). The key difference between *cis*- and *trans*-splicing is that in the latter reaction, the U1 snRNP of the spliceosome complex is apparently replaced by a SL1 snRNP. Unlike U1 snRNP, which recognizes the 5′ donor sequence in *cis*-splicing, the SL1 snRNP actually donates the 5′-most 22 nt of its RNA to the splicing reaction and is therefore partially consumed in the reaction.

Nilsen and colleagues have developed an *in vitro* splicing system for nematodes based on extracts from the pig parasitic nematode *Ascaris lumbricoides* (Hannon *et al.*, 1990; Yu *et al.*, 1993). This system has been extremely useful in further defining, biochemically, the components required for both *cis* and *trans*-splicing in nematodes (Nilsen, 1993).

If SL1 snRNP can participate with other snRNPs used in *cis*-splicing, one might expect that SL1 sequences could be donated to 3′ splice acceptor sites normally involved in *cis*-splicing, resulting in truncated and nonfunctional messages. As there is no evidence that SL1 interferes with conventional intron splicing, the two processes must be distinct, either temporally, spatially, or functionally. One possibility is that SL1 snRNP participation in a conventional spliceosome might be inefficient relative to U1 snRNP so that *cis*-splicing is favored. A spliceosome that is "stalled," because of a missing donor site, might then be available to interact with the SL snRNP, resulting in a *trans*-splicing reaction (Conrad *et al.*, 1993).

The function of the SL sequence on mRNA is unknown; there is no obvious pattern or commonality between messages that receive the SL1 sequence. SL sequences might stabilize the message or enhance its translational efficiency. For most gene products, either of these attributes might be favorable, thereby imparting a selective advantage. Under this assumption, if the 5′ UTR of a gene acquires, through mutation, an unpaired 3′ splice site, the resulting message will be *trans*-spliced to SL1 and the mutation will be fixed by selection. This leads to a stochastic accumulation of *trans*-spliced messages biased only by the under-representation of messages that cannot tolerate SL1 addition.

J. SL2 and Polycistronic Messages

The *trans*-splicing story took a new twist with the discovery of a second spliced leader RNA, known as SL2 RNA. SL2 sequences were first uncovered in the course of characterizing glyceraldehyde-3-phosphate dehydrogenase (GAPDH) mRNAs (Huang and Hirsh, 1989). There are four GAPDH genes in *C. elegans;* mRNA derived from three of these genes is predominantly *trans*-spliced to SL1, whereas that from the fourth is *trans*-spliced to SL2. SL2 is also 22 nt long and is somewhat similar to SL1; 17 of the 22 nt positions can be aligned between the two sequences if the appropriate gaps are introduced. Like SL1, SL2 originates as the 5′ terminus of a small transcript, designated SL2 RNA. Unlike SL1, there are only a handful of SL2 genes in *C. elegans* and they are dispersed in the genome.

Although both SL sequences are acquired by *trans*-splicing, these two SL sequences are generally found on distinct sets of messages. That is, the mRNA population from any given gene that undergoes *trans*-splicing will usually have either SL1 or SL2, not a mixture of both. (There are several exceptions to this rule, such as *gpd-2,* which is *trans*-spliced to both SL1 and SL2.) The general exclusivity in SL selection implies that the *trans*-splicing machinery can distinguish between different messages. The obvious candidate for such a distinction is the primary nucleotide sequence of the RNA; it is possible that the original messages contain signal sequences that specify which of the two SL RNAs will be *trans*-spliced. It had been previously demonstrated that *trans*-splicing to SL-1 requires apparently only the presence of an outron with a 3' splice site; no other obvious sequence or structural requirements can be identified (Conrad *et al.,* 1991).

The resolution to this SL leader selection paradox came from the observation by Spieth *et al.* (1993) that genes that acquire SL2 are always immediately downstream of, and in the same orientation as, an upstream transcription unit. They postulated that these juxtaposed genes may constitute a polycistronic transcription unit in which a single promoter initiates transcription that is continuous through two or more genes (Spieth *et al.,* 1993).

Like *trans*-splicing, the notion of polycistronic transcription in *C. elegans* was viewed at first with a bit of skepticism. Yet, as with *trans*-splicing, precedents for such polycistronic transcription had been found in the trypanosomes. In trypanosomes, polycistronic primary transcripts are processed to monocistronic message by *trans*-splicing reactions that recognizes a splice site between the two messages (Johnson *et al.,* 1987; Muhich and Boothroyd, 1988; Tschudi and Ullu, 1988). It appears that the same type of processing occurs in *C. elegans* except that only SL2, and not SL1, can recognize the appropriate internal splice site of cotranscribed genes. Experimental evidence for this mechanism of processing comes from transgenic animals harboring novel constructs of juxtaposed genes. Spieth *et al.* (1993) were able to convert an SL1 *trans*-spliced message to SL2 *trans*-splicing by placing the message in the downstream position of a polycistronic transcription unit.

How are these two *trans*-splicing reactions distinguished mechanistically? Unfortunately, we do not yet know the answer to this question. Genes that are *trans*-spliced to SL2 are immediately downstream of a second gene, usually separated by about 100 bp, although no sequence similarity is obvious among the characterized intergenic regions. Spieth *et al.* (1993) have suggested that the process of SL2 *trans*-splicing may be linked to message maturation and 3' end processing (cleavage and polyadenylation). An association of the SL2 snRNP with 3' processing enzymes might set the stage for SL2 *trans*-splicing and distinguish SL2- from SL1-catalyzed events. Alternatively, cleavage at the poly(A) site for the upstream message might result in an uncapped 5' terminus of the downstream message that, in turn, could be a substrate for SL2 *trans*-splicing. Surprisingly, unlike SL1, which is conserved in sequence and present in almost all nematodes examined, SL2 has only been detected in *C. elegans* and *C. briggsae* (Lee *et al.,* 1992). It is not yet known whether polycistronic transcription is similarly restricted to only some species of nematodes.

The current model for *trans*-splicing specification, then, is that the presence of an outron at the start of a gene seems to dictate SL1 *trans*-splicing, whereas polycistronic transcripts are processed to individual messages via SL2 *trans*-splicing. There are exceptions to every rule, however, and one has recently emerged in the case of SL2 *trans*-splicing. The gene *ced-9* gives rise to multiple messages, some of which are the result of bicistronic transcription initiating at a promoter preceding an upstream gene, *cyt-1,* encoding cytochrome b_{560} (Hengartner and Horvitz, 1994). The prediction is that the bicistronic transcript would be processed by *trans*-splicing of SL2 to generate the 5' end of the mature downstream message, *ced-9.* Yet, polymerase chain reaction (PCR) results show that the predominant SL sequence on this *ced-9* message is SL1, not SL2 (Hengartner and Horvitz, 1994). Unlike other SL2 processed polycistronic RNAs in which the nested messages are separated by about 100 nt, the messages in the *cyt-1/ced-9* bicistronic RNA are immediately adjacent to each other; the position of poly(A) addition to *cyt-1* transcripts overlaps the *trans*-splice acceptor sequence of *ced-9* transcripts. As a result, the 3' end cleavage of *cyt-1* message would destroy the *trans*-splice acceptor sequence of the downstream *ced-9* message, suggesting that SL acquisition would be via *trans*-splicing to the bicistronic transcript. It is possible that in such cases, SL1 is the preferred splice donor. If, however, SL1 is also capable of participating in *trans*-splicing reaction-mediated polycistronic message maturation, then other factors must influence which of the two SL snRNPs is predominantly used for any individual message.

Another complexity to the *trans*-splicing story is the emergence of variant SL RNAs in *C. elegans.* Kuwabara and Kimble (1992) showed that *tra-2* message was *trans*-spliced to SL2. Using the RACE (rapid amplification of cDNA ends) PCR method (Frohman *et al.,* 1988), they sequenced several cloned products representative of the 5' end of the *tra-2* message. In addition to the previously identified SL2 sequence (Huang and Hirsh, 1989), they also identified five novel variants that differed from the original SL2 sequence in from one to four positions. Similarly, Rubin and colleagues have shown heterogeneity in the SL2 sequences found *trans*-spliced to protein kinase C 1a messages (Land *et al.,* 1994a,b). They have identified at least five additional SL2-like genes encoding some of these variants and mapped them to dispersed sites in the genome (Table IV) (L. Ross and C. Rubin, pers. comm.). One of these five SL2-like genes could encode one of the variant SL2 sequences *trans*-spliced to *tra-2* as determined by Kuwabara and Kimble (1992).

It is possible that these SL2 variants randomly participate in *trans*-splicing reactions along with the original SL2 but are just not as abundant as SL2, due to either gene number or level of transcription. A low incidence (less than 10–20%) of heterogeneity within SL sequences on a given message would not readily be detected by directly sequencing the mRNA or sequencing a limited

Table IV
Novel Splice Leader Sequences (SLn)[a]

A. Splice Leaders on novel SL RNA genes	
SLn1, 2, 5	GGTTTTAACCCAGTTAACCAAG
SLn3	GGTTTTAACCCAAGTTAACCAAG
SLn4	GGTTTTAACCCATATAACCAAG
B. Splice leaders on RACE products	
(tra-2; pkc)	GGTTTTAACCCAGTTTAACCAAG
	GGTTTTAACCCAGTTACCAAG
	GGTTTTTACCCAGTTAACCAAG
(tra-2)	GGTTTTAACCCAGTTAACCAAG
	GGTTTAAAACCCAGTTAACAAG
(pkc)	GGTTTATACCCAGTTAACCAAG
(ckIIb)	GGTTTTAACCAGTTAACTAAG
	GTTTTAAACCCAGTTAATTGAG

[a] Data kindly provided by Charles Rubin.

number of cDNA clones. Heterogeneity may also exist for SL1 *trans*-splicing but remain undetected because of the predominately large number (110) of identical SL1 genes. The implications for SL heterogeneity on gene expression are not clear because the function of any SL sequence remains to be determined.

III. Post-transcriptional Regulation

Gene expression is often regulated post-transcriptionally by mechanisms that control message stability or translatability. Several examples of post-transcriptional regulation have been described in *C. elegans,* and each has parallels to mechanisms described in higher eukaryotes. Those described to date undoubtedly represent only a few of the variety of regulatory mechanisms operating to control gene expression in the nematode.

A. Messenger RNA Stability

An example of a general post-transcriptional control mechanism was identified from studies of three different genes: *tra-2, lin-29,* and *unc-54.* A search for suppressors of specific alleles of each of these genes converged on a single set of six genes that together define the Smg system of suppression (Hodgkin *et al.,* 1989). Smg mutant animals themselves have only a minor phenotype, affecting principally sexually dimorphic tissues of the animal [hence their name: suppressors with morphogenetic effects on genitalia (Hodgkin *et al.,* 1989)]. These Smg mutants have characteristics of general informational suppressors because their ability to suppress is allele specific but not gene specific.

Help in understanding the Smg system came from the molecular analysis available with the *unc-54* mutations. Many mutant alleles of *unc-54* have been isolated and characterized at the molecular level (Dibb *et al.*, 1985; Pulak and Anderson, 1988). The *smg* genes were able to suppress both nonsense alleles of *unc-54* and a 3'-terminal deletion that did not involve the coding region. Analysis of *unc-54* mutant message levels in either a *smg*(+) or *smg*(−) background showed that the stability of these aberrant RNAs is enhanced when the Smg system is debilitated by mutations in one of the six *smg* genes (Pulak and Anderson, 1993). In other eukaryotes, aberrant messages are more rapidly degraded than are their wild-type counterparts, suggesting a regulatory system, possibly coupled to translation, that targets these abnormal RNAs for turnover. The *unc-54* results suggest that the *smg* genes constitute a similar surveillance system in *C. elegans* that serves to prevent the accumulation of aberrant RNAs (Pulak and Anderson, 1993). Although aberrations of the Smg system have only modest effects in a wild-type genetic background, much more dramatic effects can be seen in animals carrying mutations that produce erroneous messages encoding dominant toxic products.

B. Translational Regulation

The remaining examples of post-transcriptional control in *C. elegans* are thought to affect specific subsets of genes; that is, they are not general regulatory systems as exemplified by the Smg system described above. One of the more surprising examples comes from the study of the heterochronic genes, a set of genes that control the timing of many cell fates during larval development (Ambros and Horvitz, 1984; Ambros, 1989). A key player in this genetically well-characterized pathway is the gene *lin-14* (Ambros and Horvitz, 1987; Ruvkun *et al.*, 1989), which encodes a nuclear protein (Ruvkun and Giusto, 1989). Although *lin-14* message is constant in level during development, LIN-14 protein is present in a temporal gradient; high levels are detected in late-stage embryos and L1 larvae followed by a rapid decrease to very low levels beginning in L2 larvae (Ruvkun and Giusto, 1989). It is this gradient of LIN-14 that coordinately determines the temporal pattern of many cell lineages during larval development.

The constant level of *lin-14* steady-state RNA suggested that the temporal gradient of LIN-14 resulted from control of either the translation of the message or the stability of the protein. The former possibility was more likely, as mutants of *lin-14* that prevent the downregulation of the protein at the L2 stage mapped to the 3' UTR of the *lin-14* message (Wightman *et al.*, 1991). By including these 3' UTR sequences in *lacZ* reporter gene constructs, it was shown that the 3' UTR of *lin-14* was sufficient to confer the temporal pattern of regulation to unrelated proteins (Wightman *et al.*, 1993).

A second gene, *lin-4,* was also known to be an important factor in the temporal downregulation of LIN-14 protein (Ambros, 1989; Arasu *et al.,* 1991). Interestingly, when the *lin-14* gene was cloned and characterized by Ambros and colleagues (Lee *et al.,* 1993), they found it did not encode a protein. Instead, *lin-4* produces two small RNAs (22 and 61 nt long) that are complementary to several regions in the 3' UTR of the *lin-14* message. Taken together, these results suggest that the translation of *lin-14* message is negatively regulated by an antisense interaction between *lin-4* gene products and the 3' UTR of *lin-14* mRNA (Lee *et al.,* 1993; Wightman *et al.,* 1993).

It is not yet known how, in mechanistic terms, such interactions lead to an inhibition of *lin-14* translation. Possible mechanisms include a disruption of ribosome binding to the *lin-14* mRNA and the formation of a binding site for a protein that sequesters the message in an untranslatable form or subcellular compartment. Although this is the first (and only) example in *C. elegans,* the regulation of genes by natural antisense RNA has been well documented in other systems, both prokaryotic and eukaryotic (for reviews, see Simons, 1988; Eguchi *et al.,* 1991). Synthetic antisense disruption of gene expression has been observed in *C. elegans,* with transgenic strains harboring certain *unc-22* gene constructs (Fire *et al.,* 1991), and has been used to study the function of the POU class homeodomain protein encoded by the *ceh-18* gene (Greenstein *et al.,* 1994; D. Greenstein and G. Ruvkun, pers. comm.).

In the course of studying genes in the sex determination pathway, two other cases of post-transcriptional regulation have been encountered; one involves *fem-3,* the other *tra-2.* Genetic evidence suggests that maternal *fem-3* RNA, donated to the oocyte, is translated very early in embryogenesis. Two attributes of maternal *fem-3* message seem important for its embryonic post-transcriptional regulation. First, Ahringer *et al.* (1992) have shown that this maternal message includes a longer poly(A) tract at its 3' end than *fem-3* RNA present in the adult hermaphrodite. By analogy to other systems (Wickens, 1990), they suggest that this extended poly(A) tract could function to increase the translational activity of this *fem-3* message. A second feature of the *fem-3* message is an inverted repeat sequence in the 5' UTR that potentially can base pair to form a stem–loop structure. In *Xenopus,* stem–loops can block translation of mRNAs until after fertilization, when RNA helicases become active and presumably unwind such structures (Fu *et al.,* 1991). It is possible that the *fem-3* 5' UTR repeats negatively regulate translation until they are destabilized by a helicase activity or other mechanisms.

The *tra-2* gene provides another example of post-transcriptional regulation via repeated sequences, but distinct from that seen with *fem-3.* For *tra-2,* the controlling sequence is a pair of direct repeat elements (DRE), each 28 nt long, found in the 3' UTR of the *tra-2* message (Goodwin *et al.,* 1993). The importance of DRE was uncovered in the course of defining the molecular basis of several *tra-2* gain-of-function mutations (Hodgkin and Brenner, 1977). Six of these *tra-2(gf)* mutations map to the 3' end of the gene and affect the DRE (Okkema and Kimble, 1991). Subsequently it was shown that (1) disruption of the DRE results in the association of *tra-2* RNA with larger polysomes than wild-type *tra-2* RNA, (2) DRE have no effect on *tra-2* RNA levels, (3) transfer of DRE to a reporter gene message in transgenic animals was sufficient to inhibit reporter message translation, and (4) DRE bind a factor in *C. elegans* extracts as assayed by RNA gel retardation (Goodwin *et al.*, 1993). Taken together, these results suggest that DRE constitute a binding site for a protein(s) that blocks translation of the message. The recently identified gene *laf-1* may represent this repressor (E. B. Goodwin and J. Kimble, pers. comm.). Because homozygous *laf-1* mutants are lethal, the DRE-based system of translational repression may be controlling the expression of other, as yet unidentified, genes.

The *glp-1* gene provides another example in which 3′ UTR sequences (unrelated to *tra-2* DRE) appear to regulate the translation of the message. *glp-1* RNA is maternally inherited and detectable in all blastomeres to the eight-cell stage of embryogenesis (Evans *et al.*, 1994); however, genetic studies demonstrate that early embryonic *glp-1* activity is required only in the AB lineage to mediate certain cell fate decisions (Priess *et al.*, 1987; Austin and Kimble, 1987), consistent with immunolocalization of GLP-1 protein to only the anterior blastomeres after the two-cell stage (Evans *et al.*, 1994). Injection of *in vitro* synthesized RNA, from reporter gene fusions, into the maternal gonad have shown that the 3′ UTR of *glp-1* is sufficient to confer this spatial and temporal pattern of protein expression in the embryo. This suggests that the 3′ UTR normally represses translation of maternal *glp-1* RNA in one-cell embryos and subsequently only in posterior blastomeres after the two-cell stage.

The sequences within the 3′ UTR of *glp-1* message that regulate temporal and spatial translation have been localized to specific elements (Evans *et al.*, 1994). The spatial control element contains sequences remarkably similar to nanos response elements that are required to spatially restrict the translation of *hunchback* in *Drosophila* embryos (Tautz and Pfeifle, 1989; Wharton and Struhl, 1991). As with the previous examples, it is too early to say for *C. elegans* how this element functions in mechanistic terms or whether it will be involved in the regulation of other genes. The parallels to *Drosophila* suggest regulation of *glp-1* may involve a protein related to *nanos* in the fly.

IV. Translation

Very little is known about the translational machinery of *C. elegans*. Several ribosomal proteins have been identified in random searches, but there has not been any study directed at their function. It is presumed that these factors function in nematode translation in a manner analogous to those described in other eukaryotes; however, *C. elegans* will undoubtedly use some unique mechanisms as a result of many messages sharing the same 5′-terminal sequence as a result of *trans*-splicing.

Although almost all eukaryotic proteins are initiated at a methionine codon, not all methionine codons are used to initiate translation of a protein. Clearly other factors influence the specification of the initiator methionine, such as surrounding nucleotide sequence and its relative position in the message (Kozak, 1991). Based on a systematic study of mutants in mammalian cells, Kozak assembled a consensus sequence for an optimal translational start site (GCCAC-CAUGG). She showed that deviations from this consensus at positions −3 and +4 had the strongest effects on proper initiation (the A of the AUG is defined as position +1) (Kozak, 1991).

Although there has been no systematic study of translation initiation in *C. elegans,* a comparison of translational initiation sites for 48 *C. elegans* proteins has been compiled in connection with the genome sequencing project (Table V) (P. Green, pers. comm.). The consensus sequence for the nematode shows some similarity to the Kozak consensus; all 48 proteins initiate with AUG and a purine (usually A) is in position −3. Aside from this, there is a tendency for A residues to precede the AUG, but it is difficult to derive a strong consensus sequence around the AUG.

Messages that are *trans*-spliced to splice leaders pose additional questions about the mechanism of translational initiation in nematodes. Eukaryotic mRNAs are capped at the 5′ end by a monomethylguanosine residue that is important in the recognition of mRNAs by the ribosome initiation complex; it is thought that non-*trans*-spliced messages in the nematode similarly have a monomethylguanosine cap. In contrast, several groups have shown that SL RNAs (like U RNAs) have a trimethylguanosine cap (Van Doren and Hirsh, 1988; Thomas *et al.,* 1988). *Trans*-spliced messages appear to retain the trimethylguanosine cap donated by the SL RNA (Liou and Blumenthal, 1990) and should, therefore, be poor substrates for translation if the mammalian rules apply to *C. elegans.*

A second question regarding translational initiation of *trans*-spliced messages concerns the sequence context of the initiator methionine codon. Kozak (1991)

Table V
Translational Start Sites[a]

	−7	−6	−5	−4	−3	−2	−1	1	2	3	4
A	21	13	12	29	31	20	22	48	0	0	13
C	7	10	16	11	3	10	12	0	0	0	8
G	3	11	5	5	12	8	5	0	0	48	17
U	7	14	15	3	2	10	9	0	48	0	10
Consensus	A	N	N	A/C	A/G	A	A	**A**	**U**	**G**	N

SL1: GGUUUAAUUACCCAAGUUUGAG
SL2: GGUUUUAACCCAGUUACUCAAG

[a] Raw data compiled by, and courtesy of, Phil Green.

Table VI
Codon Usage for *Caenorhabditis elegans* Genes[a]

Codon	AA[b]	Raw	Fraction	Codon	AA[b]	Raw	Fraction
UUU	F	277	28%	GAU	D	1067	60%
UUC	F	726	72%	GAC	D	705	40%
UUA	L	86	4%	UCU	S	499	26%
UUG	L	504	20%	UCC	S	433	23%
CUU	L	880	36%	UCA	S	352	18%
CUC	L	721	29%	UCG	S	266	14%
CUA	L	73	3%	AGU	S	163	9%
CUG	L	198	8%	AGC	S	190	10%
AUU	I	658	42%	CCU	P	143	10%
AUC	I	810	52%	CCC	P	77	6%
AUA	I	81	6%	CCA	P	1008	72%
				CCG	P	171	12%
AUG	M	720	100%				
				ACU	T	489	32%
GUU	V	687	41%	ACC	T	581	38%
GUC	V	600	36%	ACA	T	292	19%
GUA	V	144	8%	ACG	T	169	11%
GUG	V	254	15%				
				GCU	A	988	43%
UGU	C	273	47%	GCC	A	822	35%
UGC	C	310	53%	GCA	A	371	16%
				GCG	A	134	6%
UAU	Y	296	39%				
UAC	Y	465	61%	CGU	R	631	36%
				CGC	R	328	19%
CAU	H	317	49%	CGA	R	169	10%
CAC	H	332	51%	CGG	R	71	4%
				AGA	R	478	28%
CAA	Q	1098	69%	AGG	R	57	3%
CAG	Q	490	31%				
				GGU	G	291	15%
AAU	N	618	43%	GGC	G	107	6%
AAC	N	827	57%	GGA	G	1465	76%
				GGG	G	55	3%
AAA	K	594	28%				
AAG	K	1495	72%	GAA	E	1200	48%
				GAG	E	1321	52%
UGG	W	217	100%				

[a] Raw data compiled by, and courtesy of, Phil Green.
[b] Amino acid.

showed that changes in spacing between the AUG and the block of preceding consensus sequence strongly interfered with translation of mammalian mRNAs. In the nematode, the SL sequence is often found to be *trans*-spliced to within one or two nucleotides of the initiation AUG. Because this juxtaposed SL sequence is variably spaced relative to the AUG in different transcripts, the context around the initiation codon would likewise be variable.

How does the nematode translational machinery initiate these SL-containing messages? Presumably the SL sequence, directly or indirectly, is able to bind to the ribosomal protein complex by a mechanism that may be distinct from that of conventional mRNAs. As yet, the role of SL sequences in translation of mRNA is not known, but it has been suggested that these sequences might enhance the translation of messages, perhaps by increasing their affinity to polysomes. Understanding the relationship between SL sequences and translation should be informative in understanding the purpose of *trans*-splicing.

Genes that are abundantly expressed in organisms usually show a strong codon bias; that is, certain codons for particular amino acids are more commonly used within coding regions than others (Sharp and Li, 1987). *C. elegans* similarly shows a general bias toward the use of certain codons for some amino acids. Emmons (1988) published a codon usage table for *C. elegans* based on the limited number of sequences available at the time. The bias of codon usage in this early table has held up as the set of sequences has increased. The most recent data on codon usage in *C. elegans* were compiled as part of the genome sequencing project and are presented in Table VI (P. Green, pers. comm.).

A comparison of several gene families (e.g., actin, myosin, and collagen) showed that within a family, the codon usage was consistently biased toward the same codon preferences (C. Fields, pers. comm.). Comparisons between different families, however, showed that codon biases were sometimes drastically reduced, or even reversed, such that rare codons were consistently used within the coding region. For example, the actin and vitellogenin genes show a 200:1 preference for the use of CCA to CCU proline codons. In contrast, the gene *ama-1*, encoding the large subunit of RNA polymerase II, shows only a 5:1 preference for the use of CCA to CCU proline codons. Such codon bias differences suggest that codon asymmetry could be involved in the regulation of some genes (C. Fields, pers. comm.). It is worth noting that the codon bias of *C. elegans* is not common to all nematodes; the few genes sequenced from *C. vulgaris* suggest that this nematode has a codon bias different from that of *C. elegans* (A Fire, pers. comm.).

Acknowledgments

Thanks to Tom Blumenthal, Andy Fire, and Geraldine Seydoux for helpful comments on the text, to Phil Green for providing coding sequence and splice site data, and to the many other worm community members that allowed me to make use of their unpublished information.

References

Aamodt, E. J., Chung, M. A., and McGhee, J. D. (1991). Spatial control of gut-specific gene expression during development. *Science* **252**, 579–582.

Ahringer, J., Rosenquist, T. A., Lawson, D. N., and Kimble, J. (1992). The *Caenorhabditis elegans* sex determining gene *fem-3* is regulated post-transcriptionally. *EMBO J.* **11,** 2303–2310.

Ambros, V., and Horvitz, H. R. (1984). Heterochronic mutants of the nematode *Caenorhabditis elegans. Science* **266,** 409–416.

Ambros, V., and Horvitz, H. R. (1987). The *lin-14* locus of *Caenorhabditis elegans* controls the time of expression of specific postembryonic developmental events. *Genes Dev.* **1,** 398–414.

Ambros, V. (1989). A hierarchy of regulatory genes controls a larva-to-adult developmental switch in *C. elegans. Cell* **57,** 49–57.

Arasu, P., Wightman, B., and Ruvkun, G. (1991). Temporal regulation of *lin-14* by the antagonistic action of two other heterochronic genes, *lin-4* and *lin-28. Genes Dev.* **5,** 1825–1833.

Aroian, R. V., Levy, A. D., Koga, M., Ohshima, Y., Kramer, J. M., and Sternberg, P. W. (1993). Splicing in *Caenorhabditis elegans* does not require an AG at the 3′ splice acceptor site. *Mol. Cell. Biol.* **13,** 626–637.

Austin, J., and Kimble, J. (1987). *glp-1* is required in the germ line for regulation of the decision between mitosis and meiosis in *C. elegans. Cell* **51,** 589–599.

Austin, J., and Kimble, J. (1989). Transcript analysis of *glp-1* and *lin-12,* homologous genes required for cell interactions during development of *C. elegans. Cell* **58,** 565–571.

Bektesh, S., Van Doren, D., and Hirsh, D. (1988). Presence of the *Caenorhabditis elegans* spliced leader on different mRNAs and in different genera of nematodes. *Genes Dev.* **2,** 1277–1283.

Bird, D. M., and Riddle, D. L. (1989). Molecular cloning and sequencing of *ama-1,* the gene encoding the largest subunit of *Caenorhabditis elegans* RNA polymerase II. *Mol. Cell. Biol.* **9,** 4119–4130.

Blumenthal, T., and Thomas, T. (1988). Cis- and Trans-splicing in *C. elegans. Trends Genet.* **4,** 305–308.

Bowerman, B., Eaton, B. A., and Priess, J. R. (1992). *skn-1,* a maternally expressed gene required to specify the fate of ventral blastomeres in the early *C. elegans* embryo. *Cell* **68,** 1061–1075.

Bowerman, B., Draper, B. W., Mello, C. C., and Priess, J. R. (1993). The maternal gene *skn-1* encodes protein that is distributed unequally in early *C. elegans* embryos. *Cell* **74,** 443–452.

Brower, D. (1986). *Engrailed* gene expression in *Drosophila* imaginal discs. *EMBO J.* **5,** 2649–2656.

Bruzik, J. P., Van Doren, K., Hirsh, D., and Steitz, J. A. (1988). Trans splicing involves a novel form of small nuclear ribonucleoprotein particles. *Nature* **335,** 559–562.

Bürglin, T. R., Finney, M., Coulson, A., and Ruvkun, G. (1988). *Caenorhabditis elegans* has scores of homeobox-containing genes. *Nature* **341,** 239–243.

Bürglin, T. R., Ruvkun, G., Coulson, A., Hawkins, N. C., McGhee, J. D., Schaller, D., Wittmann, C., Müller, F., and Waterston, R. H. (1991). Nematode homeobox cluster. *Nature* **351,** 703.

Carroll, S. B., and Scott, M. P. (1985). Localization of the *fushi tarazu* protein during *Drosophila* embryogenesis. *Cell* **43,** 47–57.

Chen, L., Krause, M., Draper, B., Weintraub, H., and Fire, A. (1992). Body wall muscle formation in *Caenorhabditis elegans* embryos that lack the MyoD homolog *hlh-1. Science* **256,** 240–243.

Chuang, P.-T., Albertson, D. G., and Meyer, B. J. (1994). DPY-27: A chromosome condensation protein homolog that regulates *C. elegans* dosage compensation through association with the X chromosome. *Cell* **79,** 459–474.

Chung, J. H., Whiteley, M., and Felsenfeld, G. (1993). A 5′ element of the chicken beta-globin domain serves as an insulator in human erythroid cells and protects against position effect in *Drosophila. Cell* **74,** 505–514.

Clegg, K. B., and Piko, L. (1983). Quantitative aspects of RNA synthesis and polyadenylation in 1-cell and 2-cell mouse embryos. *J. Embryol. Exp. Morphol.* **74,** 169–182.

Conrad, R., Thomas, J., Spieth, J., and Blumenthal, T. (1991). Insertion of part of an intron into the 5′ untranslated region of a *Caenorhabditis elegans* gene converts it into a trans-spliced gene. *Mol. Cell. Biol.* **11,** 1921–1926.

Conrad, R., Liou, R. F., and Blumenthal, T. (1993). Conversion of a trans-spliced *C. elegans* gene into a conventional gene by introduction of a splice donor site. *EMBO J.* **12,** 1249–1255.

Cowan, A., and McIntosh, J. (1985). Mapping the distribution of differentiation potential for intestine, muscle and hypodermis during early development in *Caenorhabditis elegans. Cell* **41,** 923–932.

Cox, G. N., Kramer, J. M., and Hirsh, D. (1984). Number and organization of collagen genes in *Caenorhabditis elegans. Mol. Cell. Biol.* **4,** 2389–2395.

Cox, G. N., and Hirsh, D. (1985). Stage-specific patterns of collagen gene expression during development of *Caenorhabditis elegans. Mol. Cell. Biol.* **5,** 363–372.

Dibb, N. J., Brown, D. M., Karn, J., Moerman, D. G., Bolten, S. L., and Waterston, R. H. (1985). Sequence analysis of mutations that affect the synthesis, assembly and enzymatic activity of *unc-54* myosin heavy chain of *C. elegans. J. Mol. Biol.* **183,** 543–551.

Dixon, D. K., Jones, D., and Candido, E. P. M. (1990). The differentially expressed 16-kD heat shock genes of *Caenorhabditis elegans* exhibit differential changes in chromatin structure during heat shock. *DNA Cell Biol.* **9,** 177–191.

Edgar, B. A., and Schubiger, G. (1986). Parameters controlling transcriptional activation during early *Drosophila* development. *Cell* **44,** 365–372.

Edgar, L. G., and McGhee, J. D. (1986). Embryonic expression of a gut-specific esterase in *Caenorhabditis elegans. Cell* **53,** 589–599.

Edgar, L. G., and McGhee, J. D. (1988). DNA synthesis and the control of embryonic gene expression in *C. elegans. Cell* **53,** 589–599.

Edgar, L. G., Wolf, N., and Wood, W. B. (1994). Early transcription in *Caenorhabditis elegans* embryos. *Development* **120,** 443–451.

Eguchi, Y., Itoh, T., and Tomizawa, J. (1991). Antisense RNA. *Annu. Rev. Biochem.* **60,** 631–652.

Emmons, S. W. (1988). The genome. *In* "The Nematode *C. elegans*" (W. B. Wood, ed.), p. 47. Cold Spring Harbor Press, Cold Spring Harbor, New York.

Evans, T. C., Crittenden, S. L., Kodoyianni, V., and Kimble, J. (1994). Translational control of maternal *glp-1* mRNA establishes an asymmetry in the *C. elegans* embryo. *Cell* **77,** 183–194.

Felsenfeld, G., and McGhee, J. (1982). Methylation and gene control. *Nature* **296,** 602–603.

Felsenfeld, G. (1992). Chromatin as an essential part of the transcriptional mechanism. *Nature* **355,** 219–224.

Fields, C. (1990). Information content of *Caenorhabditis elegans* splice site sequences varies with intron length. *Nucleic Acids Res.* **18,** 1509–1512.

Finney, M., Ruvkun, G., and Horvitz, H. R. (1988). The *C. elegans* cell lineage and differentiation gene *unc-86* encodes a protein with a homeodomain and extended similarity to transcription factors. *Cell* **55,** 757–769.

Fire, A., Harrison, S. W., and Dixon, D. K. (1990). A modular set of *lacZ* fusion vectors for studying gene expression in *Caenorhabditis elegans. Gene* **93,** 189–198.

Fire, A., Albertson, D., Harrison, S. W., and Moerman, D. G. (1991). Production of antisense RNA leads to effective and specific inhibition of gene expression in *C. elegans* muscle. *Development* **113,** 503–514.

Forrester, W. C., Takegawa, S., Papayannopoulou, T., Stamatoyannopoulos, G., and Groudine, M. (1987). Evidence for a locus activation region: The formation of developmentally stable hypersensitive sites in globin expressing hybrids. *Nucleic Acids Res.* **15,** 10159–10177.

Frohman, M. A., Dush, M. K., and Martin, G. M. (1988). Rapid production of full length cDNAs from rare transcripts: Amplification using a single gene-specific oligonucleotide primer. *Proc. Natl. Acad. Sci. U.S.A.* **85,** 8998–9002.

Fu, L., Ye, R., Browder, L. W., and Johnston, R. N. (1991). Translational potentiation of messenger RNA with secondary structure in *Xenopus. Science* **251,** 807–810.

Garriga, G., Guenther, C., and Horvitz, H. R. (1993). Migrations of the *Caenorhabditis elegans* HSNs are regulated by *egl-43,* a gene encoding two zinc finger proteins. *Genes Dev.* **7,** 2097–2109.

Goodwin, E. B., Okkema, P. G., Evans, T. C., and Kimble, J. (1993). Translational regulation of *tra-2* by its 3' untranslated region controls sexual identity in *C. elegans. Cell* **75,** 329–339.

Greenstein, D., Hird, S., Plasterk, R. H. A., Andachi, Y., Kohara, Y., Wang, B., Finney, M., and Ruvkun, G. (1994). Targeted mutations in the *C. elegans* POU homeobox gene *ceh-18* cause defects in oocyte cell cycle arrest, gonad migration, and epidermal differentiation. *Genes Dev.* **8,** 1935–1948.

Hannon, G. J., Maroney, P. A., Kenker, J. A., and Nilsen, T. W. (1990). Trans-splicing of nematode pre-messenger RNA in vitro. *Cell* **61,** 1247–1255.

Hannon, G. J., Maroney, P. A., and Nilsen, T. W. (1991). U small nuclear ribonucleoprotein requirements for nematode cis- and trans-splicing *in vitro. J. Biol. Chem.* **266,** 22792–22795.

Hecht, R. M., Gossett, L. A., and Jeffrey, W. R. (1981). Ontogeny of maternal and newly transcribed mRNA analyzed by *in situ* hybridization during development of *Caenorhabditis elegans. Dev. Biol.* **83,** 374–379.

Hengartner, M. O., and Horvitz, H. R. (1994). *C. elegans* cell survival gene *ced-9* encodes a functional homolog of the mammalian proto-oncogene *bcl-2. Cell* **76,** 665–676.

Heschl, M. P. F., and Baillie, D. (1990). Functional elements and domains inferred from sequence comparisons of a heat shock gene in two nematodes. *J. Mol. Evol.* **31,** 3–9.

Hodgkin, J., and Brenner, S. (1977). Mutations causing transformation of sexual phenotype in the nematode *Caenorhabditis elegans. Genetics* **86,** 275–287.

Hodgkin, J., Papp, A., Pulak, R., Ambros, V., and Anderson, P. (1989). A new kind of informational suppression in the nematode *Caenorhabditis elegans. Genetics* **123,** 301–313.

Honda, S., and Epstein, H. F. (1990). Modulation of muscle gene expression in *Caenorhabditis elegans:* Differential levels of transcripts, mRNAs, and polypeptides for thick filament proteins during nematode development. *Proc. Natl. Acad. Sci. U.S.A.* **87,** 876–880.

Hope, I. A. (1994). *pes-1* is expressed during early embryogenesis in *Caenorhabditis elegans* and has homology to the fork head family of transcription factors. *Development* **120,** 505–514.

Huang, X.-Y., and Hirsh, D. (1989). A second trans-spliced RNA leader in the nematode *Caenorhabditis elegans. Proc. Natl. Acad. Sci. U.S.A.* **86,** 8640–8644.

Irniger, S., and Braus, G. H. (1994). Saturation mutagenesis of a polyadenylation signal reveals a hexanucleotide element essential for mRNA 3′ end formation in *Saccharomyces cerevisiae. Proc. Natl. Acad. Sci. U.S.A.* **91,** 257–261.

Johnson, P. J., Kooter, J. M., and Borst, P. (1987). Inactivation of transcription of UV irradiation of *T. brucei* provides evidence for a multicistronic transcription unit including a VSG gene. *Cell* **51,** 273–281.

Jones, D., Russnak, R. H., Kay, R. J., and Candido, E. P. M. (1986). Structure, expression and evolution of a heat shock gene locus in *Caenorhabditis elegans* that is flanked by repetitive elements. *J. Biol. Chem.* **261,** 12006–12015.

Kay, R. J., Boissy, R. J., Russnak, R. H., and Candido, E. P. M. (1986). Efficient transcription of a *Caenorhabditis elegans* heat shock gene pair in mouse fibroblasts is dependent on multiple promoter elements which can function bidirectionally. *Mol. Cell. Biol.* **6,** 3134–3143.

Kay, R. J., Russnak, R. H., Jones, D., Mathias, C., and Candido, E. P. M. (1987). Expression of intron-containing *C. elegans* heat shock genes in mouse cells demonstrates divergence of 3′ splice site recognition sequences between nematodes and vertebrates, and an inhibitory effect of heat shock on the mammalian spicing apparatus. *Nucleic Acids Res.* **15,** 3723–3741.

Kemphues, K. J., Kusch, M., and Wolf, N. (1988). Maternal-effect lethal mutations on linkage group II of *Caenorhabditis elegans. Genetics* **120,** 977–986.

Kennedy, B. P., Aamodt, E. J., Allen, F. L., Chung, M. A., Heschl, M. F. P., and McGhee, J. D. (1993). The gut esterase gene (*ges-1*) from the nematodes *Caenorhabditis elegans* and *Caenorhabditis briggsae. J. Mol. Biol.* **229,** 890–908.

Klein, R. D., and Meyer, B. J. (1993). Independent domains of the Sdc-3 protein control sex determination and dosage compensation in *C. elegans. Cell* **72,** 349–364.

Kooter, J. M., De Lange, T., and Borst, P. (1984). Discontinuous synthesis of mRNA in trypanosomes. *EMBO J.* **3,** 2387–2392.

Kozak, M. (1991). Structural features in eukaryotic mRNAs that modulate the initiation of translation. *J. Biol. Chem.* **266,** 19867–19870.

Kramer, J. M., Cox, G. N., and Hirsh, D. (1982). Comparisons of the complete sequences of two collagen genes from *Caenorhabditis elegans. Cell* **30,** 599–606.

Kramer, J. M., Cox, G. N., and Hirsh, D. (1985). Expression of the *Caenorhabditis elegans* collagen genes *col-1* and *col-2* is developmentally regulated. *J. Biol. Chem.* **260,** 1945–1951.

Krause, M. (1986). Actin gene expression in the nematode *Caenorhabditis elegans.* Ph.D. Thesis, University of Colorado, Boulder, Colorado.

Krause, M., and Hirsh, D. (1987). A trans-spliced leader sequence on actin mRNA in *C. elegans. Cell* **49,** 753–761.

Krause, M., Wild, M., Rosenzweig, B., and Hirsh, D. (1989). Wild-type and mutant actin genes in *Caenorhabditis elegans. J. Mol. Biol.* **208,** 381–392.

Krause, M., Fire, A., Harrison, S. W., Priess, J., and Weintraub, H. (1990). CeMyoD accumulation defines the body wall muscle cell fate during *C. elegans* embryogenesis. *Cell* **63,** 907–919.

Krause, M., Harrison, S. W., Xu, S.-Q., Chen, L., and Fire, A. (1994). Elements regulating cell- and stage-specific expression of the *C. elegans* MyoD family homolog *hlh-1. Dev. Biol.* **166,** 133–148.

Kuwabara, P. E., and Kimble, J. (1992). *tra-2* encodes a membrane protein and may mediate cell communication in the *Caenorhabditis elegans* sex determination pathway. *Mol. Biol. Cell* **3,** 461–473.

Lambie, E. J., and Kimble, J. (1991). Two homologous regulatory genes, *lin-12* and *glp-1,* have overlapping functions. *Development* **112,** 231–240.

Land, M., Islas-Trejo, A., Freedman, J. H., and Rubin, C. S. (1994a). Structure and expression of a novel, neuronal protein kinase C (PKC1B) from *Caenorhabditis elegans. J. Biol. Chem.* **269,** 9234–9244.

Land, M., Islas-Trejo, A., Freedman, J. H., and Rubin, C. S. (1994b). Origin, properties, and regulated expression of multiple mRNAs encoded by the protein kinase C1 gene of *Caenorhabditis elegans. J. Biol. Chem.* **269,** 14820–14827.

Laufer, J. A., Bazzicalupo, P., and Wood, W. B. (1980). Segregation of developmental potential in early embryos of *Caenorhabditis elegans. Cell* **19,** 569–577.

Lawrence, P., and Morata, G. (1976). Compartments in the wing of *Drosophila:* A study of the *engrailed* gene. *Dev. Biol.* **50,** 321–337.

Lawrence, P., and Struhl, G. (1982). Further studies on the *engrailed* phenotype of *Drosophila. EMBO J.* **1,** 827–833.

Lee, Y. H., Huang, X.-Y., Hirsh, D., Fox, G. E., and Hecht, R. M. (1992). Conservation of gene organization and trans-splicing in the glyceraldehyde-3-phosphate dehydrogenase-encoding genes of *Caenorhabditis briggsae. Gene* **121,** 227–235.

Lee, R. C., Feinbaum, R. L., and Ambros, V. (1993). The *C. elegans* heterochronic gene *lin-4* encodes small RNAs with antisense complementarity to *lin-14. Cell* **75,** 843–854.

Lee, D. Y., Hayes, J. J., Pruss, D., and Wolffe, A. P. (1994). A positive role for histone acetylation in transcription factor access to nucleosomal DNA. *Cell* **72,** 73–84.

Lichtsteiner, S., and Tjian, R. (1993). Cloning and properties of the *Caenorhabditis elegans* TATA-box-binding protein. *Proc. Natl. Acad. Sci. U.S.A.* **90,** 9673–9677.

Liou, R.-F., and Blumenthal, T. (1990). Trans-spliced *Caenorhabditis elegans* mRNAs retain trimethyl-guanosine caps. *Mol. Cell. Biol.* **10,** 1764–1768.

MacMorris, M., Broverman, S., Greenspoon, S., Lea, K., Madej, C., Blumenthal, T., and Spieth, J. (1992). Regulation of vitellogenin gene expression in transgenic *Caenorhabditis elegans:* Short sequences required for activation of the vit-2 promoter. *Mol. Cell. Biol.* **12,** 1652–1662.

MacMorris, M., Spieth, J., Madej, C., Lea, K., and Blumenthal, T. (1994). Analysis of the VPE sequences in the *Caenorhabditis elegans vit-2* promoter with extrachromosomal tandem array-containing transgenic strains. *Mol. Cell. Biol.* **14,** 484–491.

McGhee, J. D., and Mains, P. E. (1992). Embryonic transcription in *Caenorhabditis elegans. Semin. Dev. Biol.* **3,** 163–173.

Meedel, T. H., and Whittaker, J. R. (1978). Messenger RNA synthesis during early ascidian development. *Dev. Biol.* **66,** 410–421.

Meyer, B. J., and Casson, L. P. (1986). *Caenorhabditis elegans* compensates for the difference in X chromosome dosage between the sexes by regulating transcript levels. *Cell* **47,** 871–881.

Miller, L. M., Gallegos, M. E., Morisseau, B. A., and Kim, S. K. (1993). *lin-31,* a *Caenorhabditis elegans* HNF-3/fork head transcription factor homolog, specifies three alternative cell fates in vulval development. *Genes Dev.* **7,** 933–947.

Moore, M. J., Query, C. C., and Sharp, P. A. (1993). Splicing of precursors to mRNAs by the spliceosome. *In* "The RNA World" (R. F. Gesteland and J. F. Atkins, eds.), pp. 303–357. Cold Spring Harbor Laboratory Press, Cold Spring Harbor, New York.

Muhich, M. L., and Boothroyd, J. C. (1988). Polycistronic transcripts in trypanosomes and their accumulation during heat shock: Evidence for a precursor role in mRNA synthesis. *Mol. Cell. Biol.* **8,** 3837–3846.

Murphy, W. J., Watkins, K. P., and Agabian, N. (1986). Identification of a novel Y branch structure as an intermediate in trypanosome mRNA processing; evidence for *trans* splicing. *Cell* **47,** 517–525.

Nelson, R. G., Parsons, M., Barr, P. J., Stuart, K., Selkirk, M., and Agabian, N. (1983). Sequences homologous to the variant antigen mRNA spliced leader are located in tandem repeats and variable orphons in *Trypanosoma brucei. Cell* **34,** 901–909.

Nelson, D. W., and Honda, B. M. (1985). Genes coding for 5S ribosomal RNA of the nematode *Caenorhabditis elegans. Gene* **38,** 245–251.

Newport, J., and Kirschner, M. (1982a). A major developmental transition in early *Xenopus* embryos: I. Characterization and timing of cellular changes at the midblastula stage. *Cell* **30,** 675–686.

Newport, J., and Kirschner, M. (1982b). A major developmental transition in early *Xenopus* embryos: II. Control of the onset of transcription. *Cell* **30,** 687–696.

Nilsen, T. W. (1993). Trans-splicing of nematode pre-mRNA. *Ann. Rev. Microbiol.* **47,** 413–440.

Nishiwaki, K., Sano, T., and Miwa, J. (1993). *emb-5,* a gene required for the correct timing of gut precursor cell division during gastrulation in *Caenorhabditis elegans,* encodes a protein similar to the yeast nuclear protein SPT6. *Mol. Gen. Genet.* **239,** 313–322.

Nonet, M. L., and Meyer, B. J. (1991). Early aspects of *Caenorhabditis elegans* sex determination and dosage compensation are regulated by a zinc-finger protein. *Nature* **351,** 65–68.

Ogg, S. C., Anderson, P., and Wickens, M. P. (1990). Splicing of a *C. elegans* myosin pre-RNA in a human nuclear extract. *Nucleic Acids Res.* **18,** 143–149.

Okkema, P., and Kimble, J. (1991). Molecular analysis of *tra-2,* a sex determining gene in *C. elegans. EMBO J.* **10,** 171–176.

Okkema, P., Harrison, S. W., Plunger, V., Aryana, A., and Fire, A. (1993). Sequence requirements for myosin gene expression and regulation in *C. elegans. Genetics* **135,** 385–404.

Okkema, P. G., and Fire, A. (1994). The *C. elegans* NK-2 class homeoprotein CEH-22 is involved in combinatorial activation of gene expression in pharyngeal muscle. *Development* **120,** 2175–2186.

Priess, J. R., Schnabel, H., and Schnabel, R. (1987). The *glp-1* locus and cellular interactions in early *C. elegans* embryos. *Cell* **51,** 601–611.

Pulak, R., and Anderson, P. (1988). Structures of spontaneous deletions in *Caenorhabditis elegans. Mol. Cell. Biol.* **8,** 3748–3754.

Pulak, R., and Anderson, P. (1993). mRNA surveillance by the *Caenorhabditis elegans smg* genes. *Genes Dev.* **7,** 1885–1897.

Roberts, S. B., Emmons, S. W., and Childs, G. (1989). Nucleotide sequences of *Caenorhabditis elegans* core histone genes: Genes for different histone classes share common flanking sequence elements. *J. Mol. Biol.* **206,** 567–577.

Rosenquist, T. A., and Kimble, J. (1988). Molecular cloning and transcript analysis of *fem-3,* a sex-determination gene in *Caenorhabditis elegans. Genes Dev.* **2,** 606–616.

Ruvkun, G., and Giusto, J. (1989). The *Caenorhabditis elegans* heterochronic gene *lin-14* encodes a nuclear protein that forms a temporal developmental switch. *Nature* **338,** 313–319.

Ruvkun, G., Ambros, V., Coulson, A., Waterston, R., Sulston, J., and Horvitz, H. R. (1989). Molecular genetics of the *Caenorhabditis elegans* heterochronic gene *lin-14. Genetics* **121,** 501–516.

Sanicola, M., Ward, S., Childs, G., and Emmons, S. W. (1990). Identification of a *Caenorhabditis elegans* histone H1 gene family: Characterization of a family member containing an intron and encoding a poly(A)+ mRNA. *J. Mol. Biol.* **212,** 259–268.

Schauer, I. E., and Wood, W. B. (1990). Early *C. elegans* embryos are transcriptionally active. *Development* **110,** 1303–1317.

Schedin, P., Hunter, C. P., and Wood, W. B. (1991). Autonomy and nonautonomy of sex determination in triploid intersex mosaics of *C. elegans. Development* **112,** 833–879.

Seydoux, G., and Fire, A. (1994). Soma-germline asymmetry in the *in situ* hybridization to distributions of embryonic RNAs in *Caenorhabditis elegans*. *Development* **120**, 2823–2834.

Sharp, P. M., and Li, W. H. (1987). The codon adaptation index—a measure of directional synonymous codon usage bias, and its potential applications. *Nucleic Acids Res.* **15**, 1281–1295.

Simons, R. W. (1988). Naturally occurring anti-sense RNA control: A brief review. *Gene* **72**, 35–44.

Simpson, V. J., Johnson, T. E., and Hammen, R. F. (1986). *Caenorhabditis elegans* DNA does not contain 5-methylcytosine at any time during development or aging. *Nucleic Acids Res.* **14**, 6711–6717.

Snutch, T. P., Heschl, M. F., and Baillie, D. L. (1988). The *Caenorhabditis elegans* hsp70 gene family: A molecular genetic characterization. *Gene* **64**, 241–255.

Spieth, J., Denison, K., Kirtland, S., Cane, J., and Blumenthal, T. (1985). The *C. elegans* vitellogenin genes: Short sequences repeats in the promoter regions and homology to the vertebrate genes. *Nucleic Acids Res.* **13**, 5283–5295.

Spieth, J., MacMorris, M., Broverman, S., Greenspoon, S., and Blumenthal, T. (1988). Regulated expression of a vitellogenin fusion gene in transgenic nematodes. *Dev. Biol.* **130**, 285–293.

Spieth, J., Shim, Y. H., Lea, K., Conrad, R., and Blumenthal, T. (1991). *elt-1*, an embryonically expressed *Caenorhabditis elegans* gene homologous to the GATA transcription factor family. *Mol. Cell. Biol.* **11**, 4651–4659.

Spieth, J., Brooke, G., Kuersten, S., Lea, K., and Blumenthal, T. (1993). Operons in *C. elegans*: Polycistronic mRNA precursors are processed by trans-splicing of SL2 to downstream coding regions. *Cell* **73**, 521–532.

Storfer-Glazer, F. A., and Wood, W. B. (1994). Effects of chromosomal deficiencies on early cleavage patterning and terminal phenotype in *C. elegans* embryos. *Genetics* **137**, 499–508.

Sutton, R. E., and Boothroyd, J. C. (1986). Evidence for *trans* splicing in trypanosomes. *Cell* **47**, 527–535.

Swanson, M. S., Carlson, M., and Winston, F. (1990). SPT6, an essential gene that affects transcription in *Sacchromyces cerevisiae*, encodes a nuclear protein with an extremely acidic amino terminus. *Mol. Cell. Biol.* **10**, 4935–4941.

Tautz, D., and Pfeifle, C. (1989). A non-radioactive in situ hybridization method for the localization of specific RNAs in *Drosophila* embryos reveals a translational control of the segmentation gene *hunchback*. *Chromsoma* **98**, 81–85.

Thomas, J., Conrad, R. C., and Blumenthal, T. (1988). The *C. elegans* trans-spliced leader RNA is bound to Sm and has a trimethylguanosine cap. *Cell* **54**, 533–539.

Thomas, J., Lea, K., Zucker-Aprison, E., and Blumenthal, T. (1990). The spliceosomal snRNAs of *Caenorhabditis elegans*. *Nucleic Acids Res.* **18**, 2633–2642.

Tschudi, C., and Ullu, E. (1988). Polygene transcripts are precursors to calmodulin mRNAs in trypanosomes. *EMBO J.* **7**, 455–463.

Van der Ploeg, L. H. T., Bernards, A., Rijsewijk, R. A. M., and Borst, P. (1982). Characterization of the DNA duplication-transposition that controls the expression of two genes for the variant glycoprotein in *Trypanosoma brucei*. *Nucleic Acids Res.* **10**, 593–609.

Van Doren, K., and Hirsh, D. (1988). Trans-spliced leader RNA exists as small nuclear ribonucleoprotein particles in *Caenorhabditis elegans*. *Nature* **335**, 556–559.

Wahle, E., and Keller, W. (1992). The biochemistry of 3'-end cleavage and polyadenylation of messenger RNA precursors. *Annu. Rev. Biochem.* **61**, 419–440.

Wang, B. B., Müller-Immergluck, M. M., Austin, J., Robinson, N. T., Chisholm, A., and Kenyon, C. (1993). A homeotic gene cluster patterns the anteroposterior body axis of *C. elegans*. *Cell* **74**, 29–42.

Way, J. C., and Chalfie, M. (1989). The *mec-3* gene of *Caenorhabditis elegans* requires its own product for maintained expression and is expressed in three neuronal cell types. *Genes Dev.* **3**, 1823–1833.

Wharton, R. P., and Struhl, G. (1991). RNA regulatory elements mediate control of *Drosophila* body pattern by the posterior morphogen nanos. *Cell* **59**, 881–892.

Wickens, M. (1990). Forward, backward, how much, when: Mechanisms of poly(A) addition and removal and their role in early development. *Semin. Dev. Biol.* **3**, 399–412.

Wightman, B., Bürglin, T. R., Gatto, J., Arasu, P., and Ruvkun, G. (1991). Negative regulatory sequences in the *lin-14* 3'-untranslated region are necessary to generate a temporal switch during *Caenorhabditis elegans* development. *Genes Dev.* **5,** 1813–1824.

Wightman, B., Ha, I., and Ruvkun, G. (1993). Posttranscriptional regulation of the heterochronic gene *lin-14* by *lin-14* mediates temporal pattern formation in *C. elegans. Cell* **75,** 855–862.

Wittig, S., and Wittig, B. (1982). Function of a tRNA gene promoter depends on nucleosome position. *Nature* **297,** 31–38.

Yochem, J., Weston, K., and Greenwald, I. (1988). The *Caenorhabditis elegans lin-12* gene encodes a transmembrane protein with overall similarity to *Drosophila Notch. Nature* **335,** 547–550.

Yochem, J., and Greenwald, I. (1989). *glp-1* and *lin-12,* genes implicated in distinct cell-cell interactions in *C. elegans,* encode similar transmembrane proteins. *Cell* **58,** 553–563.

Yu, Y.-T., Maroney, P. A., and Nilsen, T. W. (1993). Functional reconstitution of U6 snRNA in nematode cis- and trans-splicing: U6 can serve as both a branch acceptor and a 5' exon. *Cell* **75,** 1049–1059.

Zarkower, D., and Hodgkin, J. (1992). Molecular analysis of the *C. elegans* sex-determining gene tra-1: A gene encoding two zinc finger proteins. *Cell* **70,** 237–249.

Zucker-Aprison, E., and Blumenthal, T. (1989). Potential regulatory elements of nematode vitellogenin genes revealed by interspecies sequence comparisons. *J. Mol. Evol.* **28,** 487–496.

CHAPTER 21

Techniques for Analyzing Transcription and Translation

Michael Krause

Laboratory of Molecular Biology
National Institute of Diabetes, Digestive, and Kidney Diseases
National Institutes of Health
Bethesda, Maryland 20892

I. Introduction

This chapter is devoted to providing information on techniques applicable to studying transcription and translation in *Caenorhabditis elegans*. These techniques are constantly evolving and being passed among workers, each making improvements or adaptations. None of the techniques discussed below are original, but, rather, have emerged from a variety of sources over the years, making it difficult to trace their origin or give credit to the originators.

Although each technique has been used successfully, for each there are alternative methods available in the literature that work equally well. In fact, depending on the available resources, you might find that an alternative technique suits your needs and facilities better than the one described below. For this reason, the procedures discussed below are usually accompanied by one or more references that will allow you to look at other, related methods. Where appropriate, there will also be a discussion of factors to consider when employing these techniques.

Most of the techniques applied to the study of higher eukaryotic gene expression are also available for the study of transcription and translation in nematodes; however, techniques based on the biochemistry and pharmacology of either synchronized embryo populations or homogeneous cell types are not, in general, feasible in *C. elegans,* because of the difficulty in isolating sufficient amounts of these samples.

One solution to the problem of embryo synchronization that would be applicable in some cases is to synchronously arrest embryos in midembryogenesis by 5-fluorodeoxyuridine treatment, as has been recently described (Stroeher *et al.,* 1994). An alternative solution, albeit a bit unattractive, is to work with the pig parasitic nematode *Ascaris lumbricoides,* which can provide biochemical amounts of cellular extracts from extremely well-synchronized embryos. It is increasingly difficult, however, to collect *Ascaris,* because these nematodes cannot be grown in culture and the infection rate among pigs is dropping.

II. Worm Growth for RNA Preparations

The starting point for transcriptional studies is most often a clean, undegraded preparation of RNA. Although the preparation of RNA from cells is usually quick and easy, the nematode does provide some troublesome nuances to consider when isolating RNA. There are two choices for growing large numbers of animals for RNA preparations: growth on plates or growth in liquid (culture methods are reviewed in detail in Chapter 1). Both require a sufficient supply of bacteria to keep pace with the rapid expansion of the nematode populations. Large preparations of bacteria can be grown in standard flasks or a fermentor (if available) and stored as a concentrated slurry at 4°C. This provides a convenient source of food that can be added to the cultures as needed.

Liquid nematode cultures yield cleaner preparations of RNA than do plates. These cultures can be a bit more variable and difficult for the novice. Good aeration is key to the success of liquid cultures. This can be accomplished by simply shaking the cultures, as one would bacterial cultures, providing they can be maintained at 15 to 25°C. Liquid culture of *C. elegans* is described by Sulston and Brenner (1974) and Sulston and Hodgkin (1988) (also see Chapter 1).

Growing large numbers of worms on plates is sometimes more convenient than liquid cultures. For high-density populations, it is advisable to increase the concentration of agar (to 2%) to prevent burrowing. Bacterial growth on plates can be increased substantially by adding a chicken egg yolk mixture to the plates. The egg yolks support rapid bacterial growth and, therefore, rapid worm growth on the plates directly. A recipe for egg plates is given in Table I.

Although agar plates are convenient, worms grown on agar yield nucleic acid preparations that are contaminated by a material that can cause problems in later manipulations. This contaminant makes it difficult to quantitate RNA samples accurately by light absorbance and can interfere with enzymes that use the RNA as a substrate, such as reverse transcriptase. (The contaminant derived from agar plate-grown worms is likewise known to inhibit restriction enzymes from cutting DNA samples.) One solution to this problem is to collect embryos by hypochlorite treatment of gravid hermaphrodites and let these embryos hatch into sterile M9 solution. Alternatively, one can grow the worms on plates made with agarose that does not produce this contaminant. To make this routinely affordable, agar plates can be overlaid with a 2.5% agarose pad.

III. RNA Preparation

Several methods for isolating RNA from *C. elegans* are found in the literature and all work equally well (for examples, see Kramer *et al.,* 1982; Blumenthal *et al.,* 1984; Rosenquist and Kimble, 1988). Most of these employ guanidinium isothiocyanate in variations of the original procedure by Chirgwin *et al.* (1979). Animals can be lysed by a variety of techniques including French press cell obliteration, Polytron homogenation, and manual grinding.

Table I
Chicken Egg Plates for Large-Scale Worm Growth

Component	Amount
2% Agar NGM plates (100 mm)	15
L-broth	50 ml
Chicken egg (yolk only)	1 yolk
Bacterial culture (OP50)	5 ml

Procedure

All items, including the outside of the eggshell, should be sterilized by either autoclaving or rinsing with ethanol. Stir and heat the L-broth to 60°C, and add one egg yolk. (The yolk can be easily separated from the white of the egg with an egg separator device available at most grocery stores; metal ones allow sterilization in an autoclave.) Bring the temperature of the stirring mixture back to 60°C for at least 10 minutes (to destroy lysozyme activity). Quickly cool the mixture to 30°C, add 5 ml of an overnight bacterial culture (strain OP50) and let sit for 15 minutes. Dispense 5 ml of egg/bacteria mixture to each 2% agar NGM plate (100 × 15 mm) and let dry in a sterile hood. The egg mixture should be dried so that is is moist but does not run when the plates are tipped on their side.

RNA Preparation Method. All labware and solutions should be clean and RNase-free, and precautions should be taken to avoid introducing contaminating RNases to the sample. Resuspend clean animals in 3 vol of 4 M guanidinium isothiocyanate (GITC, ultrapure, Bethesda Research Laboratories, 50 mM Tris–HCl (pH 7.5), 25 mM ethylenediaminetetraacetic acid (EDTA), 1% Sarkosyl (*N*-lauryl sarcosine). Freeze sample as pellets by dripping slowly into a beaker containing liquid nitrogen; store the frozen pellets at −70°C. Transfer the frozen nematode pellets to an appropriately sized mortar and pestle that has been chilled with liquid nitrogen or kept on dry ice. Lyse animals by grinding pellets into a fine powder and transfer the powder to a polypropylene tube for centrifugation and organic solvent extraction. Rinse the residual powder out of the mortar with a minimal amount of fresh GITC solution and pool with the ground lysate. Let the lysate thaw and centrifuge at 4°C and 8000g for 15 minutes to pellet debris. Extract the supernatant with an equal volume of buffer-saturated phenol and separate phases by centrifugation at 5000g for 10 minutes at 4°C. Repeat the extraction and centrifugation three times, once each with phenol, 1 : 1 phenol : chloroform, and finally chloroform alone.

Transfer the supernatant to a fresh tube and precipitate the nucleic acid by adding 0.1 vol of 3 M sodium acetate and 2.5 vol of absolute ethanol, mixing well, and storing at −20°C for at least 2 hours. Pellet RNA/DNA precipitate by centrifugation at 8000g for 15 minutes at 4°C. Briefly dry pellet and resuspend in 1 vol 10 mM EDTA. Add an equal volume of 5 M lithium chloride, mix, and store on ice for 2 hours. Collect RNA by centrifugation at 8000g for 15 minutes at 4°C. Resuspend RNA pellet in 10 mM EDTA. Precipitate RNA by adding 0.1 vol 3 M sodium acetate and 2.5 vol absolute ethanol and storing at −20°C for at least 2 hours. Pellet RNA by centrifugation at 8000g for 15 minutes at 4°C. Resuspend RNA pellet in 10 mM EDTA and store at −70°C.

IV. Northern Blot Analysis

Northern blots of RNA are routinely used to analyze transcripts in *C. elegans.* There are several things to consider before embarking on a Northern blot analysis.

Loading Controls. Northern blot analysis is often used to look at the developmental profile of message. To be confident that variations in message levels between different RNA samples reflect biology, instead of unequal loading, it is important to demonstrate equal amounts of RNA are present in each lane. In other biological systems, a common control for equal amounts of RNA is to probe for a message encoding a basal translation factor, such as elongation factor 1α (EF1α), which is ubiquitous (EF1α is often used for *Xenopus* RNA analysis; e.g., see Krieg *et al.,* 1989; Rupp and Weintraub, 1991). The EF1α-encoding gene has been cloned from *C. elegans,* but its level of expression in different tissues and developmental stages is not yet clear (M. Koga and Y. Ohshima, pers. comm.). A skeletal actin gene probe (*act-1:* Krause *et al.,* 1989) is often used to control for equal loading of RNA on blots comparing different developmental stages; however, as this actin message decreases in level during larval development, it is not a good control for this purpose. The actin probe is appropriate only when comparing different samples from either mixed populations or similarly developmentally staged populations.

For Northern blots of total RNA samples from different developmental stages, one of the best controls for equal loading is to probe for the ribosomal RNAs (e.g., using the plasmid pCe7: Files and Hirsh, 1981). For Northern blots with poly(A)+ RNA, the best probe currently available is the *C. elegans* homolog of eukaryotic initiation factor 4A, called CeIF (Roussell and Bennett, 1992). This gene appears to be ubiquitously expressed and gives rise to a 1.7-kb RNA. Perhaps the recently cloned cytoplasmic actin gene (*act-5*) will provide another probe for these controls; however, as yet it is uncharacterized (L. Schriefer, J. Waddle, and R. Waterston, pers. comm.).

Maternal RNAs. For genes that act very early in development, it is often useful to determine the maternal contributions to the embryo. There are mutants that allow one to assay the maternal contribution by comparing RNA from adult hermaphrodite animals that reflect the somatic, germ cell, and zygotic contributions. The two mutant strains routinely used for such RNA preparations are (1) *glp-4(bn2ts)*, a temperature-sensitive strain that produces very few germs cells when raised at the restrictive temperature (Beanan and Strome, 1992), and (2) *fer-1(hc1ts)*, a temperature-sensitive strain that is defective in fertilization so that animals raised at restrictive temperature produce germ cells but no embryos (Miwa and Ward, 1978). A comparison of message levels in these two mutants strains, raised at either permission or restrictive temperature, can indicate the level of maternally supplied mRNA. A probe to maternally expressed genes, such as *glp-1*, can be used to verify the RNA samples on these Northern blots (Austin and Kimble, 1989; Bowerman *et al.*, 1992).

Oocyte versus Sperm Contributions. Differences between oocyte and sperm RNA contributions to the embryo can be addressed with the *fem* (feminization of XX and XO animals) mutants. For example, *fem-3(q20sd)* XX animals raised at 25°C produce only sperm, whereas these animals raised at 15°C produce oocytes and excess sperm (Barton *et al.*, 1987).

Northern Blot Method. In this procedure, RNA is separated in a formaldehyde-contained agarose gel run in 1× Mops buffer [20 mM 4-morpholinepropanesulfonic acid (Mops), pH 7.0, 8 mM sodium acetate, 1 mM EDTA]. As formaldehyde vapors are toxic, work with formaldehyde should be done in a chemical hood; this includes preparation, running, and disposal of the gel. Typically, a 1.5% agarose gel is prepared in 1× Mops buffer in a volume that accounts for the subsequent addition of formaldehyde. After heating the solution to melt the agarose, add formaldehyde to a final concentration of 2 M and cast the gel in a chemical hood. **Do not** heat agarose solutions containing formaldehyde outside of a chemical hood because the vapors are toxic. Gels are run as submerged horizontal slab gels in 1× Mops buffer. Although some people prefer to add formaldehyde to the gel running buffer (to a final concentration of 2 M), it does not appear to improve the Northern blot results and can be omitted. Recirculation of the gel running buffer is also not required with submerged gels. If the gel is run for a long time, the buffer in each end of the apparatus can be mixed manually every few hours; short runs (2–3 hours) do not require buffer mixing.

Denatured RNA [5–30 μg total RNA or 1–5 μg poly(A) + RNA per lane] by heating for 10 minutes at 65°C in 50% formamide, 2 M formaldehyde, 1× Mops buffer. Cool samples on ice and quickly centrifuge to bring down condensed liquid; add 0.1 vol of 10× loading dye (50% glycerol, 1 mM EDTA, 0.25% bromophenol blue, 0.25% xylene cyanol). Load samples in the wells of a submerged horizontal gel; cover the gel with plastic wrap and run at 5 to 10 V/cm.

After completion of electrophoresis, remove the gel and wash with distilled, deionized water by shaking it gently in a dish. Wash the gel 4 × 5 minutes with water, followed by 2 × 30 minutes with 20× SSC (3 M sodium chloride, 0.3 M sodium citrate). Transfer the RNA from the gel to a solid support for hybridization (such as Hybond membrane, Amersham) by capillary action using a Southern/Northern blot apparatus as described in Sambrook *et al.* (1989).

V. Hybridizations

Hybridization Solution. Although many hybridization solutions are described in the literature (e.g., Kramer *et al.,* 1985; Austin and Kimble, 1989), I have found that the one described by Church and Gilbert (1984) gives consistently good signals with little background. The Church–Gilbert hybridization solution has a high concentration of detergent that often precipitates out of solution at room temperature. This does not affect the solution, which is stable at room temperature for months. Prior to use, the solution should be heated to 60°C and well mixed.

Church–Gilbert hybridization solution is prepared as a 1× stock by heating the components in a beaker while stirring. It is most convenient to have stock solutions of 20% sodium dodecyl sulfate (SDS) and 1 M phosphate buffer, pH 7.2, for making the hybridization solution. The final concentrations of components in the Church–Gilbert hybridization solution are 0.52 M phosphate buffer, pH 7.2, 7% SDS, 1 mM EDTA, 1% (w/v) bovine serum albumin (BSA, pentax fraction V). The hybridization solution can be filtered while hot to remove undissolved solids if desired.

For hybridizations, the solution is prewarmed to 60°C, and denatured probe is added to the appropriate hybridization volume (e.g., 5 ml for a 11 × 14-cm filter). For most *C. elegans* probes, hybridization at 57°C overnight will give a good, specific signal.

Wash Solution. Following hybridization, filters are washed four × 20 minutes at the hybridization temperature in 1× super blot wash [50 mM Trizma base, pH 7.8 (Sigma), 0.2 mM EDTA, 10 mM sodium pyrophosphate, 0.02% BSA,

0.02% polyvinylpyrrolidone-40, 0.02% Ficoll-400, 0.05% SDS, 0.05% Sarkosyl]. Super blot wash is made as a 10× stock solution and is stable at room temperature for months. Alternative aqueous wash solutions can be used; the high SDS and BSA concentrations in the Church–Gilbert hybridization solution result in low levels of nonspecific probe binding, so that the posthybridization washes need not be very stringent.

Probe Preparation. High-specific-activity probes can be generated by a variety of methods such as nick translation, random priming, polymerase chain reaction (PCR), primer extension, and RNA polymerase transcription from flanking plasmid vector RNA polymerase promoters (T3, T7, or SP6). For Northern blots, gene-specific, single-stranded, antisense probes are often useful for detecting low-abundance messages. For genes that are partially or completely sequenced, one can make a set of antisense primers (15–20 nucleotides long) that span the transcribed region. These can be used to prime antisense extension products; extension and cycling with Taq DNA polymerase in the presence of a ^{32}P-labeled deoxynucleotide allow one to make very high specific activity single-stranded probes. Note that this is not a logarithmic amplification by PCR; rather, for each cycle after the initial extension, there is a one molar increase in primed antisense strands compared with sense strand.

Single-Stranded Probes by PCR Method. Make a stock mix of the antisense primers for the gene of interest, each at a final concentration of 20 μM (for a 25-mer, 20 μM is equivalent to 165 ng/μl). Carry out reactions in 20-μl total volume of Taq DNA polymerase buffer without dCTP (50 mM potassium chloride, 10 mM Tris–HCl, pH 8.3, 1.5 mM magnesium chloride, 0.4% gelatin, and 1 mM each dGTP, dATP, and dTTP) with 5 μl [^{32}P]dCTP (3000 Ci/mmole), 2 μl primer mix, 1 ng template DNA, and 1 U Taq DNA polymerase (Perkin–Elmer). Although cycling conditions may vary depending on the probe sequence, primer sequences, and primer lengths, a typical reaction would use 25 cycles with denaturing at 94°C for 1 minute, annealing at 54°C for 1 minute, and extension at 72°C for 2 minutes. This relatively long extension time helps to compensate for the inefficiency of Taq DNA polymerase under these conditions in which the concentration of the radiolabeled deoxynucleotide is much lower than that of the unlabeled deoxynucleotides.

Probes can be labeled by this method to a specific activity of greater than 10^9 cpm/μg. Probes are separated from unincorporated counts by passage over a Sephadex G-50 spin column. These probes do not need to be denatured prior to use as they are single stranded. An actin gene probe made by this method can detect the three prominent actin messages [1450 nucleotides (nt), 1550 nt, and 1650 nt long] on Northern blots with 5 μg total RNA per lane, with exposure times less than 2 hours.

VI. RNase Protection

An alternative to Northern blot analysis of messages is RNase protection assays. These assays are commonly employed in tissue culture studies, but have not been widely used in *C. elegans* studies, although there are not technical limitations to their use in nematodes. Most current protocols are variants of that described by Melton *et al.* (1984); a few examples of the application of this procedure in the nematode are found in Fire *et al.* (1991), Okkema *et al.* (1993), Aroian *et al.* (1993), and Land *et al.* (1994).

RNase Protection Method. A typical reaction to detect the transcript of interest requires a ^{32}P-labeled, antisense RNA probe. These are conveniently generated by subcloning a region of the gene of interest into one of the many commercially available plasmid vectors that have T3, T7, or SP6 RNA polymerase promoters flanking the cloning site. The plasmid is linearized with the appropriate restriction enzyme, allowing one to transcribe the antisense strand in the presence of [α-^{32}P]UTP; this antisense probe transcript is then gel purified and ready for use.

Anneal the ^{32}P-labeled antisense RNA probe to total RNA (1–30 μg total RNA depending on abundance of target transcript) for 2 hours at 50°C in 50 mM Tris–HCl, pH 7.4, 0.45 M sodium chloride, 10 mM EDTA. A typical annealing reaction volume is 30 μl, overlaid with mineral oil to prevent condensation. Increase the volume to 300 μl and adjust the buffer to 40 mM Tris–HCl, pH 7.4, 0.3 M sodium chloride, 5 mM EDTA. Add 1 μl of 0.1 mg/ml RNase A (Sigma) and 300 U of RNase T1 (Bethesda Research Laboratories) (optional), and incubated the reaction at 30°C for 30 minutes. Terminate reactions by extraction with equilibrated phenol : chloroform 50 : 50 and ethanol precipitation with a carrier [such as 30 μg yeast type III RNA (Sigma) or 1 μg glycogen (Boehringer-Mannheim)]. Analyze products by electrophoresis though either native 2% agarose gels or denaturing 6 to 8% acrylamide gels, depending on the size of the protected fragments, and detection by autoradiography.

VII. S1 Mapping

S1 mapping is a convenient method used to map the 5' or 3' end of messages as well as internal splice sites. The original procedure was described by Berk and Sharp (1977) and has been detailed in Calzone *et al.* (1987) and Sambrook *et al.* (1989). Several groups have used S1 mapping to determine message endpoints in *C. elegans* (Kramer *et al.*, 1985; Graham *et al.*, 1988; Ahringer *et al.*, 1992; Kuwabara and Kimble, 1992; Okkema *et al.*, 1993).

For those messages that are *trans*-spliced to SL sequences, S1 mapping of the 5' end presents a problem. S1 mapping will identify the *trans*-splice acceptor site of the message, not the true 5' start site, because the *trans*-spliced product predominates the steady-state RNA population for most *trans*-spliced messages. This difficulty in determining the actual transcriptional start site for these messages complicates attempts to definitively identify upstream controlling elements such as the TATA box sequence. It may be possible to circumvent this problem by making transgenic lines harboring genomic constructs of the gene in which the outron splice acceptor site has been mutated, rendering the message incapable of being *trans*-spliced. This approach is labor intensive and assumes that the mutation that is introduced does not alter the normal transcriptional initiation site.

S1 Mapping Method. Efficient S1 mapping requires a radiolabeled, single-stranded DNA probe that is most often purified from a denaturing gel. This labeled DNA strand can be generated by several methods including primer extension in the presence of $[\alpha\text{-}^{32}\text{P}]$dNTP. Anneal the DNA probe and RNA (1–50 μg depending on the abundance of the target transcript) in a small volume (typically 15 μl) at 42°C overnight in 40 mM 1,4-piperazinediethanesulfonic acid (Pipes), pH 6.5, 0.4 M sodium chloride, 1 mM EDTA, and 52% formamide. Dilute the reaction on ice with 300 μl S1 mapping buffer (0.3 M sodium chloride, 50 mM sodium acetate, pH 4.5, 2 mM zinc sulfate, 5% glycerol, and 25 μg/ml single-stranded carrier DNA. Add 100 to 1000 U of S1 nuclease (Boehringer-Mannheim), and incubate the reaction at 15 to 40°C for 1 hour (the temperature and time of incubation should be titrated for each different transcript assayed). Stop the digestion by adding 80 μl of 4 M ammonium acetate, 20 mM EDTA, and 40 μg/ml yeast tRNA. Extract the reaction with equilibrated phenol: chloroform 50:50 and precipitate with sodium acetate and ethanol. Separate the digestion products on 6 to 8% denaturing acrylamide gels and detect by autoradiography.

VIII. Primer Extension

An alternative to mapping the 5′ end of a message by S1 nuclease methods is to use primer extension reactions. Although this gives the distance from the primer to the 5′ terminus of the message, it suffers the same pitfall as S1 mapping for messages that are *trans*-spliced; that is, the 5′ end of the mature message is not the true transcriptional start site of the gene. This method can be very informative, however, when working with a relatively abundant message. One can directly sequence the 5′ end of the message to determine if it is *trans*-spliced and, if so, which SL sequence is present on the message (Krause and Hirsh, 1987; Bektesh *et al.,* 1988; Conrad *et al.,* 1991).

Although the following procedure describes dideoxynucleotide sequencing of RNAs by primer extension, the same conditions can be used for primer extension alone by omitting the dideoxynucleotides and extending in the presence of deoxynucleotides only.

Primer Extension Sequencing Method. End-label 10 ng of gene-specific, antisense oligodeoxynucleotide primer with $[\gamma\text{-}^{32}\text{P}]$dATP. Anneal the labeled primer with 10 to 50 μg total RNA (or 1–5 μg poly(A) + RNA) in 12 μl volume of annealing buffer (150 mM potassium chloride, 10 mM Tris–HCl, pH 8.3) by heating it to 75°C for 2 minutes, followed by incubation at 60 to 65°C for 15 minutes. Distribute 2 μl of the annealed mixture to five separate tubes containing 1 μl of a 0.2 to 0.5 mM stock of ddATP, or ddGTP, or ddCTP, or ddTTP, or

1 μl of water (no ddNTP tube). Add 3.5 μl of reverse transcriptase sequencing buffer [20 mM Tris–HCl, pH 8.3, 6 mM magnesium chloride, 0.4 mM each dNTP, 4 U M-MLV (Moloney-Murine Leukemia Virus) reverse transcriptase (Bethesda Research Laboratories)] to each tube. Carry out primar extension sequencing by incubating reactions at 37 to 50°C for 30 minutes (higher temperatures may overcome RNA secondary structures that result in premature termination of the extension products). Terminate reactions by adding formamide loading dye, heating samples to 95°C for 2 minutes, and analyzing on 6 to 8% denaturing polyacrylamide gels with autoradiographic detection.

IX. *In Situ* Hybridization

The localization of specific mRNAs in whole animals is a valuable tool in understanding gene expression. The first application of this technique in *C. elegans* was that by Edwards and Wood (1983), who localized the relatively abundant messages for actin, collagen, and myosin in larvae and adults. The method was refined and increased in sensitivity with the availability of RNA probes. Abundant adult messages (such as actin) could be readily detected (Krause, 1986), and Schedin *et al.* (1991) used the improved methods to assay *vit* gene expression in normal and intersex animals.

Although useful for abundant messages in older animals, these *in situ* methods were not able to localize mRNAs in embryos. At the time, no genes were known to be expressed in a tissue-specific pattern during embryogenesis. This made it difficult to optimize hybridization conditions and distinguish signal from noise. Fortunately, recent advances in probe production and detection, along with the availability of several cloned, embryonically expressed genes, have made *in situ* hybridizations to *C. elegans* embryos possible (Seydoux and Fire, 1994; Evans *et al.*, 1994). A detailed explanation of one of these methods is given in Chapter 14.

X. β-Galactosidase Reporters

See Chapter 19.

XI. Antisense Inhibition

In other systems, antisense RNA has been a useful method for disrupting gene expression (see, e.g., Izant and Weintraub, 1984). Often the initiator AUG is targeted with the antisense strand, but there are no hard and fast rules for determining which regions of the message are most effective in inhibiting expression. Antisense technology has not been widely explored in *C. elegans,* although early successes are encouraging and suggest it is a viable approach for some genes. In *C. elegans* there are currently three examples of antisense-mediated inhibition of gene expression: one involves the dose-sensitive gene *unc-22* (Fire *et al.,* 1991), the second the homeobox gene *ceh-18* (D. Greenstein and G. Ruvkun, pers. comm.), and the third the maternal acting gene *par-1* (S. Gao and K. Kemphues, pers. comm.). Each of these target genes is a good substrate for antisense inhibition; *unc-22* and *ceh-18* encode products that act in dose-sensitive processes, whereas *par-1* is maternally expressed, allowing inhibition by injection of RNA directly into the gonad of hermaphrodites to affect the development of their progeny.

The ability to use antisense as a tool to study other genes that are not particularly dose sensitive or are expressed later in development will depend on many factors. For example, direct injection of antisense RNA as a method of inhibition requires that the RNA be stable and persist until the message is present, and possibly until the message is translated. For genes that are expressed in late embryogenesis, antisense RNA injected into the parental gonad will most likely have been degraded long before the targeted gene is transcribed. Although this problem of RNA stability can be overcome by generating transgenic lines harboring antisense-expressing constructs, such lines require a suitable promoter to induce a high level of expression in the appropriate temporal and spatial pattern. As yet, the available list of cloned and characterized promoters is rather limited.

XII. Reverse Transcriptase Polymerase Chain Reactions

Polymerase chain reaction-based methods of transcript analysis are very useful in studying embryonic expression in *C. elegans,* both because they are quick and because they circumvent problems in isolating large amounts of starting material, such as synchronized embryonic populations. Single embryos (or animals) at any stage of development can, in principle, be assayed for the transcription of any given gene provided suitable primers are available. PCR can be combined with many of the methods described above, such as primer extension mapping of the 5′ end of a message (Okkema *et al.,* 1993). In addition, it can be used as a semiquantitative assay to determine the expression profile of a message of interest.

A typical reverse transcriptase (RT)-PCR method that works well in *C. elegans* is outlined below (see also Barstead *et al.,* 1991; Spieth *et al.,* 1993; Garriga *et al.,* 1993; Aroian *et al.,* 1993; Hope, 1994). It is designed for use on single embryos or animals, but can be applied to any bulk RNA sample. Oligonucleotide primers to be used in the amplification of target sequences should be chosen using the same criteria as used for standard DNA PCR reactions. For any given gene, certain primer pairs work better than others; the efficiency of primer pairs is difficult to predict in advance and often must be empirically determined. Certain primer pairs may also be incompatible when used in multiplex reactions to assay more than one template simultaneously. If the gene structure is known, the PCR primer positions should be chosen such that they span an intron, preferably a large intron. This allows cDNA-derived PCR products to be distinguished from possible genomic DNA (or hnRNA)-derived products, as the two will differ in size by the length of the intervening intron(s). Very large introns may also limit the competition between cDNA and genomic templates for primers, thereby improving the sensitivity of the reaction for the detection of cDNA products.

Although this approach theoretically could be used to quantitate the relative amounts of message in different samples, in practice, it is not quantitative when starting with individual embryos and animals. Presumably these rapid, small-scale preparations contain contaminants that interfere, to a varying degree, with the RT reaction, the PCR reaction, or both. Quantitation should be possible with large-scale RNA preparations.

Single-Embryo or Worm RT-PCR Reaction. Pick one (or more) embryo(s) or worm(s) into a 5-μl drop of water in the bottom of an Eppendorf tube. Add 50 μl of GITC buffer (4 M guanidinium isothiocyanate, 50 mM Tris–HCl, pH 7.4, 50 mM EDTA, 1% Sarkosyl) and freeze at $-70°C$; thaw sample at 65°C, transfer tube to a Speed-Vac, and dry down sample. Resuspend the pellet in 100 μl of diethyl pyrocarbonate (DEPC)-treated water. Extract sample once each for 15 minutes with equilibrated phenol followed by chloroform. Add 20 μg glycogen (Boehringer-Mannheim, Catalog No. 901393) and precipitate with sodium acetate and ethanol. Resuspend the pellet in 20 μl DEPC-treated water.

This micropreparation yields total nucleic acid including RNA and genomic DNA. The DNA can be eliminated by adjusting the sample to a DNase-suitable buffer and incubating with a RNase-free DNase such as RQ1 DNase (Promega). Extract and precipitate the RNA sample as above, and resuspend in 20 μl DEPC-treated water. If you are using PCR primers that span a large intron (1 kb) and you have a relatively abundant message, you may not need to get rid of the DNA prior to RT-PCR.

Mix, on ice, 0.1 vol of micro-RNA preparation from above, 20 U RNasin (Promega), 1 U M-MLV reverse transcriptase (Bethesda Research Laboratories), and 2 ng random hexamers in RT-PCR buffer (50 mM potassium chloride, 20 mM Tris–HCl, pH 8.3, 3 mM magnesium chloride, 0.1 mg/ml gelatin) containing a final concentration of 1 mM dNTPs. Incubate at 37 to 55°C (different RNAs will have different temperature preferences) for 30 minutes, then heat-kill the enzyme at 95°C for 5 minutes.

Conditions for the PCR reaction will vary depending on target and primer sequences. Annealing temperatures usually range between 55 and 60°C and the final MgCl$_2$ concentration between 1.5 and 3 mM. A standard 50-μl reaction would include 2 μl of the reverse transcriptase reaction above combined with a pair of gene-specific primers (5 pmole each) and 1 U Taq DNA polymerase (Perkin–Elmer) in PCR buffer (50 mM potassium chloride, 20 mM Tris–HCl, pH 8.3, 2.5 mM magnesium chloride, 0.1 mg/ml gelatin) containing a final concentration of 0.2 mM dNTPs. An option is to include 0.1 μl of [^{32}P]dCTP (3000 Ci/mmole) to generate radiolabeled amplification products for autoradiographic detection.

Although amplification cycle conditions will vary depending on the target cDNAs and primers, a typical reaction is 30 to 35 cycles of denaturation at 94°C for 30 seconds, annealing at 58°C for 40 seconds, and extension at 72°C for 1 minute. A final cycle of 72°C for 10 minutes may be included to maximize full-length products if they are to be cloned. If background PCR products are a problem, the correct product can often be distinguished by Southern blot analysis with a gene-specific probe.

Spliced Leader Sequence PCR. Although the process of *trans*-splicing can cause trouble in determining transcriptional start sites, it can be very helpful in cloning cDNAs for your gene of interest. Given that 40% or more of all messages are *trans*-spliced to either SL1 or SL2, the odds are pretty good that your gene will give rise to an SL-tagged mRNA. This can be very helpful in obtaining complete 5'-end cDNAs, provided sufficient sequence information is available. Using a RT-PCR method (like that described above), one can combine a gene-specific primer with an SL primer and have a good chance of generating an amplification product that represents the complete 5' end of the message. This method is also commonly used to show that a given message is in fact *trans*-spliced (Spieth *et al.,* 1993; Hengartner and Horvitz, 1994; Hope, 1994). Table II lists some primers that have been used successfully in PCR.

Rapid Amplification of cDNA Ends (RACE) PCR. RACE PCR (Frohman *et al.,* 1988) has become a convenient method for cloning and sequencing the 5'

Table II
Useful Polymerase Chain Reaction Primers

Name	Sequence	Reference[a]
SL1	5'-GGTTTAATTACCCAAGTTTGAG-3'	1, 5, 6
SL1-RI	5'-TCTAGAATTCCGCGGTTTAATTACCCAAGTTTG-3'	2, 3
SL1-Bam	5'-AAAGGATCCTTTAATTACCCAAGTTTGAG-3'	4
SL2	5'-GGTTTTAACCCAGTTACTCAAG-3'	5, 6, 7
RACE adaptor	5'-GACTCGAGTCGACATCG-3'	8
dT^{17} adaptor	5'-GACTCGAGTCGACATCGAT^{17}-3'	2, 8, 9

1. Krause *et al.,* 1989
2. Nonet and Meyer, 1991
3. Garriga *et al.,* 1993
4. Lincke *et al.,* 1992
5. Huang and Hirsh, 1989
6. Spieth *et al.,* 1993
7. Hengartner and Horvitz, 1994
8. Frohman, *et al.,* 1988
9. Hope, 1994

and 3' terminals of mRNAs. Several groups have used the technique successfully in the nematode (Lincke *et al.*, 1992; Kuwabara and Kimble, 1992; Garriga *et al.*, 1993; Hope, 1994; Land *et al.*, 1994), and the primer and adaptor sequences are shown in Table II. Success of this protocol is more frequent when starting with efficiently selected poly(A) + RNA.

XIII. Nuclear Extracts

The analysis of nuclear factors involved in gene regulation, commonplace in other eukaryotic systems, is still in its infancy in the nematode. A few groups have isolated nuclei from *C. elegans* for the purpose of analyzing runoff transcription (Honda and Epstein, 1990; Schauer and Wood, 1990) or looking at nuclease sensitivity (Dixon *et al.*, 1990), and Nilsen's group has explored the biochemistry of splicing using *Ascaris lumbricoides* extracts (Yu *et al.*, 1993); however, the use of nuclear extracts to identify transcription factors regulating polymerase II-transcribed genes, through footprinting or gel shifts, for example, has not yet been exploited in the nematode.

One recent report of the use of nuclear extracts to identify potential regulators comes from Stroeher *et al.* (1994). They were able to detect footprints over important regions of the *ges-1* gene promoter and crosslink an embryonic factor to a regulatory element. They also demonstrated the utility of arresting embryonic development with 5-fluorodeoxyuridine (FUdR) to enrich for early embryonic factors. Hermaphrodites grown in the presence of FUdR give rise to embryos that arrest at about the 200-cell stage yet still express many of the early genes as in normal development. This provides a convenient source of developmentally staged nuclear extracts with which to study early gene expression in *C. elegans*, albeit tempered by the potential problems created by FUdR treatment.

XIV. Gel Mobility Shift Assays

The binding of proteins to specific sequences is often assayed by gel mobility shifts in which a ^{32}P-labeled oligonucleotide is retarded in mobility during gel electrophoresis when compared with free oligonucleotide. This type of assay has not been widely used in *C. elegans* to date, because the number of cloned transcription factors with defined binding site sequences is rather limited.

Proteins to be assayed for binding activity can be generated from a number of methods, for example, purified as bacterial fusion proteins or translated *in vitro* in a rabbit reticulocyte system (Promega). Typically, a 50-μl *in vitro* translation of 0.5 μg of message will generate sufficient protein to perform between 10 and 20 gel shift reactions. Complementary oligonucleotides (15–40 nucleotides long) spanning an intact, or mutant, protein binding site are synthesized. One of the strands is end-labeled with [γ-^{32}P]ATP and then annealed with a 10-fold molar excess of its complementary strand to give a final concentration of 0.1 ng/μl double-stranded oligonucleotide.

Protein and 0.1 ng labeled oligonucleotide are mixed in binding buffer [20 mM 4-(2-hydroxyethyl)-1-piperazineethanesulfonic acid (Hepes), pH 7.6, 50 mM potassium chloride, 1 mM dithiothreitol, 1 mM EDTA, 5% glycerol] in a total volume of 5 to 10 μl and incubated at 22 to 37°C for 15 minutes. A nonspecific competitor [poly(dI) : (dC), Pharmacia] is added to a concentration, previously determined by titration, that is sufficient to compete with nonspecific binding activity but not interfere with specific binding. A typical reaction might include between 0.5 and 5 μg of poly (dI) : (dC). After incubation, the reaction is separated on a native 5% acrylamide gel cast and run in gel shift TBE buffer (25 mM Tris, 25 mM boric acid, 0.5 mM EDTA). The gel is dried and bands detected by autoradiography. Appropriate controls should be included to discriminate between specific and nonspecific binding as well as the presence of unrelated proteins (e.g., present in the reticulocyte lysate) binding to the target sequence.

References

Ahringer, J., Rosenquist, T. A., Lawson, D. N., and Kimble, J. (1992). The *Caenorhabditis elegans* sex determining gene *fem-3* is regulated post-transcriptionally. *EMBO J.* **11,** 2303–2310.

Aroian, R. V., Levy, A. D., Koga, M., Ohshima, Y., Kramer, J. M., and Sternberg, P. W. (1993). Splicing in *Caenorhabditis elegans* does not require an AG at the 3′ splice acceptor site. *Mol. Cell. Biol.* **13,** 626–637.

Austin, J., and Kimble, J. (1989). Transcript analysis of *glp-1* and *lin-12*, homologous genes required for cell interactions during development of *C. elegans*. *Cell* **58,** 565–571.

Barstead, R. J., Kleinman, L., and Waterston, R. H. (1991). Cloning, sequencing and mapping of an alpha-actinin gene from the nematode *Caenorhabditis elegans*. *Cell Motil. Cytoskel.* **20,** 69–78.

Barton, M. K., Schedl, T. B., and Kimble, J. E. (1987). Gain-of-function mutations of *fem-3*, a sex determination gene in *C. elegans*. *Genetics* **115,** 107–119.

Beanen, M. J., and Strome, S. (1992). Characterization of a germ-line proliferation mutation in *C. elegans*. *Development* **116,** 755–766.

Bektesh, S., Van Doren, D., and Hirsh, D. (1988). Presence of the *Caenorhabditis elegans* spliced leader on different mRNAs and in different genera of nematodes. *Genes Dev.* **2,** 1277–1283.

Berk, A. J., and Sharp, P. A. (1977). Sizing and mapping of early adenovirus mRNAs by gel electrophoresis of S1 endonuclease-digested hybrids. *Cell* **12,** 721–732.

Blumenthal, T., Squire, M., Kirtland, S., Cane, J., Donegan, M., Spieth, J., and Sharrock, W. J. (1984). Cloning of a yolk protein gene family from *Caenorhabditis elegans*. *J. Mol. Biol.* **174,** 1–18.

Bowerman, B., Eaton, B. A., and Priess, J. R. (1992). *skn-1*, a maternally expressed gene required to specify the fate of ventral blastomeres in the early *C. elegans* embryo. *Cell* **68,** 1061–1075.

Calzone, F. J., Britten, R. J., and Davidson, E. H. (1987). Mapping of gene transcripts by nuclease protection assays and cDNA primer extension. *Methods Enzymol.* **152,** 611–632.

Chirgwin, J. M., Przybyla, A. E., MacDonald, R. J., and Rutter, W. J. (1979). Isolated of biologically active ribonucleic acid from sources enriched in ribonuclease. *Biochemistry* **18,** 5294–5299.

Church, G. M., and Gilbert, W. (1984). Genomic sequencing. *Proc. Natl. Acad. Sci. U.S.A.* **81,** 1991–1995.

Conrad, R., Thomas, J., Spieth, J., and Blumenthal, T. (1991). Insertion of part of an intron into the 5′ untranslated region of a *Caenorhabditis elegans* gene converts it into a trans-spliced gene. *Mol. Cell. Biol.* **11,** 1921–1926.

Dixon, D. K., Jones, D., and Candido, E. P. M. (1990). The differentially expressed 16-kD heat shock genes of *Caenorhabditis elegans* exhibit differential changes in chromatin structure during heat shock. *DNA Cell Biol.* **9,** 177–191.

Edwards, M. K., and Wood, W. B. (1983). Location of specific messenger RNAs in *Caenorhabditis elegans* by cytological hybridization. *Dev. Biol.* **97,** 375–390.

Evans, T. C., Crittenden, S. L., Kodoyianni, V., and Kimble, J. (1994). Translational control of maternal *glp-1* mRNA establishes an asymmetry in the *C. elegans* embryo. *Cell* **77,** 183–194.

Files, J. G., and Hirsh, D. (1981). Ribosomal DNA of *Caenorhabditis elegans*. *J. Mol. Biol.* **149,** 223–240.

Fire, A., Albertson, D., Harrison, S. W., and Moerman, D. G. (1991). Production of antisense RNA leads to effective and specific inhibition of gene expression in *C. elegans* muscle. *Development* **113,** 503–514.

Frohman, M. A., Dush, M. K., and Martin, G. M. (1988). Rapid production of full length cDNAs from rare transcripts: Amplification using a single gene-specific oligonucleotide primer. *Proc. Natl. Acad. Sci. U.S.A.* **85,** 8998–9002.

Garriga, G., Guenther, C., and Horvitz, H. R. (1993). Migrations of the *Caenorhabditis elegans* IISNs are regulated by *egl-43,* a gene encoding two zinc finger proteins. *Genes Dev.* **7,** 2097–2109.

Graham, R. W., Van Doren, K., Bektesh, S., and Candido, E. P. M. (1988). Maturation of the major ubiquitin gene transcript in *Caenorhabditis elegans* involves the acquisition of a trans-spliced leader. *J. Biol. Chem.* **263,** 10415–10419.

Hengartner, M. O., and Horvitz, H. R. (1994). *C. elegans* cell survival gene *ced-9* encodes a functional homolog of the mammalian proto-oncogene *bcl-2. Cell* **76,** 665–676.

Honda, S., and Epstein, H. F. (1990). Modulation of muscle gene expression in *Caenorhabditis elegans:* Differential levels of transcripts, mRNAs, and polypeptides for tick filament proteins during nematode development. *Proc. Natl. Acad. Sci. U.S.A.* **87,** 876–880.

Hope, I. A. (1994). *pes-1* is expressed during early embryogenesis in *Caenorhabditis elegans* and has homology to the fork head family of transcription factors. *Development* **120,** 505–514.

Huang, X.-Y., and Hirsh, D. (1989). A second trans-spliced RNA leader in the nematode *Caenorhabditis elegans. Proc. Natl. Acad. Sci. U.S.A.* **86,** 8640–8644.

Izant, J. G., and Weintraub, H. (1984). Inhibition of thymidine kinase gene expression by antisense RNA: A molecular approach to genetic analysis. *Cell* **36,** 1007–1015.

Kramer, J. M., Cox, G. N., and Hirsh, D. (1982). Comparisons of the complete sequences of two collagen genes from *Caenorhabditis elegans. Cell* **30,** 599–606.

Kramer, J. M., Cox, G. N., and Hirsh, D. (1985). Expression of the *Caenorhabditis elegans* collagen genes *col-1* and *col-2* is developmentally regulated. *J. Biol. Chem.* **260,** 1945–1951.

Krause, M. (1986). Actin gene expression in the nematode *Caenorhabditis elegans.* Ph.D. Thesis, University of Colorado, Boulder, Colorado.

Krause, M., and Hirsh, D. (1987). A trans-spliced leader sequence on actin mRNA in *C. elegans. Cell* **49,** 753–761.

Krause, M., Wild, M., Rosenzweig, B., and Hirsh, D. (1989). Wild-type and mutant actin genes in *Caenorhabditis elegans. J. Mol. Biol.* **208,** 381–392.

Krieg, P. A., Varnum, S. M., Wormington, W. M., and Melton, D. A. (1989). The mRNA encoding elongation factor 1a (EF-1a) is a major transcript at the midblastula transtion in *Xenopus. Dev. Biol.* **133,** 93–100.

Kuwabara, P. E., and Kimble, J. (1992). *tra-2* encodes a membrane protein and may mediate cell communication in the *Caenorhabditis elegans* sex determination pathway. *Mol. Biol. Cell* **3,** 461–473.

Land, M., Islas-Trejo, A., Freedman, J. H., and Rubin, C. S. (1994). Structure and expression of a novel, neuronal protein kinase C (PKC1B) from *Caenorhabditis elegans. J. Biol. Chem.* **269,** 9234–9244.

Lincke, C. R., The, I., van Groenigen, M., and Borst, P. (1992). The P-glycoprotein gene family of *Caenorhabditis elegans.* Cloning and characterization of genomic and complementary DNA sequences. *J. Mol. Biol.* **228,** 701–711.

Melton, D. A., Krieg, P. A., Rebagliati, M. R., Maniatis, T., Zinn, K., and Green, M. R. (1984). Efficient *in vitro* synthesis of biologically active RNA and RNA hybridization probes from plasmids containing a bacteriophage SP6 promoter. *Nucleic Acids Res.* **12,** 7035–7056.

Miwa, J., and Ward, S. (1978). Characterization of temperature-sensitive/fertilization-defective mutants of the nematode *C. elegans. Genetics* **88,** 285–303.

Nonet, M. L., and Meyer, B. J. (1991). Early aspects of *Caenorhabditis elegans* sex determination and dosage compensation are regulated by a zinc-finger protein. *Nature* **351,** 65–68.

Okkema, P., Harrison, S. W., Plunger, V., Aryana, A., and Fire, A. (1993). Sequence requirements for myosin gene expression and regulation in *C. elegans. Genetics* **135,** 385–404.

Rosenquist, T. A., and Kimble, J. (1988). Molecular cloning and transcript analysis of *fem-3,* a sex-determination gene in *Caenorhabditis elegans. Genes Dev.* **2,** 606–616.

Roussell, D. L., and Bennett, K. (1992). *Caenorhabditis* cDNA encodes an eIF-4A-like protein. *Nucleic Acids Res.* **20,** 3783.

Rupp, R. A. W., and Weintraub, H. (1991). Ubiquitous MyoD transcription at the midblastula transition precedes induction-dependent MyoD expression in presumptive mesoderm of *X. laevis. Cell* **65,** 927–937.

Sambrook, J., Fritsch, E. F., and Maniatis, T. (1989). Analysis and cloning of eukaryotic genomic DNA. *In* "Molecular Cloning: A Laboratory Manual" Cold Spring Harbor Laboratory Press, Cold Spring Harbor, New York.

Schauer, I. E., and Wood, W. B. (1990). Early *C. elegans* embryos are transcriptionally active. *Development* **110,** 1303–1317.

Schedin, P., Hunter, C. P., and Wood, W. B. (1991). Autonomy and nonautonomy of sex determination in triploid intersex mosaics of *C. elegans. Development* **112,** 833–879.

Seydoux, G., and Fire, A. (1994). Soma-germline asymmetry in the *in situ* hybridization to distributions of embryonic RNAs in *Caenorhabditis elegans. Development* **120,** 2823–2834.

Spieth, J., Brooke, G., Kuersten, S., Lea, K., and Blumenthal, T. (1993). Operons in *C. elegans:* Polycistronic mRNA precursors are processed by trans-splicing of SL2 to downstream coding regions. *Cell* **73,** 521–532.

Stroeher, V. L., Kennedy, B. P., Millen, K. L., Schroeder, D. F., Hawkins, M. G., Goszczynski, B., and McGhee, J. D. (1994). DNA-protein interactions in the *C. elegans* embryo: Oocyte and embryonic factors that bind to the promoter of the gut-specific *ges-1* gene. *Dev. Biol.* **163,** 367–380.

Sulston, J. E., and Brenner, S. (1974). The DNA of *Caenorhabditis elegans. Genetics* **77,** 95–104.

Sulston, J. E., and Hodgkin, J. (1988). Methods. *In* "The nematode *Caenorhabditis elegans*" (W. B. Wood, ed.), pp. 587–606, Cold Spring Harbor Laboratory, Cold Spring Harbor, New York.

Yu, Y.-T., Maroney, P. A., and Nilsen, T. W. (1993). Functional reconstitution of U6 snRNA in nematode cis- and trans-splicing: U6 can serve as both a branch acceptor and a 5′ exon. *Cell* **75,** 1049–1059.

PART IV

Genomics and Informatics

CHAPTER 22

The Physical Map of the *Caenorhabditis elegans* Genome

Alan Coulson,* Chau Huynh,† Yuko Kozono,‡ and Ratna Shownkeen*

* The Sanger Centre
Hinxton Hall
Cambridge, United Kingdom CB10 1RQ
† Department of Molecular and Cell Biology
University of California at Berkeley
Berkeley, California 94720
‡ Division of Rheumatology
University of Colorado
Denver, Colorado 80262

METHODS IN CELL BIOLOGY, VOL. 48

I. Introduction

The clone-based physical map of the 100-Mb *Caenorhabditis elegans* genome has evolved over a number of years. Although the detection of clone overlaps and construction of the map have of necessity been carried out centrally (Coulson *et al.*, 1986, 1988, 1991b), it has been essentially a community project. Without the provision of cloned markers and relevant map information by the *C. elegans* community as a whole, the map would lack the genetic anchor points and coherent structure that make it a viable entity. Currently, the map consists of 13 mapped contigs totaling in excess of 95 Mb (Fig. 1) and 2 significant unmapped contigs totaling 1.3 Mb. Telomeric clones are not yet in place. The map carries 600 physically mapped loci, of which 262 have genetic map data. With one exception, the physical extents of the remaining gaps are not known. The exception is the remaining gap on linkage group (LG) II. This has been shown to be bridged by a 225-kb *Sse*8387l fragment (C. Madej, H. Browning and S. Strome, pers. comm.).

Because the clones constituting the map are a central resource, there is essentially no necessity for individuals to construct cosmid and yeast artificial chromosome (YAC) libraries. Consequently, such protocols are not included here. Similarly, protocols for clone fingerprinting (Coulson and Sulston, 1988), which forms the basis of the determination of cosmid overlaps and the mapping of clones received from outside sources and has to be a centralized operation, and YAC linkage (Coulson *et al.*, 1988) are not given here. What follows is essentially a "user's guide" to the physical map. Details of map construction are given where required for interpretation of the map as distributed.

The physical mapping has been a collaboration between the MRC Laboratory of Molecular Biology, Cambridge, United Kingdom (now at The Sanger Centre, Cambridge, UK) and Washington University School of Medicine, St. Louis, Missouri. Inquiries regarding map interpretation, information, and materials should be addressed to alan@sanger.ac.uk or rw@nematode.wustl.edu.

II. Databases

At the time of this writing, physical map construction and editing uses the programs IMAGE and CONTIGC (Sulston *et al.*, 1988; Wobus, unpublished). The read-only version PMAP has been almost entirely superseded by incorporation of the physical map data into ACeDB (R. Durbin and J. Thierry-Mieg, unpublished, see Chapter 25 in this volume). The ACeDB display of the physical

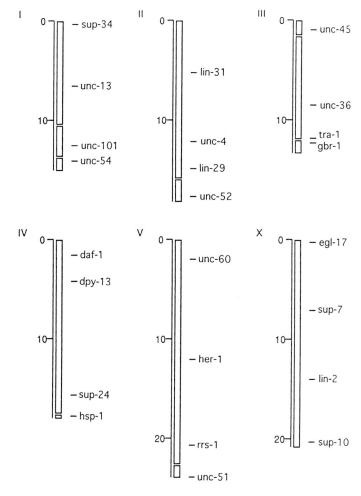

Fig. 1 ACeDB plot of the *C. elegans* physical map (data release 2-9). Scale assumes complete coverage of 110-Mb genome. Gaps between contigs are assumed to be minimal. A few markers are included for reference.

map is currently very similar to that of PMAP with the following exceptions. YACs are displayed in a separate field in ACeDB. The map locations of cDNAs and other probes (as established by positive hybridization to YACs) are not displayed in PMAP. The extent of known sequence is not displayed in PMAP. A useful function available in PMAP that is not currently incorporated into ACeDB is the ability to position computationally the "buried" class of cosmid clones (CONTASS). In the phase of global mapping when cosmid overlaps were being established by fingerprint analysis of randomly selected clones, clones that contributed no useful information to well-established regions of the map were listed as being identical or very similar to canonical clones (indicated on the display by a ∗ after the cosmid name). Although these "buried" clones can be revealed in ACeDB, no attempt is currently made to calculate their likely true position, as can be done in PMAP. (Undue reliance should not be placed on locations established by CONTASS.)

III. Interpretation of the Map

Figure 2 shows a typical ACeDB display of a region of the physical map. The various fields and the way in which the contents of those fields should be interpreted are as follows.

A. Fingerprinted Clones

The clones in this field are mostly cosmids and lambdas, with a few plasmids, P1s, and YACs. Library constructs and drug resistances are listed in Table I. The relationships of these clones have all been determined by fingerprint analysis (Coulson *et al.,* 1986). (Initial attempts were made to map YACs using the same fingerprinting scheme as was used to map smaller clones; for a variety of reasons, these attempts were unsuccessful and YACs were subsequently mapped by hybridization.) The initial framework of ordered overlapping cosmids (contigs) was developed using the following method of fingerprint analysis. Clone DNA is digested with *Hin*dIII, and the fragments are end-labeled with ^{32}P by fill-in using reverse transcriptase. The reaction is terminated, and the labeled fragments are digested with *Sau*3A1. This generates a set of labeled fragments suitable for fractionation on a 4% polyacrylamide denaturing gel (essentially as used in DNA sequencing). The mobilities, relative to standard marker bands, of the resulting autoradiograph bands are digitized. Clone relationships are established by computational searches for matching fragments (at a selected tolerance). The relationships of all the framework cosmids and all incoming clones (genetic markers, etc.) are confirmed by visual inspection and comparison of autoradiographs. As displayed, clone lengths and overlaps are proportional to the number of digitized bands derived from the fingerprint, that is, the number of *Hin*dIII sites in the clone insert. On average, the number of bands will be proportional to the true physical lengths of the inserts; however, the accuracy of this length estimate with regard to particular cosmids is poor, as it is dependent on the local distribution of *Hin*dIII sites. This fingerprinting scheme imposes an obvious constraint on what can be mapped in this way; normally a clone must contain at least two or three *Hin*dIII sites (giving four or six fingerprint bands, respectively) to map it by comparison to the entire database. A precise positioning, however, can frequently be obtained from fewer bands if the regional location has been predetermined by hybridization to a YAC grid.

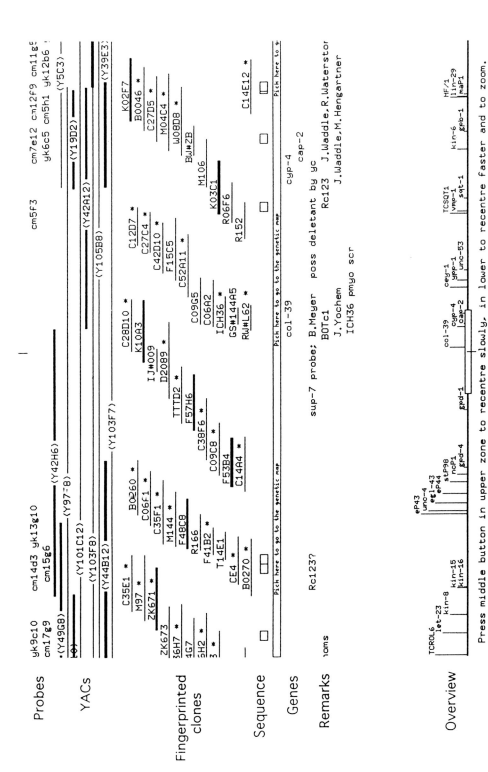

Fig. 2 ACeDB display of part of the physical map of linkage group II.

Table I
Clone Types[a]

Clone series	Vector	Comment
A	Lambda 2001	*Sau*3A1 partial
ZL	Lambda 2001	*Sau*3A1 partial, probe selected
YSL	Lambda 2001	*Sau*3A1 partial, YAC subclones
B	pJB8	*Sau*3A1 partial
C	pJB8	*Sau*3A1 ptl., microtiter array
D	pJB8	*Sau*3A1 partial, filter gridded
E	pJB8	*Sau*3A1 partial, *Eco*K⁻ host
R	pJB8	*Eco*RI partial
M	pJB8	*Mbo*I partial
ZC	pJB8	*Eco*R1 partial, probe selected
K	loristB	*Sau*3A1 partial
T	lorist2	*Sau*3A1 partial
W	lorist4	*Not*1 complete, *Sau*3A1 partial
F	lorist6	*Sau*3A1 partial
ZK		
15–56	lorist6	*Sau*3A1 partial, probe selected
57–130	lorist2	
131–164	lorist6	
165–177	lorist2	
178–192	lorist6	
193–344	lorist2	
345–354	lorist6	
355–514	lorist2	
515–552	lorist6	
553–596	lorist2	
597–616	lorist	
617–626	lorist2	
627–692	lorist6	
693–756	lorist2	
757 on	lorist6	

[a] Most clone types are defined by their initial letter(s) according to the table. In all these series, the alphabetical identifier is followed immediately by a number which either is simply serial or is a microtiter dish number and coordinate. Exceptions are (1) clones given a laboratory designation (two letters #) and, (2) cosmids from the MIT-gridded library, which have one to three identical letters followed by any letter A to H, followed by a number 1 to 12. The vector is pHC79 (amp^r) (G. Benian and R. Waterston pers. comm.; G. Ruvkun and R. Horvitz, pers. comm.). pJB8 (Ish-Horowicz and Burke, 1981) clones are amp^r; lorist (Little and Cross, 1985; Gibson *et al.*, 1987 a,b) clones are kan^r. Unless otherwise stated, the host is *Escherichia coli* 1046 or ED8767. A clone name followed by a ! indicates a duplicate fingerprint.

The heavily underlined cosmids in Fig. 2 are those that were selected to make up the subset that was gridded as representing the genome and used for contig linking by YAC hybridization (see Section III,B).

Gaps in the cosmid map are indicated by double vertical lines. These YAC "bridges" are normally allocated an arbitrary 10 fingerprint band (5 *Hin*dIII site) equivalent, except in some specific cases where such an attribution is known to be highly inappropriate.

B. Yeast Artificial Chromosomes

Cosmid contigs have been linked by hybridization of pulsed-field gel-purified YACs to grids of selected cosmids and, reciprocally, by hybridization of cosmids and other probes to gridded YACs (Coulson *et al.,* 1988). All YACs shown in this field (names bracketed as "virtual" clones to distinguish them from clones whose extent has been determined on the basis of fingerprint band content) have been mapped by hybridization to cosmid grids (unless accompanied by a remark to the contrary). YAC library origins are given in Table II. (For vector constructs and host, see Burke *et al.,* 1987 and Marchuk and Collins, 1988.) The sizes of most YACs, as determined by pulsed-field gel mobility, can be accessed in ACeDB. The sizes of most others are available on request. Because the YACs have been positioned by hybridization to a nonoverlapping subset of cosmids, their endpoints are somewhat ill-defined. YACs are generally drawn as extending to the midpoint of the most distal positively hybridizing cosmids. So, for example, in Fig. 2 the right end of Y42H6 could terminate anywhere between the very left end of K10A3 and as far right as, but not including, K03C1.

Map construction data derived from the hybridization of cosmids and other probes to YAC grids are recorded in the remarks field and are explained in that context. At certain sites it will be seen that YACs have been positioned in the absence of cosmid probes. These joins were made on the basis of hybridization data using probes derived from the sequence analysis of YAC-insert termini (Coulson *et al.,* 1991a). Again, data are recorded in the remarks field and are described in that section.

Table II
Construction of Yeast Artificial Chromosome Libraries[a]

Series	Partial digest	Vector
Y1–Y76	*Eco*RI	pYAC4
Y77–Y96	*Hpa*II	pYAC-RC
Y97	*Cla*I	pYAC-RC
Y101–Y111	*Cla*I	pYAC-RC
Y112–Y120	*Eco*RI	pYAC4

[a] The host for all libraries was AB1380.

A number of YAC names have a U or L suffix. This indicates that the YAC was isolated as the upper or lower band on a pulsed-field gel from a clone that was the result of a double transformation. Heavily underlined YACs are those that were included in the genome-representative "polytene" filter (see Section IV,E).

C. Probes

The "probes" field of the display shows the locations of probes that have been mapped by hybridization, invariably to YAC grids, most often the "polytene" filter. Currently, these probes are mostly cDNA clones derived from cDNA sequencing and mapping projects. Clones with the prefix cm are those derived from the Cambridge/St. Louis cDNA survey (Waterston *et al.*, 1992); those with the prefix yk are derived from the more extensive analysis of Kohara *et al.* (unpublished). Clones are positioned as far as possible at the midpoint of the set of positive YACs. Positive hybridizations can be revealed by clicking on the clone name. Thus (Fig. 2) clicking on yk13g10 will indicate that YACs Y49G8, Y44B12, and Y42H6 were positive hybridizations.

Probes may show secondary hybridizations to YACs from other map locations. These can be identified by reference to the polytene grid display or to the clone information window (see Chapter 25 in this volume).

D. Remarks

A wide variety of classifiable and individual remarks are found in the remarks field, in addition to gene locations and names of clone originators. Many of the individual remarks are redundant, having been generated early in the construction of the map; however, they can give clues to possible anomalies and potential problems. Further information regarding cryptic remarks can sometimes be obtained by consultation.

Classifiable remarks are as follows:

1. *cy:* Indicates a YAC or list of YACs shown as positive by hybridization to YAC grids of a cosmid or other probe to which the remark is attached. (Also cyB; B suffix indicates data derived in the St. Louis laboratory.)

2. *YWL/YWR:* Indicates a list of YACs detected by "left" end or "right" end STS probes derived from YAC termini. This does not indicate left or right end of the YAC as drawn, but as derived from the "left" or "right" universal YAC vector sequencing primers (Coulson *et al.*, 1991a). (Also, Y suffix indicates data derived in St. Louis laboratory.)

3. *PCR:* Except where there is a straightforward statement of confirmatory data, usually indicates YACs positive for a cosmid-derived STS. (Also, P prefix indicates PCR on pooled YACs; and B or Y suffix, data derived in St. Louis laboratory.)

4. *rsc:* Prefix to individual name; attached to clone used to rescue associated gene by microinjection.

5. *Rcn* (e.g., RcC9, RcD9, RcA1, RcS35). Indicates presence of a repetitive sequence of the listed class as determined by hybridization to clone grids (Naclerio *et al.,* 1992; Cangiano and La Volpe, 1993).

6. *i/s: In situ* hybridization data (see Chapter 15 in this volume).

IV. Central Resources

The following materials associated with the physical map are available on request.

A. Cosmids

Cosmids are available from the Cambridge laboratory. They are shipped in soft-agar stabs containing 20 μg/ml appropriate drug. Our experience is that in excess of 95% of clones can yield unrearranged DNA provided correct procedures are followed. Immediately on receipt of a stab, a "miniglycerol" stock should be made. This is done simply by taking an inoculum straight from the stab into 0.1 ml of growth medium (plus drug) containing 30% glycerol. This should be frozen immediately at $-70°C$ for storage. For growth, the cosmid should be streaked on the appropriate growth plate (75 μg/ml ampicillin or 50 μg/ml kanamycin) to give well-isolated colonies. For the inoculation of liquid growth, it is important to select well-isolated, small, but healthy looking colonies, and vital to avoid abnormally large, fast-growing colonies. These should be grown as a miniprep (see Section V,A) or a maxiprep (see Chapter 23 in this volume). Minipreps may offer a better chance of extracting intact DNA from recalcitrant clones. Glycerol stocks for $-70°C$ storage should also be retained from these growths.

In general, clones derived from the lorist series of vectors (based on the lambda origin of replication, which provides a more constant copy number) tend to give a better yield of DNA. Specific protocols for preparing cosmid (and YAC) DNA for microinjection are given in Chapter 19 of this volume.

B. Yeast Artificial Chromosomes

Yeast artificial chromosomes are available from the Cambridge and St. Louis laboratories. They are shipped on $-$ura slants. Miniglycerol stocks should be made as for cosmids. The protocols in Sections V,C; V,G; and V,H are for yeast/YAC miniprep and pulsed-field gel fractionation for the purification and subcloning of YACs into lambda vector.

C. Complementary DNAs

Tag-sequenced and mapped cDNA clones are available from two sources. The cm series is available from both the Cambridge and St. Louis laboratories. They are shipped as phage/agar suspension (from a plate lysate) in lambda dil. The clones are in λSHLX2 and should be plated on MC1061. This host is included when clones are mailed along with protocols. Host for "pop-out" conversion of phage to plasmid is available.

The yk series of cDNAs is available from Dr. Yuji Kohara (National Institute of Genetics, Mishima). A gridded array of 4400 of these clones, most of which have been tag sequenced and mapped, is also available.

D. Lambda Library and Hosts

Aliquots of a primary lambda library are available from the Cambridge laboratory. The library is constructed from 17-kb partial *Sau*3A1 inserts of N2 DNA in the vector lambda 2001 (Karn *et al.*, 1984). The aliquots contain about 50,000 phage. Q358 is recommended as the standard host. The more permissive CES200 (*rec*BC *sbc*B: Wyman *et al.*, 1986) has proved to be essential for recovering some regions of the genome (Spence *et al.*, 1990; Hodgkin, 1993), but DNA yields using this host are not ideal.

E. Yeast Artificial Chromosome Grids

Most of the genome is represented on a grid of 958 YACs (the polytene grid) (Coulson *et al.*, 1991b). These YACs were selected to give twofold coverage of the genome, as far as possible. Consequently, an average resolution of 100 kb is achieved for a positive probe. Mapping of the cm cDNA set using this grid indicated that about 95% of coding sequences were represented. This has been confirmed by mapping of the yk cDNA set (Y. Kohara, pers. comm.).

A supplementary (Suppoly) grid of 223 YACs has been produced to complement the original filter set. This is intended to represent regions of the genome mapped since the selection of YACs for the polytene filter and to improve coverage of some regions that were poorly represented. Some of the YACs on the Suppoly filter are incompletely characterized, and consultation may be required for interpretation. Initial results (Y. Kohara, pers. comm.) suggest that the Suppoly filter set carries most of the coding sequences not present on the original filter.

A standard low-stringency hybridization and washing protocol is given here. A protocol is also given for stripping probe from the grid under mild conditions. In this way, the filters can be used a number of times.

Gridded YACs are displayed in boldface in the physical map (Fig. 2). The key to the grid is accessible in ACeDB and is also provided as hard copy. Examination of the distribution of the gridded YACs will show that, generally, more than one YAC should be positive for a given probe. Single-colony hybridizations should therefore be viewed with suspicion, unless it is clear from the map that the relevant YAC is a sole regional representative. (A few errors and problem clones that can lead to illogical interpretation are listed on the distributed hardcopy key.) When deducing a set of cosmids likely to be relevant to a particular positive YAC grid probing, negative hybridizations should be taken into account to restrict the likely cosmid set as far as possible.

F. Sequence-Tagged Site Oligonucleotides

Oligonucleotides and/or sequences corresponding to the YAC-terminal sequence-tagged sites (STSs) produced for YAC walking are available on request (see Section III,D, remark 2, for explanation of terminology).

V. Protocols

A. Cosmid DNA Miniprep

This miniprep is based on the method of Birnboim and Doly (1979).

1. In a 15-ml culture tube, inoculate 4 ml of 2× TY containing 120 μg/ml ampicillin or 50 μg/ml kanamycin with a single colony from the plate (see text). Grow for 16 hours at 37°C with shaking.

2. To store aliquot, remove 0.5 ml into a 2-ml freezer vial containing 1 ml of sterile 50% glycerol. Vortex and freeze immediately at −70°C.

3. For extraction of cosmid DNA, remove 2 ml of culture into 2.2-ml Eppendorf tube. Spin 45 seconds (microfuge). Remove supernatant by aspiration.

4. Resuspend pellet in 250 μl of 50 m*M* glucose, 10 m*M* ethylenediaminetetraacetic acid (EDTA), 25 m*M* Tris–HCl, pH 8.0. Vortex 15 seconds to mix. Leave to stand 5 minutes at 0°C (ice/water bath).

5. Add 250 μl of 0.2 *N* NaOH, 1% sodium dodecyl sulfate (SDS, fresh). Mix by approximately 15 inversions (do not vortex). Leave to stand 5 minutes at 0°C.

6. Add 200 μl of 3 *M* sodium acetate (NaAc), pH 4.8. Mix by approximately 15 inversions (do not vortex). Leave to stand at 0°C for 60 minutes. Mix by inversion a few times.

7. Centrifuge 4 minutes at room temperature. Remove 600 μl of supernatant to 1.5-ml Eppendorf tube. Add 0.9 ml cold ethanol, mix thoroughly by inversions, and leave to stand for 20 minutes at −20°C.

8. Centrifuge 2 minutes, decant ethanol, and drain briefly. Resuspend pellet in 200 μl of 0.3 *M* NaAc, 1 m*M* EDTA. Vortex and leave to stand for 15 minutes at room temperature. Vortex again and add 400 μl of cold ethanol. Mix. Leave to stand for 20 minutes at −20°C.

9. Centrifuge 2 minutes, decant, and drain briefly. Wash the pellet once with cold ethanol, centrifuge, drain 5 minutes, and dry under vacuum. Allow to resuspend overnight at 4°C in 40 μl of TE (10 mM Tris–HCl, pH 7.4, 0.1 mM EDTA).

The yield should be around 1 to 3 μg of cosmid DNA. A larger-scale preparation is described in Chapter 23 of this volume.

B. Yeast/YAC Miniprep

1. Inoculate 20 ml −ura medium [supplemented with glucose (0.1 vol of 20%), tryptophan (0.01 vol of 5 mg/ml), and leucine (0.02 vol of 5 mg/ml)] with a fair-sized blob from a plate. Grow 24 to 26 hours at 30°C with shaking. Spin out cells (50-ml Falcon tubes) at 2000 rpm for 1 to 2 minutes.

2. Resuspend in 1.5 ml 1 M sorbitol, 0.1 M EDTA, 10 mM Tris–acetate, pH 8.0, 0.1% β-mercaptoethanol. Transfer to 2-ml Eppendorf tube. Add 0.1 ml of 2.5 mg/ml Zymolyase 100T (ICN Biomedicals). Incubate at 37°C for 1 hour. Mix by inversion occasionally.

3. Spin 1 minute in microfuge. Discard supernatant. Resuspend in 0.7 ml of 50 mM Tris–HCl, pH 7.4, 20 mM EDTA. Shake vigorously to suspend completely. (Avoid vortexing throughout the rest of the procedure.)

4. Add 35 μl of 20% SDS. Incubate at 65°C for 30 minutes. Mix occasionally.

5. Add 0.26 ml of 5 M potassium acetate, pH 4.8. Mix. Let stand at 0°C (ice/water bath) for 45 minutes.

6. Spin 5 minutes in microfuge. Remove supernatant to another 2-ml Eppendorf tube. Add 0.1 vol of 3 M NaAc and equal volume of isopropanol. Mix. Incubate 5 minutes at room temperature. Spin 1 minute. Drain.

7. Resuspend pellet in 0.5 ml of TE and 5 μl of 10 mg/ml boiled RNase. Incubate at 37°C for 90 minutes. Mix occasionally.

8. Extract twice with 0.5 ml of chloroform/phenol (50 : 50). Do not vortex but mix by finger flicking. Extract once with chloroform.

9. Add 0.1 vol of 3 M NaAc followed by 2 vol of cold ethanol. Leave at room temperature for 5 minutes. Spin 1 minute. Drain. Resuspend in 300 μl of TE; this takes about 30 minutes with agitation.

10. Add 30 μl 3 M NaAc, 700 μl cold ethanol. Leave at room temperature for 5 minutes. Spin 1 minute. Wash briefly with 70% ethanol. Spin 1 minute, drain, and vacuum dry a few minutes. Resuspend in 50 μl TE.

C. Phage DNA Miniprep

1. Grow overnight phage streaks on lambda plates layered with 100 μl of saturated cells (CES 200 or Q358 for lambda 2001 phage) in 3 ml of top agar.

2. Scrape a little portion of each streak with a toothpick into 0.5 ml of lambda dil containing CES 200 (1/10th dilution) or Q358 (1/150th dilution). Allow to

stand for 30 minutes. Add 2 ml of CY medium supplemented with 3 mM MgSO$_4$ and 30 mM Tris–HCl, pH 7.4.

3. Shake at 37°C until lysed (generally 8–10 hours). Transfer 1.5 to 2 ml of lysate to a 2-ml Eppendorf tube. Centrifuge 5 minutes.

4. Pour the supernatant into another 2-ml Eppendorf tube containing 2 μl of DNase/RNase (20 mg/ml each). Allow to stand at room temperature for 30 minutes.

5. Add 500 μl of 26% polyethylene glycol (PEG), 2.6 M NaCl. Mix by inverting several times. Allow to stand at 4°C for 1 hour to overnight.

6. Centrifuge 3 minutes in a microfuge. Discard supernatant, respin, and aspirate every bit of supernatant (PEG can cause problems later if not removed completely). Add 200 μl of 10 mM Tris–acetate, pH 8, 10 mM EDTA; keep on ice 15 minutes, then vortex to resuspend the pellet.

7. Keep on ice; add 150 μl phenol (chromatography grade). Vortex to mix thoroughly. Centrifuge 1 minute. Remove 180 μl of aqueous layer carefully into a 1.5-ml Eppendorf tube containing 20 μl of 3 M NaAc. Add 200 μl of isopropanol. Vortex to mix thoroughly. Leave at −20°C for at least 1 hour to precipitate phage DNA.

8. Centrifuge 4 minutes in microfuge. Decant supernatant carefully (invisible pellet) and drain. Wash with 1 ml of 85% ethanol, centrifuge 1 minute, decant, and drain.

9. Dry under vacuum. Resuspend in 20 to 40 μl TE, spin, and store at 4°C (or at −20°C for long storage).

D. Probing the Polytene Filters

1. Probe Labeling

See Feinberg and Vogelstein (1983, 1984).

1. Take ~50 to 100 ng of probe DNA in 16 μl of water in 0.5-ml Eppendorf tube.

2. Heat 5 minutes in boiling water. Cool on ice.

3. Add the following mix to each probe: 5 μl OLB (see Section VI); 1 μl bovine serum albumin (BSA, 10 mg/ml); 1 μl dGTC (0.5 mM); 1 μl [^{32}P]dATP (800 Ci/mmole, 10 μCi/μl); 0.5 μl Klenow polymerase.

4. Mix. Incubate at room temperature overnight.

2. Hybridization

1. Transfer probe to 5.5 ml of water in 15-ml Falcon tube. Add 50 μl of 10 mg/ml sonicated salmon sperm DNA.

2. Heat in boiling water for 5 minutes with lids slightly unscrewed. Cool on ice.

3. Add 5.5 ml of hybridization mix [100 g dextran sulfate, 160 ml of water, 30 ml of Sarkosyl NL30 (BDH, = 30% w/v sodium lauroyl sarcosinate), 300 ml 20× SCP]. Mix gently by inversion.

4. Add to filter in polythene bag, seal, and hybridize overnight at 68°C.

5. Wash the filters (four times, 20 minutes each wash) at room temperature with 0.5% SDS, 0.5× SCP warmed initially to 50°C, on orbital shaker.

6. Air-dry the filters thoroughly (at least 2 hours at room temperature), dot with ^{32}P ink, and autoradiograph using an intensifying screen at −70°C for 18 to 36 hours.

3. Stripping the Polytene Filters

To reuse, the filters can be stripped by washing at room temperature with (1) 0.2 M NaOH, 0.5 M NaCl for 10 minutes; (2) 0.5 M Tris–HCl, pH 7.4, 0.5 M NaCl for 20 minutes; (3) SSPE for 20 minutes. Air-dry.

E. Polymerase Chain Reaction Amplification of cm Series cDNA Clone Inserts

In a 0.5-ml Eppendorf tube, take small portion of lysed area of bacterial lawn and 10 μl of water, cover with mineral oil, and heat the tube at 95°C for 10 to 15 minutes. To that add a suitable mix to give final concentration of 0.2 μM each amplification primer, 200 μM each deoxynucleotide, 50 mM KCl, 10 mM Tris–HCl, pH 8.5, 1.5 mM MgCl$_2$, and 1 unit of Taq polymerase. The reaction mix is then thermally cycled 30 to 35 times. The amplification primers used are 5′-GATTTAGGTGACACTATAG (SP6 promoter-specific 19-mer, adjacent to 5′ end of cDNA insert), and 5′-TAATACGACTCACTATAGGG (T7 promoter-specific 20-mer, adjacent to 3′ end of cDNA insert).

F. YAC Plugs for Pulsed–Field Gels

1. Molds for plugs are made from strips of Perspex/Plexiglas milled and glued together to form a sheet 6 mm thick with rectangular holes. The holes are arranged in the format of a microtiter plate. For the 30-lane protocol given here, holes are 3.5 × 1.8 mm; the plugs fit into wells 3.8 × 1.5 mm (a tight fit is important). A pusher of the same cross section is necessary for extruding the plugs from the mold. In use, plug molds are formed by covering one side of the template block with transparent office tape.

2. Grow yeast cells in patches on −ura plates at 30°C for 48 hours. Collect about 1 cm^2 of cells (about 10 μl) in a small wire loop. (When handling large numbers of clones, eight loops can be clamped together at microtiter-well spacing to process multiple samples simultaneously.) Stir into 200 μl 50 mM EDTA, pH 8, in round-bottom microtiter wells (rigid plate variety, e.g., Corning). Spin, with styrofoam pad support, 3500 rpm for 2 minutes. Aspirate supernatant and

vigorously vortex plate to soften the pellets. Add 10 μl 50 mM EDTA, pH 8, to each well and vortex very gently.

3. The following steps should be done up to one row at a time, to allow about 5 minutes between adding solution I and adding the agarose. Add 6 μl solution I and vortex very gently. Wait 5 minutes. Add 40 μl 1% LGT agarose in 0.1 M EDTA, held at 42°C. Mix immediately by pumping in and out of a yellow tip. Avoid air bubbles. Transfer to mold. (Agitate briefly while ejecting to liberate air bubbles. Any that rise to the surface should be removed.)

4. Allow plugs to harden at 4°C for a few minutes. Remove tape from the mold. Push the plugs into 100 μl of solution II in flat-bottom wells. Seal edges of the plate and lid with Parafilm. Incubate at 37°C for 24 hours.

5. Aspirate the solution (protect plug from aspiration with a small spatula). Add 150 μl solution III. Seal the plate and incubate at 50°C for at least 24 hours.

6. Aspirate the solution, add 200 μl 0.5 M EDTA, pH 9, and store at 4°C. Use within a few days if possible.

7. Prior to putting the plugs into the gel, wash them twice in 1 ml 0.05$\times$ TBE. The second wash can be overnight if necessary. (This can conveniently be done in a Nunc 24-well multidish.)

8. We use a Southern waltzer turntable apparatus (Southern *et al.,* 1987). These take 250-ml, 22-cm-diameter circular gels. Gels are 0.7% agarose in 0.5$\times$ TBE. After the gel has set (best left for several hours at 4°C), pipet 5 ml of running buffer around the comb region. Withdraw the comb and ease any air bubbles from the wells with the pipet tip. Insert the plugs into the gel wells using a pair of small bent spatulas. The plugs must fit firmly for good resolution. For YACs up to about 600 kb, we run for 22 hours at 160 V with a switch time of 50 seconds.

SCE: 1 M sorbitol, 0.1 M Na citrate, 0.06 M EDTA, pH 7.
Solution I: 1 ml SCE, 1 mg zymolyase 100T, 50 μl β mercaptoethanol
Solution II: 2 ml 0.5 M EDTA, pH 9, 150 μl β-mercaptoethanol.
Solution III: 2 ml 0.5 M EDTA, pH 9, 67 μl Sarkosyl NL30, 2 mg proteinase K.

G. Subcloning YACs to Lambda

J. Sulston (unpublished).

1. Make plugs as above but for 0.5-cm lanes, from about 10 mg yeast cells. Run the pulsed-field gel as above. Stain in 500 ml water plus 50 μl 10 mg/ml ethidium bromide for 1 hour. Wash in 1 liter 0.5$\times$ TBE 1 hour.

2. Cut slices on long-wave UV box. Wash each slice in 1 ml water for 15 minutes. Wash in 1 ml S buffer for 1 hour.

3. Remove to microtiter well with 0.2 ml S buffer and 0.01 unit or 0.005 unit *Sau*3A1. Incubate overnight at 20°C.

4. Remove into 1 ml TBE for 1 hour. Combine related YAC slices, melt at 65°C, and add 0.2 ml of cold TE. Mix and immediately add 0.2 ml of cold phenol. Vortex, spin, and remove supernatant. Reduce the volume by isobutanol extraction to about 0.25 ml. Add NaCl to 0.1 *M*, 3 μg glycogen carrier, and 0.6 ml ethanol. Freeze, spin, wash, and dry. Resuspend in 4 μl TE plus loading dye. Run, with size markers, on a 0.5% LGT 20-ml minigel under 30 ml TBE for 2 hours at 12 mA.

5. Stain with ethidium bromide and cut out 12 to 20-kb region based on size markers. (Experiment product will not be visible.) Melt at 65°C; add an equal volume of cold TE and 2 vol of phenol. Vortex, spin, and remove aqueous layer. Repeat extraction. Add 1 μg glycogen and 4 μl 1 *M* NaCl, and reduce the volume to about 40 μl with isobutanol. Add 2 vol ethanol, freeze, spin, wash, and dry. Disperse in 1.5 μl TE.

6. For ligation, introduce in turn into a 1- to 5-μl Micropet (Clay Adams Inc) 0.3 μl of slice extract, 0.3 μl lambda 2001 arms (about 8 ng), and 0.3 μl ligation mix (see below). Mix by gently blowing into a yellow tip and returning to the capillary. Seal the Micropet. (This can be done by flaming and sealing the distal end, allowing the reaction mix to be sucked in as the capillary cools, then flaming the proximal end.) Incubate at 15°C overnight.

7. Expel the reaction into an appropriate fraction of packaging mix. Plate on CES200. A total titer of over 500 is satisfactory. Titers up to 10,000 have been observed. The phage should be positively screened with the original YAC and negatively screened with an adjacent yeast chromosome. This is important to eliminate fragments of yeast genomic DNA and 2-μm circles that are found throughout the pulsed-field gel.

S buffer: 100 m*M* NaCl, 10 m*M* Tris–Cl, pH 7.4, 10 m*M* MgCl$_2$, 100 μg/ml BSA.

3× ligation mix: 200 m*M* Tris–Cl, pH 7.4, 15 m*M* MgCl$_2$, 15 m*M* dithiothreitol, 3 m*M* ATP, 1 unit/5μl T4 ligase (Boehringer).

VI. General Recipes

−*Ura medium* (per liter): 8 g yeast nitrogen base without amino acids (Difco), 11 g casamino acids (Difco), 55 mg adenine, 55 mg tyrosine.

2× TY medium (per liter): 16 g tryptone, 10 g yeast extract, 5 g NaCl.

Lambda dil (per liter): 10 ml 1 *M* Tris–HCl, pH 7.4, 5 ml 1 *M* MgSO$_4$, 11.7 g NaCl, 1 g gelatin.

CY medium (per liter): 10 g casamino acids, 5 g yeast extract, 3 g NaCl, 2 g KCl. Adjust to pH 7.0.

20× SCP (per liter): 116.88 g NaCl, 107 g Na$_2$HPO$_4$·2H$_2$O, 7.44 g EDTA. Adjust to pH 6.2 with concentrated HCl.

20× SSPE (per 500 ml): 104 g NaCl, 15.6 g NaH$_2$PO$_4$·2H$_2$O, 3.7 g EDTA, 25 ml of 4 *N* NaOH.

OLB: 50 units pd(N)$_6$.Na$^+$ (Pharmacia) oligonucleotides, 370 μl water, 185 μl TE, 926 μl 2 *M* 4-(2-hydroxyethyl)-1-piperazineethanesulfonic acid (Hepes), pH 6.6 (NaOH titrated), 363 μl of (1.25 *M* Tris–HCl, pH 8.0, 0.125 *M* MgCl$_2$), 7 μl of 2-mercaptoethanol.

10× TBE (per liter): 108 g Tris base, 55 g boric acid, 9.3 g EDTA.

References

Birnboim, H. C., and Doly, J. (1979). A rapid alkaline extraction procedure for screening recombinant plasmid DNA. *Nucleic Acids Res.* **7**, 1513–1523.

Burke, D., Carle, G., and Olson, M. (1987). Cloning of large segments of exogenous DNA into yeast by means of artificial chromosome vectors. *Science* **236**, 806–812.

Cangiano, G., and La Volpe, A. (1993). Repetitive DNA sequences located in the terminal portion of the *Caenorhabditis elegans* chromosomes. *Nucleic Acids Res.* **21**, 1133–1139.

Coulson, A., Sulston, J., Brenner, S., and Karn, J. (1986). Toward a physical map of the genome of the nematode Caenorhabditis elegans. *Proc. Natl. Acad. Sci. U.S.A.* **83**, 7821–7825.

Coulson, A., Waterston, R., Kiff, J., Sulston, J., and Kohara, Y. (1988). Genome linking with yeast artificial chromosomes. *Nature* **335**, 184–186.

Coulson, A., and Sulston, J. (1988). Genome mapping by restriction fingerprinting. *In* "Genome Analysis-A Practical Approach" (K. Davies, ed.), pp. 19–39. IRL Press, Oxford, U.K.

Coulson, A., Kozono, Y., Shownkeen, R., and Waterston, R. (1991a). The isolation of insert-terminal YAC fragments by genomic sequencing. *Technique* **3**, 17–23.

Coulson, A., Kozono, Y., Lutterbach, B., Shownkeen, R., Sulston, J., and Waterston, R. (1991b). YACs and the *C. elegans* genome. *Bioessays* **13**, 413–417.

Feinberg, A. P., and Vogelstein, B. (1983). A technique for radiolabelling DNA restriction fragments to high specific activity. *Anal. Biochem.* **132**, 6–13. and (1984) *Anal. Biochem.* **137**, 266–267.

Gibson, T., Coulson, A., Sulston, J., and Little, P. (1987a). Lorist2, a cosmid with transcriptional terminators insulating vector genes from interference with the insert: Effect on DNA yield and cloned insert frequency. *Gene* **53**, 275–281.

Gibson, T., Rosenthal, A., and Waterston, R. (1987b). Lorist6, a cosmid vector with *Bam*HI, *Not*I, *Sca*I and *Hind*III cloning sites and altered neomycin phosphotransferase gene expression. *Gene* **53**, 283–286.

Hodgkin, J. (1993). Molecular cloning and duplication of the nematode sex-determining gene *tra-1*. *Genetics* **133**, 543–560.

Ish-Horowicz, D., and Burke, J. (1981). Rapid and efficient cosmid cloning. *Nucleic Acids Res.* **9**, 2989–2998.

Karn, J., Matthes, H. W. D., Gait, M. J., and Brenner, S. (1984). *Gene,* **32**, 217–224.

Little, P., and Cross, S. (1985). A cosmid vector that facilitates restriction enzyme mapping. *Proc. Natl. Acad. Sci. U.S.A.* **82**, 3159–3163.

Marchuk, D., and Collins, F. (1988). pYAC-RC, a yeast artificial chromosome vector for cloning DNA cut with infrequently cutting restriction endonucleases. *Nucleic Acids Res.* **16**, 7743.

Naclerio, G., Cangiano, G., Coulson, A., Levitt, A., Ruvulo, V., and La Volpe, A. (1992). Molecular and genomic organisation of clusters of repetitive DNA sequences in *Caenorhabditis elegans*. *J. Mol. Biol.* **226**, 159–168.

Southern, E. M., Anand, R., Brown, W., and Fletcher, D. (1987). A model for the separation of large DNA molecules by crossed field gel electrophoresis. *Nucleic Acids Res.* **15**, 5925–5943.

Spence, A., Coulson, A., and Hodgkin, J. (1990). The product of *fem-1*, a nematode sex-determining gene, contains a motif found in cell cycle control proteins and receptors for cell-cell interactions. *Cell* **60**, 981–990.

Sulston, J., Mallet, F., Staden, R., Durbin, R., Horsnell, T., and Coulson, A. (1988). Software for genome mapping by fingerprinting techniques. *CABIOS,* **4,** 125–132.

Waterston, R., Martin, C., Craxton, M., Hyunh, C., Coulson, A., Hillier, L., Durbin, R., Green, P., Shownkeen, R., Halloran, N., Metzstein, M., Hawkins, T., Wilson, R., Berks, M., Du, Z., Thomas, K., Thierry-Mieg, J., and Sulston, J. (1992). A survey of expressed genes in *Caenorhabditis elegans. Nature Genetics* **1,** 114–123.

Wyman, A., Wertman, K., Barker, D., Helms, C., and Petri, W. (1986). Factors which equalise the representation of genome segments in recombinant libraries. *Gene* **49,** 263–271.

CHAPTER 23

Genomic DNA Sequencing Methods

Anthony Favello,* LaDeana Hillier,* and Richard K. Wilson*,†

* Genome Sequencing Center
† Department of Genetics
Washington University School of Medicine
St. Louis, Missouri 63108

I. Introduction

Understanding the organization and function of the *Caenorhabditis elegans* genome requires an understanding of its primary structure. An organism's genetic material can be studied and analyzed through several methodologies, one of which is genomic sequencing. Unlike cDNA sequencing, genomic sequencing deciphers both the coding and noncoding regions of DNA. The method currently in use for large-scale DNA sequence analysis of the *C. elegans* genome employs a random or "shotgun" strategy (Wilson *et al.,* 1994). This involves using the physical map of the genome, in which overlapping cosmid or yeast artificial chromosome (YAC) clones have been ordered along the six chromosomes. These genomic clones are fragmented by mechanical forces to generate random subclones which are sequenced and assembled by computer.

Our present strategy calls for approximately 700 random subclones to be prepared and sequenced for each cosmid clone. This number of subclones provides nearly complete fivefold coverage of the cosmid, thus eliminating most of the need for library screening and primer-directed sequencing. The subclones are assembled using the xbap program (Dear and Staden, 1991). After the shotgun phase is complete, the cosmid is "finished" by closing gaps, resolving compressions, and double stranding. The final sequence is then analyzed by computer to find genes and regions of homology with other genomes and finally submitted to the public sequence databases. By systematically sequencing overlapping cosmids and portions of YACs, an entire genome can be completed.

II. Methods

A. From Cosmids to Subclones

When sequencing *C. elegans* cosmid clones, the first few steps are critical to success. As cosmid clones must be handled carefully to prevent the deletion and rearrangement to which they are prone, freezer stocks of cosmids (typically received as stabs) should be prepared immediately. Cosmid DNA is prepared using alkaline lysis and cesium chloride gradient ultracentrifugation. This preparation must be performed carefully, because use of shortcuts can result in contaminated or nonrandom M13 subclone libraries. In addition, to ensure that the correct clone is in hand and that a deletion or rearrangement event has not occurred, cosmid DNA is fingerprinted and compared with the original mapping results, which are available in ACeDB (R. Durbin and J. Thierry-Mieg, unpublished). Once the appropriate cosmids have been prepared, the subclone library is constructed through sonication, size fractionation, end repair, and ligation (Bankier and Barrell, 1983). Though these steps are very straightforward, they are nonetheless important to the shotgun sequencing strategy. For example, fraction size determination is critical in reducing the number of potential chimeric clones and for ensuring complete coverage of a cosmid.

1. Preparation of Cosmid DNA

1. Start from a glycerol freezer stock; these should be made immediately on receiving a stab from the Cambridge laboratory (using a sterile loop, transfer cells to 100 μl 2$\times$ (16 g Bacto-tryptone, 10 g yeast extract, 5 g NaCl) YT + 100 μl sterile glycerol, vortex, place at $-80°C$). Streak the clone on a YT plate with the appropriate antibiotic (50 μg/ml ampicillin for pJB8 cosmids, 70 μg/ml kanamycin for lorist cosmids). Use individual colonies to inoculate two or three 250-ml cultures in 2$\times$ YT medium with the appropriate antibiotic, using 1-liter flasks.

2. When good cultures are obtained (16–24 hours), collect cells by centrifugation for 5 minutes at 7000 rpm in 250-ml centrifuge bottles. *Note:* Cells may be frozen at $-80°C$ at this point.

3. Vortex to resuspend the cell pellet in 6 ml GET buffer (50 mM glucose, 10 mM ethylenediaminetetraacetic acid (EDTA), 25 mM Tris–HCl, pH 8.0). Transfer to 30-ml centrifuge tube. Keep on ice.

4. Add 8 ml sodium dodecyl sulfate (SDS)/NaOH (1% SDS, 0.2 M NaOH) and gently invert each bottle 15 times to mix. Incubate 7.5 minutes on ice. The mixture should become very viscous.

5. Add 6 ml 3 M NaOAc, pH 4.8 and gently invert each bottle 15 times to mix. Incubate 30 minutes on ice.

6. Clear the lysate by centrifugation at 12,000 rpm for 20 minutes at 4°C.

7. Transfer the clear supernatant into a 50-ml centrifuge tube. Remove any flocculent material with a large pipet tip. Add 2 vol of absolute ethanol, mix, and centrifuge at 2000 rpm for 5 minutes at room temperature.

8. Discard supernatant and wash DNA with 20 ml 80% ethanol. Centrifuge at 3000 rpm for 5 minutes at room temperature.

9. Discard supernatant and invert for 5 minutes to dry (be careful that DNA pellet does not slide out of the tube). Cap loosely and dry under vacuum for 1 hour.

10. Dissolve DNA pellet in 2.5 ml TE buffer (10 mM Tris–HCl, 1 mM EDTA, pH 8.0), and let sit overnight at 4°C.

11. Add 2.9 g ultrapure cesium chloride, cap, and mix by inversion until all of the CsCl has dissolved. Add 250 μl ethidium bromide (10 mg/ml) and mix.

12. Centrifuge samples at 3000 rpm for 10 minutes. Avoiding the protein–ethidium aggregate, transfer the DNA–CsCl solution to 2.8-ml ultracentrifuge tubes. Seal the tubes and place in the TL-100 rotor (Beckman Instruments, Fullerton, CA).

13. Centrifuge the samples at 70,000 rpm for 16 hours at 20 to 25°C.

14. Visualize ethidium-stained DNA bands under long-wave UV light source. Vent the tube by piercing at the top with a 20-gauge needle. Slowly and carefully, remove the lower, denser cosmid/plasmid DNA band using a 1-cc syringe fitted with a 21-gauge needle. Do not try to remove every bit of the band, or sheared *Escherichia coli* DNA may also be pulled down.

15. Transfer the samples to clean 2.8-ml ultracentrifuge tubes, fill with TE buffer + CsCl (29 g CsCl in 25 ml TE buffer), seal, and place in the TL-100 rotor.

16. Centrifuge the samples at 100,000 rpm for 4 hours at 20 to 25°C.

17. Visualize ethidium-stained DNA bands as before. Carefully remove the cosmid/plasmid DNA band to a 1.5-ml microcentrifuge tube and add distilled water to 0.5 ml.

18. Extract twice with 0.5 ml water-saturated *n*-butanol to remove ethidium bromide. To the final aqueous phase, add 1 ml absolute ethanol. Precipitate the DNA for 15 minutes at room temperature.

19. Centrifuge at 13,000 rpm for 20 minutes in a microcentrifuge to pellet the DNA. Discard supernatant. Wash once with 1 ml 70% ethanol. Dry DNA pellets for a few minutes under vacuum.

20. Dissolve DNA pellets in 40 μl TE buffer.

21. Quantitate the DNA using fluorometry; check cosmid size by agarose gel electrophoresis versus a known standard.

2. Cosmid Fingerprinting

The initial mapping of *C. elegans* cosmid clones was performed by sequential restriction digestion using *Hin*dIII and *Sau*3A, with cosmids orientated, overlapped, and placed into contiguous segments according to the unique fingerprint of each clone (see Chapter 22 in this volume). Prior to constructing M13 libraries and DNA sequencing, it is useful to repeat this analysis for a cosmid and compare the resulting fingerprint with the initial map data. This exercise provides a simple means for ensuring that the correct cosmid has been received and that a deletion (e.g., missing bands) or rearrangement (e.g., bands of incorrect size) has not occurred.

1. Save 50 to 100 ng of DNA from a cosmid prep. Run 1 μl on a 0.7% agarose gel to check approximate size, presence of *E. coli* DNA, RNA, and so on.

2. Make up fingerprint mix 1 (for 25 samples) as follows and keep on ice: [α^{32}P]dATP (800 Ci/mmole), 2–3 μl; distilled, deionized water (ddH$_2$O), 40 μl; 10× medium salt buffer, 10 μl; RNase A (10 mg/ml), 1 μl; 0.5 mM ddGTP, 2.5 μl; *Hin*dIII (10 units/μl), 2 μl; AMV reverse transcriptase, 1 μl. The 10× medium salt buffer contains 500 mM NaCl, 5 ml of 1 M stock; 100 mM Tris–HCl (pH 7.5), 0.5 ml of 2 M stock; 100 mM MgCl$_2$, 1 ml of 1 M stock; 10 mM dithiothreitol (DTT), 1 ml of 0.1 M stock; ddH$_2$O, to 10 ml.

3. Place 2 μl cosmid DNA (50–100 ng) in 0.6-ml microcentrifuge tubes. Add 2 μl mix 1 to each sample. Tap to mix and incubate at 37°C for 45 minutes.

4. Transfer samples to 65°C and incubate for 25 minutes to inactivate reverse transcriptase. Cool on ice.

5. Make up fingerprint mix 2 and keep on ice: ddH$_2$O, 20 μl; 10× medium salt buffer, 2 μl; *Sau*3AI (20–30 units/μl), 2 μl.

6. Add 2 μl mix 2 to each sample. Tap to mix and incubate at 37°C for 2 hours.

7. Add 4 μl dye/EDTA/formamide to each sample. Tap to mix and heat at 100°C for 10 minutes. Load 4 μl of each sample on a 7 M urea, 4% polyacrylamide gel. Every fifth lane on the gel should contain 1 μl of λ DNA/*Sau*3AI markers (see below). The gel should be bonded to the unnotched plate.

λ *DNA/Sau3A I markers:* Make fresh every 3 months. Combine ddH$_2$O, 35 μl; 10× medium salt buffer, 5 μl; λ DNA (BRL, 0.3 μg/μl), 2.5 μl; *Sau*3AI (20 units/μl), 1 μl. Incubate at 37°C for 1 hour. Then add 10 mM dGTP, 2 μl; 10 mM dTTP, 2.5 μl; AMV reverse transcriptase, 1 μl; [α-^{35}S]dATP (1000 Ci/mmole), 4 μl. Incubate at 37°C for 30 minutes. Store at −20°C. To use, add 1 μl to 4 μl of dye/formamide/EDTA. Heat at 100°C for 10 minutes. Load 4 μl per well.

8. Electrophorese the samples at 30 W constant power for about 1.75 hours (until bromophenol blue (BPB) dye is about 1 cm from the bottom of the gel).

9. Separate the plates. Fix the gel in 10% acetic acid for 15 minutes. Wash the gel in tap water for 30 minutes, and dry for about 30 minutes on top of an open gel dryer (80°C).

10. Autoradiograph overnight at room temperature.

3. DNA Sonication and Repair

1. Prior to beginning the shearing experiment, set up the sonicator with the cup horn probe. Fill the cup with ice-cold water.

2. In a 1.5-ml microcentrifuge tube, prepare a solution of DNA to be sheared as follows: DNA (5 μg), x μl; 10$\times$ mb buffer, 6 μl; ddH$_2$O, to 60 μl. Keep the DNA on ice.

10$\times$ mb (mung bean nuclease) buffer: 300 mM NaOAc, pH 5.0, 100 μl of 3 M NaOAc, pH 5.0; 500 mM NaCl, 100 μl of 5 M NaCl; 10 mM ZnCl$_2$, 200 μl of 50 mM ZnCl$_2$; 50% glycerol, 500 μl of glycerol; 100 μl of ddH$_2$O. *Note:* Prepare fresh 50 mM ZnCl$_2$, then prepare fresh 10$\times$ mb buffer.

3. Set the sonicator power switch to "on," set the timer to "hold," and set the power to "10." *Important:* Pulse the sonicator twice for 40 seconds to warm it up.

4. Set the power to "3". Clamp the sample tube so that it is 1 to 3 mm above the opening in the probe. Sonicate twice for 6 seconds.

5. Place the DNA back on ice. Load 1 μl on a 0.7% agarose gel to ensure good shearing. Repeat sonication if necessary.

6. Repair the ends of the sheared DNA by incubation with mung bean nuclease as follows: DNA, 59 μl; mung bean nuclease, 0.3 μl (Pharmacia, 130 units/μl). Incubate at 30°C for 30 minutes.

7. Add 140 μl distilled water, 20 μl 1 M NaCl, and 200 μl water-saturated phenol. Vortex vigorously and place on ice for 5 minutes. Centrifuge 10 minutes to separate phases, and transfer aqueous phase to a 1.5-ml microcentrifuge tube.

8. Add 2.5 vol (500 μl) absolute ethanol, mix, and place at −80°C for 15 minutes. Pellet the DNA by centrifugation, wash once with 70% ethanol, and dry briefly under vacuum

9. Dissolve the sheared DNA in 25 μl water and add 5 μl glycerol/BP/XC loading dye (0.25% BP, 0.25% XC, 30% glycerol). Load 15 μl in each of two wells on a 0.8% (1$\times$ TAE) low-melting agarose gel. Electrophorese at 90 mA for approximately 90 minutes.

10. Photograph the gel under long-wave UV and excise slices containing DNA fragments of 1 to 2 kb. Cut away all excess agarose. Place the gel slices in 1.5-ml microcentrifuge tubes. Melt the agarose at 65°C for 5 minutes, vortex, and place at 65°C for an additional 3 minutes. Aliquot 0.25 ml into microcentrifuge tubes, add an equal volume of water, vortex, and place at room temperature for 2 minutes. Add 0.5 ml water-saturated phenol and vortex vigorously. Place on ice for 5 minutes, vortex, and place at −80°C for at least 15 minutes.

11. Spin the frozen sample in a microcentrifuge for 5 minutes. Transfer the upper phase to a clean tube and add 0.5 vol of phenol. Vortex vigorously, spin for 5 minutes, and transfer upper phase to a clean tube.

12. Extract the sample once with water-saturated ether. To the final aqueous phase, add 0.1 vol 1 M NaCl and 2 vol ethanol. Place at $-80°C$ for at least 15 minutes.

13. Centrifuge 15 minutes at room temperature to pellet DNA. Wash once with 70% ethanol and dry briefly under vacuum.

14. Dissolve the purified sheared DNA fragments in 25 μl TE buffer and carefully quantitate the concentration with the fluorometer.

4. M13 Vector Preparation and Ligations

The sheared DNA fragments are ligated into the M13mp18 sequencing vector. This vector is ideally suited to a large-scale sequencing project, as the known universal priming site facilitates computer assembly and orientation of subclones. Furthermore, the double-stranded replicative form of M13 is useful for closing sequence gaps and sequencing the complementary strand because the universal and reverse primers can be used to sequence the same subclone.

1. To prepare cloning vector, set up the following restriction digest: M13mp18 RF DNA (5 μg), x μl; 10× SmaI buffer, 20 μl; ddH$_2$O, y μl; SmaI (10 units/μl), 1 μl; Total = 200 μl. Incubate at room temperature for 2 hours. Analyze 1 μl on an agarose gel to confirm linearization.

2. Add 1 μl 5 M NaCl and 125 μl 95% ethanol and place at $-80°C$ for at least 15 minutes. Pellet the DNA by centrifugation for 30 minutes. Wash once with 1 ml 70% ethanol and dry briefly under vacuum.

3. Dissolve the DNA pellet in 46 μl 1× phosphatase buffer (supplied with enzyme). Add 40 units calf alkaline intestinal phosphatase (Boehringer, 10 units/μl). Mix gently and incubate at 37°C for 1 hour.

4. Add 25 μl phenol; vortex vigorously. Centrifuge 5 minutes to separate phases, and transfer the aqueous phase to a new tube. Repeat the extraction once more with 50 μl phenol : chloroform. Extract once with 50 μl water-saturated ether. Add 1 μl 5 M NaCl and 125 μl 95% ethanol, mix, and place at $-80°C$ for 15 minutes. Pellet the DNA by centrifugation for 30 minutes, wash once with 1 ml 70% ethanol, and dry briefly under vacuum.

5. At this point, it is advisable to purify the linear M13 DNA by agarose gel electrophoresis. Dissolve each 5 μg sample in 20 μl TE buffer and add 2 μl BP–XC–glycerol dye; load 11 μl per well on a 0.7% low-gelling-temperature agarose gel. Electrophorese until the tracking dyes are well separated. Excise the linear M13 bands and elute DNA as described for sheared cosmid fragments. Dissolve the final pellet in TE buffer to an approximate concentration of 20 ng/μl. Check the DNA concentration by spectrophotometry.

6. Set up library ligation reactions as follows: M13mp18 DNA, SmaI, CIP, 1 μl (20 ng); sheared, repaired DNA, x μl (200 ng); 10× ligation buffer, 1 μl;

10 mM ATP, 1 μl; ddH$_2$O, y μl; T4 DNA ligase (5 units/μl), 1 μl. Total = 10 μl. Incubate overnight at room temperature. Store at $-20°C$.

10$\times$ ligation buffer (make fresh each time): ddH$_2$O, 30 μl; 1 M Tris–HCl, pH 7.5, 50 μl; 1 M MgCl$_2$, 10 μl; 1 M DTT, 10 μl.

5. Electrotransformation of *Escherichia coli*

1. Prepare an appropriate dilution of the ligation mix to be used. When the ligation contains approximately 20 ng of M13 vector, this will be about 1:25. To increase transformation efficiency, denature the ligase by heating at 65°C for 7 minutes (after heating, place at room temperature for 5 minutes).

2. For each transformation, chill a sterile electroporation cuvette. Remove electrocompetent cells from the $-80°C$ freezer and thaw on ice. For each M13 transformation, prepare a sterile tube containing 25 μl IPTG (isopropyl-β-D-thio-galactopyranoside) (25 mg/ml in water), 25 μl X-Gal (5-bromo-4-chloro-3-indolyl-β-D-galactopyranoside)(25 mg/ml in dimethylformamide), and 3 ml YT top agar; place in the 45°C water bath. YT plates should be prewarmed at 37°C for several hours (if water remains on plates, there is a danger of cross-contamination). For each plasmid transformation, prepare a sterile tube containing 1 ml SOC medium. If pUC plasmids are used, L + Amp plates should be prespread with 25 μl IPTG and 25 μl X-Gal.

3. Mix 25 μl electrocompetent cells with 1 to 2 μl diluted ligation mix. This may be done in the cuvette. Tap the cuvette on the benchtop to remove bubbles. Keep the cuvette on ice.

4. Follow the manufacturer's instructions for use of the electroporator device. For the *E. coli* Pulser (Bio-Rad), switch the unit on, and set the proper voltage by pressing the "Raise" and "Lower" buttons simultaneously. For 0.1-cm cuvettes, set to 1.80 kV; for 0.2-cm cuvettes, set to 2.50 kV. Insert the cuvette in the holder and slide the holder into the tray.

5. Press the pulse buttons simultaneously until the tone is heard.

6. Remove the cuvette from the Pulser. Using a flattened pipet tip, immediately transfer the sample to the tube containing SOC or YT top agar. For M13 transfections, plate immediately on YT plates. For plasmid transformations, place the tube at 37°C for 5 to 30 minutes; plate 100 μl on L + Amp plates. Incubate at 37°C overnight.

B. M13 Shotgun Sequencing

Our present sequencing strategy uses a random or "shotgun" approach to achieve extensive sequence coverage of a cosmid. Approximately 700 M13 subclones are prepared, generally providing a nearly complete representation of the cosmid. High-quality template DNA is critical to producing reliable sequence data, and we have tested numerous methods before deciding on our current method of DNA preparation. This method is quick, safe, and cost efficient and ensures consistent, reproducible template.

1. Preparation of M13 DNA

1. Start with an overnight culture or glycerol stock of JM101 to inoculate fresh 2× YT (1 ml per subclone). Grow to early log phase (approximately 1 hour). Alternatively, a frozen overnight culture of JM101 1:100 can be diluted in 2× YT (100 ml for each batch of 96).

2. Transfer 0.8 ml of the JM101 culture to each of 96 1.2-ml minitubes (one rack or box).

3. Wearing clean gloves, pick M13 plaques using sterile toothpicks. Drop each toothpick into a culture tube; remove after all 96 have been picked. Cover the rack of tubes with the provided cover. Incubate at 37°C for 6 to 15 hours with vigorous shaking.

4. Centrifuge the cultures at 3500 rpm for 15 minutes to pellet the cells (set the brake on "Low"). While the cells are pelleting, use a 12-channel pipetter to add 120 μl 20% polyethylene glycol (PEG), 2.5 M NaCl to each tube in a second 96-tube rack.

5. Using the 12-channel pipetter, carefully transfer 0.6 ml (e.g., 3 × 200 μl) phage supernatant to the rack of 96 tubes. (*Note:* If each row of tips is put back in the rack, they can be reused in step 6.) Cover the tubes with a Beckman 96-cap cover and invert several times to mix. Leave at room temperature for 15 minutes.

6. During PEG precipitation, use the 12-channel pipetter to place 25 μl sterile 80% glycerol in each well of a standard 96-well plate (Corning "Cell Wells"). Then transfer an additional 50 μl of each phage supernatant to the 96-well plate that contains glycerol. Pipet up and down to mix the supernatant with the glycerol and place this archive plate at −80°C.

7. Centrifuge the samples at 3500 rpm for 15 minutes to pellet the phage.

8. When centrifugation is finished, carefully discard the supernatant. This is best done by placing an empty, bottomless tube box over all of the tubes and then quickly dumping the supernatant into the sink. Place the inverted tubes on a paper towel for a few minutes to drain. With the tubes still inverted, place them on a dry paper towel in the centrifuge carrier. Spin the inverted tubes at 500 rpm for 5 minutes to remove all traces of supernatant. The phage pellets will stay in the bottoms of the tubes.

9. Add 20 μl TTE buffer (0.25% v/v Triton X-100, 10 mM Tris–HCl, 1 mM EDTA, pH 8.0) to each tube. Seal the tubes with foil tape and vortex vigorously on the multitube vortexer. Give the samples a quick spin in the centrifuge to return liquid to the bottoms of tubes.

10. Heat samples at 80°C for 10 minutes in a water bath. Lift the tubes out of the rack before placing in the water bath.

11. Spin the samples briefly to return liquid to the bottoms of the tubes and transfer to a 96-well plate. Add 30 μl water.

2. DNA Sequencing Reactions

This procedure is for use with the Applied Biosystems 373A DNA sequencer. Either universal or reverse sequencing primer may be used. Reliable sequence data of up to 400 bp can be produced when the reactions are run on a 34-cm 4.75% polyacrylamide gel.

1. Set up reactions in 0.6-ml microcentrifuge tubes (for PE 480 Thermal Cycler) or in a 96-well microtube plate (for PE 9600 Thermal Cycler), as follows:

	A	C	G	T
5× SequiTherm buffer	1 μl	1 μl	2 μl	2 μl
dNTP/ddXTP mix	1 μl	1 μl	2 μl	2 μl
dye–primer (0.4 pmole/μl)	1 μl	1 μl	2 μl	2 μl
DNA template (ca. 100 ng/μl)	1 μl	1 μl	2 μl	2 μl
SequiTherm DNA polymerase (0.28 units/μl)	1 μl	1 μl	2 μl	2 μl
Total	5 μl	5 μl	10 μl	10 μl

Note: For multiple samples, master mixes containing all components except the DNA template may be prepared. The master mixes may be stored at −20°C for several days.

2. Preheat the thermal cycler to 95°C.

3. Using a step-cycle file (e.g., maximum rate of temperature change between setpoints), perform thermal cycling as follows: 95°C for 4 seconds, 55°C* for 10 seconds, 70°C for 60 seconds, for 5 cycles; then 95°C for 4 seconds, 70°C for 60 seconds, for an additional 10 cycles. *Note:* When using the reverse primer (RP), annealing temperature should be 50°C. At the conclusion of thermal cycling, the samples should be kept at 4°C until ethanol precipitation.

4. Remove samples from reaction tubes and transfer to a 1.5-ml microcentrifuge tube containing 3 μl 5 M NH$_4$OAc, pH 7.4, and 80 μl ethanol. Combine the A, C, G, and T reactions for each DNA template. Mix and place on ice for at least 15 minutes.

5. Pellet the fluorescence-labeled reaction products by centrifugation at 13,000g for 15 minutes at room temperature. Wash once with 250 μl 70% ethanol. Dry briefly under vacuum.

6. Dissolve each sample in 5 μl formamide/50 mM EDTA (5:1, v/v), heat at 95°C for 3 minutes, and load on sequencing gel.

10× SequiTherm buffer: 500 mM Tris–HCl, pH 9.3, 25 mM MgCl$_2$.

dNTP mixes: (a) Prepare 20 mM dNTP stocks: 20 μl 100 mM dNTP + 80 μl TE (10:0.1, pH 8.0). (b) Prepare stock dNTP mixes (for 200 reactions):

dATP mix: 1.25 μl 20 mM dATP, 5.0 μl each 20 mM dCTP, dGTP, dTTP, 184.75 μl TE

dCTP mix: 1.25 μl 20 mM dCTP, 5.0 μl each 20 mM dATP, DGTP, dTTP, 184.75 μl TE dGTP mix: 2.50 μl 20 mM dGTP, 10.0 μl each 20 mM dATP, dCTP, dTTP, 367.50 μl TE

dTTP mix: 2.50 μl 20 mM dTTP, 10.0 μl each 20 mM dATP, dCTP, dGTP, 367.50 μl TE

ddXTP mixes:

ddATP (3.0 mM): 100 μl of 5 mM ddATP + 67 μl of TE (Σ = 167 μl)

ddCTP (1.5 mM): 50 μl of 5 mM ddCTP + 117 μl of TE (Σ = 167 μl)

ddGTP (0.25 mM): 16.7 μl of 5 mM ddGTP + 317.3 μl of TE (Σ = 334 μl)

ddTTP (2.5 mM): 167 μl of 5 mM ddTTP + 167 μl of TE (Σ = 334 μl)

dNTP/ddXTP working mixes (for 100 reactions): Mix stock dNTP mix with stock ddXTP mix in a 1:1 ratio:

50 μl dATP + 50 μl ddATP

50 μl dCTP + 50 μl ddCTP

100 μl dGTP + 100 μl ddGTP

100 μl dTTP + 100 μl ddTTP

SequiTherm DNA polymerase (Epicentre Technologies): SequiTherm DNA polymerase (5 units/μl), 48 μl; 5× cycle sequencing buffer, 120 μl; ddH$_2$O, 672 μl. Total = 840 μl (per 96 samples).

Loading solution: Mix 5 parts deionized formamide with 1 part 50 mM EDTA, pH 8.0.

3. Processing and Assembly

The ABI 373A DNA sequencers can be loaded with 36 samples for 10-hour runs twice a day. The sequence data are collected and analyzed by a Macintosh computer with software that calls the DNA base sequence and creates individual sample files. In the genome sequencing project, the sample files that contain both the sequence and the digital trace data are transferred from the Macintosh to a Sun computer. Once on the Sun, the sample files are processed by a series of programs (L. Hillier, J. Parsons, and S. Dear, unpublished) which compress the files, move files to appropriate directories (one directory per cosmid project), mask marginal data, remove M13 and cosmid vector sequences, and segregate poor-quality data. The data are then automatically assembled into contiguous blocks (contigs) of overlapping subclone reads using the bap program (Dear and Staden, 1991). The program also generates a series of statistics that allow data quality to be monitored. Once all 700 clones have been processed, one can begin the task of editing the sequences and closing the remaining gaps using a range of more directed methods.

C. Finishing Cosmid Sequences

1. Initial Finishing Steps

Finishing a cosmid involves a combination of computer work and bench work. The initial finishing steps take place on the computer using the xbap program. xbap is a modified Staden package used for assembling, editing, and managing each cosmid project (Dear and Staden, 1991; Gleeson and Staden, 1991). In xbap, several hundred sequences can be assembled into contigs in a matter of minutes on a Sun SPARCstation. The contigs can be viewed and edited, bringing up the original trace data to resolve conflicts (Gleeson and Hillier, 1991). Additional tools are provided for finding regions of poor quality or regions yet to be sequenced on both strands, screening for restriction enzymes, and checking for consistency of read pairs (when templates have been sequenced in both the forward and reverse directions). The first steps in finishing involve identifying the major contigs, finding the insert ends, and extending reads at contig ends in an effort to close gaps. The original reads are masked to allow no more than 400 bp to be considered for initial assembly. Once assembled, the reads may be unmasked manually to reveal additional data. This is useful for subclones that are present at regions of low or single-strand coverage or at the ends of contigs. Once the ends of major contigs have been extended, the "Find Internal Joins" (FIJ) tool can be used to look for small or marginal overlaps between existing contigs. Some of these overlaps will represent good matches which can be edited and joined together. Another useful step often performed is to add data from overlapping cosmids. This is done using the "stealdata" program (L. Hillier and S. Dear, unpublished). Here, a file of shared reads from the overlapping cosmid(s) is generated and can be used to incorporate reads from one cosmid into the other. These data are often valuable for closing gaps and resolving problems caused by sequence compressions and repeats.

The next step involves looking at both ends of each contig and generating a list of subclones which, if extended by additional sequencing, may produce the data needed to join one contig with another. A software tool ("finish") has been developed that automatically generates this list of subclones for all of the contigs in a cosmid project (G. Marth, unpublished). The end subclones are then resequenced, either with reverse primer (RP) or with universal primer (UP), on a gel designed to produce a longer read (XL).

2. XL Reads, RP Reads, and Primer-Directed Sequencing

Once a list of subclones has been generated, closure of gaps can be accomplished with extra long (XL) and reverse primer (RP) reads. The XL reads involve choosing a subclone that reads into a gap and resequencing it with UP. These reactions are then loaded on an ABI 373A sequencer that has been modified to increase the well-to-read distance to 48 cm (standard distance is

24 cm). By adjusting the gel percentage to 4.0%, a 16-hour run often yields read lengths greater than 700 bp. These extra data generated by XL reads are often sufficient to close many of the remaining gaps.

Reverse primer reads can also be used to close gaps. As the M13 subclones have an average insert size of 1.4 kb, one can choose a subclone that, when sequenced with RP, should yield data that assemble 1.4 kb away from the original read in the opposite orientation. Thus, by calculating distances, it is often possible to produce a read that spans a specific region. Using polymerase chain reactions (PCR) and single-stranded M13 DNA as template with UP and RP, one can generate a double-stranded copy of the subclone insert suitable for sequencing with RP. The PCR protocol for M13 inserts follows.

a. PCR Amplification of Subclone Inserts

1. PCR may be performed using either 1 μl of phage supernatant or 1 μl of single-stranded M13 DNA. To each sample, add 49 μl of PCR mix: ddH$_2$O, 30.5 μl; 10× PCR buffer, 5 μl; 1.25 mM dNTPs, 8 μl; −40 UP (12 μM), 2.5 μl; −40 RP (12 μM), 2.5 μl; Taq DNA polymerase, 0.5 μl. Total = 49 μl per sample.

10× PCR buffer: 500 mM KCL, 100 mM Tris–HCl, pH 8.3 (23°C), 15 mM MgCl$_2$, 0.1% (w/v) gelatin.

2. It is a good idea to make a little more mix than will be needed. For example, for amplifying 24 samples, prepare sufficient mix for 25 samples. If using the DNA Thermal Cycler, overlay each reaction with 80 μl of light mineral oil. Cap all tubes tightly.

3. Spin the 96-well plate assembly briefly to mix. Preheat the thermal cycler to 95°C. Place the sample tubes in the preheated block and begin the thermal cycler program. Use a step-cycle file (e.g., maximum rate of temperature change between setpoints) with the following parameters:

PE 480 Thermal Cycler: 94°C for 30 seconds, 55°C for 30 seconds, 72°C for 60 seconds, for 35 cycles.

PE 9600 Thermal Cycler: 92°C for 10 seconds, 55°C for 60 seconds, 72°C for 60 seconds, for 35 cycles.

At the conclusion of thermal cycling, the samples should be kept at 4°C until PEG precipitation.

4. Remove samples from reaction tubes and transfer to a 1.5-ml microcentrifuge tube containing 8 μl 5 M NaCl, 8 μl TE buffer, 14 μl 40% PEG-8000, 10 mM MgCl$_2$. (If samples have been overlaid with mineral oil, avoid transferring any oil.) Vortex the samples and leave at room temperature for 15 minutes.

5. Pellet the amplification reaction products by centrifugation at 13,000g for 15 minutes at room temperature. Carefully remove all of the supernatant by aspiration. Wash twice with 250 μl 95 to 100% ethanol. Dry briefly under vacuum.

6. Dissolve each sample in 12 μl TE buffer.

b. RP Sequencing

The sequencing reaction is essentially the same as the UP sequencing reaction with the noted changes in thermal cycling conditions. Use 1 μl of the purified PCR product in the A and C reactions and 2 μl in the G and T reactions.

The XL and RP reads are also useful for completing the complementary strand sequence of the cosmid. If an area requiring double stranding has a subclone reading into it, this clone can be extended using the modified ABI 373A. Subclones located 1 to 1.4 kb away can be amplified by PCR and sequenced with RP to generate its complement in the single-stranded area. A list of all of the M13 subclones needed for double stranding can be generated by the "finish" program.

If XL and RP reads fail to close gaps, or if the aforementioned modification of the ABI 373A is not available, custom oligonucleotide primers can be synthesized for additional sequence reads or PCR amplification. Lists of sequencing primers may be generated from within xbap using the "Oligo Selection Tool" (originally "OSP"; Hillier and Green, 1991).

After the primers have been synthesized, they may be used with one of two dye-labeled terminator chemistries to extend the sequence. The first terminator chemistry uses a set of dideoxynucleotides labeled with rhodamine derivatives and Taq DNA polymerase. The Taq chemistry can use either single- or double-stranded template, but, due to uneven incorporation of the terminators, typically produces data of lesser quality. The other terminator chemistry uses a set of dideoxynucleotides labeled with fluorescein derivatives and Sequenase T7 DNA polymerase. Although this second terminator requires single-stranded template, it typically produces data of much higher quality. An additional advantage of the Sequenase terminator chemistry is that postreaction purification steps to remove unincorporated dye terminators are not necessary. Both methods are designed for the use of custom, unlabeled sequencing primers. In addition to the obvious difference in enzyme characteristics, the two methods often have different applications. For example, Taq terminators can be used when only double-stranded product is available (e.g., a region between two contigs that exists only as PCR product). Sequenase terminators, on the other hand, offer a powerful means for resolving the compression artifacts that result from secondary structure.

3. Compression Resolution

In addition to their use for extending clone reads with custom primers, the terminator chemistries are useful for resolving compressions. The AT-rich genomic sequence of *C. elegans* contains a large number of minihairpins (GC[N]$_{1-5}$GC) which produce compression artifacts. Typically, the artifact obscures the sequence on only one strand, so a read from the opposite strand usually allows the compression to be resolved; however, compressions that obscure the sequence on both strands are common. To resolve these regions, one can choose a subclone that contains the compression and resequence using universal primer with one of the two terminator chemistries. The Sequenase terminator chemistry is especially useful for compression resolution, presumably because of the thio-lated deoxynucleotides that are included in the reaction. Note that for use of the Sequenase terminator chemistry, an ABI 373A sequencer must be equipped with a five-color (530/545/560/580/610) filter wheel.

a. Sequenase Dye-Terminator Reactions

1. For each sample, set up an annealing reaction in 1.5-ml microcentrifuge tubes as follows: $10\times$ Mn^{2+} buffer, 2 μl; $10\times$ Mops buffer, 2 μl; ssDNA (2 μg), 2 μl; primer (3.2 pmole/μl), 1 μl; ddH$_2$O, 4 μl. Total = 11 μl.

2. Incubate at 55 to 65°C for 5 minutes, then place at room temperature for 15 minutes. Briefly centrifuge to collect condensation.

3. Add the following reagents to each annealing reaction:

	Standard	XL reads
2 mM [α-S]dNTPs	0 μl	3 μl
ddH$_2$O	1 μl	0 μl
ABI's dye-terminator/[α-S]dNTPs mix	7 μl	5 μl
Sequenase v.2 (1:4 dilution, 3.25 units/μl	1 μl	1 μl

Note: When sequencing multiple samples, make a premix of the above reagents; add 9 μl of the premix to each sample.

4. Mix gently and incubate at 37°C for 10 minutes.

5. To each reaction, add 20 μl of 9.5 M ammonium acetate and 100 μl of ethanol. Mix and place on ice for 10 minutes (cover to protect from light).

6. Pellet reaction products by centrifugation at 13,000g for 15 minutes at room temperature. Wash twice with 300 μl of 70% ethanol; dry briefly under vacuum.

7. Dissolve each sample in 5 μl of formamide/50 mM EDTA (5:1, v/v), heat at 95°C for 3 minutes, and load on sequencing gel. *Note:* Remember to select the 530/545/560/580 filter set on the ABI 373A sequencer prior to beginning data collection.

10$\times$ Mn^{2+} buffer: 50 mM MnCl$_2$, 150 mM sodium isocitrate.

10$\times$ Mops buffer: 400 mM 4-morpholinepropanesulfonic acid (Mops), pH 7.5, 500 mM NaCl, 100 mM MgCl$_2$.

2 mM [α-S]dNTPs: Store at pH 7.2 in Tris–EDTA.

Dye-terminator/[α-S]dNTPs mix: Purchase from ABI (Catalog No. 401489); store at −20°C.

mT7 DNA polymerase (Sequenase v.2) with pyrophosphatase: From USB; 13 units/μl Sequenase, 0.012 units/μl pyrophosphatase.

b. Taq Dye-Terminator Reactions

1. Prepare a reaction premix using the various buffers and reagents as follows:

	4× Mix	20× Mix
5× TACS	16 μl	80 μl
dNTP mix	4 μl	20 μl
DyeDeoxy A Terminator	4 μl	20 μl
DyeDeoxy C Terminator	4 μl	20 μl
DyeDeoxy G Terminator	4 μl	20 μl
DyeDeoxy T Terminator	4 μl	20 μl
AmpliTaq DNA polymerase	2 μl	10 μl

Note: Premixes may be stored in the dark at 4°C for several days.

2. Set up reactions in 0.6-ml GeneAmp tubes (for PE 480 Thermal Cycler) or in 0.2-ml MicroAmp tubes (for PE 9600 Thermal Cycler), as follows: reaction premix, 9.5 μl; ssDNA template, 5.0 μl (use 1 μg dsDNA or 0.7 μg PCR product); primer (0.8 μM), 1.0 μl (use 3.2 μM for dsDNA or PCR product); water, x μl. Total = 20.0 μl. If using the DNA Thermal Cycler, overlay each reaction with 50 μl of light mineral oil. Cap all tubes tightly.

3. Preheat the thermal cycler to 95°C.

4. Using a step-cycle file (e.g., maximum rate of temperature change between setpoints), perform thermal cycling as follows:

PE 480 Thermal Cycler: 96°C for 30 seconds, 50°C for 15 seconds, 60°C for 4 minutes, for 25 cycles.

PE 9600 Thermal Cycler: 96°C for 15 seconds, 50°C for 1 second, 60°C for 4 minutes, for 25 cycles.

At the conclusion of thermal cycling, the samples should be kept at 4°C.

5. Prior to electrophoresis, excess dye-terminator must be removed from the reactions. This is best done using Centri-Sep spin columns (Princeton Separations, Princeton, NJ) as follows:

a. Gently tap the column to settle the resin in the bottom of the column.

b. Remove the top cap and add 750 μl of water to the column.

c. Replace the cap and invert several times to swell the resin. Allow the resin to hydrate for at least 30 minutes. After hydration, the columns may be stored at 4°C for a few days. Remove any air bubbles by inverting the column and allowing the gel to settle again. Remove the top cap first, then the bottom cap. Allow the column to drain completely by gravity.

d. Insert the column into a collection tube and centrifuge in a swinging-bucket rotor at 2400 rpm for 2 minutes.

e. Discard the collection tube and the effluent. Insert the column into a second collection tube.

f. Load the 20-μl sample directly to the center of the bed of the column.

g. Centrifuge at 2400 rpm for 2 minutes. The reaction products will pass through the column into the collection tube. The column, containing unincorporated dye-terminator, may be discarded.

h. Dry the sample for a few minutes under vacuum.

i. Dissolve each dry pellet in 5 μl of formamide/50 mM EDTA (5:1, v/v). Heat at 95°C for 3 minutes and load on the sequencing gel.

5× TACS buffer: 400 mM Tris–HCl, 100 mM ammonium sulfate, pH 9.0, 10 mM MgCl$_2$.

dNTP mix: 750 μM dITP, 150 μM dATP, 150 μM dCTP, 150 μM dTTP.

4. Problem Solving

After a cosmid is contiguous and double stranded, the finisher must work to identify and resolve repeated sequences. Repeats represent the single most difficult aspect of large-scale sequencing. There are several types of repeats, each with its own unique problems. Tandem repeats are arranged sequentially in the same orientation, often with some small amount of unique sequence inbetween. Interspersed repeats are sequences that occur with a large amount of intervening sequence. Inverted repeats consist of a sequence that has an inverted copy of itself occurring a few to a few hundred base pairs downstream. All three types of repeats are of varying length and copy number and can be perfect copies with no differences in their sequence.

Interspersed repeats are the easiest to resolve. With longer repeats ($>$ 400 bp), problems can occur during the initial assembly if reads are put into the database in the wrong place. By unmasking extra data or running an XL read on the clones in question, they can usually be extended beyond the repeat area and assembled where they belong.

A similar strategy can sometimes be applied to tandem repeats. Problems occur when the reads are matched with the wrong copy of the repeat. By extending the reads, either on the computer or with XL reactions, some unique flanking sequence can usually be found. With large repeats, or a large number of tandem copies of a repeat, it may not be possible to find unique flanking sequences simply by extending the read. In these cases, RP reactions can be very useful by providing sequence data from the other end of the M13 insert, a region that may not be contained within the repeat. Although the UP and RP reads from the same clone are not contiguous, they are physically linked and can be properly assembled on that basis. In addition, PCR can be used to size the repeat region (e.g., estimate the number of tandem copies).

Inverted repeats are the most difficult problem to resolve, especially when cosmid subclones have been generated in M13 vectors. Some inverted repeats presumably form a hairpin structure which is unstable in the single-stranded infectious form of M13. Hence, inverted repeats are often present at the end of a contig with all subclones at that point reading away from the gap for approximately 700 bp (e.g., half of the average insert size). If the repeat segment is short ($<$ 200 bp) or the intervening loop relatively long ($>$ 500 bp), subclones usually can be found that may be extended into or through the gap with XL or RP reads. Inverted repeats of intermediate size (200–500 bp) are unstable in M13;

however, PCR can be used to amplify the repeat region. The resulting PCR product can be cloned in a plasmid vector or sequenced directly. The current method of choice is to clone the PCR product into a TA cloning vector (Holton and Graham, 1990). The TA vector has a single-base 3' overhang ("T") which is compatible with the single-base 5' overhang ("A") added by Taq DNA polymerase. The TA vector also has the universal and reverse priming sites so the PCR product can be sequenced from both ends using dye-primers. TA subcloning is performed using essentially the protocols previously described for ligation, transformation, and plating. In this case colonies, rather than plaques, are picked and DNA is isolated using the following small-scale plasmid preparation.

1. Pellet cells from 1.5 ml of overnight cultures by centrifuging for 15 seconds; discard the supernatant.

2. Add 150 μl of ET buffer (25 mM Tris–HCl, pH 8.0, 10 mM EDTA) + RNase A [add 10 μl of 10 mg/ml RNase A (DNase-free) per 1 ml of ET buffer]. Mix on the multitube vortexer for 3 to 4 minutes.

3. Add 150 μl of freshly prepared lysis solution (1 ml of 10 M NaOH, 5 ml of 10% SDS, 44 ml of ddH$_2$O). Mix gently by inverting a few times (do not vortex). Leave at room temperature for 5 minutes.

4. Add 150 μl of 2.55 M KOAc, pH 4.8 (10 ml 3 M KOAc, pH 4.8 + 1.7 ml ddH$_2$O), invert twice to mix. Leave on ice 5 minutes.

5. Centrifuge for 5 minutes to pellet chromosomal DNA and cell debris. Remove supernatant (400 μl) to a clean tube.

6. To each aqueous phase, add an equal volume of phenol:chloroform (1:1). Vortex for 10 seconds and centrifuge for 5 minutes to separate phases. Transfer the aqueous phase to a clean tube.

7. Add 1 ml of absolute ethanol and mix by inversion. Place on ice for 10 minutes.

8. Centrifuge 10 minutes to pellet plasmid DNA. Discard supernatant.

9. Wash the DNA pellet once with 1 ml of 70% ethanol. Dry briefly under vacuum.

10. Resuspend the DNA pellet in 80 μl of TE buffer. Analyze 1 μl on a mini-agarose gel.

The TA subclones are then sequenced with UP or RP using the DNA sequencing methods described above. These two reactions will produce sequence reading into the gap that can subsequently be used for oligo selection and terminator reactions. In this way, a template is produced and sequenced on both strands that will span the gap caused by the presence of the inverted repeat.

Large inverted repeats (500 bp to 1 kb) often prove resistant to amplification by PCR. In these cases, oligonucleotides must be chosen from unique flanking sequence on both sides of the repeat and used to screen a plasmid subclone library. Although this can be done by hybridization, pooling schemes followed by PCR to identify subclones in the repeat region are more reliable. For example, the sonicated DNA fragments that were used to produce the original M13 library can be used again to generate a library in pUC18. Alternatively, a pUC library can be made from larger random fragments of the cosmid. After transformation, a few hundred colonies may be picked to microtiter trays, grown up, and pooled to facilitate rapid DNA preparation and screening by PCR. Typically, four 96-well trays (e.g., 384 subclones) are used to produce 4 plate pools, 8 row pools, and 12 column pools. Using these 24 pools, plasmid is prepared by the small-scale alkaline lysis procedure (see above), and the resulting DNAs are screened by PCR and analyzed by agarose gel electrophoresis. PCR screening involves the use of one custom primer (flanking the repeat region) and one vector primer. The presence of a unique PCR product in one of each type of pool indicates a subclone in the repeat region. Furthermore, the size of the product indicates how much of that subclone covers the repeat region. Once a few subclones have been identified, one can go back to the microtiter plate wells that contain the original cultures and purify DNA for sequencing.

D. Analysis

1. BLAST

Once the sequence is complete, it can be compared against the public databases using the BLAST programs (Altschul *et al.,* 1990) to look for similarities to existing genes and for cDNAs, tRNAs, snRNAs and known repetitive elements. In the *C. elegans* genome project, sequences are also searched for tRNAs using "trnascan" (Fichant and Burks, 1991) and for local inverted and tandem repeats using programs written by R. Durbin (unpublished). MSPcrunch is used for removing biased composition and redundant matches from BLAST output, and Blixem is a multiple-alignment viewer used to scan and evaluate BLAST alignments (E. Sonnhammer and R. Durbin, manuscript submitted).

2. Genefinder

Additionally, likely genes can be predicted using the program Genefinder (Hillier and Green, unpublished), which uses a statistically rigorous evaluation of likelihoods to locate splice sites and define exons and a dynamic programming algorithm to parse these into predicted genes. *C. elegans* cDNA data are useful for confirming predicted splice patterns. Once sequences have been analyzed, the data can be submitted for entry into the ACeDB nematode database (R. Durbin and J. Thierry-Mieg, unpublished), which presents the sequence in the context of other available information about the worm.

III. Summary

Sequence analysis of cosmids from *C. elegans* and other organisms currently is best done using the random or "shotgun" strategy (Wilson *et al.,* 1994). After shearing by sonication, DNA is used to prepare M13 subclone libraries which provide good coverage and high-quality sequence data. The subclones are assembled and the data edited using software tools developed especially for *C. elegans* genomic sequencing. These same tools facilitate much of the subsequent work to complete both strands of the sequence and resolve any remaining ambiguities. Analysis of the finished sequence is then accomplished using several additional computer tools including Genefinder and ACeDB. Taken together, these methods and tools provide a powerful means for genome analysis in the nematode.

References

Altschul, S. F., Gish, W., Miller, W., Myers, E. W., and Lipman, D. J. (1990). Basic local alignment search tool. *J. Mol. Biol.* **215,** 403–410.

Bankier, A. T., and Barrell, B. G. (1983). Shotgun DNA sequencing. *In* "Techniques in the Life Sciences" (R. A. Flavell, ed.), Vol. B5, pp. 1–34. Elsevier Scientific Publishers, County Clare, Ireland.

Dear, S. and Staden, R. (1991). A sequence assembly and editing program for efficient management of large projects. *Nucleic Acids Res.* **19,** 3907–3911.

Fichant, G. A., and Burks, C. (1991). Identifying potential tRNA genes in genomic DNA sequences. *J. Mol. Biol.* **220,** 659–671.

Gleeson, T., and Hillier, L. (1991). A trace display and editing program for data from fluorescence based sequencing machines. *Nucleic Acids Res.* **19,** 6481–6483.

Gleeson, T. J., and Staden, R. (1991). An X windows and UNIX implementation of our sequence analysis package. *Comput. Appl. Biosci.* **7,** 398.

Hillier, L., and Green, P. (1991). OSP: A computer program for choosing PCR and DNA sequencing primers. *PCR Methods Appl.* **1,** 124–128.

Holton, T. A. and Graham, M. W. (1990). A simple and efficient method for direct cloning of PCR products using ddT-tailed vectors. *Nucleic Acids Res.* **19,** 1156.

Wilson, R., Ainscough, R., Anderson, K., Baynes, C., Berks, M., Bonfield, J., Burton, J., Connell, M., Copsey, T., Cooper, J., Coulson, A., Craxton, M., Dear, S., Du, Z., Durbin, R., Favello, A., Fraser, A., Fulton, L., Gardner, A., Green, P., Hawkins, T., Hillier, L., Jier, M., Johnston, L., Jones, M., Kershaw, J., Kirsten, J., Laister, N., Latreille, P., Lightning, J., Lloyd, C., Mortimore, B., O'Callaghan, M., Parsons, J., Percy, C., Rifken, L., Roopra, A., Saunders, D., Shownkeen, R., Sims, M., Smaldon, N., Smith, A., Smith, M., Sonnhammer, E., Staden, R., Sulston, J., Thierry-Mieg, J., Thomas, K., Vaudin, M., Vaughan, K., Waterston, R., Watson, A., Weinstock, L., Wilkinson-Sproat, J., and Wohldman, P. (1994). 2.2 Mb of contiguous nucleotide sequence from chromosome III of *C. elegans. Nature* (*London*) **368,** 32–38.

CHAPTER 24

Large-Scale Complementary DNA Sequencing Methods

Lucinda L. Fulton, * **LaDeana Hillier,** * **and Richard K. Wilson** *,†

* Genome Sequencing Center
† Department of Genetics
Washington University School of Medicine
St. Louis, Missouri

I. Introduction

Sequence analysis of cDNA clones is a useful means for characterizing genes in *Caenorhabditis elegans* and investigating gene expression at specific stages of development. As we have previously described, single-pass sequencing of random cDNA clones has proven to be a powerful method for gene identification (Waterston *et al.,* 1992). Sequencing strategies for cDNA clones will vary depending on the length of the cDNA and the vector in which it has been cloned. Further considerations include whether a single-pass or "tag" sequence is adequate or if the complete sequence of a cDNA is desired.

To provide high efficiency when cloning cDNAs, bacteriophage lambda vectors are typically used. Although a large number of clones are recovered, the cDNA is present as a small portion of a very large recombinant lambda clone. Depending on the vector that was used for library construction, it is often difficult to separate the cDNA insert from the cloning vector prior to DNA sequencing. As outlined in Fig. 1, several approaches can be considered to provide a template for DNA sequencing. First, it is possible to simply purify lambda DNA and sequence directly using labeled primer, although this approach typically does not produce data of very high quality. A more desirable approach is to subclone the cDNA insert into a plasmid. If unique restriction sites are present flanking the insert, the cDNA is easily excised and subcloned into the appropriate plasmid. Some lambda vectors contain rare-cleavage restriction sites flanking the cloning site,

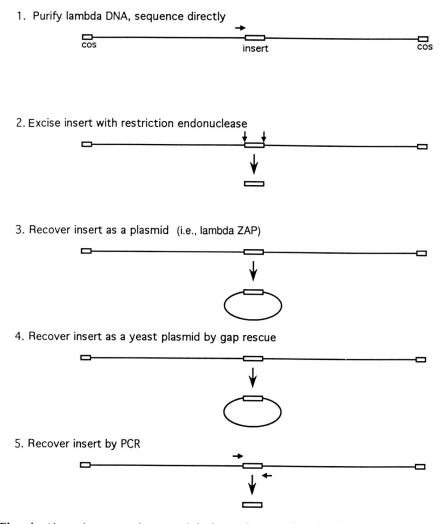

Fig. 1 Alternative approaches to subcloning and sequencing cDNAs from bacteriophage lambda clones.

thereby providing an effective means for excising the cDNA insert. The most convenient and commonly used strategy is based on "automatic subcloning." Bacteriophage lambda vectors such as Lambda ZAP (Stratagene, San Diego, CA) have been developed that contain plasmid sequences flanking the cloning site; an autoexcision mechanism allows the cDNA insert to be recovered as a plasmid clone (Short *et al.,* 1988). This may also be accomplished using the gap rescue method in yeast cells (Erickson and Johnston, 1993). Once available as a plasmid clone, the cDNA may be sequenced directly using primers from both ends or with either the deletional or random strategies directly using primers from both ends or with either the deletional or random strategies. Small cDNA inserts (5 kb or less) can be amplified by polymerase chain reaction (PCR) using vector-specific primers on either side of the cloning site. The resulting PCR products can be sequenced using any of the three aforementioned strategies. This PCR approach has proven very powerful for rapid tag sequencing of large numbers of cDNA clones.

As mentioned above, a useful approach for surveying gene repertoire and gene expression in specific types of tissues or cell cultures is single-pass or "tag" sequencing of cDNA clones. Here, data collected from a single sequence run are taken from one end of the cDNA clone, typically using a dye-labeled primer that anneals in flanking vector sequence. With the high capacity of automated sequencing instruments such as the Applied Biosystems 373A, a large number of tag sequences can be generated rapidly. In this chapter, we describe methods for PCR amplification and single-pass fluorescent sequencing of *C. elegans* cDNAs. To produce the highest-quality data while maintaining throughput at a maximum, the PCR templates are purified by polyethylene glycol (PEG) precipitation. Cycle sequencing with dye-labeled primers is the method of choice for sequencing.

We also describe methods for complete sequencing of *C. elegans* cDNAs. The exonuclease III deletion method of Henikoff (1987) is especially useful for cDNAs in the size range 2 to 6 kb, and the multiple cloning sites of some of the newer lambda vectors typically provide an adequate choice of restriction enzymes for unidirectional deletion. A second method for complete sequencing of cloned cDNAs is the random of "shotgun" strategy (see Chapter 23 in this volume). Although this may be generally preferred for cDNAs larger than 5 kb, it is possible to stitch several small cDNAs together prior to shotgun subcloning (Andersson *et al.,* 1994). For cDNA sequencing in general, several excellent sources of additional reading and alternate protocols are available. These include the comprehensive methods manuals of Sambrook *et al.* (1989) and Ausubel *et al.* (1987–1994).

II. Methods

A. From mRNA to cDNA Clones

A variety of methods are available for construction of cDNA libraries in general, and these are described in detail elsewhere (Sambrook *et al.,* 1989). For

C. elegans in particular, an excellent procedure for construction of expression libraries was described by Barstead and Waterston (1989). In addition, one could consider using one of the bacteriophage lambda vectors which allows autoexcision to facilitate subsequent DNA sequence analysis.

B. Storage and Growth of cDNA Clones

Once a cDNA library has been chosen, it is helpful to organize the individual clones in a 96-well format (one cDNA clone per well). The individual cDNA clones are easier to work with in such an array and multichannel pipetters can be used to ensure accuracy and decrease the amount of time spent pipetting the clones from one tray to another. A 96-well format also decreases the amount of space needed to store the clones.

1. Array and Storage of cDNA Clones

Complementary DNA clones are stored easily as agarose plugs in 96-well microtiter plates. Although there are several ways to make such trays, one procedure is as follows:

1. Prepare SM buffer containing 0.6% agarose and sterilize by autoclaving.
2. Sterilize glycerol by autoclaving separately.
3. Melt the SM/0.6% agarose in a microwave oven.
4. Heat the glycerol as well.
5. Mix the SM/agarose and the hot glycerol in 7 : 3 (to yield a final concentration of glycerol of 30%).
6. Quickly dispense 0.1 ml of the mixture into the wells of a 96-well microtiter plate and let stand to solidify.
7. Plates can be stored at 4°C until use.
8. cDNA clones from glycerol stocks or fresh plates can be stabbed into the agarose/glycerol plug. The cDNAs can be stored like this for months at −80°C.

SM buffer: NaCl, 5.8 g; MgSO₄·7 H₂O, 2.0 g; 1 *M* Tris–HCl (pH 7.5), 50 ml; 2% gelatin solution, 5 ml. Add water to 1 liter. Autoclave to sterilize.

2. Growth of Phage Clones for Template Preparation

Once a means of storage of the cDNAs has been determined, the process of growing the phage clones to allow template production for PCR can begin. A stock of competent host bacterial cells can be prepared and stored at 4°C. To prepare the bacteria (MC1061), inoculate 50 ml of 2× YT, 0.2% maltose plus the appropriate antibiotic in a 250-ml sterile flask. Incubate overnight at 37°C on a shaker. Transfer the overnight culture to a 50-ml tube and centrifuge the bacteria at 3000 rpm for 10 minutes at room temperature. Discard the supernatant and resuspend the cell pellet in 10 mM $MgSO_4$ (one-fourth volume of the original culture). Store at 4°C. This stock can be used for up to 1 month.

The bacteriophage are amplified by infection of the bacterial host followed by plating on TB agarose in individual wells of a 96-well microtiter tray. This system works best if a 12- or 8-channel pipetter can be used to make all the transfers. The protocol for this is as follows:

1. During the incubation, melt 50 ml of TB top agarose and cool to 45°C in a water bath.

2. Add 125 μl of TB agarose to each well of a 96-well microtiter tray. Warm in the 37°C incubator until use in step 4.

3. Add 10 μl of distilled water to each well in an empty 96-well microtiter tray. Using an 8- or 12-channel pipetter, stab each well of the glycerol/SM tray that contains the cDNAs. Move the pipet tips to the water-containing tray and pipet up and down to transfer the clones. Add 10 μl of bacteria in $MgSO_4$ buffer to each well and adsorb phage to cells by incubating at 37°C for 15 minutes.

4. After the incubation, add 25 μl of TB top agarose to row A of the microtiter tray containing the bacteria and phage. Pipette up and down a few times to mix. Then transfer the mixture to row A of the microtiter tray containing the TB agarose. Repeat this step for the remaining rows.

5. Let the tray stand at room temperature for 5 minutes to allow the TB top agarose to solidify.

6. Incubate at 37°C overnight. After the incubation, plaques should be visible in each well of the microtiter tray. Elute the phage by adding 20 μl of distilled water to each well.

7. At this point, cover the tray with a plastic plate sealer (Costar, Cambridge, MA) or aluminum tape (R. S. Hughes, Sunnyvale, CA) to prevent evaporation and store at 4°C for several hours before attempting the PCR.

2× YT: Bacto-tryptone, 16 g; yeast extract, 10 g; NaCl, 5 g. Adjust volume to 1 liter and autoclave.

TB agarose: Bacto-tryptone, 10 g; agarose, 10 g; NaCl, 5 g. Adjust volume to 1 liter and autoclave. This is usually stored in a volume of 100 ml/bottle.

TB top agarose: Bacto-tryptone, 10 g; agarose, 7 g; NaCl, 5g. Adjust volume to 1 liter and autoclave. This is usually stored in a volume of 50 ml/bottle. *Note:* Remember to always use agarose, as agar will inhibit PCR.

C. PCR Amplification of cDNA Inserts

The clones are now ready to be used as templates for PCR. The DNA template for the PCR is not isolated from the phage; instead, template is produced by a brief lysis of the phage heads. The concentration of phage in each well is dependent on the concentration of the original SM/glycerol stock, and will vary from clone to clone. For best results with the PCR procedure, the amount of phage that produces satisfactory PCR amplification should be determined by titration of a few clones. Typically, this will be 5 μl, 1 μl, and 1 μl of a 1:10 dilution.

1. Add the phage to the amplification vessel (tubes or microtiter wells, depending on the thermal cycler to be used) and bring the volume up to 5 μl using sterile water. The phage heads are lysed by heating at 95°C for 5 minutes in the thermal cycler.

2. To each sample, add 5 μl 10× PCR buffer, 8 μl 1.25 mM dNTPs, 1 μl 10 μM primer A, 1 μl 10 μM primer B, 1 μl Taq DNA polymerase (5 units/μl), 29 μl sterile water. Total per sample = 45 μl. For best results, prepare a master mix of these components and add 45 μl to each DNA sample. It is a good idea to make a little more mix than you actually need.

3. Spin the samples briefly to mix. Preheat the thermal cycler to 95°C. Place the samples in the preheated block and begin the appropriate cycling program. The following program is used in our laboratory for the PE 9600 Thermal Cycler: 95°C for 60 seconds, 52°C for 120 seconds, 72°C for 120 seconds, for 35 cycles. Then incubate at 72°C for 10 minutes. At the conclusion of thermal cycling, load 5 μl of each sample on a 0.7% agarose gel with an appropriate molecular size marker to check for successful amplification before proceeding to the next step. The samples can be stored at 4°C.

Notes. (a) If PCR yields spurious bands, raise the annealing temperature in the thermal cycling program to correct this problem. (b) If PCR fails, the phage titer may be low; another round of phage growth may be necessary to increase the amount of template. This growth can be done by repeating the plating process previously described. Mix 10 μl of the phage mixture from this new plate with the competent cells instead of the phage from this new plate. The rest of the procedure remains the same. This substitution allows the phage to be amplified again. Once this second plate (2×) has been made, another PCR can be performed. With some libraries, the titer of the glycerol stock may be very low, and a few successive growths may be necessary before the PCR will produce sufficient product.

4. Once sufficient PCR product is in hand, the samples are purified by polyethylene glycol (PEG) precipitation. To do this, add to each sample 8 μl of TE buffer, 8 μl of 5 M NaCl, and 16 μl of 40% PEG-8000, 10 mM MgCl$_2$. Vortex briefly to mix and incubate at room temperature for at least 15 minutes.

5. Pellet the DNA by centrifugation at 13,000g for 15 minutes. (If the PCR was performed in the 96-well format, the samples may be precipitated in a 96-well tray and pelleted by centrifugation at 3500 rpm for 30 minutes using a Beckman GPKR centrifuge.)

6. To remove the PEG mixture, invert the 96-well tray on a paper towel and spin for 3 minutes at 300 rpm in a Beckman GPKR centrifuge. If tubes are used,

aspiration should be used to remove all of the PEG. At this point a series of two 70% ethanol washes, 200 μl each, may be done to clean up the DNA; however, this wash step may be omitted with good sequencing results.

7. Resuspend each sample in 20 μl of TE buffer and vortex. Check yield by loading 2 μl of a few samples on a 0.7% agarose gel.

The samples are now ready to be sequenced or can be stored at $-20°C$ for several months.

10× PCR buffer: 500 mM KCl, 100 mM Tris–HCl (pH 8.3), 15 mM MgCl$_2$, 0.1% (w/v) gelatin.

D. Direct Single-Pass DNA Sequencing

The following procedure may then be used to read 300 to 400 bases from one end of the insert. These data are then used to search the public databases for similarities. The success rate for this method typically runs between 80 and 90%. The loss is usually due to human error, pipetting errors that occur during the sequencing protocol, or clones that do not readily amplify by PCR. The procedure described here is designed for use with the Applied Biosystems 373A DNA sequencer. The appropriate dye-labeled primers should be used, depending on how the cDNA library was constructed. SequiTherm (Epicenter Technologies, Madison, WI) is the enzyme used in the protocol.

1. Reactions are set up using 0.6-ml GeneAmp tubes (for the Perkin–Elmer 480 DNA Thermal Cycler) or 0.2-ml MicroAmp tubes (for the PE 9600 Thermal Cycler), as follows:

	A	C	G	T
5× SequiTherm buffer	1 μl	1 μl	2 μl	2 μl
dNTP/ddXTP mix	1 μl	1 μl	2 μl	2 μl
Dye-primer (0.4 pmole/μl)	1 μl	1 μl	2 μl	2 μl
SequiTherm DNA polymerase (0.28 units/μl)	1 μl	1 μl	2 μl	2 μl
DNA template	1 μl	1 μl	2 μl	2 μl
Total	5 μl	5 μl	10 μl	10 μl

For multiple sample, mixes may be made containing all reagents except the DNA template. Master mixes may be stored at $-20°C$ for several days.

3. PCR conditions for cycle sequencing are as follows:

PE 480 DNA Thermal Cycler: 95°C for 30 seconds, 55°C* for 30 seconds, 70°C for 60 seconds, for 15 cycles. Then 95°C for 30 seconds, 70°C for 60 seconds, for an additional 15 cycles.

PE 9600 Thermal Cycler: 95°C for 4 seconds, 55°C* for 10 seconds, 70°C for 60 seconds, for 15 cycles. Then 95°C for 4 seconds, 70°C for 60 seconds, for an additional 15 cycles.

When sequencing with T7, T3, Universal, or Reverse dye-primer, the listed cycling conditions work well; however, when using the SP6 dye-primer, the annealing temperature should be lowered to 50°C. After the sequencing PCR, samples should be kept at 4°C until ethanol precipitation.

4. To the A well of each sample add the following: 3 μl of 5 M NH$_4$OAc (pH 7.4) and 100 μl of 100% ethanol. Add the A reaction into the C, G, and T reactions for each DNA template. Mix and pellet the reactions products by centrifuging for 30 minutes at 3500 rpm using a Beckman GPKR.

5. Wash the pellets once with 200 μl of 70% ethanol. Spin 15 minutes at 3500 rpm using the Beckman GPKR. Dry briefly under vacuum.

6. Dissolve each sample in 5 μl of formamide/50 mM ethylenediamine tetra-acetic acid (EDTA, 5:1, v/v), heat at 95°C for 3 minutes, and load on sequencing gel.

Notes.   (a) If all of the sequencing reactions fail, there may be a problem with one of the reagents. Bad enzyme will produce some sequence data and die off early or produce no data at all. Always be sure to double-check that the correct primer is being used with the current vector. If the wrong primer is used, there will be primer peaks but no sequence after them. (b) Gel problems are another cause of sequence failures. If this occurs, the peaks produced will be too closely spaced or will contain a high background. Fresh gel solutions should always be used. (c) Another problem that results in high background is the presence of PEG left over from the precipitation step. Sequence data will be produced, but the traces will be noisy and contain base calling errors due to the high background. If this occurs, the PCR and PEG precipitations must be repeated.

E. Complete cDNA Sequencing

Complementary DNA clones that are selected from libraries by traditional screening methods (Sambrook *et al.,* 1989) or recovered through single-pass surveys can be completely sequenced using a variety of strategies; however, two main approaches can be considered. For smaller cDNAs (2–5 kb), the deletional method is very useful. Enzyme kits containing exonuclease III, mung bean nuclease, and DNA ligase can be purchased from several suppliers (an excellent kit is available from New England Biolabs, Beverly, MA). The procedure described below provides a series of deletional subclones over the entire length of the cDNA. The insert size of the deletional subclones can be determined by agarose gel electrophoresis and sequenced in order of size. For larger clones (>5 kb), the shotgun strategy is preferred, especially if the cDNA insert can be recovered as a plasmid clone or excised from the lambda vector using restriction endonucleases.

1. Detectional Sequencing

a. Restriction Digestion

For deletions up to 1.5 kb from the unprotected end, start with 10 μg of template DNA. For deletions up to 3 kb, start with 20 μg of DNA. If the two restriction enzymes are not fully active under the same buffer conditions, or if repair of one site is required to generate a protected end, sequential digests will be necessary. Often it is possible to perform a low-ionic-strength digest first, then increase salt concentration and add the second enzyme. If repair is necessary, use the T4 DNA polymerase method described earlier, but substitute 0.5 mM α-thio-deoxyribonucleoside triphosphates and omit the kinase step.

1. Set up the restriction digest as follows: template DNA, x μl (10 μg); 10× buffer, 5 μl, ddH$_2$O, y μl, restriction enzyme(s), z μl (20 units of each). Total = 50 μl. Incubate at the appropriate temperature for 1 to 2 hours. Load 1 μl on an agarose gel to ensure complete digestion.

2. When linearization is complete, add 5 μl of 1% sodium dodecyl sulfate (SDS), 0.2 M EDTA to the digest. Then, add 50 μl of phenol (TE buffer-saturated):chloroform (1:1). Vortex vigorously.

3. Centrifuge the samples for a few minutes to separate phases. Remove the aqueous (top) phase to another tube.

4. Add 50 μl of chloroform, vortex, and repeat step 3.

5. To the final aqueous phase, add 0.1 vol 5 M NaCl and 2 vol of absolute ethanol. Mix thoroughly and incubate on ice for 15 minutes.

6. Pellet the DNA by centrifugation for 15 minutes at room temperature. Discard the ethanol supernatant and wash the pellet with 400 μl of 70% ethanol. Dry briefly under vacuum.

7. Dissolve the DNA pellet in 30 μl of 1× exo III buffer. Load 1 μl on an agarose gel to verify DNA concentration.

10× exo III buffer: 660 mM Tris–HCl, pH 8.0, 6.6 mM MgCl$_2$.

b. Exonuclease III Digestion

In general, when 5 μg of template DNA is incubated with 100 units of exonuclease III, approximately 300 bp is removed per minute. For deletions up to 1.5 kb, time points should be taken from the reaction every 50 seconds. For deletions of 1.5 to 3 kb, template DNA should be predigested for 5 minutes prior to removing time points. For larger deletions, increase predigestion time accordingly. It is important to remember that the degradation rate of exonuclease III will vary considerably with different lots and vendors.

1. Dilute 5 μl of template DNA to a final volume of 60 μl with 1× exo III buffer. Place the sample in a 37°C water bath.

2. Add 2 μl of 10× mbn buffer and 8 μl of sterile, distilled water to each of six microcentrifuge tubes, labeled MB1 through MB6, and place the tubes on ice.

10× mbn buffer: 500 mM NaOAc, pH 5.0, 300 mM NaCl, 10 mM ZnSO$_4$.

3. Add 100 units of exonuclease III to the 5 μg DNA sample and mix gently.

4. Every 10 seconds, remove a 2-μl aliquot from the exonuclease III reaction and add it to the contents of an "MB" tube until five aliquots have been added

to that tube (i.e., MB1 has ten 50-second time points, MB2 has sixty 100-second time points, etc.). When the fifth aliquot has been added, transfer the "MB" tube to a dry ice bath. *Note:* In the procedure described here, "50-second time points" consist of five 10-second time points. This helps to ensure production of deletion subclones with sufficient overlap.

5. After all time points have been taken, incubate all of the "MB" tubes at 68°C for 15 minutes.

6. Chill the samples on ice for 5 minutes, then centrifuge briefly to collect condensate.

7. Add 3 units of mung bean nuclease to each tube and incubate at 30°C for 30 minutes.

8. To each "MB" tube, add 19 μl of 1× TE buffer and 40 μl of phenol (TE buffer-saturated):chloroform (1:1). Vortex vigorously.

9. Centrifuge the samples for a few minutes to separate phases. Remove the aqueous (top) phases to new tubes.

10. Add 40 μl of chloroform to each sample, vortex, and repeat step 9.

11. To the final aqueous phases, add 0.1 vol of 5 M NaCl and 2 vol of absolute ethanol. Mix thoroughly and incubate on ice for 15 minutes.

12. Pellet the DNA by centrifugation for 15 minutes at room temperature. Discard the ethanol supernatant and wash the pellet with 200 μl of 70% ethanol. Dry briefly under vacuum.

13. Dissolve each DNA pellet in 10 μl of TE buffer. Load 5 μl of each sample on an agarose gel to determine fragment sizes and DNA concentration. Be sure to include a molecular weight standard of known concentration on the gel.

c. Religation of the Subclones

Set up ligation reactions as follows: DNA sample, x μl (approximately 100 ng); 10× ligase buffer, 2.5 μl; ddH$_2$O, y μl; T4 DNA ligase, z μl (NEB, 150 units, see Note). Total + 23.5 μl. Incubate the reactions overnight at 15°C.

10× ligase buffer 500 mM Tris-HCl, pH 7.8, 100 mM MgCl$_2$, 200 mM dithiothreitol, 10 mM ATP.

Note: T4 DNA ligase from different vendors will affect results. Good results have been obtained using ligase from New England Biolabs (use 150 NEB units) and Boehringer-Mannheim (use 2 Weiss units).

d. Transformation, Screening, and Sequencing

Transformation of *Escherichia coli* with the religated subclones can be performed using the standard CaCl$_2$ method or by electroporation (see Chapter 23 in this volume). For electroporation, 1 ng of DNA should produce a sufficient number of colonies for pUC-based recombinants. The methods described above for plasmid minipreps can be used to prepare DNA and assay for subclones with the appropriate size insert. As the universal priming site is typically adjacent to the site of deletion, the subclones may be sequenced using the cycle sequencing method described above.

2. Shotgun Sequencing

For complete sequencing of cDNA clones using the shotgun approach, see the procedures described in Chapter 23.

F. Analysis

For tag sequencing projects, once several cDNA sequences have been completed, they can be compared against the public databases using the BLAST programs (Altschul *et al.,* 1990) to look for similarities to existing genes. For larger cDNAs which have been sequenced completely, there are several computer tools one can use to analyze the sequence. For example, the Staden package contains xbap, which provides for sequence assembly, editing, and primer selection. Also, the xnip program can be used to search for restriction sites and analyze open reading frames. Other programs are available both in the public domain and commercially (e.g., Intelligenetics, DNA Star, Applied Biosystems). Once sequences have been analyzed, the data can be submitted for entry into the ACeDB nematode database (R. Durbin and J. Thierry-Mieg, unpublished), which presents the sequence in the context of other available information about the worm. (*Note:* For additional information on ACeDB submission, contact Richard Durbin: rd@sanger.ac.uk.)

III Summary

Complementary DNA libraries are useful tools for uncovering genes of interest in *C. elegans* and finding specific homologies to genes in other organisms (Waterston *et al.,* 1992; McCombie *et al.,* 1992). When working with existing cDNA libraries, be sure to carefully choose which libraries would be most beneficial to the type of research being done. Some libraries may be specific for genes that are present in lower copy numbers, whereas others may be of a more general nature. It is important to fully understand the source and construction of the library you will be working with. Once an appropriate library has been chosen, work may begin to isolate a specific cDNA and sequence it completely or to survey many cDNAs by single-pass DNA sequencing. Whatever the project, it is important to develop a specific strategy for both the sequencing and the organization of the clones being characterized. The strategies and procedures we have outlined in this chapter have proven effective for rapid and comprehensive cDNA characterization.

References

Altschul, S. F., Gish, W., Miller, W., Meyers, E. W., and Lipman, D. J. (1990). Basic local alignment search tool. *J. Mol. Biol.* **215,** 403–410.

Andersson, B., Povinelli, C., Wentland, M., Muzny, D., and Gibbs, R. (1994). Adaptor-based uracil DNA glycosylase cloning simplifies shotgun library construction for large scale sequencing. *Anal. Biochem.* **218,** 300–308.

Ausubel, F. M., Brent, R., Kingston, R. E., Moore, D. D., Seidman, J. G., Smith, J. A., and Struhl, K. (1987–1994). "Current Protocols in Molecular Biology" Vol. 1 and 2. Current Protocols, Inc. (J. Wiley & Sons), New York.

Barstead, R. J. and Waterston, R. H. (1989). The basal component of the nematode dense body is vinculin. *J. Biol. Chem.* **264,** 10177–10179.

Erickson, J. R., and Johnston, M. (1993). Direct cloning of yeast genes from an ordered set of lambda clones in *Saccharomyces cerevisiae* by recombination *in vivo. Genetics* **134,** 151–157.

Henikoff, S. (1987). Unidirectional digestion with exonuclease III creates targeted breakpoints for DNA sequencing. *Methods Enzymol.* **155,** 156–165.

McCombie, W. R., Adams, M. A., Kelley, J. M., FitzGerald, M. G., Utterback, T. R., Khan, M., Dubnick, M., Kerlavage, A. R., Venter, J. C., and Fields, C. (1992). *Caenorhabditis elegans* expressed sequence tags identify gene families and potential disease gene homologues. *Nature Genetics* **1,** 124–131.

Sambrook, J., Fritsch, E. F., and Maniatis, T. (1989). "Molecular Cloning: A Laboratory Manual" Vol. 1, 2, and 3. Cold Spring Harbor Press, Cold Spring Harbor, New York.

Short, J. M., Fernandez, J. M., Sorge, J. A., and Huse, W. D. (1988). Lambda ZAP: A bacteriophage lambda expression vector with *in vivo* excision properties. *Nucleic Acids Res.* **16,** 7583–7600.

Waterston, R., Martin, C., Craxton, M., Huynh, C., Coulson, A., Hillier, L., Durbin, R., Green, P., Shownkeen, R., Halloran, N., Metzstein, M., Hawkins, T., Wilson, R., Berks, M., Du, Z., Thomas, K., Thierry-Mieg, J., and Sulston, J. (1992). A survey of expressed genes in *Caenorhabditis elegans. Nature Genetics* **1,** 114–123.

CHAPTER 25

ACeDB and Macace

Frank H. Eeckman[*] and Richard Durbin[†]

[*] LBL Human Genome Center
Berkeley, California
[†] The Sanger Centre
Hinxton Hall
Cambridge, United Kingdom

I. Introduction

ACeDB (A *Caenorhabditis elegans* Data Base) is a data management and display system that contains a wide range of genomic and other information about *C. elegans.* This chapter provides an overview of ACeDB for the *C. elegans* user, focusing in particular on the Macintosh version Macace. Previous reviews of ACeDB include those of Thierry-Mieg and Durbin (1992) and Durbin and Thierry-Mieg (1994), which describe the general properties of the whole system, and that by Dunham *et al.* (1994), which discussed the use of ACeDB for physical map data collection and assembly.

ACeDB was developed by Jean Thierry-Mieg and Richard Durbin primarily for the *C. elegans* project, when the genomic sequencing project was just beginning in 1990. The original aim was to create a single database that integrated the genetic and physical maps with both genomic sequence data and the literature references. The forerunner of ACeDB was the program CONTIG9 (Sulston *et al.,* 1988), which was developed to maintain and edit the physical map. CONTIG9 served researchers around the world by providing critical on-line access to the current physical map as it was being constructed (Coulson *et al.,* 1986). This policy of immediate access allowed members of the worm community to see the same data as the people making the map, and proved very successful in maximizing use of the map. The same approach was adopted as a template for ACeDB. These two principles, developing a comprehensive database for all types of genomic and related data and providing public access to the data in the same form as used by the data-collecting laboratories, have continued to underlie developments of ACeDB.

Over the last 5 years, a wide range of genome projects relating to other organisms have taken the ACeDB program and used it to develop databases for their own data. ACeDB has been used both in public projects designed to redistribute public data in a coordinated fashion and laboratory-based projects for collecting new data. Others, such as the *C. elegans* ACeDB, have used the database for both purposes. The reason it has been possible to adapt ACeDB so widely is that its flexible data structure allows new types of objects and new types of information about these objects to be added easily.

This chapter describes (1) how to obtain ACeDB and documentation for it, (2) how to access and use the information in ACeDB, and (3) how to use ACeDB as a laboratory-based data managing system. Some of what we discuss is specific to the nematode database, but other information applies to the basic computer software program and, hence, to any database using the ACeDB program.

II. System Information and Requirements

A. Availability and System Requirements

Originally, ACeDB was developed for UNIX workstations, and it now runs on machines from many manufacturers. A Macintosh-specific version (Macace), developed by Frank H. Eeckman, Richard Durbin, and Cyrus Harmon, uses the standard Macintosh graphical system. The UNIX version uses X-windows for its graphical interface. Where there is a shared UNIX computer on a local network, it is possible to run ACeDB from either an X-terminal, a Macintosh (MacX), or a PC running an X-terminal emulator program.

ACeDB is distributed primarily by anonymous ftp (file transfer program), which allows users to copy the database onto their own local computer. As a result, people can have full rapid access to all the data, but they must have fairly powerful computing systems and a nonnegligible amount of hard disk space. Updates are released periodically and are announced via an e-mail mailing list and through the ACeDB and *C. elegans* news groups (see below). For the UNIX version, these updates can be obtained by anonymous ftp and added to the local database by a simple command inside ACeDB (see below). During every update, the Macintosh version is typically recopied in its entirety. ACeDB is distributed from the following anonymous ftp sites:

1. The main distribution site for the UNIX version and the official documentation is

   ncbi.nlm.nih.gov in directory ~ftp/repository/acedb.

2. Alternative sites include:

   cele.mrc-lmb.cam.ac.uk in ~ftp/pub/acedb,
   lirmm.lirmm.fr in ~ftp/pub/acedb,
   bioinformatics, weizmann.ac.il in ~ftp/pub/databases/acedb.

3. Macace is distributed from:

   genome.lbl.gov in ~ftp/pub/macace,
   cele.mrc-lmb.cam.ac.uk in ~ftp/pub/acedb/macace,

or via the World Wide Web,

   http://www-hgc.lbl.gov/Genome/macace.html.

The UNIX version has been compiled and run on many workstation types. Active support is available for SGI (Irix), DEC (OSF), or PC486 level machines, as well as for SUN workstations with either SunOS or Solaris operating systems. For PC486 level users, Linux serves as a useful freeware UNIX port for Intel 80×86 machines and is an alternative operating system to DOS, Windows, or OS/2. Although all these machines provide virtual memory, 32 MByte of random access memory (RAM) is desirable (half of which will be used by the operating system and graphics), with more being advisable if many processes are to be run simultaneously. The worm database takes 150 MByte of disk space at the time of this writing, and some extra space is needed during transfer and loading of the data. Printing graphics or other data from UNIX machines generates a postscript file, which can then be printed by most UNIX printer systems. To install the UNIX version, obtain from any of these sites the files README, NOTES, and INSTALL. NOTES describes which other files you should get and how to use the INSTALL script.

The minimal configuration requirements for Macace are a Macintosh IIci running System 7.x, with 16 MByte of memory, a 270-MByte hard disk, and a 14-in. color monitor. Alternatively, a 100 series Powerbook can be used. We do not recommend this type of system though. A good value-for-money system is the Quadra 630 with 16 MByte of RAM and a 500-MByte hard disk. For new purchases we recommend a PowerMac with a minimum of 24 MByte of RAM and a 500/1000-MByte hard drive and a 17-in. multisynch monitor. Macace runs as a native PowerPC program. For printing one can use any Quickdraw printer, although we recommend a 600-dpi laser printer. Macace can run with virtual memory.

To install Macace, use Fetch (© Trustees of Dartmouth College, 1994) or any MacBinary II-compatible ftp program to retrieve the self-extracting archive from the addresses given above. Make sure you have enough disk space to accommodate both the packed and the unpacked archive. Consult the README file to find out how much space is needed. Double-click the mouse on the archive, and Macace will self-extract and install itself on your hard disk. There is no need to restart the machine.

In addition to local copies of the entire database, there is a network version of the ACeDB code written by Guy Decoux (Moulon, France) for the World Wide Web (WWW). This has been used to establish a number of WWW servers and can be accessed using standard viewer programs such as Mosaic and Netscape from workstations, Macintoshes, or PCs attached to the Internet. The primary server is at Moulon (http://moulon.inra.fr), with another major node at the USDA National Agricultural Library (http://probe.nalusda.gov:8000).

B. Information about ACeDB

There are several user manuals for ACeDB. Perhaps the best general introduction is a guide from Bruno Gaeta of the Australian National Genome Information Service, ANGIS. This guide is available either as a compressed postscript file or as a Macintosh Microsoft Word document compressed using the compression program Stuffit. Other useful and fairly up-to-date user guides have been written by Mary O'Callaghan (user_guide.moc) and for the *Arabidopsis thaliana* database (AAtDB). These, together with a wide variety of other information about ACeDB, can be found on the NAL WWW server (http://probe.nalusda.gov:8000). For those readers without WWW access, both the ANGIS manual and a more general package of documentation (wdoc.tar.Z) are available in the standard ftp archives (see above).

There is also a newsnet newsgroup devoted to ACeDB called bionet.software.acedb. Update announcements are sent to this news group and to the general worm news group, bionet.celegans. There is also an explicit e-mail mailing list for updates for people who do not read news groups. To have yourself added to (or removed from) this list, send e-mail to rd@sanger.ac.uk. To add/remove yourself to a Macace-specific mailing list, send e-mail to FHEeckman@lbl.gov.

C. Communicating with the Authors

To communicate with the authors and other developers, we recommend using the news group bionet.software.acedb. The authors can also be reached directly at rd@sanger.ac.uk and mieg@kaa.cnrs-mop.fr. Macace will have a bug report facility on the LBL WWW server (http://www-hgc.lbl.gov/Genome/macace.html). We hope to bring this on-line mid-1995. You will need a WWW application that supports the forms protocol to use this facility, such as a recent version of Mosaic or Netscape. If you do not have access to such an application, please send e-mail to FHEeckman@lbl.gov.

III. Basic Use of ACeDB: Browsing and Searching

To start the UNIX version you can probably type "acedb" at the command line. If not, consult the person who installed your version of the program and/ or someone who knows about UNIX; there are lots of ways to set things up. To start the Macintosh application, double-click on it.

A. Browsing

Two windows should be visible when you start: the main window, which lists classes and contains Template and Text Search fields, and a Keyset window listing objects (Fig. 1). To browse, select an object from the Keyset window, and click twice on it (left mouse button in UNIX). This brings up another window with more information about the object. Displays can either show text information or display a map, depending on the type of object. In general, other named objects on maps or bold objects in text displays can also be displayed themselves by double-clicking.

1. Mouse Functions in Xace and Macace

A UNIX mouse has three buttons: left, middle, and right. Each button has certain associated functionality with which UNIX users are familiar. PC mice have two buttons. Refer to one of the user guides on how to simulate the third button when running Linux. The Macintosh has a mouse with one button. MacX lets one assign keystrokes to simulate middle and right mouse buttons. In Macace, we simulate the middle mouse button using the shift key, and eliminate the need for the right mouse button.

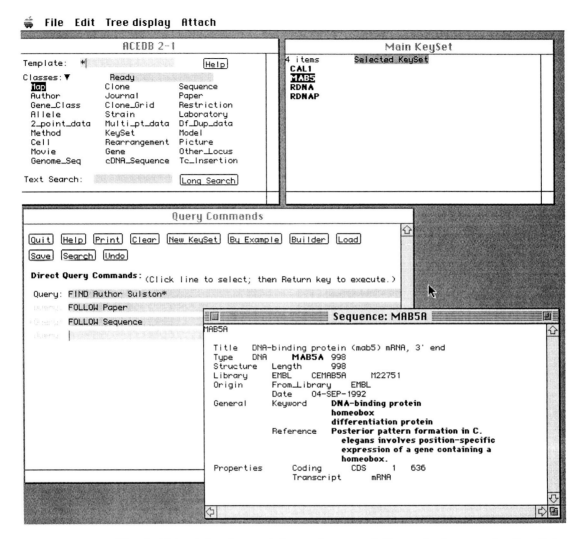

Fig. 1 Main window, keyset window, and query tool. The result of a query that lists all the sequences in the database reported by J. Sulston is shown in the keyset window. The procedure is described in the text (Section III,B). One of the sequences is shown as a text display.

Left Mouse Button. The left mouse button is used to select items. To find out more about an item click on it twice. There is no real double-clicking in ACeDB in the sense that the clicks have to come within a certain time interval. Clicking on the same item twice in a row, with any time interval, will open up another display. The (only) mouse button on the Macintosh serves the role of this left mouse button in UNIX.

Middle Mouse Button. The middle mouse button can be used to control scroll and zoom of map displays. Clicking the middle mouse button shows a line which will become the new center line for the display when the button is released, perhaps after dragging. The middle mouse action is mimicked by holding the shift key down while using the mouse on the Macintosh; however, it is also possible to scroll and zoom all the maps in other ways (by dragging a scroll icon and using buttons).

Right Mouse Button. The right mouse button accesses the popup menus in UNIX. On the Macintosh all the menus are in the menubar, so there is no need to use this feature. Some pickable items on maps have customized menus (e.g., genes on the genetic map); on the Macintosh, these menus appear in the menubar once the item has been selected.

To exit from ACeDB in the UNIX version you must select Quit from the popup menu in the main window, using the right mouse button. On the Macintosh, Quit is in the File menu. Similarly, in Macace you can print or get help in any window using the Print . . . and Help options from the File menu. Under UNIX, most windows have a Print option near the top of their menu. They also have a Help option there. Help on UNIX may either call an internal help package or connect to one using WWW/Mosaic. Some versions of Macace use the new help facility under System 7.5. Unfortunately you cannot always rely on the help package to be completely up to date. If you want to help update the help file you can send mail to the authors with proposed changes!

B. Searching

By a series of clicks and resulting new displays you can rapidly obtain much of the data in the database. This is the simplest way to find data in ACeDB, but it can be longwinded. Often you will want to find data in other ways, either because you already know the names of the objects you are interested in, or because you know some of their properties. This section shows you how to use this sort of information.

1. Template Searches

Template searches are done using the template text entry box in the main window. To perform a template search, carry out the following steps: highlight the class with the mouse, click in the template box so it turns yellow, type in the name or part of the name in the template box, then press the Return or Enter key. You can use the wild card character "*" to match any string of letters. The special character "?" matches a single letter. Wild cards can be used anywhere in the name. So, for example, "D*" matches all names beginning with D, and "A*J" matches all names starting with A and ending with J. The case of the template characters does not matter, as names in ACeDB are not normally case sensitive; however, they can be made case sensitive on a class-specific basis by editing wspec/options.wrm.

2. Text Searches

Text searches provide a simple but powerful method to find objects in ACeDB related to some keyword or topic in which you are interested. They use the Text Search text entry box in the main window. A heterogeneous set of objects can be retrieved this way. Basic text searches look for a string match using all names in the database, plus most text. To do this, click in the box next to Text Search so it turns yellow, and type in the string. It can contain wild cards, just like the template described in the previous section, but it is better to be more rather than less specific. Hit Return. You will have to wait a few seconds, then the list of matching objects will appear in the main keyset window. If you press the Long Search button instead, the program will also search all the abstracts and any other long pieces of text stored in the database. This will take considerably longer to execute.

3. Query Searches

Queries are the most powerful way to search the database. They are also the most complex to use. Writing a successful query statement requires some understanding of the internal structure of the database. For example, one has to know what the different classes are and how information is organized within those classes. One also has to understand the query syntax. We present an example query that attempts to find all the sequences in the database reported by J. Sulston. Use the following sequence: Use the pull-down menu and select the Query option. Into the yellow box next to the title Query, type

FIND Author Sulston*

To perform the query you must press the return key. This will search out all the authors whose name starts with Sulston, and show them in a keyset window. A new query box will then appear and you could type a second query command:

FOLLOW Paper

This gives all the papers referred to from the current set of objects, in this case, all papers by the Sulstons. Next type

FOLLOW Sequence

It is also possible to get the same result by concatenating all the statements on one line:

FOLLOW Author Sulston*; FOLLOW Paper; FOLLOW Sequence.

At any point, if a query does not work the way you want, you can press the UNDO button to return to the previous state.

As this example shows, in simple cases queries can seem fairly intuitive, though this does not always make the correct query easy to find. In general, we advise that you use simple queries and combine them, rather than try to design very complex queries (we do this ourselves). It is also good to try to adapt existing queries that you know work. Apart from the brief example here, there are examples in several of the manuals, and there are files of examples that come with the database. You can load in these examples using the Load button and save working examples you have constructed yourself using Save.

In addition to the basic tool for queries described here, your version of ACeDB may also have other query construction tools in the main menu, such as Query Builder and Query by Examples. These are designed to give more guidance, but are not as flexible.

C. Keysets

All the ways of searching for objects described in the last section work by generating a list of objects, normally in the Main KeySet window. Such a list of objects is called a *keyset*. Apart from clicking on objects in a keyset to display them, there are other things you can do with them; keysets play an important role in ACeDB. First, we describe operations you can perform from the Keyset menu (popup in Xace, menubar in Macace).

The three dump options allow data to be exported from ACeDB in different formats. Ace Dump exports all the text information about each object in the keyset in the standard paragraph format, which we will return to later in the chapter. This is the main way to extract large sets of data from ACeDB. Name Dump just creates a list of all the names of the objects in the list, with their classes. Sequence Dump dumps out any DNA sequences in the list in FASTA format, which is a standard format used by many sequence analysis packages.

The first two blocks of options let you edit and combine keysets. The Copy operation makes a new keyset window with a copy of the current keyset in it. This can be useful for keeping several lists on the screen. The Add-Remove Keys option lets you interactively edit the current list by clicking on objects — try it: it gives instructions. The Save option lets you save useful lists inside the database as objects in their own right, but for this you need write access to the database, as described later in the chapter.

The AND, OR, MINUS, and XOR options all allow you to combine to keysets in various ways. To use them you should have two keysets displayed, perhaps one made by Copy (or the NEW KeySet option from the query tool). One of these will have a pink box at the top saying Selected KeySet. Only one keyset at a time can be the selected keyset; in general it will be the last one you clicked in. To combine two keysets, taking only those things in both keysets, make one the selected keyset, then go to the other and choose AND from its menu. This is easy in UNIX, where you can use the right button to pop up a menu in it. On the Macintosh, you must select the title bar of the second keyset, then the KeySet menu. If you click in the window itself, then it becomes the selected keyset, defeating your operation. This unnatural operation may be superseded in a future release. The principle, however, is that the actions combine the current keyset, to which the menu belongs, with the selected keyset, defined by the pink box.

The concept of a selected keyset is used several other places in the program. For example, the DNA analysis tools allows you to search for sequence motifs in a list of sequences, where the list is taken from the selected keyset. Also, many of the map displays let you highlight a set of objects, and again the set is defined by the selected keyset. In general, wherever the program requires a set of objects it uses the selected keyset. The principle behind this is that there is a flexible set of tools to construct an arbitrary keyset, and this can be used in many ways.

At the bottom of the keyset menu are a number of convenience items. The Show as Text option lets you show the current selected item in its text form, even if the default display for it would be in a map. This can be useful for genes, rearrangements, clones, and sequences, all of which are displayed in maps by default (see next section). The Show Related Biblio option shows a bibliography of all the papers referred to in all the objects in the current list (including any paper objects in it). This can be useful for printing out (see above about printing). The Find Neighbors option replaces the current list by all the objects referred to from objects in the current list. This is a way to find related objects, but often the list expands very rapidly.

D. Tables

Finally, there is another powerful tool in ACeDB that lets you construct tables similar to a spreadsheet, defining successive columns in terms of queries on previous columns. These tables can also be dumped out in text form for external programs, for example, for transferring to a Macintosh or PC spreadsheet program. Again, as with the Query tool, you can save and load table definitions from external files, and the standard release comes with some examples. It is beyond the scope of this chapter to give a full description of how to specify tables. If you want to use this feature, please read further documentation from the WWW server.

IV. *Caenorhabditis elegans* Data and Map Displays

The main *C. elegans* database combines information from many sources. The primary sources are the following:

1. The genomic sequence and the physical map from the Cambridge/St. Louis genome consortium

2. The CGC strain list, mailing list, and bibliography from the CGC in Minnesota (Theresa Stiernagle and Bob Herman)

3. The genetic map, genetic map data, gene list, and laboratory registration list from the CGC outpost in Cambridge (Sylvia Martinelli and Jonathan Hodgkin)

4. The *Worm Breeder's Gazette* and Worm Meeting contents information from Minnesota, and text mostly via the WCS (some now from direct submissions)

5. Worm bibliographic entries from Medline and DNA sequence entries from EMBL/Genbank (via Cambridge)

6. Sequence and map information on cDNA EST's from Yuji Kohara, the parts list and lineage from the worm book (Wood, 1988)

7. Neural synaptic information from John White, Eileen Southgate and Nichol Thomson

8. Tc1 insertion site information from Ronald Pasterk

9. Expression information from Ian Hope

10. Restriction enzyme information from REBASE

There are also a large number of corrections, fixes, and individual pieces or groups of data from many individual worm researchers.

Here we show you how to get at the main types of data described above and make the best use of them. This section is fairly specific for the *C. elegans* database, though it does introduce the main types of graphical displays.

A. Genetic Map and Mapping Data

To display a genetic map, you can either select the Map class in the main window and then pick a map explicitly, or pick a gene or rearrangement, which by default will be displayed in its context in the genetic map. If you do the latter, the gene will be highlighted on the map; if you want to see the text data for it, you can just click on it again. Normally the last item you clicked is highlighted, and a brief description of it will be shown in the light blue band at the top of the display. Other related items may also be highlighted, in different colors, depending on the relationship.

The Zoom In, Zoom Out, and Whole buttons are self-explanatory. To move up or down, either use the middle mouse function as described earlier or drag the green slider with the left mouse function. If you use the middle mouse function to the left of the green slider, you can not only drag it up and down, but can also change the magnification by an arbitrary factor. You can also configure the magnification directly, and some of the parameters of other columns, by clicking on the green labels at the bottom of the window.

In general, a map display is a set of columns containing different types of data (Fig. 2). You can control which columns are visible by using the Columns menu and clicking the different columns on and off. By default most columns are on. For chromosomes with many rearrangements, you will probably want to turn off the Rearrangements column, unless you are specifically interested in them, in which case you will have to make the window very wide. If you turn on the Ordered Genes column, the genes will split into two sets. The ones on the left have been chosen on the basis that their order is unambiguously determined

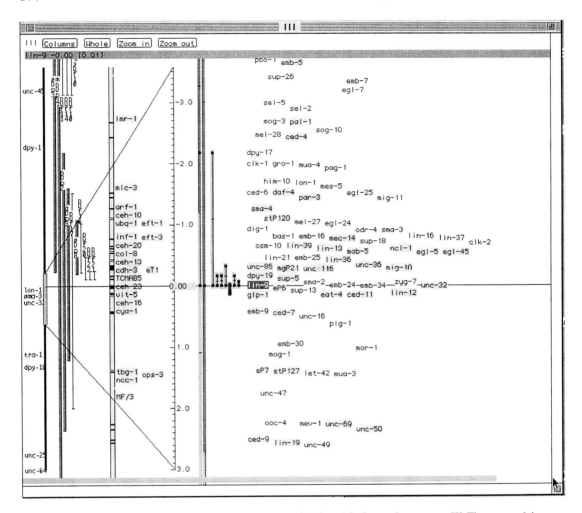

Fig. 2 Genetic map display of the central region of *C. elegans* chromosome III. The extent of chromosome is shown by the black bar on the left-hand side. The visible part is indicated by the length of the slider bar (green on color displays). To the left of the scale bar, the light gray bar (yellow) represents contigs and provides a link to the physical map. The function GMap Data for *lin-9* has been illustrated by the recombination data shown to the right of the scale bar. See text for a more detailed description.

with respect to each other; some arbitrary choices were made in this process of selection. The purpose of the Reversed Physical column is to show inconsistencies between the genetic and physical maps. These are indicated by small red marks next to the yellow bar representing the physical map (Contigs column). If you double click on this bar you will display the physical map, centered on the point where you clicked. This will be described below.

One of the most useful features of the genetic map is the ability to show all the CGC map data for a gene. If you click on a gene, and press the GMap Data button, you will see two new columns appearing containing 2point and Multipoint map data objects. Rectangles and lines on these indicate the other markers used and confidence information. Note that for 2point data it is not uncommon for single data items to be outside their confidence intervals. Horizontal lines on Multipoint objects indicate where there are recombinants. You can click twice on either type of object to see the corresponding data in text form. To show the dependence of the gene position on the data, you can display a likelihood distribution, using the menu attached to the gene itself. The resulting histogram assumes that all other gene positions are correct (not always justified!). The red lines are absolute limits on left and right positions based on multipoint, deficiency/ duplication, and physical mapping. In the new version of ACeDB you can show likelihood histograms for multiple genes simultaneously. There are other functions in the GMap Data menu, but the most important one for normal use is the one to clear data when the columns get too full. The others all have to do with global operations used when constructing the map.

B. Clones and the Physical Map

The default display for a clone is the horizontal physical map. So if you want to see the physical map around a clone, select the Clone class in the main window, then type the name of the clone in the Template box (see above), and hit return. The horizontal physical map display is the oldest display in ACeDB. It is based on the display of the CONTIG9 program used for assembling the nematode physical map and is rather specific for the nematode data.

As with the genetic map, you can scroll the horizontal map either with the middle/shift button or by picking and dragging the green slider at the bottom. Attached to this slider is a reduced-size map showing just the cloned loci, to give some impression of relative position. In general, if you click on an object, related or attached objects are also highlighted. If you double-click, you display the object itself either as text or on another type of map display.

The upper half of the display is divided into three zones (Fig. 3). The top zone is used to display a series of names which indicate cDNA probes from the cDNA EST sequencing projects that have been placed on the map by hybridization to yeast artificial chromosomes (YACs). Clicking on these will highlight the positive YACs. Note that clones starting with YK in the uppercase are not real clones, but rather groups of clones from Yuji Kohara that he has clustered on the basis of their sharing identical 3' EST sequences. Below the probe data are two sets of lines representing clones. The upper, long ones with names beginning with Y are the YACs, and the lower, shorter ones are the cosmids. Certain cosmids are shown with an asterisk after their names. These clones are canonical for others that have been "buried." You can see the names of the buried clones by double-clicking on a cosmid with an asterisk after its name. Clones present on filter hybridization grids are indicated by a bold line. Gaps between cosmid contigs that had to be bridged with YACs are indicated by double vertical

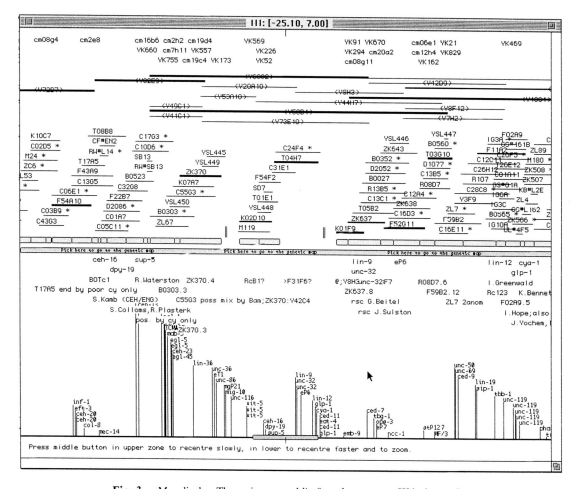

Fig. 3   pMap display. The region around *lin-9* on chromosome III is shown. See text for description.

lines. These gaps are of unknown size; they have been drawn five units wide by convention.

Below the clones are a number of regions of attached information. Yellow bars represent DNA sequences corresponding to a clone in this region. Short sequences probably come from a cDNA probe, whereas long ones are likely to come from a genomic cosmid. Clicking on the sequence displays it (see below for sequence display). Note that sometimes many cDNA boxes can fall on top of one another, so you cannot reach them all in this way. Below the clones is a green bar that acts like a button to bring up the genetic map, centered by interpolation at (approximately) the corresponding position. Just below this are the names of genes or other loci that have been attached to the map. Finally, there are text comments attached to the clones. Some of these describe rescue experiments; most are private notes written by Alan Coulson when constructing the map.

C. The Clone Grid

The clone grid display was designed to allow data entry for the results of hybridization experiments against the "polytene" filter grids made available by the physical mapping project. It is accessed through the menu option Clone_Grid in the ACeDB main window. The only grids of general interest are POLY1 and SUP_POLY, which are the original "polytene" filter and the more recent supplementary one designed to fill known gaps. This facility can be used by anyone using the polytene filters to locate genes by hybridization.

If you double-click on one of the grid objects you will see an image symbolizing the array of clones. There are two modes, controlled by buttons in the header region. In Map mode you can double-click on a square and go to the corresponding position in the physical map. In Edit mode you can edit a hybridization pattern by clicking. Then, if you switch to Map mode, clicking on positive (colored) squares will cluster them, so that the position you go to in the physical map display will be determined by the overlap region of all the positive YACs, which will be highlighted in magenta.

If you have write access to the database (see final section of the chapter), you can save this hybridization pattern with an object in the Clone class corresponding to the probe. It will then be permanently displayed in the appropriate position on the physical map, once the physical map has been recalculated. This is how all the hybridization data for the sequencing consortium cDNAs were entered.

D. Sequence Display (fMap)

The Sequence class listed in the main window is very large, because in addition to the sequences from the genomic project, it contains cDNA EST sequences, worm sequences from EMBL/Genbank, and entries for Swissprot and PIR protein sequences that match any of these. Normally it is better to start from the Genome_Seq or cDNA_Sequence subclass, which are at the end of the list of classes in the main window. The Genome_Seq subclass contains all the primary cosmid clones that are being sequenced by the consortium.

When you display a sequence object by double-clicking on it, you bring up a sequence display window (Fig. 4). This is in many ways the most complex window in the ACeDB package. By default it shows features and annotation for the sequence, but as with the Genetic map display, there are many possible columns that can be turned on and off, including ones for the DNA sequence itself and a three-frame translation. In addition to zooming and scrolling exactly as with the genetic map, you can also use the Reverse-Complement option to look at the other strand. In addition, there are menus for controlling the display of the DNA, and for accessing various analysis tools. These tools operate within the

Active Zone, which is in general a subregion of the sequence being displayed. You can change the extent of the active zone by typing in new values in the text entry box at the top. The extent of the active zone is shown in blue adjacent to the yellow summary bar.

One of the analytical tools within the fMap is the Genefinder package written by Phil Green (unpublished). It is accessed by its own menu. If you click on the Genefinder button, you will see a number of new columns showing all stop codons (horizontal lines) and start codons (yellow boxes) in the three forward frames, regions of high coding potential (gray boxes) also by frame, and predicted splice sites, depicted by a hook symbol whose length indicates degree of confidence. These can help suggest alternatives to the predicted splicing pattern. There are also facilities built into ACeDB for interactive editing of predicted splicing patterns, but these are beyond the scope of this chapter. We are currently preparing a WWW manual for using Genefinder, which should be available from the The Sanger Centre (http://www.sanger.ac.uk) and should also be integrated into the on-line documentation in future releases of ACeDB.

Another of the tools starts a separate Analysis window. This gives access to various forms of simple sequence analysis. The analysis can be applied either to the sequence currently being displayed, in which case all actions just apply to the active zone (see above), or to a keyset of sequences (see Section III,C). The most useful function is the motif search. This can act either in DNA or AA (amino acid) mode. In AA mode, searches will act on a six-frame translation of DNA sequence. To use the motif search, just type a pattern into the yellow text entry box, and hit return. Hits will be shown in text further down the window and symbolically on the displayed sequence. The motif can be either a string of IUPAC symbols (i.e., for DNA a, c, g, t plus n for any base, r for purine, etc.) or a known motif name from the Motif class. At present, ACeDB recognizes most restriction enzyme names as known motifs. An important feature is that you can allow mismatches for motif matches, using the Max Mismatch button. The Show Gels button brings up another window, which displays predicted agarose gels for arbitrary motif/restriction enzyme combinations cutting within the active zone of the currently displayed sequence.

V. Concepts

A. Underlying Approach

Databases fall into three broad categories: flat-file, relational, and object oriented. Some of the simpler personal computer-type databases are flat-file systems, where all the information is stored in a set of records. Most large database systems are relational, and the information is represented in a series of tables. Relational systems are very powerful and have extensive transaction and query facilities; however, they are best suited for information that comes in regular structures. They are not very well suited for the heterogeneous types and amounts

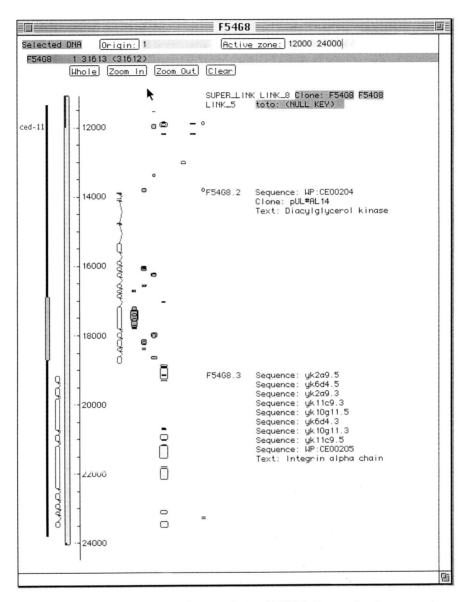

Fig. 4 Sequence display for part of the genomic cosmid F54G8. Two predicted genes are shown: F54G8.2 on the forward strand and F54G8.3 on the reverse strand. The light blue boxes to the right of the F54G8.2 gene structure represent matches to protein in three reading frames, helping to identify this as a putative diacylglycerol kinase. There are some larger yellow boxes opposite F54G8.3 showing DNA matches to cDNA EST sequences. Protein homology information for F54G8.3 (to α-integrins) is visible only if you reverse-complement and look at the other strand. Further information about the matches and predicted gene products can be obtained by clicking on the items; a single click gives brief information in the light blue bar in the header; a double-click displays the object itself. Many items have their own menus; for example, from the menu for a predicted gene you can request display or export of the gene translation.

of information encountered in biology. This type of information is best represented in an object-oriented system, where all the information pertaining to one object is stored together in an extendable data structure. Object-oriented databases are a rather new phenomenon, and the field of databases is dominated largely by relational systems. Because of increasing demands for more flexible database managers, however, the newer relational systems are incorporating object-oriented extensions and the distinction between the two types of database managers is becoming blurred.

People often ask, Is ACeDB objected oriented? The truth is that although ACeDB incorporates many features of object-oriented systems, it would probably not be regarded as a true object-oriented system by the computer science community. For example, ACeDB stores information in objects organized in classes. Class definitions determine what can be stored in an object and how the information is displayed; however, the classes themselves are not hierarchically organized and there is no inheritance of attributes. Classes do not include methods and the program is written in a non-object-oriented language (ANSI C). On the other hand, the hierarchy of classes is replaced by a hierarchical system for the arrangement of information within each class. This is a very natural representation for biological information, where elaborations of detail may be available in different directions for different objects, but in most cases very little is known. Another main advantage of ACeDB over a conventional system is the ability to redefine the "schema" without rebuilding the database. In the next section, we briefly describe how data are arranged in ACeDB and then illustrate how to modify data.

B. Data Structures

The information in ACeDB is stored in objects that are organized in classes. Each object belongs to only one class. The classes represent categories of information such as maps, clones, sequences, authors, journals, papers, alleles, strains, and laboratories. These classes are "visible" and are shown in the main window. There is also a set of internal, nonvisible classes used by the program to organize further information. Examples of these are Text and Longtext. The user need not be concerned with these nonvisible classes. All classes have a template or model that defines how information is stored in objects from that class. The model consists of a hierarchical arrangement of "tags" and "values." An example of the model for the class Author is given below:

```
?Author Full_name Text
        Laboratory UNIQUE ?Laboratory XREF Staff
        Old_lab ?Laboratory
        Address     Mail Text
          E_mail Text
          Phone Text
          Fax Text
        Paper ?Paper
```

In the ACeDB display the tags are shown in plain font, and the value or data slots in bold. Words in italics are modifiers and which are not described further here. There are two kinds of "values": straight information (e.g., the Full_name, which is a Text object), and pointers to other objects (e.g., Paper whose value is ?Paper, a pointer to a separate Paper object). Pointers to items in other classes are indicated by an initial question mark. These pointers are the links connecting different pieces of data in the database.

To make this a bit more specific, here is the object tree for Author Sulston JE:

> Sulston JE
> Full_name John Sulston
> Laboratory **CB**
> Address Mail The Sanger Centre
>   Hinxton Hall
>   Cambridge CB10 1RQ
>   U.K.
>   E_mail jes@sanger.ac.uk
>   Phone 44–1223–884244
>   Fax 44–1223–494919
> **Paper → 111**

The values associated with the Paper tag are collapsed in this view, as indicated by the arrow. If you double-click the collapsed outline it will expand and list the titles of the 111 papers in the database that list John Sulston as an author. Note that Sulston JE is an object in the class Author. All the pointers that are part of this object are outlined in bold font. For example, the laboratory CB is a pointer to an object CB in the class Laboratory.

Models can be found in the file models.wrm in the /wspec directory (or folder). All the tags are listed in the file tags.wrm in the /wspec directory.

VI. Using ACeDB to Store One's Own Data

In most cases it seems rather unlikely that you will want to make changes to the ACeDB database. You may not have a need for anything other than the official updates as they are released. It is possible, however, to use the program to set up your own private database containing local data and, also, to add information into your copy of the public database. We recommend that if you want to do the latter, it is better to have a separate database of your own information as well. There are methods we describe below to dump these data out into files that can be read into your copy of the public database. The main reason for doing things this way is that if you ever have to rebuild your main database (e.g., if you receive a new release of Macace, or if there is a new major version of Xace), then you still have your own data, and can simply read that in again. Also, this avoids the problem where the public updates can overwrite changes that you have made locally. Note that you will always be able to load the public updates, even if you have edited your database. In this respect adding objects into it will not corrupt it.

ACeDB is a very flexible program and many changes and adaptations can be implemented without changing the code. For example, it is possible to add new classes and tags, even to an existing database, without invalidating any existing data. We do not discuss changes in the code itself. Although the source code is available at ftp sites, it is complex and we strongly recommend that you consult the authors before starting to change it.

If you wish to make changes to ACeDB, you should familiarize yourself with the user's guide and the installation guide. You do not need to be a UNIX or Macintosh expert, but you should be familiar with the basics of a hierarchical file system and you should know how to create and edit files, for example, with a word processor on the Macintosh. In either case, what is described below is in essence identical on both systems and you will be able to transport your changes (both data and structural) from one system to another.

A. Write Access

To add or remove objects from the database you need to have write access. Write access is organized in macrotransactions called *sessions*. A session is initiated by selecting the menu item "Write Access" and is terminated by doing a global save. In UNIX, Write Access and Save are in the pulldown menu in the main window. In the Macintosh version, they are in the file menu. The changes made during any one session are valid for that session, but will not be permanent unless you do a global save in the manner described above. If you quit the program without saving, you will be asked if you want to save the changes you have made. If you reply No, then the database will remain unchanged for the next session. At any time, one person at most can have write access to the database. This prevents possible confusion if two separate processes update the same object.

Under UNIX you can only get write access if your login name appears in the specification file wspec/passwd.wrm, which can be edited by the user owning the database. If your login name is not in this file, the option Write Access and associated items do not appear in the main menu. On the Macintosh, when you select Write Access, a password dialog will appear. Type in your password. Macace is distributed with the default password acedb. To change the password, edit the resource fork with a resource editor such as ResEdit and change string #500.

B. Editing Data

Once you have write access you can create and edit data. There are two basic ways to do this. The first is interactive, via the graphical user interface provided by ACeDB; This is intuitive but cumbersome for large amounts of data. The second and in many ways most important is via a standard file interchange format, .ace files.

1. Interactive Method

The interactive method for adding new data to the database is useful for making small changes. Select the Add/Alias/Rename menu option in the main window menu. A small window will appear that allows you to select a class and type in a name for your object. You can access existing objects or create new ones. You can also rename existing objects, or delete them, using the menu options. When you hit the return key, a new window will appear with all the information about the object that you want to access. If you are creating a new object, the window will be empty except for the name of the object.

To edit an object interactively, first display it in text form, for example, as described above from the Add/Alias/Rename window. Select Update from the menu. In Update mode an expanded template is added to existing data, showing all the types of information you can add to the object. To add information, double-click one of the light blue boxes; it should turn yellow and you can then type in the data and hit return. For pointer fields you can also double-click on the object you want to point to, if it is shown in another window. To change a field, just double-click on it, and edit the field. To delete data, select the field with a single click, and choose Delete from the menu. You can also delete tags, which will remove the whole branch of the tree following them. When you have completed editing your object, you can save the changes. You can also cancel by closing the editing window.

2. The .ace File Method

The interactive methods described above are convenient for making small changes and additions, but cumbersome for entering large amounts of data. To do this it is better to use another mechanism to update the database, via external data files written in .ace (dot-ace) format. A tool accessed from the Read .ace Files option in the menu parses these files into the database, giving error messages and status feedback as appropriate. It should be straightforward to use. Note that the Open File options recognize only file names ending in the string .ace (hence the name); please do not forget this.

The .ace file format is what you get if you dump data from the keyset window using the Ace Dump menu option. The best way to learn is to look at examples made in this way. The basic principles are as follows: The file is organized in paragraphs, which are separated by at least one blank line. Each paragraph refers to one object, and the first line contains the class name, followed by the object name. On each new line a tag and data for that object can be entered. If the data contain spaces, they should be enclosed in double quotes. If you wish to continue the data onto the next line, use a backslash at the end of the line. Anything following the pair of characters "//" is treated as a comment.

If a data line starts with "-D" before the tag, then the information on the line will be deleted, rather than added. As discussed above, if you delete a tag, the whole branch of data following that tag will be deleted. It is also possible to delete a whole object by placing "-D" before the class name at the beginning of the paragraph, in which case no data lines are needed. Finally, you can rename objects by placing "-R" before the class name and following the old object name with the new one. Together, these additions allow arbitrary edits on a database to be performed via .ace files.

C. Transferring Data between Databases

The way to transfer data from one ACeDB database to another is to dump out the data as an .ace file, and read it in. Dumping out .ace files is also an easy way to compare the contents of two databases. A program, called acediff, in the distribution facilitates this process.

VII. Conclusion

This chapter has only given a brief introduction to ACeDB, and it is sure to be out of date soon. The most important information provided here is the pointers to electronic information available on the Internet, including where to obtain the database. There are many significant developments in both software and *C. elegans* data that are best accessed by consulting the documentation available at the ftp sites and the NAL WWW site or the records of the bionet.software.acedb newsgroup.

Acknowledgments

In addition to the work by the orignal authors and others mentioned in this chapter, the current state of the ACeDB project depends on a large number of people who have contributed software, ideas, and data. These include Danielle Thierry-Mieg, Ulrich Sauvage, Simon Kelley, Erik Sonnhammer, Friedemann Wobus, Detlef Wolf, and Suzanna Lewis. We also thank Gerry Rubin at the University of California at Berkeley and Ed Theil and John McCarthy at LBL for their support of the development of Macace. We thank Julie Ahringer for commenting on the manuscript. The Sanger Centre is supported by the Wellcome Trust and the MRC.

References

Coulson, A. R., Sulston, J. E., Brenner, S., and Karn J. (1986). Towards a physical map of the genome of the nematode *C. elegans. Proc. Natl. Acad. Sci. U.S.A.* **83,** 7821–7825.
Dunham, I., Durbin, R., Thierry-Mieg, J., and Bentley, D. (1994). Physical mapping projects and ACEDB. *In* "Guide to Human Genome Computing" (M. Bishop, ed.), pp. 111–158. Academic Press, San Diego.

Durbin, R., and Thierry-Mieg, J. (1994). The ACEDB genome database. *In* "Computational Methods in Genome Research", (Sandor Suhai, ed.). Plenum, New York.

Sulston, J., Mallett, F., Staden, R., Durbin, R., Horsnell, T., and Coulson, A. (1988). Software for genome mapping by fingerprinting techniques. *CABIOS* **4,** 125–132.

Thierry-Mieg, J., and Durbin, R. (1992). ACeDB, a *C. elegans* database. *Cahiers IMABIO* **5,** 15–24.

Wood, W. B. (1988). "The Nematode *Caenorhabditis elegans.*" Cold Spring Harbor Laboratory Press, Cold Spring Harbor, NY.

CHAPTER 26

The Worm Community System, Release 2.0 (WCSr2)

Laura M. Shoman, * **Ed Grossman,** ‡ **Kevin Powell,** †
Curt Jamison, * **and Bruce R. Schatz** ‡

* Community Systems Laboratory
Graduate School of Library and Information Science and
‡ National Center for Supercomputing Applications
Beckman Institute
University of Illinois, Urbana–Champaign
Urbana, Illinois 61801
† Digital Library Initiative
51 Grainger Engineering Library
Urbana, Illinois 61801

I. Introduction

The Worm Community System (WCS) is a digital library that contains knowledge about *Caenorhabditis elegans,* and a software environment that enables the user to interact with the community library across the international computer network, the Internet. The functions of the software environment enable the user to browse, search, and retrieve the existing knowledge of the community. In addition, users may add data and literature to the library for timely dissemination to the research community and for private collaboration with colleagues at local or remote sites. This capacity for dynamically updating information should help to better propagate knowledge across the community. This chapter provides a survey of the system's history, features, and requirements, and describes basic uses of the system.

II. System Information and Requirements

A. History

The first version of WCS (WCSr1) was funded by the National Science Foundation as a research model, a prototype of a research community electronic collaboratory (National Research Council, 1993; Pool, 1993). WCSr1, distributed in 1991, ran in more than 25 laboratories. The second version (WCSr2), described below, was also funded by NSF and was released in the summer of 1994 as an X-windows application that runs on Sun workstations, and, through X-windows emulators, on Apple Macintosh and DOS personal computers. The initial application was developed at the University of Arizona in Tucson, starting in 1989. In 1993, the project relocated to the University of Illinois, Urbana–Champaign (UIUC).

B. Overview and Content

The WCS contains a variety of data objects (such as documents, genes, clones, and lineages) within one application. Relationships between the concepts in these data types are indicated by links. These links are created initially by the system when new data are incorporated, building on the current store of information. In addition, links can be created by individual users to define new relationships among the data, thereby creating new knowledge. Links also provide one method for navigating through the data. The purpose of the system is to support the display and recording of patterns in the information space, where the patterns are formed by links between objects and represent important relationships.

Information in WCS attempts to span the range of all that a researcher might find useful, including formal and informal literature and data. The literature includes abstracts from most of the *Caenorhabditis* Genetic Center bibliography, full text of all articles from the complete *Worm Breeder's Gazette* (the *C. elegans* community newsletter), and abstracts from the most recent worm meetings. The data include genomic data from the MRC/WUSTL mapping and sequencing project (genes, maps, sequences), community data from the Minnesota stock center (stains, people), and the beginnings of cellular data (cells, lineages).

Part of the WCS software is run from a computer in the local laboratory. Data are accessed "live" and in real time across the Internet from a server at UIUC. This model of computing allows for relatively instantaneous updates of the data as new objects are added by users, and does not require massive amounts of disk storage at each local site. The software environment provides for transparency, hiding from the user the complexities of handling the different physical locations and the different data types and supplying a simple uniform set of commands for the library of community knowledge.

As a tool, WCSr2 complements ACeDB. Although WCSr2 and ACeDB are both hypermedia-based biological databases, they differ in a number of ways. WCSr2 is a community system. To that end, it allows interactive creation and editing of new objects by end users within the system. It also supports editorial and privacy controls, allowing users to restrict access to data and to determine how reliable a particular piece of data is. Finally, while ACeDB distributes its database with the software, WCSr2 has a client-server architecture with a central database. This allows all users immediate access to new data, instead of relying on periodic updates of the database.

C. Availability and System Requirements

Current information about WCS can be found on the Community Systems Laboratory (CSL) server, anonymous ftp csl.ncsa.uiuc.edu (141.142.221.11). From the WCSr2 subdirectory, get README. Additional documentation may also be available (e.g., the users' manual in a variety of formats, and a quick start sheet). Directions to the binary code and additional, up-to-date system information are given in the README file. The following information pertains to WCSr2.

Workstation Requirements. Sites will need to have an Internet connection from a Sun workstation to access the CSL server. The data, search engines, thesaurus server, etc., reside on the CSL server at UIUC. The following machines are suggested for workstations: SparcStation 5, SparcStation LX, SparcStation 10, or SparcStation 20. Tolerable, but very slow performance can be achieved on SparcStations 2, 1+, and IPX. The "minimum recommended configuration" would be a SparcStation2 with at least 32 Mbyte of random access memory

(RAM). These workstations should run version 4.1.x of Sun's operating system, or Solaris 2.3 or later. At the time of this writing, WCSr2 had not been tested on earlier versions of Solaris. The Sun station should run at least 32 Mbyte of RAM.

There are several factors, local and regional, that affect the performance of the system in each laboratory. These factors include the local hardware configuration and network at each institution, the level of traffic on the Internet, and the nature of search or retrieval being performed. For example, searching data for a broad term that will retrieve hundreds of "hits" may take up to a minute, perhaps longer, depending on various factors as indicated above. Retrieving the cell lineage or other graphical displays will take longer, in part because of the size of the data traveling across the Internet.

The search query is sent to the CSL server in Illinois, and then data responsive to the search are sent back to your local workstation—the data are not stored locally on your workstation. This system design is different from the earlier release of WCS and from current releases of ACeDB. A central location for data allows the community to access the most current data and provides for immediate dissemination of information (at the level desired by the author) to the community.

X-Windows Platform. The local software requires an X-windows environment and, in addition to that environment, will take up approximately 10 Mbyte of space on a hard drive. This disk space requirement may increase over releases, but no dramatic increase is anticipated. On Sun workstations, CSL staff have used both X11R5 and OpenWindows (the Sun product) with good results.

Nodes. Users have run WCS on microcomputer nodes, using the local Sun workstation as a server. The Apple Macintosh or PC clone must be connected with Ethernet to the Sun workstation that, in turn, is connected to the CSL server over the Internet. WCS is an X-windows application and cannot be run on a Macintosh or PC clone without an X-windows environment. Macintosh users have used Apple's product, MacX. DOS-based machines have used PC-Xview for Windows, a product from Network Computing Devices, to good effect. A Macintosh node running off the server should have a mininum of 8 MBytes of RAM. The Mac should be in the 68040 processor family. Higher-end 68030 Macs will run MacX acceptably if no other applications are running. A DOS-based node should have a minimum of 8 Mbytes of RAM. The processor should be a 486/66.

Monitor Resolution. On either machine (Mac or DOS) the monitor should have a resolution of 1024×768 pixels. Apple's 16-in. monitor has a resolution of 800×600 pixels and is considered acceptable by some users. Color is not used in WCS.

Input Devices. The interface requires a keyboard and a mouse (or trackball) input device.

Printing. Printing can be done from the Sun server transparently, using the existing printing configuration through X-windows. Printing directly from a Macintosh is done through MacX.

III. Concepts and Conventions

A. Information Space

The data in this digital library exist in an information space: all the information consists of objects, which are also called information units (iu or ius, plural), which are interconnected by relationship links to form the space (Fig. 1). This information space is much like a web. The information units are points within the web; links are the threads of the web, giving definition to the space while being a part of the web itself.

B. Types

Object types, sometimes referred to as data types, include 2- and 3-factor data, deficiencies, genetic rearrangements (e.g., translocations), strain names, gene names, chromosomes, contigs, clones, sequences, cells (lineage history), documents, images, persons, and laboratories. A user can add new data that are "recognized" by the system as fitting into one of these preexisting categories. A user might, for example, enter a new gene or a document. The system will then present the user with the appropriate form to complete, and the data will be incorporated into the system. In addition, the system will "type-check" each entry within the form to confirm, for example, that the new gene name is unique or that it contains a clone that references an actual clone on the physical map.

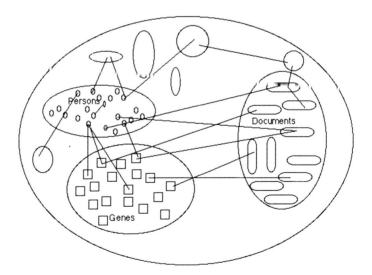

Fig. 1 The Information Space is created by linked objects, linked initially by the system as new data are entered and then by users as they traverse the space and make their own connections, developing new knowledge as new relationships are discovered.

C. Navigating Information Space

A user may enter the space of existing objects by first issuing a search to retrieve objects and then navigating links from these objects to other related objects. A user can also share objects with the community, adding them to the space by first issuing a command to create objects and then completing the form presented by the system. A user may also create links between objects—between a new object and existing objects, or between two (or more) existing objects.

Commands can be issued on a selected object. The basic commands for manipulating the information units are the same for all objects in the system. Once commands have been learned for one object type, the same commands can be used on any object or collection of objects (sets). Commands are issued through the command buttons (e.g., Search All and Search This Type in Fig. 2) and popup menus (Utilities and Type Selection menu in Fig. 2 and other menus presented on other windows). See Fig. 2 and below.

D. Interface Conventions

The WCS uses a graphical user interface. The Search Window (Fig. 2) is the starting point. The display on the local monitor may vary from the illustrated

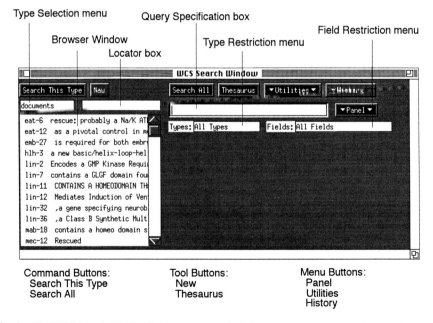

Fig. 2 The WCS Search Window is the gateway to the information space. A graphical user interface of boxes, buttons, windows, and menus, WCS allows novice computer users an opportunity to explore and exploit the information space.

display due to equipment differences; however, the general principles discussed here apply to all kinds of displays.

The Search Window contains elements common throughout the rest of the application: popup menus, objects, buttons, and scroll windows. To perform a function, for example, issue a command to an object or enter data into a field, the object, box, or field must be selected. To select an object or a field, click on it once. A selected item will be highlighted in some way, either by a rectangular outline or a reverse highlight (white characters on black background). In the case of a box or a field, the cursor must be in that space before data can be entered; you can type into a boxed field as well. Depending on the function being performed, data may be added by (1) typing characters, (2) copy and paste functions, or (3) selecting data from popup menus. Popup menus in the Search Window include the Type Selection menu, and the Type and Field Restriction menus. The user can type queries or names of known objects in the Query Specification box and the Locator box. Buttons in windows indicate Tools, Commands, or popup Menus that list commands. Tool buttons are Thesaurus and History; Command buttons include Search All and Search this Type; the Menu buttons are Panel and Utilities. Scroll bars, on the right side of the Browser Window, for example, allow movement through each window. As information is added to a window, scroll bars may appear on the right side, or on the bottom (to permit scrolling left and right across an image or lineage).

IV. Browsing and Searching

A. Browsing

The Browser is made up of those fields and windows on the left side of the Search Window: the Type Selection menu, the Locator box, and the Browser Window (see Fig. 2). The Browser is the quickest way to locate information by object type. The Browser is also used when new data are being added (see Section V on Sharing). To use the Browser, click and hold on the Type Section menu to display a list of all of the types known by WCS. Highlight the data type to be browsed to select it. The selected type appears in the Type Selection menu, and the list of objects of that type appears in the Browser Window. If you know the name of a particular object, type the name in the Locator box. The Browser Window will scroll to the object (presuming it is in the object store). To retrieve the object, click on the name in the Browser Window or finish typing the name in the Locator box and press the Return/Enter key.

B. Searching

The right side of the Search Window can be used to build powerful, complex queries using nested boolean searches and restricting the types of data and fields that will be searched. The Query Specification box and the Type and Field Restriction menus make up a functioning unit called a Panel (see below). In addition, the buttons Thesaurus and History are found on the right side of the Search Window. These will be explained below.

The broadest search is performed by typing words in the Query Specification box and then clicking on Search All (or pressing the Return key). The application first removes prefixes and suffixes, and then looks for the matching string of characters in the documents and forms. The results of the search appear in a new window labeled Set of IUs (a set of information units). If no matches exist for the search query, a dialog box will appear. The set is actually an object; the commands invoked on a single object can be invoked on a set as well. For example, one such command will retrieve all of the items that are somehow related (through links) to all of the objects in the set. See Fig. 3 for a sample search session.

To restrict the search to one type of data, select the type from the Type Selection menu, enter the word(s) in the Query Specification box, and click on Search This Type. To restrict the search to one or more types of data, and one

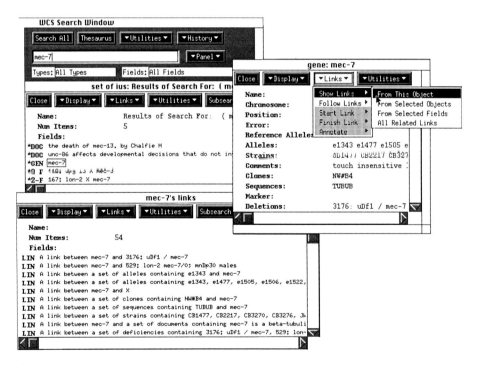

Fig. 3 Search WCS by typing a query (mec-7) and clicking the Search All button. The results are seen in the set of information units: Results of Search For: (mec-7). The results include documents, the gene object itself, and 2-factors. The gene object is selected and retrieved. Links from the gene object are shown in the set of 54 objects. Any of these objects can be retrieved for further study.

Query Specification box   Type Restriction menu   popup menu of known types

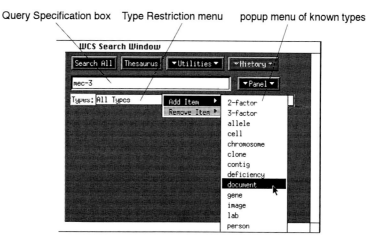

Fig. 4 Restricting the type of data to be searched allows the user to focus on a specific source, be it a document from a particular journal, a certain allele, or a particular author. The Type Restriction menu and Field Restriction menu found in the Panel provide this flexibility.

or more corresponding fields within the data type, use the Panel (Fig. 4). Panels consist of (1) a Query Specification box, (2) a Type Restriction menu, (3) a Field Restriction menu, and (4) boolean search tools (parentheses and boolean boxes).

Specify the query. Use the Type Restriction menu to restrict the type(s) of objects to be searched. Fields within that data type may also be restricted, to further focus the search. The Panel can also be used to "stack" queries. Panels are added to the query structure by clicking on the Panel button on the Search Window. For example, one can search for *mec-7, mec-3* and "touch" by using panels to focus each search. Boolean searches can be constructed by adding parentheses (Fig. 5).

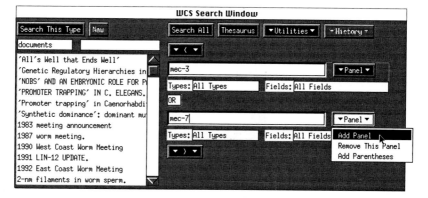

Fig. 5 Complex and powerful queries are manageable using multiple Panels and incorporating parenthetical Boolean statements within a search query.

C. Thesaurus

The thesaurus provides a list of terms associated with the search term(s) used in the most recent query and may thus be helpful in suggesting additional terms to search for. The Thesaurus command button is located on the Search Window, and clicking on the button brings up the Thesaurus Window (Fig. 6). The Result Terms are not synonyms for the Query Terms, but, rather, terms that occur within the same sentence or abstract. A search performed from the Thesaurus Window is performed within all data types, not on those types that may have been specified in the previous query. The Thesaurus also provides an additional field, New Query Term, allowing the user to add a term not listed in the other windows.

D. Links

Data within the information space are linked. Following links among the information units is one method of navigating through the information space (see Figs. 3 and 7). After a search has retrieved a set of objects, one can follow links among the objects or show a list of the objects related to a specific item within the set. To show or follow the links of a specific object, select the object. Use the Links menu to show or follow links. Showing the links from an object

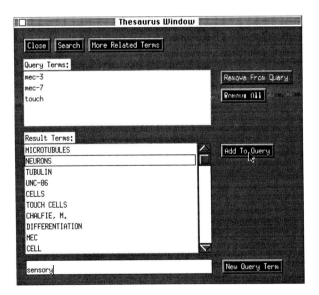

Fig. 6 The Thesaurus provides the user with a listing of terms related to the search query. Result Terms are words or phrases associated with the Query Terms and may be useful, suggesting different terms and strategies for searching. The terms may be names of genes or people, or may be topical in nature.

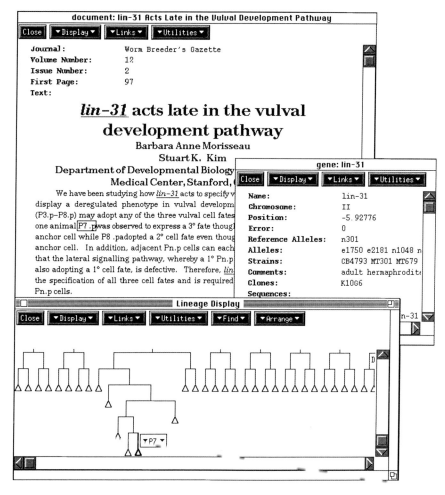

Fig. 7 Following Links: lin-31, and P7.p within the document are links to the objects themselves. Fields within the gene may also be live links to other objects.

provides a set of objects related to the selected object (as in Fig. 3). Following the links opens each object (see Fig. 7).

E. Other Display Features

The History menu keeps track of the most recent 20 windows opened. The user can select from that list to return to a particular object.

Documents may have figures, tables, or line drawings associated with them (Fig. 8). To retrieve any existing images, display the document. The Display menu item Show Images will be enabled if figures accompany the selected docu-

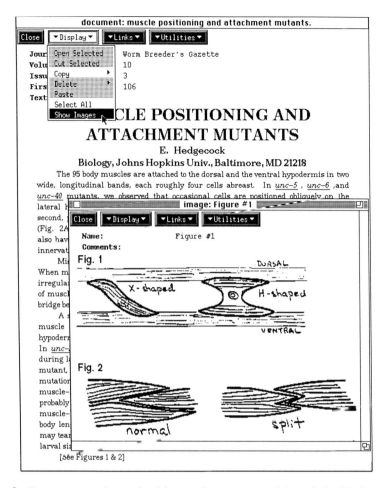

Fig. 8 Documents may have related images that are retrieved through the Display menu.

ment. Images may also be retrieved as objects of a set or by showing or following links from a document.

Cells are displayed as a lineage display, as in Fig. 9. The lineage allows the user to view data in a variety of ways. A user can browse the entire lineage representation. Using the Arrange menu, the display can be manipulated, providing flexibility and dynamic interaction with the data. Every branch point and terminal branch are live objects that can be linked arbitrarily to other objects, including selected text in documents, selected fields in genes, and clones. There is a sample gray-scale image of the organism that can be retrieved with the Find Image command. Such images illustrate a cell at some level of development.

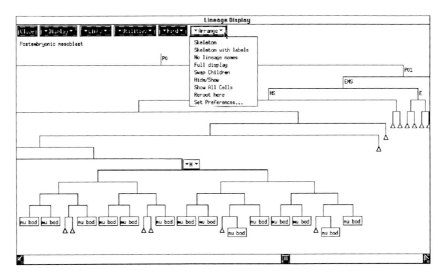

Fig. 9 The Cell Lineage display allows a user to view graphic information on a particular cell and then interact with the data, following development of the cells through generations, linking cells to other objects within the system, and viewing images of the organism.

V. Sharing Data

As a national prototype of an electronic community system, WCS provides the worm community with an unparalleled opportunity to share information, including informal and formal research, and community folklore. An individual in one laboratory can create a new object and create links between the new object and existing objects. An individual at a different laboratory (even on a different continent) can retrieve that information practically instantaneously, and can use it to create new relationships among other objects within the space. This ability to share data is balanced by a feature that allows the author of the new object to control how the new object is distributed. Collaboration across the country can now occur, with security and privacy features protecting the team effort until sharing is deemed appropriate by the owner.

A. Login and Object Ownership

Select Login from the Utilities menu in the Search Window. A window will open, requesting name and password. The user should enter data in the Name field, last name first and then first initial. Review the listing in the window below the Name field. If the user's name appears in that list, a password has been assigned by the system. Contact CSL for the password needed to log in, sending e-mail to wcs@csl.ncsa.uiuc.edu, requesting the password. Once an individual logs in, that person controls read/write privileges and retains editorial control over any objects he or she has created.

B. Linking Objects

Login is also required to make links between existing data. For example, when reviewing search results, a user might see certain patterns, relationships, or connections between different data. The user may make links between those objects. To link two objects, use the Links menu to Start a link at one object and Finish a link at the other.

C. Creating a New Object

Use the New button to create a new object after picking its type from the Type Selection menu. A new object window for that type will appear. If a document is being created, the individual who has logged in is presumed to be the first author. To enter a value-object in a field, select the field. The value can be entered in two ways: by typing or by copy-and-paste. If typing text, the characters entered are type-checked. If a clone name is entered in a name field of an allele, the system will respond with an error message. Multiple objects can be entered into a single field, type-checked as a set by tabbing after entering each object. If the data typed in fields other than the new object's Name field represent other objects already within the system, a link is automatically generated between the object being created and the existing object.

Copying and pasting an existing object into a new object will also create an immediate link. To copy and paste, retrieve the data to be embedded and select Copy from the Display menu (Fig. 10). The allele object has been copied. Click on the new object window, and make sure the appropriate field (where you want to paste the object) is selected, highlighted with a cursor or box. The allele field is selected in the gene:test-1 object. Select Paste from the Display menu. The name of the existing object will appear in the highlighted field.

A user may also create and save a set of objects. In the Utilities menu, select New Set. A new window will open, a Set of IUs with no items in it. When an object is found of particular interest, use the Display menu to copy the object and paste it into the New Set window.

D. Publishing New Objects

When creating a new object, the owner has the opportunity to restrict who reads and writes to the object. The level of privacy or security can be adjusted by the owner at any time. The default is that all users may read objects that are added to the system, but not write to them.

When creating a new object, select Permissions from the Utilities menu. The Permissions window will be displayed (Fig. 11). Assigning a user Writer privilege

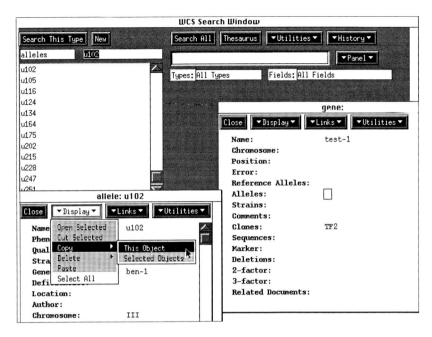

Fig. 10 Creating a new object (gene:test-1), using current objects from the system (e.g., allele: u102, clone: TF2). Copy-and-Paste functions allow a user to create new objects without extensive keyboard work.

automatically grants them reading privilege. Assigning a user Reader privilege assigns that individual reading privileges and denies reading privileges to all users not in the Reader list. Other users may not retrieve the object.

Much like the "real" community, the virtual community system provides for moderating and curating of data. As can be seen on the Permissions window, the default is that new data are posted to WCS, without review or moderation. As the community uses the system to disseminate information, however, levels of review will be implemented. A moderated object will be sent to a moderator who may apply some criteria yet to be developed to screen each submission. Criteria may be general, not necessarily editorial in nature. For example, the *Worm Breeders' Gazette* is a moderated journal. Submissions are sent to a central clearinghouse and informal screening ensures articles conform to a certain type. A curated object is reviewed by an evaluating individual or group to ensure not only that it meets certain editorial guidelines, but that the data are appropriate. The criteria that the community chooses to use and the individuals that will fill these vital roles have not been identified. Technologically, the mechanisms are available within WCS to provide various levels of quality of research to the community, from informal data to peer review. The community can develop the appropriate standards and implement the technology.

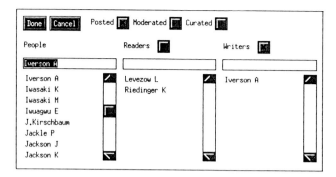

Fig. 11 An author of a new object can restrict publication of that object, allowing only collaborators or selected individuals to read and/or write to the new object. The Permission window displays the level of privilege provided to individuals. The default setting allows all users to read objects. No one but the author/owner can write to an object (edit, amend, delete), unless otherwise specified by the owner.

VI. Discussion

Research communities encounter and incorporate new technologies in the pursuit of knowledge as a matter of course. For example, full texts and abstracts have been available on-line through various commercial services for decades, and have been used by scientist and scholar from the beginning. The Internet and its predecessors, ARPANET and NSFnet, have long supported the transfer of data between researchers. Although the initial impetus for the ARPANET was to run remote jobs on supercomputers, the primary uses of the network were communication, collaboration, and data exchange among advanced research laboratories working for the Department of Defense. The decentralized network typology and evolution of the loosely regulated anarchy of the Internet grew out of ARPANET.

On-line services provide an alternate method of distribution of material that is simultaneously published in paper form. The issues of quality control in on-line services do not focus on the quality of the material being distributed on-line. Peer review and quality control for content are unrelated to the availability of the abstract or article in the on-line environment—the article has received editorial approval (and perhaps is available in print) before the information is made available on-line. Quality generally refers to the methods of indexing, integrity of data input, and usability of the service.

At the other end of the spectrum, the proliferation of USENET newsgroups, ftp sites, gopher hosts, mailing lists, and other Internet services has led to exponential growth in informal communication, information that is not subjected to any kind of peer or critical review before being "posted." There may be some form of moderation prior to posting, meaning that there is a human being who reviews the post for "appropriate, subject-related content," but who does not look at the quality of the data. Traditional channels of informal communication in the worm community include regional and international meetings and the *Worm Breeder's Gazette*. These channels were supplemented in July 1994 with the introduction of a USENET newsgroup, bionet.celegans.

In addition to informal channels, the Internet has also served as a testbed for several experiments, including electronic journals and biological databases such as GenBank. Unlike commercial on-line services, these electronic journals are not the digitized files of printed journals or abstracts made available on the Internet, but are written, edited, and distributed entirely on the Internet. Some experiments have attempted to incorporate various levels of quality control; others are clearly vanity press publications.

In the case of GenBank, the quality and duplication of data have been major concerns. GenBank supports direct submission through electronic data publishing (Cinkosky *et al.*, 1991), but the volume of submissions has required development of submission tools and methods specifically to reduce the level of redundancy, thereby improving quality of data. Tremendous resources have been devoted to the cleanup and management of the database by Los Alamos National Laboratory and the National Center for Biotechnology Information.

Further discussion of the changes in scientific research and of the many problems accompanying changes in the delivery of scholarly and scientific information is available elsewhere and is outside the scope of this chapter (see, for example, Gardner, 1990; Harnad, 1992a,b; Harrison *et al.*, 1991; Hoke, 1994a,b; Hunt, 1990; Langschied, 1994; Okerson, 1991, 1993; Olson, 1994). As can be seen by the few examples presented here, however, the incorporation of technological advances into the research process is not new and not without periods of experimentation and adjustment. That this chapter appears as part of the community literature is a reflection of the adjustment process. Whether the community will incorporate the system within its information-sharing patterns by using the system's electronic publishing features is part of the ongoing experiment.

The WCS supports a mechanism of electronic publishing, one that provides for various levels of quality control through a variety of methods. Policies for using these are to be established by the community. The first level is access: one must run the WCS front-end application to access and read WCS material. The second level is at a password level: to enter data, or to create links, a user must have a password and must log into the system. The third level of quality control is accomplished by the automated assignment of authorship to a particular item: once logged into the system, a user is recognized as the author of the object created and the user name is shown in the author field of a document (as one example). Higher levels of quality control, through moderation, curation, and peer review, can be accommodated.

As implemented in the software, the quality-control methods build on the contemporary model of quality control within the community, where curation is done by people at the MRC and at The Sanger Centre, and moderation of informal publication is done by the editors of the *Worm Breeder's Gazette.*

Privacy control also models the community: research and collaboration are organized around groups in laboratories, not necessarily individuals.

At present there are no "WCS guidelines for authors," and there is no restriction of data that can be added (except that noted above concerning object types). Any implementation of peer review would require cooperation between the developers and leadership within the worm community. The lack of formal guidelines and peer review mimics the current state of the community, which has monitored itself and has provided a level of socialization to new members that guides research and publication practices. To date, the sample of added data has been too small to tell what publication niche will be filled by WCS.

The changes in technology exemplified in the WCS provide opportunities and challenges to the scientific community, and solutions will evolve out of discussion and collaboration between laboratories and the developers.

VII. The Future

The goal of WCSr1 was to bring up an electronic community system of interlinked data and literature for *C. elegans* available across the network. The goal of the current WCSr2 is to support collaboration within the community, enabling entry and publishing of data and links across the network. Future releases will explore the ability of a network information system to provide a facility for "dry-lab biology," where experiments can be run electronically by analyzing correlations between units in the information space. This will involve expanding the data sets to include other model organisms and central archives such as GenBank, GDB, and Medline. Although these are largely available on the Internet today, the database items are stored as flat text, rather than as structured objects with powerful search functions, relationship links, graphical displays, and analysis programs (Mount and Schatz, 1994). The WCS is thus not only a national model of the future of genome databases and science information systems (Courteau, 1991; Pool, 1993), but also a harbinger of the new paradigm in biology prophesied by Walter Gilbert (Gilbert, 1991).

Acknowledgments

The Worm Community System was partially funded by the National Science Foundation under Grants IRI-90-15407, IRI-92-57252, and BIR-93-19844. Other support was provided by the University of Arizona and the University of Illinois. In addition, the National Library of Medicine provided a copy of the IRX search software, which was then modified and adapted for WCS. Scott Hudson provided his user interface tool kit as the foundation for the "front end" of the system, implemented much of the release 1 version, and provided significant design advice for release 2. Terry Friedman wrote much of the original "back end" of the system. John Calley developed the lineage display. Hsinchun Chen created the Thesaurus functions. Samuel Ward provided support of many kinds for WCS at the University of Arizona.

Jean Thierry-Mieg and Richard Durbin have kindly provided the genome data from ACeDB. Theresa Stiernagle and Bob Herman provided stock data and they edit the *Worm Breeder's Gazette*, which CSL then digitally encodes. In earlier days of this project, these data and much additional help were provided by the former curator of the stock center, Mark Edgley. Finally, we are grateful for the many comments from the users of WCS.

References

Cinkosky, M. J., Fickett, J. W., and Gilna, P. (1991). Electronic data publishing and GenBank. *Science* **252,** 1273–1277.

Courteau, J. (1991). Genome databases. *Science* **254,** 201–207.

Gardner, W. (1990). The electronic archive: Scientific publishing the the 1990s. *Psychol. Sci.* **1**(6), 333–341.

Gilbert, W. (1991). Towards a paradigm shift in biology. *Nature* **349,** 99.

Harnad, S. R. (1992a). Interactive publication: Extending the American Physical Society's discipline-specific model for electronic publishing. *Serials Rev.* **18**(1–2), 58–61.

Harnad, S. R. (1992b). PSYCOLOQUY; a model forum for "scholarly skywriting." *Serials Rev.* **18**(1–2), 60.

Harrison, T. M., Stephen, T., and Winter, J. (1991). Online journals: Disciplinary designs for electronic scholarship. *The Public-Access Computer Systems Review* **2**(1), 25–28.

Hoke, F. (1994a). Scientists predict Internet will revolutionize research. *The Scientist* May 2, 1994 [Online], 8(9). Available: gopher.cic.net, /e-serials/alphabetic/s/the-scientist/the-scientist-940502.

Hoke, F. (1994b). New Internet capabilities fueling innovative science. *The Scientist* May 16, 1994 [Online], 8(10). Available: gopher.cic.net, /e-serials/alphabetic/s/the-scientist/the-scientist-940516.

Hunt, E. (1990). People, pitfalls and the electronic archive. *Psychol. Sci.* **1**(6), 346–349.

Langschied, L. (1994). Electronic journal forum: VPIEJ-L: An online discussion group for electronic journal publishing concerns. *Serials Rev.* **20**(1), 89–94+.

Mount, D. W., and Schatz, B. R. (1994). A genomic database for Escherichia coli: Total information on a given organism. *In* "Biocomputing: Informatics and Genome Projects" (D. W. Smith, ed.), pp. 249–267. Academic Press, San Diego.

National Research Council (U.S.). Committee on a National Collaboratory: Establishing the User-Developer Partnership (1993). National collaboratories: applying information technology for scientific research. National Academy Press, Washington, D.C.

Okerson, A. (1991). The electronic journal: What, whence, and when? *The Public-Access Computer Systems Review* **2**(1), 5–24.

Okerson, A. (1993). Electronic journal publishing on the Net. Developments and issues. *In* "New Technologies and New Directions: Proceedings from the Symposium on Scholarly Communication, University of Iowa, November 14–16, 1991" (G. R. Boynton and S. D. Creth, eds.), pp. 51–64. Meckler, Westport, Connecticut.

Olson, J. (1994). "Electronic Journal Literature: Implications for Scholars" Mecklermedia, Westport, Connecticut.

Pool, R. (1993). Computing in science—Beyond databases and e-mail. *Science* **261,** 841–843.

Appendix A: Additional Information and Resources

I. *Caenorhabditis* Genetics Center (CGC)

> 250 Biological Sciences Center
> 1445 Gortner Avenue
> St. Paul, MN 55108–1095
> (612) 625–2265
> Fax: (612) 625–5754
> e-mail: *stier@molbio.cbs.umn.edu*
> (Curator: Theresa Stiernagle)
> (Director: Robert K. Herman)

The *Caenorhabditis* Genetics Center, which is funded by a contract from the National Center for Research Resources, serves three main functions for the worm community.

1. The CGC serves as a central repository for mutant *C. elegans* strains. Certain standard bacterial strains and wild *C. elegans* isolates are also available. The CGC fills strain orders on written (or e-mail) request. Users are reminded to acknowledge the CGC and National Institutes of Health (NIH) when publishing experimental work resulting from use of received strains.

2. The CGC publishes and distributes, three times a year, the *Worm Breeder's Gazette* (WBG), which contains abstracts of work in progress by *C. elegans* laboratories. The WBG also contains updates of the *C. elegans* bibliography and serves as a community newsletter for announcing upcoming meetings, job advertisements, and so on. Subscriptions are currently $30 per volume (six issues over 2 years) for U.S. and Canadian subscribers (slightly more for international subscribers).

3. The CGC coordinates the updating of the genetic map and acts as a clearinghouse for genetic nomenclature. This function is subcontracted to Jonathan Hodgkin at the MRC Laboratory of Molecular Biology (LMB) in Cambridge, England. Mapping data are sent to MRC LMB where they are used in the

assembly of map updates. Updated versions of genetic map data are available through the *C. elegans* database (ACeDB). A hard-copy version is published biennially as a WBG issue.

Many of the CGC files (strain list, CGC Bibliography, WBG subscriber directory) are available on the Internet using Gopher (gopher elegans.cbs.umn.edu).

II. Internet and Other Computer Resources

A. Useful ftp Sites

Cosmid sequence data from the *C. elegans* genome project:

> ftp site: ftp.sanger.ac.uk.
> directory: pub/databases/C. elegans_sequences

The latest version of the Macace database:

> anonymous ftp site: ftp.genome.lbl.gov
> or via World Wide Web: http://www-hgc.lbl.gov/Genome/macace.html

See Chapter 25 for more information.
The latest version of the Worm Community System:

> anonymous ftp site: ftp.csl.ncsa.uiuc.edu

B. Sites Accessible via Gopher

Use the path Other Gophers/North America/USA/massachusetts/Massachusetts General Hospital/Molecular Biology/Caenorhabditis information to access a variety of important *C. elegans* information. A few useful items are listed below, but this list is likely to grow through time.

1. ACeDB, A *Caenorhabditis* Data Base: This version does not provide genetic map data and cosmid map, but it does allow you to do literature searches which include both regular journal articles and WBG and Worm Meeting abstracts. In fact, the complete text of relevant WBG and Worm Meeting abstracts can be pulled up using this system.

2. *C. elegans* protocols: This folder contains a variety of additional and updated *C. elegans* protocols which have been contributed by a number of *C. elegans* laboratories.

3. Strains and Alleles (University of Texas): Within this folder are the strain lists of several laboratories including the *Caenorhabditis* Genetics Center. In addition, an "Announcements" folder serves as a community bulletin board.

C. *C. elegans* Electronic Discussion Group

1. To Subscribe (Access Using Your Own Account)

In Europe, Africa, or Central Asia, send the one-line message

> SUB bionet-news.bionet.celegans
> TO: MXT@dl.ac.uk

In the Americas or the Pacific Rim, send the one-line message

> subscribe celegans
> TO: biosci-server@net.bio.net

2. To Cancel Your Subscription

Change the above to either UNSUB or unsubscribe, respectively.

3. To Post a Message

Using a newsreader interface, simply post a message into bionet.celegans. Be sure to set your "distribution" to "world" or else the message might not leave your site. To post by e-mail, mail your message to one of the following addresses depending on your location. These addresses are for posting messages only. Please do not send subscription requests to the posting addresses.

> Europe, Africa, Central Asia: celegans@daresbury.ac.uk
> Americas and Pacific Rim: celegans@net.bio.net

4. To Reply to a Message

Using a newsreader interface, simply use the reply or follow-up command on your newsreader to send either private or public replies. If you are using e-mail (Internet), replies to messages that you receive will *not* be automatically returned to the group. Your reply must contain either of the two newsgroup posting addresses above in your message header if you want to share it with everyone on the group.

5. To Look at Archives of the List

Use Newswatcher or other interface and look for bionet.celegans. Via Gopher, use net.bio.net as your Gopher server and look in the CELEGANS directory. For more information on using the system, request BIOSCI FAQ from biosci-help@net.bio.net.

Administrative questions about the system should be sent to biosci-help@net.bio.net in the US or biosci@daresbury.ac.uk. in the United Kingdom.

III. Other Useful Information

The guide to *C. elegans* nomenclature conventions can be found in Horvitz, H. R., Brenner, S., Hodgkin, J., and Herman, R. K. (1979). A uniform genetic nomenclature for the nematode *Caenorhabditis elegans. Mol. Gen. Genet.* **175:**129–133.
Also see *Worm Breeder's Gazette* **10**(1):1–5 (1987).

Appendix B: *Caenorhabditis* Genetics Center—Laboratory Designations

AB	aa	Bird, A., CSIRO, Adelaide, Australia
AE	at	Sluder, A., University of Georgia, Athens
AF	sz	Fodor, A., Hungarian Academy of Science, Szeged
AL	ic	Alfonso, A., University of Iowa, Iowa City
AS	id	Spence, A., University of Toronto, Ontario
AT	yj	Politz, S., Worcester Polytechnic Institute, Worcester, MA
AV	me	Villeneuve, A., Stanford University Medical School, Stanford, CA
BA	hc	Ward, S., University of Arizona, Tucson
BC	s	Baillie, D., Simon Fraser University, Burnaby, BC
BE	sc	Edgar, B., University of California, Santa Cruz
BG	nw	Goodwin, B., Northwestern University, Chicago, IL
BH	hb	Honda, B., Simon Fraser University, Burnaby, BC
BL	in	Blumenthal, T., Indiana University, Bloomington
BM	bb	Mitchell, D., Boston Biomedical Research Institute, Boston, MA
BS	oz	Schedl, T., Washington University, St. Louis, MO
BW	ct	Wood, B., University of Colorado, Boulder
CB	e	Hodgkin, J., MRC, Cambridge, England
CD	dc	Johnson, C., NemaPharm, Inc., Cambridge, MA
CF	mu	Kenyon, C., University of California, San Francisco
CH	rq	Kramer, J., Northwestern University Medical School, Chicago, IL
CL	dv	Link, C., University of Denver, Denver, CO
CW	fc	Morgan, P., Case Western Reserve University, Cleveland, OH
CX	ky	Bargmann, C., University of California, San Francisco
DA	ad	Avery, L., University of Texas Southwestern Medical Center, Dallas
DB	rv	Bird, D., University of California, Riverside
DD	d	Otsuka, T., Illinois State University, Normal
DF	ny	Fitch, D., New York University, New York
DG	tn	Greenstein, D., Vanderbilt University, Nashville, TN
DH	b	Hirsh, D., Columbia University, New York
DM	ra	Moerman, D., University of British Columbia, Vancouver
DP	ed	Pilgrim, D., University of Alberta, Edmonton
DR	m	Riddle, D., University of Missouri, Columbia
DS	tx	Shakes, D., University of Houston, Houston, TX
DT	jb	Stinchcomb, D., Synergen Inc., Boulder, CO
DZ	ez	Zarkower, D., University of Minnesota, Minneapolis
EA	ls	Aamodt, E., Louisiana State University Medical Center, Shreveport

EE	up	Bucher, B., University of Pennsylvania, Philadelphia
EF	ab	Ferguson, C., University of Chicago, Chicago, IL
EG	ox	Jorgensen, E., Salt Lake City, UT
EH	lw	Shaw, J., University of Minnesota, St. Paul
EJ	dx	Lambie, E., Dartmouth College, Hanover, NH
EL	om	Maine, E., Syracuse University, Syracuse, NY
EM	bx	Emmons, S., Albert Einstein University, Bronx, NY
ER	jd	Walthall, B., Georgia State University, Altanta
EU	or	Bowerman, B., University of Oregon, Eugene
FF	f	Thierry-Mieg, D., CRBM du CNRS, Montpellier, France
FH	ec	Meneely, P., Fred Hutchinson Cancer Research Center, Seattle, WA
FK	ks	Ohshima, Y., Kyushu University, Kukuoka, Japan
FR	sw	Muller, F., University of Fribourg, Fribourg, Switzerland
FS	tf	Roberts, T., Florida State University, Tallahassee
GB	sf	Benian, G., Emory University, Atlanta, GA
GE	t	Schnabel, R. & H., Max-Planck-Institut, Tubingen, Germany
GG	g	Von Ehrenstein, G., Max-Planck Institute, Gottingen, Germany
GR	mg	Ruvkun, G., Massachussetts General Hospital, Boston
GS	ar	Greenwald, I., Columbia University, New York
GT	a	Dusenbery, D., Georgia Institute of Technology, Atlanta
HE	su	Epstein, H., Baylor College of Medicine, Houston, TX
HH	hs	Hecht, R., University of Houston, Houston, TX
HK	kh	Kagawa, H., Okayama University, Okayama, Japan
HR	sb	Mains, P., University of Calgary, Alberta
IA	ij	Johnstone, I., University of Glasgow, Glasgow, Scotland
IM	ur	Wadsworth, B., University of Medicine and Dentistry of New Jersey, Piscataway
JC	ut	Katsura, I., University of Tokyo, Tokyo
JJ	zu	Priess, J., Fred Hutchinson Cancer Research Center, Seattle, WA
JK	q	Kimble, J., University of Wisconsin, Madison
JL	fm	Lissemore, J., John Carroll University, University Heights, OH
JM	ca	McGhee, J., University of Calgary, Alberta
JP	gn	Nelson, G., Jet Propulsion Laboratory, Caltech, Pasadena, CA
JR	w	Rothman, J., University of Wisconsin, Madison
JT	sa	Thomas, J., University of Washington, Seattle
JW	je	Way, J., Rutgers University, Piscataway, NJ
KB	um	Bennett, K., University of Missouri, Columbia
KC	wx	Chow, K., Hong Kong, University of Science and Technology, Clear Water Bay, Kowloo
KE	ha	Edwards, K., Haverford College, Haverford, PA
KK	it	Kemphues, K., Cornell University, Ithaca, NY
KM	gv	Krause, M., NIH Laboratory of Molecular Biology, Bethesda, MD
KP	nu	Kaplan, J., Massachusetts General Hospital, Boston
KR	h	Rose, A., University of British Columbia, Vancouver
LC	pa	Loer, C., Lafayette College, Easton, PA
LK	gs	Manser, J., Harvey Mudd College, Claremont, CA
LR	rk	Rokeach, L., University of Montreal, Quebec
LT	wk	Padgett, R., Waksman Institute, Piscataway, NJ
LU	lr	De Stasio, B., Lawrence University, Appleton, WI
LV	wc	Venolia, L., Williams College, Williamstown, MA
MB	ib	Burnell, A., St. Patrick's College, Maynooth, Ireland
MC	gc	Crowder, M., Washington University School of Medicine, St. Louis, MO

MH	ku	Han, M., University of Colorado, Boulder
MJ	k	Miwa, J., NEC Fundamental Research Laboratories, Tsukuba, Japan
MK	hx	Klass, M., University of Houston, Houston, TX
ML	mc	Labouesse, M., Strasbourg Cedex, France
MM	an	Hamelin, M., Merck Research Laboratories, Rahway, NJ
MP	lb	Wolinsky, E., New York University Medical School, New York
MQ	qm	Hekimi, S., McGill University, Montreal, Quebec
MT	n	Horvitz, B., MIT, Cambridge, MA
MW	wm	Wickens, M., University of Wisconsin, Madison
NA	gb	Bazzicalupo, P., IIGB, Naples, Italy
NC	wd	Miller, D., Duke University Medical Center, Durham, NC
NE	rp	Pertel, R., FDA, Washington, DC
NF	tk	Nishiwaki, K., NEC Fundamental Research Laboratories, Tsukuba, Japan
NG	gm	Garriga, G., University of California Berkeley
NH	ay	Stern, M., Yale University, New Haven, CT
NJ	rh	Hedgecock, E., Johns Hopkins University, Baltimore, MD
NL	pk	Plasterk, R., NKI, Amsterdam, The Netherlands
NM	js	Nonet, M., Washington University, St. Louis, MO
NS	nr	Server, F., Cambridge NeuroScience Research, Cambridge, MA
NT	uc	Perry, M., University of Toronto, Ontario, Canada
NW	ev	Culotti, J., Mount Sinai Hospital Research Institute, Toronto, Ontario
NY	yn	Li, C., Boston University, Boston, MA
PA	hv	Trent, C., Western Washington University, Bellingham
PB	bd	Baird, S., Wright State University, Dayton, OH
PC	ub	Candido, P., University of British Columbia, Vancouver
PD	cc	Fire, A., Carnegie Institution, Baltimore, MD
PH	hf	Hartman, P., Texas Christian University, Fort Worth
PJ	j	Jacobson, L., University of Pittsburgh, Pittsburgh, PA
PK	cr	Kuwabara, P., MRC-LMB, Cambridge, England
PR	p	Russell, D., University of Pittsburgh, Pittsburgh, PA
PS	sy	Sternberg, P., California Institute of Technology, Pasadena
RB	ok	Barstead, R., Oklahoma Medical Research Foundation, Oklahoma City
RC	g	Cassada, R., Universität Freiburg, Freiburg, Germany
RE	v	Ellis, R., University of Michigan, Ann Arbor
RG	ve	Rougvie, A., University of Minnesota, St. Paul
RM	md	Rand, J., Oklahoma Medical Research Foundation, Oklahoma City
RW	st	Waterston, B., Washington University, St. Louis, MO
SC	lm	Miller, L., Santa Clara University, Santa Clara, CA
SD	ga	Kim, S., Stanford University Medical School, Stanford, CA
SL	eb	L'Hernault, S., Emory University, Atlanta, GA
SP	mn	Herman, B., University of Minnesota, St. Paul
SQ	zk	Siddiqui, S., Toyohashi University, Toyohashi, Japan
SS	bn	Strome, S., Indiana University, Bloomington
SW	se	Weintraub, H., FHCRC, Seattle, Washington
TB	ch	Burglin, T., Biozentrum, Basel, Switerland
TD	tc	Lew, K., Forsyth Dental Center, Boston, MA
TJ	z	Johnson, T., University of Colorado, Boulder
TK	kn	Ishii, N., Tokai University School of Medicine Tokai, Japan
TM	sj	Honda, S., Jet Propulsion Laboratory, Pasadena, CA
TN	cn	Hosono, R., Kanazawa University, Kanazawa, Ishikawa, Japan
TR	r	Anderson, P., University of Wisconsin, Madison

TT	tb	Babu, P., Tata Institute, Bombay, India
TU	u	Chalfie, M., Columbia University, New York
TW	cj	Collins, J., University of New Hampshire, Durham
TY	y	Meyer, B., University of California, Berkeley
UC	la	Mancillas, J., University of California, Los Angeles
UK	ln	Nawrocki, L., University College, London
UL	le	Hope, I., University of Leeds, Leeds, England
UT	mm	Van der Kooy, D., University of Toronto, Toronto, Ontario
UW	wb	Woods, R., University of Winnipeg, Winnipeg, Manitoba
VD	sn	Van Doren, K., Syracuse University, Syracuse, NY
VT	ma	Ambros, V., Dartmouth College, Hanover, NH
WG	au	Grant, W., CSIRO, Armidale, NSW, Australia
WJ	sh	Sharrock, W., University of Minnesota, St. Paul
WR	oh	Morgan, B., College of Wooster, Wooster, OH
WS	op	Hengartner, M., Cold Spring Harbor Laboratory, Cold Spring Harbor, NY
WW	xx	Samoiloff, M., University of Manitoba Winnipeg
YK	ms	Kohara, Y., National Institute of Genetics, Mishima, Japan
ZB	bz	Driscoll, M., Rutgers University, Piscataway, NJ
ZZ	x	Lewis, J., University of Texas, San Antonio

Appendix C: Gene Names and Descriptions

I. Registered and Provisional Gene Names in Current Use

Name	Laboratory	Description or Explanation
abl	CB	ABL (mammalian oncogene) related
ace	PR	AcetylCholinEsterase abnormality
act	RW	ACTin
aex	JT	Aboc, EXpulsion (defecation) defective
age	TJ	AGEing abnormality
ali	CB	ALae Inconspicuous
ama	DR	AMAnitin resistance abnormality
anc	CB	ANChorage of nuclei abnormal
aph	JJ	Anterior PHarynx defective
apl	NY	Amyloid Precursor-Like
apx	JJ	Anterior Pharynx in eXcess
arf	CB	ADP Ribosylation Factor related
arp	RW	Actin-Related Protein
atn	RW	alpha-AcTiNin family
avr	CD	AVermectin Resistance abnormal
bas	LC	Biogenic Amine Synthesis related
ben	TU	BENomyl resistance abnormal
bli	CB	BLIstered
bor	RC	BORdering behavior abnormal
cad	PJ	CAthepsin D deficient
caf	PH	CAFfeine resistance abnormal
cah	CB	Cyclase Associated protein Homolog
cal	CB	CALmodulin related
can	NJ	CAN cell abnormality
cap	RW	CAP-Z protein related
cat	CB	CATecholamine abnormality
cdh	BW	CaDHerin family
ced	CB	CEll Death abnormality
ceh	GR	*C. Elegans* Homeobox
ces	MT	CEll death Selection abnormal
cey	PD	*C. Elegans* Y box related

cha	PR	CHoline Acetyltransferase
che	CB	CHEmotaxis abnormal
cib	GE	Changed Identity of Blastomeres
clb	CH	CoLlagen, Basement membrane associated
clk	MQ	CLocK (biological timing) abnormal
clr	CB	CLeaR
cod	PS	COpulation Defective
col	DH	COLlagen
cpr	CB	Cysteine PRotease related
crt	CB	CalRe Ticulin
cut	NA	CUTiclin
cya	CB	CYclin A
cyb	CB	CYclin B
cyp	MT	CYcloPhilin related
cyt	CB	CYTochrome
daf	DR	DAuer larva Formation abnormal
deb	RW	DEnse Body component
dec	JT	DEfecation Cycle abnormal
deg	TU	DEGeneration of certain neurons
dif	CB	DIFferentiation, embryonic abnormality
dig	MT	DIsplaced Gonad
dpy	CB	DumPY
dyf	SP	DYe-Filling abnormality
eat	DA	EATing (pharyngeal pumping) abnormal
eft	PC	Elongation FacTor
egf	CB	EGF (epidermal growth factor) motif related
egl	MT	EGg-Laying Abnormal
eha	CB	Egg laying Hormone of *Aplysia*, related
eln	CB	ELoNgation factor
elt	BL	Erythrocyte-Like Transcription factor
emb	GG	EMBryogenesis abnormal
enu	CB	ENhancer of Uncoordinated behavior
epi	NJ	EPithelialization abnormal
exc	NJ	EXCretory canal defective
exp	JT	EXPulsion (defecation) defective
fab	KP	Foraging behavior ABnormal
fem	CB	FEMinization
fer	BA	FERtilization (sperm) defective
flp	NY	FMRF-amide-Like Peptide
flr	JC	FLuoride Resistance abnormal
flu	CB	FLUorescence of gut abnormal
fog	CB	Feminization Of Germ line
gap	CB	GAP-43 related
gbr	CB	GABA Receptor related
ges	JM	Gut ESterase
ggl	EH	Gut GranuLe abnormality
gld	BS	Germ Line Differentiation abnormal
glh	KB	Germ Line Helicase
glp	JK	Germ Line Proliferation abnormal
glv	EJ	Germ Line maturation and Vulval induction defective
goa	PS	G protein, class O, Alpha subunit

gon	CB	GONad development abnormal
gpa	PS	G Protein, Alpha subunit
gpb	PS	G Protein, Beta subunit
gpd	DH	Glyceraldehyde-3-Phosphate Dehydrogenase
gro	CB	GROwth rate abnormal
gsa	FK	G protein, class S, Alpha subunit
gst	GS	Glutathione *S*-Transferase
gum	EJ	GUt Morphology abnormal
gus	NA	GlUcuronidaSe
gut	EH	GUT differentiation abnormal
ham	MT	HSN Abnormal Migration
hch	CB	HatCHing abnormality
her	CB	HERmaphroditization
him	CB	High Incidence of Males
his	EM	HIStone
hlh	PD	Helix–Loop–Helix family
hsp	BC	Heat Shock Protein
hum	CB	Heavy chain, Unconventional Myosin
inf	CB	INitiation Factor
int	CF	INTegrin related
itr	CB	Inositol Triphosphate Receptor family
itt	TJ	Increased ThermoTolerance
kin	CB	protein KINase
kra	HK	Ketamine Response Abnormal
kup	BL	Kinase UPstream (cotranscribed with kinase)
lag	JK	*Lin-12* And *Glp-1* related
lar	CB	LAnnate Resistance affected
lep	EM	LEPtoderan male tail
let	KR	LEThal
lev	ZZ	LEVamisole resistance abnormal
lgx	GS	*Lin-12* and *Glp-1* X-hybridizing
lin	CB	LINeage abnormal
lmb	CB	LaMinin B related
lmr	CB	LaMinin Receptor related
lon	CB	LONg
lrp	GS	LDL RecePtor related
lrx	GS	LRp X-hybridizing
mab	CB	Male ABnormaL
mah	TN	MAHi (=paralyzed in Japanese)
mai	BL	Mitochondrial ATPase Inhibitor related
mau	MQ	MAternal effect Uncoordinated
mec	TU	MEChanosensory abnormality
mei	KK	MEIotic abnormality
mel	KK	Maternal Effect Lethal
mes	SS	Maternal Effect Sterile
mev	TK	MEthyl Viologen (paraquat) resistance abnormal
mex	JJ	Muscle in EXcess
mig	CB	MIGration of cells abnormal
mlc	TR	Myosin Light Chain
mog	JK	Masculinization of Germ line
mor	CB	MORphological abnormality

mpk	CB	MAP-Kinase related
msp	BA	Major Sperm Protein
mtl	CB	MeTaLothionein related
mua	NJ	MUscle cell Attachment abnormal
mup	NJ	MUscle cell Positioning abnormal
mut	TR	MUTator
myb	CB	MYB (mammalian oncogene) related
myo	CB	MYOsin (heavy chain)
ncc	CB	Nematode Cell Cycle associated
ncl	CB	NuCLeoli abnormal
nhr	AE	Nuclear Hormone Receptor family
nob	BW	kNOB-like posterior (NO Backside)
nop	KK	NO Pseudocleavage
nuc	CB	NUClease abnormality
oar	BS	Oocyte ARrest in diakenesis defect
odc	CB	Ornithine DeCarboxylase
odr	CX	ODoRant response abnormality
ooc	SP	OOCyte formation abnormal
ops	CB	OPSin related
osm	PR	OSMotic avoidance abnormality
ost	CB	OSTeonectin related
oxy	TM	OXYgen sensitivity abnormal
pag	CB	PAttern of reporter Gene expression abnormal
pal	CF	Posterior ALae of males abnormal
par	KK	embryonic PARtitioning abnormal
pat	RW	Paralyzed Arrest at Twofold stage
pbo	JT	PBOc defective (defecation)
pel	JR	Pharynx and ELongation defective
pes	UL	Patterned Expression Site
pgl	SS	P-GranuLe abnormality
pgp	NL	P-GlycoProtein family
pha	GE	PHArynx development abnormal
phm	DA	PHaryngeal Muscle defect
pie	JJ	Pharynx and Intestine in Excess
plg	CB	copulatory PLuG formation
pop	JJ	POsterior Pharynx abnormal
prk	CB	PIM (mammalian oncogene) Related Kinase
pry	CF	PolyRaY
pvp	NJ	PVP (neuron) abnormal
rab	CB	RAB family
rad	SP	RADiation sensitivity abnormal
ram	SB	RAy Morphology abnormal
rec	KR	RECombination abnormality
rhl	CB	RNA HeLicase related
ric	RM	Resistance to Inhibitors of Cholinesterase
rol	CB	ROLler
rpc	CB	RNA Polymerase, type 3 (C)
rpl	DH	Ribosomal Protein, Large subunit
rpo	DR	RNA POlymerase
rrn	CB	Ribosomal RNA
rrp	MH	Related to Rap and ras Proteins

rrs	CB	Ribosomal RNA, Small
rsn	BL	RNA, Small Nuclear
rtm	BH	RNA, Transfer, M = methionine
rtr	CB	RNA, Transfer, R = arginine
rtw	CB	RNA, Transfer, W = tryptophan
rtx	CB	RNA, Transfer, X – selenocysteine
ryr	CB	RYanodine Receptor related
sch	CB	Sodium CHannel related
sdc	TY	Sex determination and Dosage Compensation
sdm	CB	Superoxide Dismutase, Mn class
sel	GS	Suppressor/Enhancer of *Lin-12*
sem	MT	SEx Muscle abnormality
sip	CB	Stress-Induced Protein
skn	JJ	SKiN (hypodermis) in excess
sli	PS	Suppressor of LIneage defect
sls	CB	Spliced Leader Sequence (SL1, SL2)
sma	CB	SMAll
smg	CB	Suppressor with Morphogenetic effect on Genitalia
smu	SP	Suppressor of *Mec* and *Unc*
snb	CB	SyNaptoBrevin related
sns	PR	SeNSory abnormality
snt	CB	SyNapto Tagmin related
sod	CB	SuperOxide Dismutase
sog	EL	Suppressor of Glp-1
spa	CB	Sodium/Potassium ATPase
spe	BA	SPErmatogenesis abnormal
sqt	BE	SQuaT
src	CB	SRC (vertebrate oncogene) related
srf	AT	SuRFace antigen
srl	BC	Suppressor of Roller Lethality
ssg	CB	Spermatogenesis-Specific Gene
ssp	BA	Sperm-Specific Product
stu	CB	STErile UNcoordinated
sud	GE	SUpernumerary Divisions in embryo
sum	GS	SUppressor of Multivulva phenotype
sup	CB	SUPpressor
sur	MH	SUppressor of activated *Ras*
sus	DR	SUppressor of Suppressor
suv	SD	SUppressor of Vulvaless
syh	CB	amino-acyl tRNA SYnthetase, Histidyl
tab	TU	Touch response ABnormal
tax	GT	chemoTAXis abnormal
tba	CB	TuBulin, Alpha
tbb	CB	TuBulin, Beta
tbg	CB	TuBulin, Gamma
tbx	CB	T-BoX related
tmy	CB	TropoMYosin
tnc	CB	TropoNin C
toh	CB	TOllisH (tolloid related)
tpa	MJ	TPA resistance abnormal
tra	CB	TRAnsformer

ttx	PR	ThermoTaXis abnormal
ubc	PC	UBiquitin Conjugating enzyme
ubq	PC	UBiQuitin
unc	CB	UNCoordinated
uts	CB	Unidentified TransSpliced transcript
uvt	BL	Unidentified ViTellogenin-linked transcript
uxt	TY	Unidentified seX-linked Transcript
vab	CB	Variable Abnormal morphology
vet	BW	Very Early Transcript
vex	PS	Vulval EXecution abnormal
vit	BL	Vitelline membrane protein related
wnt	CF	WNT (wingless/int) related
xol	TY	XO Lethal
ypp	CB	tYrosine PhosPhatase
zen	JR	Zygotic epidermal ENclosure defective
zyg	DH	ZYGote defective

====== ## II. Retired Gene Names (Synonymous with Existing Gene Classes)

Name	Lab	Description or Explanation
acr	CB	AcetylCholine Receptor (see *lev-1*)
ber	CB	BERgerac strain-specific defect (see *zyg-12*)
crf	GR	*C. elegans* Receptor Finger-corticosteroid receptor family
isx	BA	InterSeX (see *fem*)
lan	CB	LANnate resistance abnormal (see *unc-18, ric-1*)
raf	CB	RAF (mammalian oncogene) related (see *lin-45*)
tcf	TN	TriChlorFon resistance abnormal (see *unc-41*)
tmr	CB	TetraMisole Resistance abnormal (see *lev*)

SUBJECT INDEX

A

Ablation
  laser ablation, 114, 206, 225–248
  photoablation, 248–249
ACeDB, 534–536, 568, 584–604
  browsing and searching, 587–592
  computer requirements, 585–586
  database
    concepts, 598–601
    contents, 592–598
  Web sites regarding, 585–587, 598, 604
  Worm Community System, comparison, 609, 610
  writing to, 597, 601–604
acediff 604
ace-1 gene, 128, 134
Acetaldehyde, mutagenesis, 40, 42–43
Acetylcholine, 188
Acetylcholine receptor agonists, mutant studies, 189
act gene, 517
Actin gene probe, 516–517, 519
Actin genes, 495, 505
age-1 gene, 189
Alkaline phosphatase-mediated detection, 331, 333
Altered duplication, 136–137
ama-1 gene, 189, 505
ama-2 gene, 189
α-Amanitin, 189, 192, 197, 313
Amino acids, codons, 505
Anesthetics, 189, 397
Antibodies
  monoclonal antibodies, 377–379, 382–383
  to nematode antigens, 377–383
  polyclonal antibodies, 377, 379–380
  staining, 316–317, 365–366, 371–372, 374–376
Antigens, immunofluorescence, 365–389
Antihelmintics, 200
Antinematode compounds, 188, 193, 200
Antisense inhibition, 522–523
Antisense primers, 519
Antisense probes, 519, 520
Antisense RNA, 61, 475, 501, 523, 580
Antistatic devices, serial thin sections, 429
Ascaris lumbricoides, 496, 526

Ascaris suum, sperm, 274, 288–295, 298
Assembly pathway, 98
Associative learning, 207
Automatic subcloning, 573
Avidin conjugates, 25
avr-14 gene, 189
avr-15 gene, 189
Axenization method, 12–14, 26

B

Bacteria, for nematode culture, 18–19, 21, 24–25
Bacteriophage, clones, 574–575
Bacteriophages, DNA, miniprep, 544–545
Balancers, *see* Genetic balancers
Basal translation factor, 516
Behavioral plasticity, 205–222
  mechanosensation, 214–221
  olfactory adaptation, 211
  taste adaptation, 209
  taste conditioning, 213
  thermotaxis, 211–213
ben-1 gene, 189
Bergerac strain, 51–52
  genetic mapping, 82–95
Bioactive compounds, interactions with gene products, 187–201
Biochemical purification, 437, 440
Biotin, labeling with, 25
Biotin–dUTP, 341
Blastomeres, 303–320
  culture, 306–308, 312
  cytochemistry, 314–317
  drug treatments, 312–313
  isolation, 304, 308–312
  radioactive labeling, 313–314
  solutions used, 317–320
BLAST, 568
Blixem, 568

C

Caenorhabditis elegans, see also specific strains
  cell biology
    blastomeres, 303–320

641

VOLUMES IN SERIES

Founding Series Editor
DAVID M. PRESCOTT

Volume 1 (1964)
Methods in Cell Physiology
Edited by David M. Prescott

Volume 2 (1966)
Methods in Cell Physiology
Edited by David M. Prescott

Volume 3 (1968)
Methods in Cell Physiology
Edited by David M. Prescott

Volume 4 (1970)
Methods in Cell Physiology
Edited by David M. Prescott

Volume 5 (1972)
Methods in Cell Physiology
Edited by David M. Prescott

Volume 6 (1973)
Methods in Cell Physiology
Edited by David M. Prescott

Volume 7 (1973)
Methods in Cell Biology
Edited by David M. Prescott

Volume 8 (1974)
Methods in Cell Biology
Edited by David M. Prescott

Volume 9 (1975)
Methods in Cell Biology
Edited by David M. Prescott

Volume 10 (1975)
Methods in Cell Biology
Edited by David M. Prescott

Volume 11 (1975)
Yeast Cells
Edited by David M. Prescott

Volume 12 (1975)
Yeast Cells
Edited by David M. Prescott

Volume 13 (1976)
Methods in Cell Biology
Edited by David M. Prescott

Volume 14 (1976)
Methods in Cell Biology
Edited by David M. Prescott

Volume 15 (1977)
Methods in Cell Biology
Edited by David M. Prescott

Volume 16 (1977)
Chromatin and Chromosomal Protein Research I
Edited by Gary Stein, Janet Stein, and Lewis J. Kleinsmith

Volume 17 (1978)
Chromatin and Chromosomal Protein Research II
Edited by Gary Stein, Janet Stein, and Lewis J. Kleinsmith

Volume 18 (1978)
Chromatin and Chromosomal Protein Research III
Edited by Gary Stein, Janet Stein, and Lewis J. Kleinsmith

Volume 19 (1978)
Chromatin and Chromosomal Protein Research IV
Edited by Gary Stein, Janet Stein, and Lewis J. Kleinsmith

Volume 20 (1978)
Methods in Cell Biology
Edited by David M. Prescott

Advisory Board Chairman
KEITH R. PORTER

Volume 21A (1980)
**Normal Human Tissue and Cell Culture, Part A: Respiratory, Cardiovascular,
   and Integumentary Systems**
Edited by Curtis C. Harris, Benjamin F. Trump, and Gary D. Stoner

Volume 31 (1989)
Vesicular Transport, Part A
Edited by Alan M. Tartakoff

Volume 32 (1989)
Vesicular Transport, Part B
Edited by Alan M. Tartakoff

Volume 33 (1990)
Flow Cytometry
Edited by Zbigniew Darzynkiewicz and Harry A. Crissman

Volume 34 (1991)
Vectorial Transport of Proteins into and across Membranes
Edited by Alan M. Tartakoff

Selected from Volumes 31, 32, and 34 (1991)
Laboratory Methods for Vesicular and Vectorial Transport
Edited by Alan M. Tartakoff

Volume 35 (1991)
Functional Organization of the Nucleus: A Laboratory Guide
Edited by Barbara A. Hamkalo and Sarah C. R. Elgin

Volume 36 (1991)
***Xenopus laevis:* Practical Uses in Cell and Molecular Biology**
Edited by Brian K. Kay and H. Benjamin Peng

Series Editors
LESLIE WILSON AND PAUL MATSUDAIRA

Volume 37 (1993)
Antibodies in Cell Biology
Edited by David J. Asai

Volume 38 (1993)
Cell Biological Applications of Confocal Microscopy
Edited by Brian Matsumoto

Volume 39 (1993)
Motility Assays for Motor Proteins
Edited by Jonathan M. Scholey

Volume 40 (1994)
A Practical Guide to the Study of Calcium in Living Cells
Edited by Richard Nuccitelli

ISBN 0-12-564149-4

90018

9 780125 641494